WORLD HEALTH ORGANIZATION
INTERNATIONAL AGENCY FOR RESEARCH ON CANCER

IARC Monographs on the Evaluation of Carcinogenic Risks to Humans

VOLUME 97

1,3-Butadiene, Ethylene Oxide and Vinyl Halides (Vinyl Fluoride, Vinyl Chloride and Vinyl Bromide)

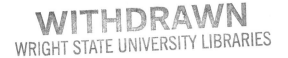
This publication represents the views and expert opinions
of an IARC Working Group on the
Evaluation of Carcinogenic Risks to Humans,
which met in Lyon,

5–12 June 2007

2008

IARC MONOGRAPHS

In 1969, the International Agency for Research on Cancer (IARC) initiated a programme on the evaluation of the carcinogenic risk of chemicals to humans involving the production of critically evaluated monographs on individual chemicals. The programme was subsequently expanded to include evaluations of carcinogenic risks associated with exposures to complex mixtures, life-style factors and biological and physical agents, as well as those in specific occupations.

The objective of the programme is to elaborate and publish in the form of monographs critical reviews of data on carcinogenicity for agents to which humans are known to be exposed and on specific exposure situations; to evaluate these data in terms of human risk with the help of international working groups of experts in chemical carcinogenesis and related fields; and to indicate where additional research efforts are needed.

The lists of IARC evaluations are regularly updated and are available on Internet: http://monographs.iarc.fr/

This programme has been supported by Cooperative Agreement 5UO1CA33193 awarded since 1982 by the United States National Cancer Institute, Department of Health and Human Services. Additional support has been provided since 1986 by the European Commission, Directorate-General EMPL (Employment, and Social Affairs), Health, Safety and Hygiene at Work Unit, and since 1992 by the United States National Institute of Environmental Health Sciences.

Published by the International Agency for Research on Cancer,
150 cours Albert Thomas, 69372 Lyon Cedex 08, France
©International Agency for Research on Cancer, 2008

Distributed by WHO Press, World Health Organization, 20 Avenue Appia, 1211 Geneva 27, Switzerland
(tel.: +41 22 791 3264; fax: +41 22 791 4857; e-mail: bookorders@who.int).

IARC Library Cataloguing in Publication Data

1,3-Butadiene, Ethylene oxide and Vinyl Halides (Vinyl Fluoride, Vinyl Chloride and Vinyl Bromide)/ IARC Working Group on the Evaluation of Carcinogenic Risks to Humans (2007 : Lyon, France)

(IARC monographs on the evaluation of carcinogenic risks to humans ; v. 97)

1. Butadienes – adverse effects   2. Carcinogens   3. Ethylene oxide – adverse effects
4. Vinyl Compounds – adverse   5. Neoplasms – chemically induced
I. IARC Working Group on the Evaluation of Carcinogenic Risks to Humans   II. Series

ISBN 978 92 832 1297 3   (NLM Classification: W1)
ISSN 1017-1606

PRINTED IN FRANCE

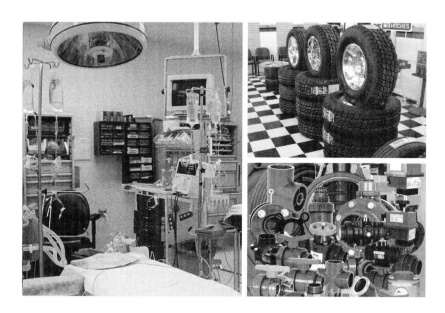

1 Ethylene oxide is an effective fumigant and sterilant for microbial organisms. It is used to treat hospital equipment, disposable and reusable medical items, drugs, packaging materials, scientific equipment and many other items.

2 The largest single use for 1,3-butadiene is in the production of styrene-butadiene rubber for tyres and tyre products.

3 Vinyl chloride is used primarily in the manufacture of polyvinyl chloride.

Cover design: Georges Mollon, IARC

CONTENTS

NOTE TO THE READER

The term 'carcinogenic risk' in the IARC Monographs series is taken to mean that an agent is capable of causing cancer under some circumstances. The Monographs evaluate cancer hazards, despite the historical presence of the word 'risks' in the title.

Inclusion of an agent in the Monographs does not imply that it is a carcinogen, only that the published data have been examined. Equally, the fact that an agent has not yet been evaluated in a monograph does not mean that it is not carcinogenic.

The evaluations of carcinogenic risk are made by international working groups of independent scientists and are qualitative in nature. No recommendation is given for regulation or legislation.

Anyone who is aware of published data that may alter the evaluation of the carcinogenic risk of an agent to humans is encouraged to make this information available to the Carcinogen Identification and Evaluation Group, International Agency for Research on Cancer, 150 cours Albert Thomas, 69372 Lyon Cedex 08, France, in order that the agent may be considered for re-evaluation by a future Working Group.

Although every effort is made to prepare the monographs as accurately as possible, mistakes may occur. Readers are requested to communicate any errors to the Carcinogen Identification and Evaluation Group, so that corrections can be reported in future volumes.

IARC MONOGRAPHS ON THE EVALUATION OF CARCINOGENIC RISKS TO HUMANS

VOLUME 97
1,3-BUTADIENE, ETHYLENE OXIDE AND VINYL HALIDES (VINYL FLUORIDE, VINYL CHLORIDE AND VINYL BROMIDE)

Lyon, 5–12 June 2007

LIST OF PARTICIPANTS

Working Group Members[*]

Marc Baril, Robert Sauvé Research Institute on Health and Occupational Safety (IRSST), 505 boulevard de Maisonneuve Ouest, Montreal, Quebec H34 3C2, Canada

Pier Alberto Bertazzi[1], Department of Occupational and Environmental Health and EPOCA Epidemiology Research Center, University of Milan & Foundation IRCCS, OM Polyclinic, Mangiagalli and Regina Elena, Via San Barnaba 8, 20122 Milan, Italy

James A. Bond, Chemico-Biological Interactions, 25 Rabbitbrush Road, Santa Fe, NM 87506-7782, USA (*not present for evaluations*)

David Coggon[2], MRC Epidemiology Resource Centre, University of Southampton, Southampton SO16 6YD, United Kingdom (*Subgroup Chair, Cancer in Humans*)

David Eastmond[3], Environmental Toxicology Graduate Program, University of California, Riverside, 2109 Biological Sciences Building, Riverside, CA 92521-0314, USA

Adnan Elfarra, Department of Comparative Biosciences, School of Veterinary Medicine, University of Wisconsin-Madison, 2015 Linden Drive, Madison, WI 53706, USA

---

[1] Dr Bertazzi chairs a department that has a research contract with Plastics Europe, whose member companies manufacture the chemicals reviewed at this meeting. The value of the contract is less than 5% of the department's research budget.

[2] Dr Coggon has received travel support from the plastics industry to attend advisory group meetings for the study disclosed by Dr Bertazzi. Dr Coggon also has received travel support from the chemical industry to attend another recent scientific meeting. Neither Dr Coggon nor his department received professional compensation for these activities.

[3] Dr Eastmond's laboratory received research support on a topic unrelated to this meeting from Dow Chemical Company and from Bayer AG (a former subsidiary that is now Lanxess Corporation). The funds were received in 1997 but not used until recently. The funds do not support Dr Eastmond's salary and comprise less than 10% of the laboratory's overall funding. Dow Chemical manufactures or uses 1,3-butadiene, ethylene oxide, and vinyl chloride. Lanxess manufactures polybutadiene rubber.

Rogene Henderson, Lovelace Respiratory Research Institute, 2425 Ridgecrest Dr. SE, Albuquerque, NM 87108, USA

Charles William Jameson, National Institute of Environmental Health Sciences, National Institutes of Health, PO Box 12233, 79 Alexander Drive, Research Triangle Park, NC 27709, USA

Timo Kauppinen, Finnish Institute of Occupational Health, Topeliuksenkatu 41 a A, 00250 Helsinki, Finland (*Subgroup Chair, Exposure Data*)

Kannan Krishnan[4], Department of Environmental and Occupational Health, Human Toxicology Research Group, University of Montreal, Montreal, Canada

Hans Kromhout, Environmental Epidemiology Division, Institute for Risk Assessment Sciences (IRAS), Utrecht University, PO Box 80.178, Jenalaan 18d, 3508 TD Utrecht, The Netherlands

Marie-Jeanne Marion, National Institute of Health and Medical Research (INSERM), 151 Cours Albert Thomas, 69424 Lyon cedex 03, France

Ron Melnick, Environmental Toxicology Program, National Institute of Environmental Health Sciences, 111 Alexander Drive, PO Box 12233, Research Triangle Park, NC 27709, USA (*Subgroup Chair, Mechanistic and Other Relevant Data*)

Franz Oesch, Institute of Toxicology, University of Mainz, Obere Zahlbacherstrasse 67, 55131 Mainz, Germany

Kimmo Peltonen, Chemistry and Toxicology Unit, Finnish Food Safety Authority (EVIRA), Mustialankatu 3, 00790 Helsinki, Finland

Roberta Pirastu, Department of Animal and Human Biology, University La Sapienza, P.le A. Moro 5, 00185 Rome, Italy

Jerry M. Rice[5], Georgetown University Medical Center, Department of Oncology, Box 571465, Lombardi Comprehensive Cancer Center, Level LL, Room S150, 3800 Reservoir Road NW, Washington, DC 20057-1465, USA (*Subgroup Chair, Cancer in Experimental Animals*)

Paul A. Schulte, Education and Information Division, National Institute for Occupational Safety and Health (NIOSH/CDC), Robert A. Taft Laboratories, Mail Stop C14, 4676 Columbia Parkway, Cincinnati, OH 45226-1998, USA (*unable to attend*)

Leslie Stayner, University of Illinois at Chicago, School of Public Health (M/C 923), 1603 West Taylor Street, Room 971, Chicago, IL 60612, USA (*Meeting Chair*)

Paolo Vineis, Department of Epidemiology & Public Health, Imperial College, St Mary's Campus, London W2 1PG, United Kingdom

Vernon Walker, Lovelace Respiratory Research Institute, 2425 Ridgecrest Dr SE, Albuquerque, NM 87108, USA

---

[4] Dr Krishnan receives research support from Exxon Mobil Corporation through a grant administered by the Natural Sciences and Engineering Research Council of Canada. These industry funds comprise less than 5% of his research group's overall funding. Until 2004 Dr Krishnan performed a small amount of consulting work for the American Chemistry Council on topics unrelated to this meeting.

[5] Dr Rice helped organize and received industry travel support to attend a symposium on butadiene and chloroprene health risks in September 2005.

Elizabeth M. Ward, Epidemiology and Surveillance Research, American Cancer Society, 250 Williams Street, Atlanta, GA 30303-1002, USA

Invited Specialists

Elizabeth Delzell[6], University of Alabama at Birmingham, Department of Epidemiology, School of Public Health, 1665 University Boulevard, 517 Ryals Building, Birmingham, AL 35294-0022, USA

Tommaso A. Dragani[7], Research Unit 'Polygenic Inheritance', IRCCS Foundation, National Tumour Institute, Via G. Venezian 1, 20133 Milan, Italy

Mary Jane Teta[8], Health Sciences Exponent, Inc., 8 Dogwood Court, Middlebury, CT 06762, USA

Representative

US Environmental Protection Agency

Jennifer Jinot, U.S. Environmental Protection Agency, Mailcode 8623D, 1200 Pennsylvania Avenue NW, Washington, DC 20460, USA

Observers

Observer for the European Council of Vinyl Manufacturers

Jean-Claude Besson[9], Arkema, 04600 Saint-Auban, France

Observer for the European Council of Vinyl Manufacturers

Marc Boeckx[10], Prevention and Protection Department, Tessenderlo Group, Heilig Hartlaan 21, 3980 Tessenderlo, Belgium

Observer for the International Institute of Synthetic Rubber Producers, Inc.

R. Jeffrey Lewis, ExxonMobil Biomedical Sciences, Inc., Epidemiology & Health Surveillance Section, 1545 Route 22 East, PO Box 971, Room LF 264, Annandale, NJ 08801-0971, USA

---

[6] Dr Delzell's research on 1,3-butadiene and other chemicals has been supported by funds provided to her university by the International Institute of Synthetic Rubber Producers, the Health Effects Institute, CEFIC (the European Chemical Industry Council), and the American Chemistry Council. Dr Delzell is also serving as a consultant to several companies with interests in vinyl chloride, including Modine Manufacturing Company and Cooper Industries Inc.

[7] Dr Dragani served as a consultant to EniChem (now Syndial). He has discussed serving as a consultant to Solvay on a future court case involving vinyl chloride.

[8] Dr Teta is retired from the Dow Chemical Company and owns shares in that company. Dr Teta serves as a consultant to the American Chemistry Council. Her scientific publications have been funded by the American Chemistry Council and by Union Carbide Corporation (now a subsidiary of Dow Chemical). Clients of her employer, Exponent Inc, include companies that have interests in the chemicals considered at this meeting.

[9] Dr Besson is employed by Arkema (a manufacturer of vinyl chloride) and is also supported by the European Council of Vinyl Manufacturers.

[10] Dr Boeckx is employed by Tessenderlo Group (a manufacturer of vinyl chloride) and also chairs the Medical Committee of the European Council of Vinyl Manufacturers, where he conducts their world register of liver angiosarcoma cases.

IARC Secretariat

Andrea Altieri, *IARC Monographs* programme (*Co-Rapporteur, Cancer in Humans*)

Robert Baan, *IARC Monographs* programme (*Rapporteur, Mechanistic and Other Relevant Data*)

Véronique Bouvard, *IARC Monographs* programme (*Co-Rapporteur, Mechanistic and Other Relevant Data*)

Vincent James Cogliano, *IARC Monographs* programme (*Head of Programme*)

Fabrizio Giannandrea, Lifestyle, Environment and Cancer Group

Fatiha El Ghissassi, *IARC Monographs* programme (*Co-Rapporteur, Mechanistic and Other Relevant Data*)

Yann Grosse, *IARC Monographs* programme (*Responsible Officer; Rapporteur, Cancer in Experimental Animals*)

Julia Heck, Lifestyle, Environment and Cancer Group

Jane Mitchell, *IARC Monographs* programme (*Editor*)

Nikolai Napalkov, *IARC Monographs* programme

Béatrice Secretan, *IARC Monographs* programme (*Rapporteur, Exposure Data*)

Kurt Straif, *IARC Monographs* programme (*Rapporteur, Cancer in Humans*)

Administrative assistance

Sandrine Egraz

Brigitte Kajo

Michel Javin

Martine Lézère

Helene Lorenzen-Augros

Post-meeting assistance

Dorothy Russell

PREAMBLE

IARC MONOGRAPHS ON THE EVALUATION OF CARCINOGENIC RISKS TO HUMANS

PREAMBLE

The Preamble to the *IARC Monographs* describes the objective and scope of the programme, the scientific principles and procedures used in developing a *Monograph*, the types of evidence considered and the scientific criteria that guide the evaluations. The Preamble should be consulted when reading a *Monograph* or list of evaluations.

A. GENERAL PRINCIPLES AND PROCEDURES

1. Background

Soon after IARC was established in 1965, it received frequent requests for advice on the carcinogenic risk of chemicals, including requests for lists of known and suspected human carcinogens. It was clear that it would not be a simple task to summarize adequately the complexity of the information that was available, and IARC began to consider means of obtaining international expert opinion on this topic. In 1970, the IARC Advisory Committee on Environmental Carcinogenesis recommended '...that a compendium on carcinogenic chemicals be prepared by experts. The biological activity and evaluation of practical importance to public health should be referenced and documented.' The IARC Governing Council adopted a resolution concerning the role of IARC in providing government authorities with expert, independent, scientific opinion on environmental carcinogenesis. As one means to that end, the Governing Council recommended that IARC should prepare monographs on the evaluation of carcinogenic risk of chemicals to man, which became the initial title of the series.

In the succeeding years, the scope of the programme broadened as *Monographs* were developed for groups of related chemicals, complex mixtures, occupational exposures, physical and biological agents and lifestyle factors. In 1988, the phrase 'of chemicals' was dropped from the title, which assumed its present form, *IARC Monographs on the Evaluation of Carcinogenic Risks to Humans*.

Through the *Monographs* programme, IARC seeks to identify the causes of human cancer. This is the first step in cancer prevention, which is needed as much today as when

IARC was established. The global burden of cancer is high and continues to increase: the annual number of new cases was estimated at 10.1 million in 2000 and is expected to reach 15 million by 2020 (Stewart & Kleihues, 2003). With current trends in demographics and exposure, the cancer burden has been shifting from high-resource countries to low- and medium-resource countries. As a result of *Monographs* evaluations, national health agencies have been able, on scientific grounds, to take measures to reduce human exposure to carcinogens in the workplace and in the environment.

The criteria established in 1971 to evaluate carcinogenic risks to humans were adopted by the Working Groups whose deliberations resulted in the first 16 volumes of the *Monographs* series. Those criteria were subsequently updated by further ad-hoc Advisory Groups (IARC, 1977, 1978, 1979, 1982, 1983, 1987, 1988, 1991; Vainio *et al.*, 1992; IARC, 2005, 2006).

The Preamble is primarily a statement of scientific principles, rather than a specification of working procedures. The procedures through which a Working Group implements these principles are not specified in detail. They usually involve operations that have been established as being effective during previous *Monograph* meetings but remain, predominantly, the prerogative of each individual Working Group.

2. Objective and scope

The objective of the programme is to prepare, with the help of international Working Groups of experts, and to publish in the form of *Monographs*, critical reviews and evaluations of evidence on the carcinogenicity of a wide range of human exposures. The *Monographs* represent the first step in carcinogen risk assessment, which involves examination of all relevant information in order to assess the strength of the available evidence that an agent could alter the age-specific incidence of cancer in humans. The *Monographs* may also indicate where additional research efforts are needed, specifically when data immediately relevant to an evaluation are not available.

In this Preamble, the term 'agent' refers to any entity or circumstance that is subject to evaluation in a *Monograph*. As the scope of the programme has broadened, categories of agents now include specific chemicals, groups of related chemicals, complex mixtures, occupational or environmental exposures, cultural or behavioural practices, biological organisms and physical agents. This list of categories may expand as causation of, and susceptibility to, malignant disease become more fully understood.

A cancer 'hazard' is an agent that is capable of causing cancer under some circumstances, while a cancer 'risk' is an estimate of the carcinogenic effects expected from exposure to a cancer hazard. The *Monographs* are an exercise in evaluating cancer hazards, despite the historical presence of the word 'risks' in the title. The distinction between hazard and risk is important, and the *Monographs* identify cancer hazards even when risks are very low at current exposure levels, because new uses or unforeseen exposures could engender risks that are significantly higher.

In the *Monographs*, an agent is termed 'carcinogenic' if it is capable of increasing the incidence of malignant neoplasms, reducing their latency, or increasing their severity or multiplicity. The induction of benign neoplasms may in some circumstances (see Part B, Section 3a) contribute to the judgement that the agent is carcinogenic. The terms 'neoplasm' and 'tumour' are used interchangeably.

The Preamble continues the previous usage of the phrase 'strength of evidence' as a matter of historical continuity, although it should be understood that *Monographs* evaluations consider studies that support a finding of a cancer hazard as well as studies that do not.

Some epidemiological and experimental studies indicate that different agents may act at different stages in the carcinogenic process, and several different mechanisms may be involved. The aim of the *Monographs* has been, from their inception, to evaluate evidence of carcinogenicity at any stage in the carcinogenesis process, independently of the underlying mechanisms. Information on mechanisms may, however, be used in making the overall evaluation (IARC, 1991; Vainio *et al.*, 1992; IARC, 2005, 2006; see also Part B, Sections 4 and 6). As mechanisms of carcinogenesis are elucidated, IARC convenes international scientific conferences to determine whether a broad-based consensus has emerged on how specific mechanistic data can be used in an evaluation of human carcinogenicity. The results of such conferences are reported in IARC Scientific Publications, which, as long as they still reflect the current state of scientific knowledge, may guide subsequent Working Groups.

Although the *Monographs* have emphasized hazard identification, important issues may also involve dose–response assessment. In many cases, the same epidemiological and experimental studies used to evaluate a cancer hazard can also be used to estimate a dose–response relationship. A *Monograph* may undertake to estimate dose–response relationships within the range of the available epidemiological data, or it may compare the dose–response information from experimental and epidemiological studies. In some cases, a subsequent publication may be prepared by a separate Working Group with expertise in quantitative dose–response assessment.

The *Monographs* are used by national and international authorities to make risk assessments, formulate decisions concerning preventive measures, provide effective cancer control programmes and decide among alternative options for public health decisions. The evaluations of IARC Working Groups are scientific, qualitative judgements on the evidence for or against carcinogenicity provided by the available data. These evaluations represent only one part of the body of information on which public health decisions may be based. Public health options vary from one situation to another and from country to country and relate to many factors, including different socioeconomic and national priorities. Therefore, no recommendation is given with regard to regulation or legislation, which are the responsibility of individual governments or other international organizations.

3. Selection of agents for review

Agents are selected for review on the basis of two main criteria: (a) there is evidence of human exposure and (b) there is some evidence or suspicion of carcinogenicity. Mixed exposures may occur in occupational and environmental settings and as a result of individual and cultural habits (such as tobacco smoking and dietary practices). Chemical analogues and compounds with biological or physical characteristics similar to those of suspected carcinogens may also be considered, even in the absence of data on a possible carcinogenic effect in humans or experimental animals.

The scientific literature is surveyed for published data relevant to an assessment of carcinogenicity. Ad-hoc Advisory Groups convened by IARC in 1984, 1989, 1991, 1993, 1998 and 2003 made recommendations as to which agents should be evaluated in the *Monographs* series. Recent recommendations are available on the *Monographs* programme website (http://monographs.iarc.fr). IARC may schedule other agents for review as it becomes aware of new scientific information or as national health agencies identify an urgent public health need related to cancer.

As significant new data become available on an agent for which a *Monograph* exists, a re-evaluation may be made at a subsequent meeting, and a new *Monograph* published. In some cases it may be appropriate to review only the data published since a prior evaluation. This can be useful for updating a database, reviewing new data to resolve a previously open question or identifying new tumour sites associated with a carcinogenic agent. Major changes in an evaluation (e.g. a new classification in Group 1 or a determination that a mechanism does not operate in humans, see Part B, Section 6) are more appropriately addressed by a full review.

4. Data for the *Monographs*

Each *Monograph* reviews all pertinent epidemiological studies and cancer bioassays in experimental animals. Those judged inadequate or irrelevant to the evaluation may be cited but not summarized. If a group of similar studies is not reviewed, the reasons are indicated.

Mechanistic and other relevant data are also reviewed. A *Monograph* does not necessarily cite all the mechanistic literature concerning the agent being evaluated (see Part B, Section 4). Only those data considered by the Working Group to be relevant to making the evaluation are included.

With regard to epidemiological studies, cancer bioassays, and mechanistic and other relevant data, only reports that have been published or accepted for publication in the openly available scientific literature are reviewed. The same publication requirement applies to studies originating from IARC, including meta-analyses or pooled analyses commissioned by IARC in advance of a meeting (see Part B, Section 2c). Data from government agency reports that are publicly available are also considered. Exceptionally, doctoral theses and other material that are in their final form and publicly available may be reviewed.

Exposure data and other information on an agent under consideration are also reviewed. In the sections on chemical and physical properties, on analysis, on production and use and on occurrence, published and unpublished sources of information may be considered.

Inclusion of a study does not imply acceptance of the adequacy of the study design or of the analysis and interpretation of the results, and limitations are clearly outlined in square brackets at the end of each study description (see Part B). The reasons for not giving further consideration to an individual study also are indicated in the square brackets.

5. Meeting participants

Five categories of participant can be present at *Monograph* meetings.

(a) The Working Group is responsible for the critical reviews and evaluations that are developed during the meeting. The tasks of Working Group Members are: (i) to ascertain that all appropriate data have been collected; (ii) to select the data relevant for the evaluation on the basis of scientific merit; (iii) to prepare accurate summaries of the data to enable the reader to follow the reasoning of the Working Group; (iv) to evaluate the results of epidemiological and experimental studies on cancer; (v) to evaluate data relevant to the understanding of mechanisms of carcinogenesis; and (vi) to make an overall evaluation of the carcinogenicity of the exposure to humans. Working Group Members generally have published significant research related to the carcinogenicity of the agents being reviewed, and IARC uses literature searches to identify most experts. Working Group Members are selected on the basis of (a) knowledge and experience and (b) absence of real or apparent conflicts of interests. Consideration is also given to demographic diversity and balance of scientific findings and views.

(b) Invited Specialists are experts who also have critical knowledge and experience but have a real or apparent conflict of interests. These experts are invited when necessary to assist in the Working Group by contributing their unique knowledge and experience during subgroup and plenary discussions. They may also contribute text on non-influential issues in the section on exposure, such as a general description of data on production and use (see Part B, Section 1). Invited Specialists do not serve as meeting chair or subgroup chair, draft text that pertains to the description or interpretation of cancer data, or participate in the evaluations.

(c) Representatives of national and international health agencies often attend meetings because their agencies sponsor the programme or are interested in the subject of a meeting. Representatives do not serve as meeting chair or subgroup chair, draft any part of a *Monograph,* or participate in the evaluations.

(d) Observers with relevant scientific credentials may be admitted to a meeting by IARC in limited numbers. Attention will be given to achieving a balance of Observers from constituencies with differing perspectives. They are invited to observe the meeting and should not attempt to influence it. Observers do not serve as meeting chair or subgroup chair, draft any part of a *Monograph*, or participate in the evaluations. At the meeting, the meeting chair and subgroup chairs may grant Observers an opportunity to speak, generally after they have observed a discussion. Observers agree to respect the Guidelines for Observers at *IARC Monographs* meetings (available at http://monographs.iarc.fr).

(e) The IARC Secretariat consists of scientists who are designated by IARC and who have relevant expertise. They serve as rapporteurs and participate in all discussions. When requested by the meeting chair or subgroup chair, they may also draft text or prepare tables and analyses.

Before an invitation is extended, each potential participant, including the IARC Secretariat, completes the WHO Declaration of Interests to report financial interests, employment and consulting, and individual and institutional research support related to the subject of the meeting. IARC assesses these interests to determine whether there is a conflict that warrants some limitation on participation. The declarations are updated and reviewed again at the opening of the meeting. Interests related to the subject of the meeting are disclosed to the meeting participants and in the published volume (Cogliano *et al.*, 2004).

The names and principal affiliations of participants are available on the *Monographs* programme website (http://monographs.iarc.fr) approximately two months before each meeting. It is not acceptable for Observers or third parties to contact other participants before a meeting or to lobby them at any time. Meeting participants are asked to report all such contacts to IARC (Cogliano *et al.*, 2005).

All participants are listed, with their principal affiliations, at the beginning of each volume. Each participant who is a Member of a Working Group serves as an individual scientist and not as a representative of any organization, government or industry.

6. Working procedures

A separate Working Group is responsible for developing each volume of *Monographs*. A volume contains one or more *Monographs*, which can cover either a single agent or several related agents. Approximately one year in advance of the meeting of a Working Group, the agents to be reviewed are announced on the *Monographs* programme website (http://monographs.iarc.fr) and participants are selected by IARC staff in consultation with other experts. Subsequently, relevant biological and epidemiological data are collected by IARC from recognized sources of information on carcinogenesis, including data storage and retrieval systems such as PubMed. Meeting participants who are asked to prepare preliminary working papers for specific sections are expected to supplement the IARC literature searches with their own searches.

For most chemicals and some complex mixtures, the major collection of data and the preparation of working papers for the sections on chemical and physical properties, on analysis, on production and use, and on occurrence are carried out under a separate contract funded by the US National Cancer Institute. Industrial associations, labour unions and other knowledgeable organizations may be asked to provide input to the sections on production and use, although this involvement is not required as a general rule. Information on production and trade is obtained from governmental, trade and market research publications and, in some cases, by direct contact with industries. Separate production data on some agents may not be available for a variety of reasons (e.g. not collected or made public in all producing countries, production is small). Information on uses may be obtained from published sources but is often complemented by direct contact with manufacturers. Efforts are made to supplement this information with data from other national and international sources.

Six months before the meeting, the material obtained is sent to meeting participants to prepare preliminary working papers. The working papers are compiled by IARC staff and sent, prior to the meeting, to Working Group Members and Invited Specialists for review.

The Working Group meets at IARC for seven to eight days to discuss and finalize the texts and to formulate the evaluations. The objectives of the meeting are peer review and consensus. During the first few days, four subgroups (covering exposure data, cancer in humans, cancer in experimental animals, and mechanistic and other relevant data) review the working papers, develop a joint subgroup draft and write summaries. Care is taken to ensure that each study summary is written or reviewed by someone not associated with the study being considered. During the last few days, the Working Group meets in plenary session to review the subgroup drafts and develop the evaluations. As a result, the entire volume is the joint product of the Working Group, and there are no individually authored sections.

IARC Working Groups strive to achieve a consensus evaluation. Consensus reflects broad agreement among Working Group Members, but not necessarily unanimity. The chair may elect to poll Working Group Members to determine the diversity of scientific opinion on issues where consensus is not readily apparent.

After the meeting, the master copy is verified by consulting the original literature, edited and prepared for publication. The aim is to publish the volume within six months of the Working Group meeting. A summary of the outcome is available on the *Monographs* programme website soon after the meeting.

B. SCIENTIFIC REVIEW AND EVALUATION

The available studies are summarized by the Working Group, with particular regard to the qualitative aspects discussed below. In general, numerical findings are indicated as they appear in the original report; units are converted when necessary for easier comparison. The Working Group may conduct additional analyses of the published data and use them in their assessment of the evidence; the results of such supplementary analyses are given in square brackets. When an important aspect of a study that directly impinges on its interpretation should be brought to the attention of the reader, a Working Group comment is given in square brackets.

The scope of the *IARC Monographs* programme has expanded beyond chemicals to include complex mixtures, occupational exposures, physical and biological agents, lifestyle factors and other potentially carcinogenic exposures. Over time, the structure of a *Monograph* has evolved to include the following sections:

1. Exposure data
2. Studies of cancer in humans
3. Studies of cancer in experimental animals
4. Mechanistic and other relevant data
5. Summary
6. Evaluation and rationale

In addition, a section of General Remarks at the front of the volume discusses the reasons the agents were scheduled for evaluation and some key issues the Working Group encountered during the meeting.

This part of the Preamble discusses the types of evidence considered and summarized in each section of a *Monograph*, followed by the scientific criteria that guide the evaluations.

1. Exposure data

Each *Monograph* includes general information on the agent: this information may vary substantially between agents and must be adapted accordingly. Also included is information on production and use (when appropriate), methods of analysis and detection, occurrence, and sources and routes of human occupational and environmental exposures. Depending on the agent, regulations and guidelines for use may be presented.

(a)   General information on the agent

For chemical agents, sections on chemical and physical data are included: the Chemical Abstracts Service Registry Number, the latest primary name and the IUPAC systematic name are recorded; other synonyms are given, but the list is not necessarily comprehensive. Information on chemical and physical properties that are relevant to identification, occurrence and biological activity is included. A description of technical products of chemicals includes trade names, relevant specifications and available information on composition and impurities. Some of the trade names given may be those of mixtures in which the agent being evaluated is only one of the ingredients.

For biological agents, taxonomy, structure and biology are described, and the degree of variability is indicated. Mode of replication, life cycle, target cells, persistence, latency, host response and clinical disease other than cancer are also presented.

For physical agents that are forms of radiation, energy and range of the radiation are included. For foreign bodies, fibres and respirable particles, size range and relative dimensions are indicated.

For agents such as mixtures, drugs or lifestyle factors, a description of the agent, including its composition, is given.

Whenever appropriate, other information, such as historical perspectives or the description of an industry or habit, may be included.

(b)   Analysis and detection

An overview of methods of analysis and detection of the agent is presented, including their sensitivity, specificity and reproducibility. Methods widely used for regulatory purposes are emphasized. Methods for monitoring human exposure are also given. No critical evaluation or recommendation of any method is meant or implied.

(c)   Production and use

The dates of first synthesis and of first commercial production of a chemical, mixture or other agent are provided when available; for agents that do not occur naturally, this information may allow a reasonable estimate to be made of the date before which no human exposure to the agent could have occurred. The dates of first reported occurrence of an exposure are also provided when available. In addition, methods of synthesis used in past and present commercial production and different methods of production, which may give rise to different impurities, are described.

The countries where companies report production of the agent, and the number of companies in each country, are identified. Available data on production, international trade and uses are obtained for representative regions. It should not, however, be inferred that those areas or nations are necessarily the sole or major sources or users of the agent. Some identified uses may not be current or major applications, and the coverage is not necessarily comprehensive. In the case of drugs, mention of their therapeutic uses does not necessarily represent current practice nor does it imply judgement as to their therapeutic efficacy.

(d)   Occurrence and exposure

Information on the occurrence of an agent in the environment is obtained from data derived from the monitoring and surveillance of levels in occupational environments, air, water, soil, plants, foods and animal and human tissues. When available, data on the generation, persistence and bioaccumulation of the agent are also included. Such data may be available from national databases.

Data that indicate the extent of past and present human exposure, the sources of exposure, the people most likely to be exposed and the factors that contribute to the exposure are reported. Information is presented on the range of human exposure, including occupational and environmental exposures. This includes relevant findings from both developed and developing countries. Some of these data are not distributed widely and may be available from government reports and other sources. In the case of mixtures, industries, occupations or processes, information is given about all agents known to be present. For processes, industries and occupations, a historical description is also given, noting variations in chemical composition, physical properties and levels of occupational exposure with date and place. For biological agents, the epidemiology of infection is described.

(e)   Regulations and guidelines

Statements concerning regulations and guidelines (e.g. occupational exposure limits, maximal levels permitted in foods and water, pesticide registrations) are included, but they may not reflect the most recent situation, since such limits are continuously reviewed and modified. The absence of information on regulatory status for a country should not be taken to imply that that country does not have regulations with regard to the exposure. For biological agents, legislation and control, including vaccination and therapy, are described.

2. Studies of cancer in humans

This section includes all pertinent epidemiological studies (see Part A, Section 4). Studies of biomarkers are included when they are relevant to an evaluation of carcinogenicity to humans.

(a)   Types of study considered

Several types of epidemiological study contribute to the assessment of carcinogenicity in humans — cohort studies, case–control studies, correlation (or ecological) studies and intervention studies. Rarely, results from randomized trials may be available. Case reports and case series of cancer in humans may also be reviewed.

Cohort and case–control studies relate individual exposures under study to the occurrence of cancer in individuals and provide an estimate of effect (such as relative risk) as the main measure of association. Intervention studies may provide strong evidence for making causal inferences, as exemplified by cessation of smoking and the subsequent decrease in risk for lung cancer.

In correlation studies, the units of investigation are usually whole populations (e.g. in particular geographical areas or at particular times), and cancer frequency is related to a summary measure of the exposure of the population to the agent under study. In correlation studies, individual exposure is not documented, which renders this kind of study more prone to confounding. In some circumstances, however, correlation studies may be more informative than analytical study designs (see, for example, the *Monograph* on arsenic in drinking-water; IARC, 2004).

In some instances, case reports and case series have provided important information about the carcinogenicity of an agent. These types of study generally arise from a suspicion, based on clinical experience, that the concurrence of two events — that is, a particular exposure and occurrence of a cancer — has happened rather more frequently than would be expected by chance. Case reports and case series usually lack complete ascertainment of cases in any population, definition or enumeration of the population at risk and estimation of the expected number of cases in the absence of exposure.

The uncertainties that surround the interpretation of case reports, case series and correlation studies make them inadequate, except in rare instances, to form the sole basis for inferring a causal relationship. When taken together with case–control and cohort studies, however, these types of study may add materially to the judgement that a causal relationship exists.

Epidemiological studies of benign neoplasms, presumed preneoplastic lesions and other end-points thought to be relevant to cancer are also reviewed. They may, in some instances, strengthen inferences drawn from studies of cancer itself.

(b)   Quality of studies considered

It is necessary to take into account the possible roles of bias, confounding and chance in the interpretation of epidemiological studies. Bias is the effect of factors in study design or execution that lead erroneously to a stronger or weaker association than in fact exists between an agent and disease. Confounding is a form of bias that occurs when the relationship with disease is made to appear stronger or weaker than it truly is as a result of an association between the apparent causal factor and another factor that is associated with either an increase or decrease in the incidence of the disease. The role of chance is related to biological variability and the influence of sample size on the precision of estimates of effect.

In evaluating the extent to which these factors have been minimized in an individual study, consideration is given to a number of aspects of design and analysis as described in the report of the study. For example, when suspicion of carcinogenicity arises largely from a single small study, careful consideration is given when interpreting subsequent studies that included these data in an enlarged population. Most of these considerations apply equally to case–control, cohort and correlation studies. Lack of clarity of any of these aspects in the reporting of a study can decrease its credibility and the weight given to it in the final evaluation of the exposure.

Firstly, the study population, disease (or diseases) and exposure should have been well defined by the authors. Cases of disease in the study population should have been identified in a way that was independent of the exposure of interest, and exposure should have been assessed in a way that was not related to disease status.

Secondly, the authors should have taken into account — in the study design and analysis — other variables that can influence the risk of disease and may have been related to the exposure of interest. Potential confounding by such variables should have been dealt with either in the design of the study, such as by matching, or in the analysis, by statistical adjustment. In cohort studies, comparisons with local rates of disease may or may not be more appropriate than those with national rates. Internal comparisons of frequency of disease among individuals at different levels of exposure are also desirable in cohort studies, since they minimize the potential for confounding related to the differ-ence in risk factors between an external reference group and the study population.

Thirdly, the authors should have reported the basic data on which the conclusions are founded, even if sophisticated statistical analyses were employed. At the very least, they should have given the numbers of exposed and unexposed cases and controls in a case–control study and the numbers of cases observed and expected in a cohort study. Further tabulations by time since exposure began and other temporal factors are also important. In a cohort study, data on all cancer sites and all causes of death should have been given, to reveal the possibility of reporting bias. In a case–control study, the effects of investigated factors other than the exposure of interest should have been reported.

Finally, the statistical methods used to obtain estimates of relative risk, absolute rates of cancer, confidence intervals and significance tests, and to adjust for confounding should have been clearly stated by the authors. These methods have been reviewed for case–control studies (Breslow & Day, 1980) and for cohort studies (Breslow & Day, 1987).

(c)   Meta-analyses and pooled analyses

Independent epidemiological studies of the same agent may lead to results that are difficult to interpret. Combined analyses of data from multiple studies are a means of resolving this ambiguity, and well-conducted analyses can be considered. There are two types of combined analysis. The first involves combining summary statistics such as relative risks from individual studies (meta-analysis) and the second involves a pooled analysis of the raw data from the individual studies (pooled analysis) (Greenland, 1998).

The advantages of combined analyses are increased precision due to increased sample size and the opportunity to explore potential confounders, interactions and modifying effects that may explain heterogeneity among studies in more detail. A disadvantage of combined analyses is the possible lack of compatibility of data from various studies due to differences in subject recruitment, procedures of data collection, methods of measure-ment and effects of unmeasured co-variates that may differ among studies. Despite these limitations, well-conducted combined analyses may provide a firmer basis than individual studies for drawing conclusions about the potential carcinogenicity of agents.

IARC may commission a meta-analysis or pooled analysis that is pertinent to a particular *Monograph* (see Part A, Section 4). Additionally, as a means of gaining insight from the results of multiple individual studies, ad-hoc calculations that combine data from different studies may be conducted by the Working Group during the course of a *Mono-graph* meeting. The results of such original calculations, which would be specified in the text by presentation in square brackets, might involve updates of previously conducted analyses that incorporate the results of more recent studies or de-novo analyses. Irrespective of the source of data for the meta-analyses and pooled analyses, it is im-portant that the same criteria for data quality be applied as those that would be applied to individual studies and to ensure also that sources of heterogeneity between studies be taken into account.

(d)   Temporal effects

Detailed analyses of both relative and absolute risks in relation to temporal variables, such as age at first exposure, time since first exposure, duration of exposure, cumulative exposure, peak exposure (when appropriate) and time since cessation of exposure, are reviewed and summarized when available. Analyses of temporal relationships may be useful in making causal inferences. In addition, such analyses may suggest whether a carcinogen acts early or late in the process of carcinogenesis, although, at best, they allow only indirect inferences about mechanisms of carcinogenesis.

(e)   Use of biomarkers in epidemiological studies

Biomarkers indicate molecular, cellular or other biological changes and are increasingly used in epidemiological studies for various purposes (IARC, 1991; Vainio et al., 1992; Toniolo et al., 1997; Vineis et al., 1999; Buffler et al., 2004). These may include evidence of exposure, of early effects, of cellular, tissue or organism responses, of individual susceptibility or host responses, and inference of a mechanism (see Part B, Section 4b). This is a rapidly evolving field that encompasses developments in genomics, epigenomics and other emerging technologies.

Molecular epidemiological data that identify associations between genetic polymorphisms and interindividual differences in susceptibility to the agent(s) being evaluated may contribute to the identification of carcinogenic hazards to humans. If the polymorphism has been demonstrated experimentally to modify the functional activity of the gene product in a manner that is consistent with increased susceptibility, these data may be useful in making causal inferences. Similarly, molecular epidemiological studies that measure cell functions, enzymes or metabolites that are thought to be the basis of susceptibility may provide evidence that reinforces biological plausibility. It should be noted, however, that when data on genetic susceptibility originate from multiple comparisons that arise from subgroup analyses, this can generate false-positive results and inconsistencies across studies, and such data therefore require careful evaluation. If the known phenotype of a genetic polymorphism can explain the carcinogenic mechanism of the agent being evaluated, data on this phenotype may be useful in making causal inferences.

(f)   Criteria for causality

After the quality of individual epidemiological studies of cancer has been summarized and assessed, a judgement is made concerning the strength of evidence that the agent in question is carcinogenic to humans. In making its judgement, the Working Group considers several criteria for causality (Hill, 1965). A strong association (e.g. a large relative risk) is more likely to indicate causality than a weak association, although it is recognized that estimates of effect of small magnitude do not imply lack of causality and may be important if the disease or exposure is common. Associations that are replicated in several studies of the same design or that use different epidemiological approaches or under different circumstances of exposure are more likely to represent a causal relationship than isolated observations from single studies. If there are inconsistent results among investigations, possible reasons are sought (such as differences in exposure), and results of studies that are judged to be of high quality are given more weight than those of studies that are judged to be methodologically less sound.

If the risk increases with the exposure, this is considered to be a strong indication of causality, although the absence of a graded response is not necessarily evidence against a causal relationship. The demonstration of a decline in risk after cessation of or reduction in exposure in individuals or in whole populations also supports a causal interpretation of the findings.

A number of scenarios may increase confidence in a causal relationship. On the one hand, an agent may be specific in causing tumours at one site or of one morphological type. On the other, carcinogenicity may be evident through the causation of multiple tumour types. Temporality, precision of estimates of effect, biological plausibility and coherence of the overall database are considered. Data on biomarkers may be employed in an assessment of the biological plausibility of epidemiological observations.

Although rarely available, results from randomized trials that show different rates of cancer among exposed and unexposed individuals provide particularly strong evidence for causality.

When several epidemiological studies show little or no indication of an association between an exposure and cancer, a judgement may be made that, in the aggregate, they show evidence of lack of carcinogenicity. Such a judgement requires firstly that the studies meet, to a sufficient degree, the standards of design and analysis described above. Specifically, the possibility that bias, confounding or misclassification of exposure or outcome could explain the observed results should be considered and excluded with reasonable certainty. In addition, all studies that are judged to be methodologically sound should (a) be consistent with an estimate of effect of unity for any observed level of exposure, (b) when considered together, provide a pooled estimate of relative risk that is at or near to unity, and (c) have a narrow confidence interval, due to sufficient population size. Moreover, no individual study nor the pooled results of all the studies should show any consistent tendency that the relative risk of cancer increases with increasing level of exposure. It is important to note that evidence of lack of carcinogenicity obtained from several epidemiological studies can apply only to the type(s) of cancer studied, to the dose levels reported, and to the intervals between first exposure and disease onset observed in these studies. Experience with human cancer indicates that the period from first exposure to the development of clinical cancer is sometimes longer than 20 years; latent periods substantially shorter than 30 years cannot provide evidence for lack of carcinogenicity.

3. Studies of cancer in experimental animals

All known human carcinogens that have been studied adequately for carcinogenicity in experimental animals have produced positive results in one or more animal species

(Wilbourn *et al.*, 1986; Tomatis *et al.*, 1989). For several agents (e.g. aflatoxins, diethyl-stilbestrol, solar radiation, vinyl chloride), carcinogenicity in experimental animals was established or highly suspected before epidemiological studies confirmed their carcinogenicity in humans (Vainio *et al.*, 1995). Although this association cannot establish that all agents that cause cancer in experimental animals also cause cancer in humans, it is biologically plausible that agents for which there is *sufficient evidence of carcinogenicity* in experimental animals (see Part B, Section 6b) also present a carcinogenic hazard to humans. Accordingly, in the absence of additional scientific information, these agents are considered to pose a carcinogenic hazard to humans. Examples of additional scientific information are data that demonstrate that a given agent causes cancer in animals through a species-specific mechanism that does not operate in humans or data that demonstrate that the mechanism in experimental animals also operates in humans (see Part B, Section 6).

Consideration is given to all available long-term studies of cancer in experimental animals with the agent under review (see Part A, Section 4). In all experimental settings, the nature and extent of impurities or contaminants present in the agent being evaluated are given when available. Animal species, strain (including genetic background where applicable), sex, numbers per group, age at start of treatment, route of exposure, dose levels, duration of exposure, survival and information on tumours (incidence, latency, severity or multiplicity of neoplasms or preneoplastic lesions) are reported. Those studies in experimental animals that are judged to be irrelevant to the evaluation or judged to be inadequate (e.g. too short a duration, too few animals, poor survival; see below) may be omitted. Guidelines for conducting long-term carcinogenicity experiments have been published (e.g. OECD, 2002).

Other studies considered may include: experiments in which the agent was administered in the presence of factors that modify carcinogenic effects (e.g. initiation–promotion studies, co-carcinogenicity studies and studies in genetically modified animals); studies in which the end-point was not cancer but a defined precancerous lesion; experiments on the carcinogenicity of known metabolites and derivatives; and studies of cancer in non-laboratory animals (e.g. livestock and companion animals) exposed to the agent.

For studies of mixtures, consideration is given to the possibility that changes in the physicochemical properties of the individual substances may occur during collection, storage, extraction, concentration and delivery. Another consideration is that chemical and toxicological interactions of components in a mixture may alter dose–response relationships. The relevance to human exposure of the test mixture administered in the animal experiment is also assessed. This may involve consideration of the following aspects of the mixture tested: (i) physical and chemical characteristics, (ii) identified constituents that may indicate the presence of a class of substances and (iii) the results of genetic toxicity and related tests.

The relevance of results obtained with an agent that is analogous (e.g. similar in structure or of a similar virus genus) to that being evaluated is also considered. Such results may provide biological and mechanistic information that is relevant to the

understanding of the process of carcinogenesis in humans and may strengthen the biological plausibility that the agent being evaluated is carcinogenic to humans (see Part B,
Section 2f).

(a)   Qualitative aspects

An assessment of carcinogenicity involves several considerations of qualitative importance, including (i) the experimental conditions under which the test was performed,
including route, schedule and duration of exposure, species, strain (including genetic
background where applicable), sex, age and duration of follow-up; (ii) the consistency of
the results, for example, across species and target organ(s); (iii) the spectrum of neoplastic
response, from preneoplastic lesions and benign tumours to malignant neoplasms; and
(iv) the possible role of modifying factors.

Considerations of importance in the interpretation and evaluation of a particular study
include: (i) how clearly the agent was defined and, in the case of mixtures, how
adequately the sample characterization was reported; (ii) whether the dose was monitored
adequately, particularly in inhalation experiments; (iii) whether the doses, duration of
treatment and route of exposure were appropriate; (iv) whether the survival of treated
animals was similar to that of controls; (v) whether there were adequate numbers of
animals per group; (vi) whether both male and female animals were used; (vii) whether
animals were allocated randomly to groups; (viii) whether the duration of observation was
adequate; and (ix) whether the data were reported and analysed adequately.

When benign tumours (a) occur together with and originate from the same cell type as
malignant tumours in an organ or tissue in a particular study and (b) appear to represent a
stage in the progression to malignancy, they are usually combined in the assessment of
tumour incidence (Huff et al., 1989). The occurrence of lesions presumed to be preneoplastic may in certain instances aid in assessing the biological plausibility of any
neoplastic response observed. If an agent induces only benign neoplasms that appear to be
end-points that do not readily undergo transition to malignancy, the agent should nevertheless be suspected of being carcinogenic and requires further investigation.

(b)   Quantitative aspects

The probability that tumours will occur may depend on the species, sex, strain,
genetic background and age of the animal, and on the dose, route, timing and duration of
the exposure. Evidence of an increased incidence of neoplasms with increasing levels of
exposure strengthens the inference of a causal association between the exposure and the
development of neoplasms.

The form of the dose–response relationship can vary widely, depending on the
particular agent under study and the target organ. Mechanisms such as induction of DNA
damage or inhibition of repair, altered cell division and cell death rates and changes in
intercellular communication are important determinants of dose–response relationships
for some carcinogens. Since many chemicals require metabolic activation before being

converted to their reactive intermediates, both metabolic and toxicokinetic aspects are important in determining the dose–response pattern. Saturation of steps such as absorption, activation, inactivation and elimination may produce non-linearity in the dose–response relationship (Hoel *et al.*, 1983; Gart *et al.*, 1986), as could saturation of processes such as DNA repair. The dose–response relationship can also be affected by differences in survival among the treatment groups.

(*c*)   *Statistical analyses*

Factors considered include the adequacy of the information given for each treatment group: (i) number of animals studied and number examined histologically, (ii) number of animals with a given tumour type and (iii) length of survival. The statistical methods used should be clearly stated and should be the generally accepted techniques refined for this purpose (Peto *et al.*, 1980; Gart *et al.*, 1986; Portier & Bailer, 1989; Bieler & Williams, 1993). The choice of the most appropriate statistical method requires consideration of whether or not there are differences in survival among the treatment groups; for example, reduced survival because of non-tumour-related mortality can preclude the occurrence of tumours later in life. When detailed information on survival is not available, comparisons of the proportions of tumour-bearing animals among the effective number of animals (alive at the time the first tumour was discovered) can be useful when significant differences in survival occur before tumours appear. The lethality of the tumour also requires consideration: for rapidly fatal tumours, the time of death provides an indication of the time of tumour onset and can be assessed using life-table methods; non-fatal or incidental tumours that do not affect survival can be assessed using methods such as the Mantel-Haenzel test for changes in tumour prevalence. Because tumour lethality is often difficult to determine, methods such as the Poly-K test that do not require such information can also be used. When results are available on the number and size of tumours seen in experimental animals (e.g. papillomas on mouse skin, liver tumours observed through nuclear magnetic resonance tomography), other more complicated statistical procedures may be needed (Sherman *et al.*, 1994; Dunson *et al.*, 2003).

Formal statistical methods have been developed to incorporate historical control data into the analysis of data from a given experiment. These methods assign an appropriate weight to historical and concurrent controls on the basis of the extent of between-study and within-study variability: less weight is given to historical controls when they show a high degree of variability, and greater weight when they show little variability. It is generally not appropriate to discount a tumour response that is significantly increased compared with concurrent controls by arguing that it falls within the range of historical controls, particularly when historical controls show high between-study variability and are, thus, of little relevance to the current experiment. In analysing results for uncommon tumours, however, the analysis may be improved by considering historical control data, particularly when between-study variability is low. Historical controls should be selected to resemble the concurrent controls as closely as possible with respect to species, gender and strain, as well as other factors such as basal diet and general laboratory environment, which may affect tumour-response rates in control animals (Haseman *et al.*, 1984; Fung *et al.*, 1996; Greim *et al.*, 2003).

Although meta-analyses and combined analyses are conducted less frequently for animal experiments than for epidemiological studies due to differences in animal strains, they can be useful aids in interpreting animal data when the experimental protocols are sufficiently similar.

4. Mechanistic and other relevant data

Mechanistic and other relevant data may provide evidence of carcinogenicity and also help in assessing the relevance and importance of findings of cancer in animals and in humans. The nature of the mechanistic and other relevant data depends on the biological activity of the agent being considered. The Working Group considers representative studies to give a concise description of the relevant data and issues that they consider to be important; thus, not every available study is cited. Relevant topics may include toxico-kinetics, mechanisms of carcinogenesis, susceptible individuals, populations and life-stages, other relevant data and other adverse effects. When data on biomarkers are in-formative about the mechanisms of carcinogenesis, they are included in this section.

These topics are not mutually exclusive; thus, the same studies may be discussed in more than one subsection. For example, a mutation in a gene that codes for an enzyme that metabolizes the agent under study could be discussed in the subsections on toxico-kinetics, mechanisms and individual susceptibility if it also exists as an inherited poly-morphism.

(a)   Toxicokinetic data

Toxicokinetics refers to the absorption, distribution, metabolism and elimination of agents in humans, experimental animals and, where relevant, cellular systems. Examples of kinetic factors that may affect dose–response relationships include uptake, deposition, biopersistence and half-life in tissues, protein binding, metabolic activation and de-toxification. Studies that indicate the metabolic fate of the agent in humans and in experi-mental animals are summarized briefly, and comparisons of data from humans and animals are made when possible. Comparative information on the relationship between exposure and the dose that reaches the target site may be important for the extrapolation of hazards between species and in clarifying the role of in-vitro findings.

(b)   Data on mechanisms of carcinogenesis

To provide focus, the Working Group attempts to identify the possible mechanisms by which the agent may increase the risk of cancer. For each possible mechanism, a representative selection of key data from humans and experimental systems is sum-marized. Attention is given to gaps in the data and to data that suggests that more than one mechanism may be operating. The relevance of the mechanism to humans is discussed, in particular, when mechanistic data are derived from experimental model systems. Changes in the affected organs, tissues or cells can be divided into three non-exclusive levels as described below.

(i)   *Changes in physiology*

Physiological changes refer to exposure-related modifications to the physiology and/or response of cells, tissues and organs. Examples of potentially adverse physiological changes include mitogenesis, compensatory cell division, escape from apoptosis and/or senescence, presence of inflammation, hyperplasia, metaplasia and/or preneoplasia, angiogenesis, alterations in cellular adhesion, changes in steroidal hormones and changes in immune surveillance.

(ii)   *Functional changes at the cellular level*

Functional changes refer to exposure-related alterations in the signalling pathways used by cells to manage critical processes that are related to increased risk for cancer. Examples of functional changes include modified activities of enzymes involved in the metabolism of xenobiotics, alterations in the expression of key genes that regulate DNA repair, alterations in cyclin-dependent kinases that govern cell cycle progression, changes in the patterns of post-translational modifications of proteins, changes in regulatory factors that alter apoptotic rates, changes in the secretion of factors related to the stimulation of DNA replication and transcription and changes in gap–junction-mediated intercellular communication.

(iii)   *Changes at the molecular level*

Molecular changes refer to exposure-related changes in key cellular structures at the molecular level, including, in particular, genotoxicity. Examples of molecular changes include formation of DNA adducts and DNA strand breaks, mutations in genes, chromosomal aberrations, aneuploidy and changes in DNA methylation patterns. Greater emphasis is given to irreversible effects.

The use of mechanistic data in the identification of a carcinogenic hazard is specific to the mechanism being addressed and is not readily described for every possible level and mechanism discussed above.

Genotoxicity data are discussed here to illustrate the key issues involved in the evaluation of mechanistic data.

Tests for genetic and related effects are described in view of the relevance of gene mutation and chromosomal aberration/aneuploidy to carcinogenesis (Vainio *et al.*, 1992; McGregor *et al.*, 1999). The adequacy of the reporting of sample characterization is considered and, when necessary, commented upon; with regard to complex mixtures, such comments are similar to those described for animal carcinogenicity tests. The available data are interpreted critically according to the end-points detected, which may include DNA damage, gene mutation, sister chromatid exchange, micronucleus formation, chromosomal aberrations and aneuploidy. The concentrations employed are given, and mention is made of whether the use of an exogenous metabolic system *in vitro* affected the test result. These data are listed in tabular form by phylogenetic classification.

Positive results in tests using prokaryotes, lower eukaryotes, insects, plants and cultured mammalian cells suggest that genetic and related effects could occur in mammals. Results from such tests may also give information on the types of genetic effect produced and on the involvement of metabolic activation. Some end-points described are clearly genetic in nature (e.g. gene mutations), while others are associated with genetic effects (e.g. unscheduled DNA synthesis). In-vitro tests for tumour promotion, cell transformation and gap–junction inter-cellular communication may be sensitive to changes that are not necessarily the result of genetic alterations but that may have specific relevance to the process of carcinogenesis. Critical appraisals of these tests have been published (Montesano *et al.*, 1986; McGregor *et al.*, 1999).

Genetic or other activity manifest in humans and experimental mammals is regarded to be of greater relevance than that in other organisms. The demon-stration that an agent can induce gene and chromosomal mutations in mammals *in vivo* indicates that it may have carcinogenic activity. Negative results in tests for mutagenicity in selected tissues from animals treated *in vivo* provide less weight, partly because they do not exclude the possibility of an effect in tissues other than those examined. Moreover, negative results in short-term tests with genetic end-points cannot be considered to provide evidence that rules out the carcinogenicity of agents that act through other mechanisms (e.g. receptor-mediated effects, cellular toxicity with regenerative cell division, peroxisome proliferation) (Vainio *et al.*, 1992). Factors that may give misleading results in short-term tests have been discussed in detail elsewhere (Montesano *et al.*, 1986; McGregor *et al.*, 1999).

When there is evidence that an agent acts by a specific mechanism that does not involve genotoxicity (e.g. hormonal dysregulation, immune suppression, and formation of calculi and other deposits that cause chronic irritation), that evidence is presented and reviewed critically in the context of rigorous criteria for the operation of that mechanism in carcinogenesis (e.g. Capen *et al.*, 1999).

For biological agents such as viruses, bacteria and parasites, other data relevant to carcinogenicity may include descriptions of the pathology of infection, integration and expression of viruses, and genetic alterations seen in human tumours. Other observations that might comprise cellular and tissue responses to infection, immune response and the presence of tumour markers are also considered.

For physical agents that are forms of radiation, other data relevant to carcinogenicity may include descriptions of damaging effects at the physiological, cellular and molecular level, as for chemical agents, and descriptions of how these effects occur. 'Physical agents' may also be considered to comprise foreign bodies, such as surgical implants of various kinds, and poorly soluble fibres, dusts and particles of various sizes, the patho-genic effects of which are a result of their physical presence in tissues or body cavities. Other relevant data for such materials may include characterization of cellular, tissue and physiological reactions to these materials and descriptions of pathological conditions other than neoplasia with which they may be associated.

(c)   Other data relevant to mechanisms

A description is provided of any structure–activity relationships that may be relevant to an evaluation of the carcinogenicity of an agent, the toxicological implications of the physical and chemical properties, and any other data relevant to the evaluation that are not included elsewhere.

High-output data, such as those derived from gene expression microarrays, and high-throughput data, such as those that result from testing hundreds of agents for a single end-point, pose a unique problem for the use of mechanistic data in the evaluation of a car-cinogenic hazard. In the case of high-output data, there is the possibility to overinterpret changes in individual end-points (e.g. changes in expression in one gene) without con-sidering the consistency of that finding in the broader context of the other end-points (e.g. other genes with linked transcriptional control). High-output data can be used in assessing mechanisms, but all end-points measured in a single experiment need to be considered in the proper context. For high-throughput data, where the number of observations far exceeds the number of end-points measured, their utility for identifying common mechan-isms across multiple agents is enhanced. These data can be used to identify mechanisms that not only seem plausible, but also have a consistent pattern of carcinogenic response across entire classes of related compounds.

(d)   Susceptibility data

Individuals, populations and life-stages may have greater or lesser susceptibility to an agent, based on toxicokinetics, mechanisms of carcinogenesis and other factors. Examples of host and genetic factors that affect individual susceptibility include sex, genetic poly-morphisms of genes involved in the metabolism of the agent under evaluation, differences in metabolic capacity due to life-stage or the presence of disease, differences in DNA re-pair capacity, competition for or alteration of metabolic capacity by medications or other chemical exposures, pre-existing hormonal imbalance that is exacerbated by a chemical exposure, a suppressed immune system, periods of higher-than-usual tissue growth or regeneration and genetic polymorphisms that lead to differences in behaviour (e.g. addiction). Such data can substantially increase the strength of the evidence from epidemiological data and enhance the linkage of in-vivo and in-vitro laboratory studies to humans.

(e)   Data on other adverse effects

Data on acute, subchronic and chronic adverse effects relevant to the cancer eval-uation are summarized. Adverse effects that confirm distribution and biological effects at the sites of tumour development, or alterations in physiology that could lead to tumour development, are emphasized. Effects on reproduction, embryonic and fetal survival and development are summarized briefly. The adequacy of epidemiological studies of repro-ductive outcome and genetic and related effects in humans is judged by the same criteria as those applied to epidemiological studies of cancer, but fewer details are given.

5. Summary

This section is a summary of data presented in the preceding sections. Summaries can be found on the *Monographs* programme website (http://monographs.iarc.fr).

(a)   Exposure data

Data are summarized, as appropriate, on the basis of elements such as production, use, occurrence and exposure levels in the workplace and environment and measurements in human tissues and body fluids. Quantitative data and time trends are given to compare exposures in different occupations and environmental settings. Exposure to biological agents is described in terms of transmission, prevalence and persistence of infection.

(b)   Cancer in humans

Results of epidemiological studies pertinent to an assessment of human carcino-genicity are summarized. When relevant, case reports and correlation studies are also summarized. The target organ(s) or tissue(s) in which an increase in cancer was observed is identified. Dose–response and other quantitative data may be summarized when available.

(c)   Cancer in experimental animals

Data relevant to an evaluation of carcinogenicity in animals are summarized. For each animal species, study design and route of administration, it is stated whether an increased incidence, reduced latency, or increased severity or multiplicity of neoplasms or pre-neoplastic lesions were observed, and the tumour sites are indicated. If the agent produced tumours after prenatal exposure or in single-dose experiments, this is also mentioned. Negative findings, inverse relationships, dose–response and other quantitative data are also summarized.

(d)   Mechanistic and other relevant data

Data relevant to the toxicokinetics (absorption, distribution, metabolism, elimination) and the possible mechanism(s) of carcinogenesis (e.g. genetic toxicity, epigenetic effects) are summarized. In addition, information on susceptible individuals, populations and life-

stages is summarized. This section also reports on other toxic effects, including reproductive and developmental effects, as well as additional relevant data that are considered
to be important.

6. Evaluation and rationale

Evaluations of the strength of the evidence for carcinogenicity arising from human
and experimental animal data are made, using standard terms. The strength of the mechanistic evidence is also characterized.

It is recognized that the criteria for these evaluations, described below, cannot
encompass all of the factors that may be relevant to an evaluation of carcinogenicity. In
considering all of the relevant scientific data, the Working Group may assign the agent to
a higher or lower category than a strict interpretation of these criteria would indicate.

These categories refer only to the strength of the evidence that an exposure is
carcinogenic and not to the extent of its carcinogenic activity (potency). A classification
may change as new information becomes available.

An evaluation of the degree of evidence is limited to the materials tested, as defined
physically, chemically or biologically. When the agents evaluated are considered by the
Working Group to be sufficiently closely related, they may be grouped together for the
purpose of a single evaluation of the degree of evidence.

(a)   Carcinogenicity in humans

The evidence relevant to carcinogenicity from studies in humans is classified into one
of the following categories:

Sufficient evidence of carcinogenicity: The Working Group considers that a causal
relationship has been established between exposure to the agent and human cancer.
That is, a positive relationship has been observed between the exposure and cancer in
studies in which chance, bias and confounding could be ruled out with reasonable
confidence. A statement that there is *sufficient evidence* is followed by a separate
sentence that identifies the target organ(s) or tissue(s) where an increased risk of
cancer was observed in humans. Identification of a specific target organ or tissue does
not preclude the possibility that the agent may cause cancer at other sites.

Limited evidence of carcinogenicity: A positive association has been observed between
exposure to the agent and cancer for which a causal interpretation is considered by the
Working Group to be credible, but chance, bias or confounding could not be ruled out
with reasonable confidence.

Inadequate evidence of carcinogenicity: The available studies are of insufficient quality,
consistency or statistical power to permit a conclusion regarding the presence or
absence of a causal association between exposure and cancer, or no data on cancer in
humans are available.

Evidence suggesting lack of carcinogenicity: There are several adequate studies covering
the full range of levels of exposure that humans are known to encounter, which are
mutually consistent in not showing a positive association between exposure to the
agent and any studied cancer at any observed level of exposure. The results from
these studies alone or combined should have narrow confidence intervals with an
upper limit close to the null value (e.g. a relative risk of 1.0). Bias and confounding
should be ruled out with reasonable confidence, and the studies should have an
adequate length of follow-up. A conclusion of *evidence suggesting lack of carcinogenicity* is inevitably limited to the cancer sites, conditions and levels of exposure,
and length of observation covered by the available studies. In addition, the possibility
of a very small risk at the levels of exposure studied can never be excluded.

In some instances, the above categories may be used to classify the degree of evidence related to carcinogenicity in specific organs or tissues.

When the available epidemiological studies pertain to a mixture, process, occupation
or industry, the Working Group seeks to identify the specific agent considered most likely
to be responsible for any excess risk. The evaluation is focused as narrowly as the available data on exposure and other aspects permit.

(b)   Carcinogenicity in experimental animals

Carcinogenicity in experimental animals can be evaluated using conventional bioassays, bioassays that employ genetically modified animals, and other in-vivo bioassays
that focus on one or more of the critical stages of carcinogenesis. In the absence of data
from conventional long-term bioassays or from assays with neoplasia as the end-point,
consistently positive results in several models that address several stages in the multistage
process of carcinogenesis should be considered in evaluating the degree of evidence of
carcinogenicity in experimental animals.

The evidence relevant to carcinogenicity in experimental animals is classified into one
of the following categories:

Sufficient evidence of carcinogenicity: The Working Group considers that a causal
relationship has been established between the agent and an increased incidence of
malignant neoplasms or of an appropriate combination of benign and malignant
neoplasms in (a) two or more species of animals or (b) two or more independent
studies in one species carried out at different times or in different laboratories or
under different protocols. An increased incidence of tumours in both sexes of a single
species in a well-conducted study, ideally conducted under Good Laboratory
Practices, can also provide *sufficient evidence*.

A single study in one species and sex might be considered to provide *sufficient
evidence of carcinogenicity* when malignant neoplasms occur to an unusual degree
with regard to incidence, site, type of tumour or age at onset, or when there are strong
findings of tumours at multiple sites.

Limited evidence of carcinogenicity: The data suggest a carcinogenic effect but are limited for making a definitive evaluation because, e.g. (a) the evidence of carcinogenicity is restricted to a single experiment; (b) there are unresolved questions regarding the adequacy of the design, conduct or interpretation of the studies; (c) the agent increases the incidence only of benign neoplasms or lesions of uncertain neoplastic potential; or (d) the evidence of carcinogenicity is restricted to studies that demonstrate only promoting activity in a narrow range of tissues or organs.

Inadequate evidence of carcinogenicity: The studies cannot be interpreted as showing either the presence or absence of a carcinogenic effect because of major qualitative or quantitative limitations, or no data on cancer in experimental animals are available.

Evidence suggesting lack of carcinogenicity: Adequate studies involving at least two species are available which show that, within the limits of the tests used, the agent is not carcinogenic. A conclusion of *evidence suggesting lack of carcinogenicity* is inevitably limited to the species, tumour sites, age at exposure, and conditions and levels of exposure studied.

(c)   Mechanistic and other relevant data

Mechanistic and other evidence judged to be relevant to an evaluation of carcinogenicity and of sufficient importance to affect the overall evaluation is highlighted. This may include data on preneoplastic lesions, tumour pathology, genetic and related effects, structure–activity relationships, metabolism and toxicokinetics, physicochemical parameters and analogous biological agents.

The strength of the evidence that any carcinogenic effect observed is due to a particular mechanism is evaluated, using terms such as 'weak', 'moderate' or 'strong'. The Working Group then assesses whether that particular mechanism is likely to be operative in humans. The strongest indications that a particular mechanism operates in humans derive from data on humans or biological specimens obtained from exposed humans. The data may be considered to be especially relevant if they show that the agent in question has caused changes in exposed humans that are on the causal pathway to carcinogenesis. Such data may, however, never become available, because it is at least conceivable that certain compounds may be kept from human use solely on the basis of evidence of their toxicity and/or carcinogenicity in experimental systems.

The conclusion that a mechanism operates in experimental animals is strengthened by findings of consistent results in different experimental systems, by the demonstration of biological plausibility and by coherence of the overall database. Strong support can be obtained from studies that challenge the hypothesized mechanism experimentally, by demonstrating that the suppression of key mechanistic processes leads to the suppression of tumour development. The Working Group considers whether multiple mechanisms might contribute to tumour development, whether different mechanisms might operate in different dose ranges, whether separate mechanisms might operate in humans and experimental animals and whether a unique mechanism might operate in a susceptible group.

The possible contribution of alternative mechanisms must be considered before concluding that tumours observed in experimental animals are not relevant to humans. An uneven level of experimental support for different mechanisms may reflect that disproportionate resources have been focused on investigating a favoured mechanism.

For complex exposures, including occupational and industrial exposures, the chemical composition and the potential contribution of carcinogens known to be present are considered by the Working Group in its overall evaluation of human carcinogenicity. The Working Group also determines the extent to which the materials tested in experimental systems are related to those to which humans are exposed.

(d)   Overall evaluation

Finally, the body of evidence is considered as a whole, in order to reach an overall evaluation of the carcinogenicity of the agent to humans.

An evaluation may be made for a group of agents that have been evaluated by the Working Group. In addition, when supporting data indicate that other related agents, for which there is no direct evidence of their capacity to induce cancer in humans or in animals, may also be carcinogenic, a statement describing the rationale for this conclusion is added to the evaluation narrative; an additional evaluation may be made for this broader group of agents if the strength of the evidence warrants it.

The agent is described according to the wording of one of the following categories, and the designated group is given. The categorization of an agent is a matter of scientific judgement that reflects the strength of the evidence derived from studies in humans and in experimental animals and from mechanistic and other relevant data.

Group 1:   The agent is *carcinogenic to humans*.

This category is used when there is *sufficient evidence of carcinogenicity* in humans. Exceptionally, an agent may be placed in this category when evidence of carcinogenicity in humans is less than *sufficient* but there is *sufficient evidence of carcinogenicity* in experimental animals and strong evidence in exposed humans that the agent acts through a relevant mechanism of carcinogenicity.

Group 2.

This category includes agents for which, at one extreme, the degree of evidence of carcinogenicity in humans is almost *sufficient*, as well as those for which, at the other extreme, there are no human data but for which there is evidence of carcinogenicity in experimental animals. Agents are assigned to either Group 2A (*probably carcinogenic to humans*) or Group 2B (*possibly carcinogenic to humans*) on the basis of epidemiological and experimental evidence of carcinogenicity and mechanistic and other relevant data. The terms *probably carcinogenic* and *possibly carcinogenic* have no quantitative significance and are used simply as descriptors of different levels of evidence of human carcinogenicity, with *probably carcinogenic* signifying a higher level of evidence than *possibly carcinogenic*.

Group 2A: The agent is *probably carcinogenic to humans*.

This category is used when there is *limited evidence of carcinogenicity* in humans and *sufficient evidence of carcinogenicity* in experimental animals. In some cases, an agent may be classified in this category when there is *inadequate evidence of carcinogenicity* in humans and *sufficient evidence of carcinogenicity* in experimental animals and strong evidence that the carcinogenesis is mediated by a mechanism that also operates in humans. Exceptionally, an agent may be classified in this category solely on the basis of *limited evidence of carcinogenicity* in humans. An agent may be assigned to this category if it clearly belongs, based on mechanistic considerations, to a class of agents for which one or more members have been classified in Group 1 or Group 2A.

Group 2B: The agent is *possibly carcinogenic to humans*.

This category is used for agents for which there is *limited evidence of carcinogenicity* in humans and less than *sufficient evidence of carcinogenicity* in experimental animals. It may also be used when there is *inadequate evidence of carcinogenicity* in humans but there is *sufficient evidence of carcinogenicity* in experimental animals. In some instances, an agent for which there is *inadequate evidence of carcinogenicity* in humans and less than *sufficient evidence of carcinogenicity* in experimental animals together with supporting evidence from mechanistic and other relevant data may be placed in this group. An agent may be classified in this category solely on the basis of strong evidence from mechanistic and other relevant data.

Group 3:   The agent is *not classifiable as to its carcinogenicity to humans*.

This category is used most commonly for agents for which the evidence of carcinogenicity is *inadequate* in humans and *inadequate* or *limited* in experimental animals.

Exceptionally, agents for which the evidence of carcinogenicity is *inadequate* in humans but *sufficient* in experimental animals may be placed in this category when there is strong evidence that the mechanism of carcinogenicity in experimental animals does not operate in humans.

Agents that do not fall into any other group are also placed in this category.

An evaluation in Group 3 is not a determination of non-carcinogenicity or overall safety. It often means that further research is needed, especially when exposures are widespread or the cancer data are consistent with differing interpretations.

Group 4:   The agent is *probably not carcinogenic to humans*.

This category is used for agents for which there is *evidence suggesting lack of carcinogenicity* in humans and in experimental animals. In some instances, agents for which there is *inadequate evidence of carcinogenicity* in humans but *evidence suggesting lack of carcinogenicity* in experimental animals, consistently and strongly supported by a broad range of mechanistic and other relevant data, may be classified in this group.

(*e*)   *Rationale*

The reasoning that the Working Group used to reach its evaluation is presented and discussed. This section integrates the major findings from studies of cancer in humans, studies of cancer in experimental animals, and mechanistic and other relevant data. It includes concise statements of the principal line(s) of argument that emerged, the conclusions of the Working Group on the strength of the evidence for each group of studies, citations to indicate which studies were pivotal to these conclusions, and an explanation of the reasoning of the Working Group in weighing data and making evaluations. When there are significant differences of scientific interpretation among Working Group Members, a brief summary of the alternative interpretations is provided, together with their scientific rationale and an indication of the relative degree of support for each alternative.

References

Bieler, G.S. & Williams, R.L. (1993) Ratio estimates, the delta method, and quantal response tests for increased carcinogenicity. *Biometrics*, **49**(3), 793–801

Breslow, N.E. & Day, N.E. (1980) *Statistical Methods in Cancer Research*, Vol. 1, *The Analysis of Case–Control Studies* (IARC Scientific Publications No. 32), Lyon, IARC

Breslow, N.E. & Day, N.E. (1987) *Statistical Methods in Cancer Research*, Vol. 2, *The Design and Analysis of Cohort Studies* (IARC Scientific Publications No. 82), Lyon, IARC

Buffler, P., Rice, J., Baan, R., Bird, M. & Boffetta, P., eds (2004) *Mechanisms of Carcinogenesis: Contributions of Molecular Epidemiology* (IARC Scientific Publications No. 157), Lyon, IARC

Capen, C.C., Dybing, E., Rice, J.M. & Wilbourn, J.D. (1999) *Species Differences in Thyroid, Kidney and Urinary Bladder Carcinogenesis* (IARC Scientific Publications No. 147), Lyon, IARC

Cogliano, V.J., Baan, R.A., Straif, K., Grosse, Y., Secretan, M.B., El Ghissassi, F. & Kleihues, P. (2004) The science and practice of carcinogen identification and evaluation. *Environmental Health Perspect.*, **112**(13), 1269–1274

Cogliano, V., Baan, R., Straif, K., Grosse, Y., Secretan, B., El Ghissassi, F. & Boyle, P. (2005) Transparency in IARC Monographs. *Lancet Oncol.*, **6**(10), 747

Dunson, D.B., Chen, Z. & Harry, J. (2003) A Bayesian approach for joint modeling of cluster size and subunit-specific outcomes. *Biometrics*, **59**(3), 521–30

Fung, K.Y., Krewski, D. & Smythe, R.T. (1996) A comparison of tests for trend with historical controls in carcinogen bioassay. *Can. J. Statist.*, **24**, 431–454

Gart, J.J., Krewski, D., Lee, P.N., Tarone, R.E. & Wahrendorf, J. (1986) *Statistical Methods in Cancer Research*, Vol. 3, *The Design and Analysis of Long-term Animal Experiments* (IARC Scientific Publications No. 79), Lyon, IARC

Greenland, S. (1998) Meta-analysis. In: Rothman, K.J. & Greenland, S., eds, *Modern Epidemiology,* Philadelphia, Lippincott Williams & Wilkins, pp. 643–673

Greim, H., Gelbke, H.-P., Reuter, U., Thielmann, H.W. & Edler, L. (2003) Evaluation of historical control data in carcinogenicity studies. *Hum. exp. Toxicol.*, **22**, 541–549

Haseman, J.K., Huff, J. & Boorman, G.A. (1984) Use of historical control data in carcinogenicity studies in rodents. *Toxicol. Pathol.*, **12**(2), 126–135

Hill, A.B. (1965) The environment and disease: Association or causation? *Proc. R. Soc. Med.*, **58**, 295–300

Hoel, D.G., Kaplan, N.L. & Anderson, M.W. (1983) Implication of nonlinear kinetics on risk estimation in carcinogenesis. *Science*, **219**, 1032–1037

Huff, J.E., Eustis, S.L. & Haseman, J.K. (1989) Occurrence and relevance of chemically induced benign neoplasms in long-term carcinogenicity studies. *Cancer Metastasis Rev.*, **8**, 1–21

IARC (1977) *IARC Monographs Programme on the Evaluation of the Carcinogenic Risk of Chemicals to Humans*. Preamble (IARC intern. tech. Rep. No. 77/002)

IARC (1978) *Chemicals with Sufficient Evidence of Carcinogenicity in Experimental Animals –* IARC Monographs *Volumes 1–17* (IARC intern. tech. Rep. No. 78/003)

IARC (1979) *Criteria to Select Chemicals for* IARC Monographs (IARC intern. tech. Rep. No. 79/003)

IARC (1982) *IARC Monographs on the Evaluation of the Carcinogenic Risk of Chemicals to Humans*, Suppl. 4, *Chemicals, Industrial Processes and Industries Associated with Cancer in Humans* (IARC Monographs, Volumes 1 to 29), Lyon, IARC

IARC (1983) *Approaches to Classifying Chemical Carcinogens According to Mechanism of Action* (IARC intern. tech. Rep. No. 83/001)

IARC (1987) *IARC Monographs on the Evaluation of Carcinogenic Risks to Humans*, Supplement 7, *Overall Evaluations of Carcinogenicity: An Updating of* IARC Monographs *Volumes 1 to 42*, Lyon, IARC

IARC (1988) *Report of an IARC Working Group to Review the Approaches and Processes Used to Evaluate the Carcinogenicity of Mixtures and Groups of Chemicals* (IARC intern. tech. Rep. No. 88/002)

IARC (1991) *A Consensus Report of an IARC Monographs Working Group on the Use of Mechanisms of Carcinogenesis in Risk Identification* (IARC intern. tech. Rep. No. 91/002)

IARC (2004) *IARC Monographs on the Evaluation of Carcinogenic Risks to Humans*, Vol. 84, *Some Drinking-water Disinfectants and Contaminants, including Arsenic*, Lyon, IARC, pp. 39–267

IARC (2005) *Report of the Advisory Group to Recommend Updates to the Preamble to the* IARC Monographs (IARC Int. Rep. No. 05/001)

IARC (2006) *Report of the Advisory Group to Review the Amended Preamble to the* IARC Monographs (IARC Int. Rep. No. 06/001)

McGregor, D.B., Rice, J.M. & Venitt, S., eds (1999) *The Use of Short- and Medium-term Tests for Carcinogens and Data on Genetic Effects in Carcinogenic Hazard Evaluation* (IARC Scientific Publications No. 146), Lyon, IARC

Montesano, R., Bartsch, H., Vainio, H., Wilbourn, J. & Yamasaki, H., eds (1986) *Long-term and Short-term Assays for Carcinogenesis—A Critical Appraisal* (IARC Scientific Publications No. 83), Lyon, IARC

OECD (2002) *Guidance Notes for Analysis and Evaluation of Chronic Toxicity and Carcinogenicity Studies* (Series on Testing and Assessment No. 35), Paris, OECD

Peto, R., Pike, M.C., Day, N.E., Gray, R.G., Lee, P.N., Parish, S., Peto, J., Richards, S. & Wahrendorf, J. (1980) Guidelines for simple, sensitive significance tests for carcinogenic effects in long-term animal experiments. In: *IARC Monographs on the Evaluation of the Carcinogenic Risk of Chemicals to Humans*, Suppl. 2, *Long-term and Short-term Screening Assays for Carcinogens: A Critical Appraisal*, Lyon, IARC, pp. 311–426

Portier, C.J. & Bailer, A.J. (1989) Testing for increased carcinogenicity using a survival-adjusted quantal response test. *Fundam. appl. Toxicol.*, **12**(4), 731–737

Sherman, C.D., Portier, C.J. & Kopp-Schneider, A. (1994) Multistage models of carcinogenesis: An approximation for the size and number distribution of late-stage clones. *Risk Anal.*, **14**(6), 1039–1048

Stewart, B.W. & Kleihues, P., eds (2003) *World Cancer Report,* Lyon, IARC

Tomatis, L., Aitio, A., Wilbourn, J. & Shuker, L. (1989) Human carcinogens so far identified. *Japan. J. Cancer Res.*, **80**, 795–807

Toniolo, P., Boffetta, P., Shuker, D.E.G., Rothman, N., Hulka, B. & Pearce, N., eds (1997) *Application of Biomarkers in Cancer Epidemiology* (IARC Scientific Publications No. 142), Lyon, IARC

Vainio, H., Magee, P., McGregor, D. & McMichael, A., eds (1992) *Mechanisms of Carcinogenesis in Risk Identification* (IARC Scientific Publications No. 116), Lyon, IARC

Vainio, H., Wilbourn, J.D., Sasco, A.J., Partensky, C., Gaudin, N., Heseltine, E. & Eragne, I. (1995) [Identification of human carcinogenic risk in IARC Monographs.] *Bull. Cancer*, **82**, 339–348 (in French)

Vineis, P., Malats, N., Lang, M., d'Errico, A., Caporaso, N., Cuzick, J. & Boffetta, P., eds (1999) *Metabolic Polymorphisms and Susceptibility to Cancer* (IARC Scientific Publications No. 148), Lyon, IARC

Wilbourn, J., Haroun, L., Heseltine, E., Kaldor, J., Partensky, C. & Vainio, H. (1986) Response of experimental animals to human carcinogens: An analysis based upon the *IARC Monographs* Programme. *Carcinogenesis*, **7**, 1853–1863

GENERAL REMARKS

This ninety-seventh volume of *IARC Monographs* contains evaluations of the carcinogenic hazard to humans of 1,3-butadiene, ethylene oxide and some vinyl halides (vinyl fluoride, vinyl chloride and vinyl bromide). The most recent previous evaluations of these industrial gases were published in Supplement 7 (IARC, 1987) for vinyl chloride, Volume 60 (IARC, 1994) for ethylene oxide, Volume 63 (IARC, 1995) for vinyl fluoride and Volume 71 (IARC, 1999) for 1,3-butadiene and vinyl bromide. Newer epidemiological and mechanistic studies have since been published and are evaluated in this volume.

Numbers of exposed workers

No estimates of numbers of exposed workers worldwide are available. National estimates have been reported for the USA (National Occupational Exposure Survey, NOES) and for the member states of the European Union (CAREX information system on occupational exposure to carcinogens).

NOES was a nationwide observational survey that was conducted in a sample of 4490 establishments from 1981 to 1983. The target population was defined as employees working in establishments or job sites in the USA that employed eight or more workers in a category defined in the list of Standard Industrial Classifications. Generally, these classifications mainly covered construction, manufacturing, transportation, private and business services and hospital industries. The NOES sampled little or no activity in agriculture, mining, wholesale/retail trade, finance/real estate or government operations. NOES addressed recordable potential exposure that had to meet two criteria: (1) a chemical, physical or biological agent or trade-name product had to be observed in sufficient proximity to an employee such that one or two physical phases of that agent or product probably came into contact or entered the body of the employee; and (2) the duration of the potential exposure had to meet the minimal duration guidelines, i.e., it must have presented a potential exposure for at least 30 min per week (on an annual average) or be used at least once per week for 90% of the weeks or the work year (NOES, 1997).

The CAREX information system was designed to provide selected exposure data and documented estimates of the number of workers exposed to carcinogens by country, carcinogen and industry for 15 Member States of the European Union. CAREX includes data on agents that have been evaluated by the IARC (all agents in Groups 1 and 2A as of February 1995, and selected agents in Group 2B) and on ionizing radiation that were displayed across 55 industrial classes. The minimal criterion for exposure was defined agent by agent. In general, workers were considererd to have been exposed if a specified background level was exceeded. Occupational exposures for 1990–93 were estimated in two phases. Firstly, estimates were generated by the CAREX system on the basis of data from national labour forces and estimates of exposure prevalence from two reference countries (Finland and the USA) that had the most comprehensive data available on exposures to these agents. Thereafter, these estimates were refined for selected countries (Finland, France, Germany, Italy, the Netherlands, Spain, Sweden, the United Kingdom) by national experts with regard to the perceived exposure patterns in their own countries compared with those of the reference countries (Kauppinen et al., 2000).

The figures of NOES and CAREX are not comparable because definitions of exposure, data collection and estimation methods were different. The inclusion or exclusion of workers exposed only occasionally, or to very low levels that were close to the background levels, may strongly influence the estimates. The NOES estimates (from 1981 to 1983) and CAREX estimates (from 1990 to 1993) are also fairly old and the extent of exposure may have changed considerably since then.

Classification of lymphomas

The diagnosis and classification of haematopoietic and lymphopoietic malignancies are extremely complex and have undergone successive changes over the course of time. The original classification was based largely on morphology of the tumour cells and this was reflected in the 9th International Classification of Diseases (ICD-9) categories 200–208 (WHO, 1975). The more recent WHO classification (Jaffe et al., 2001) considers more recent developments in cytogenetics and molecular biology and has little overlap with the ICD-9 classification (WHO, 1975). Also a distinction between ICD-9 200 and 202 is probably not meaningful in the light of the WHO re-classification. It has to be noted that this WHO classification was superseded in 2008 (Swerdlow et al., 2008).

The major change in the WHO classification is that lymphocytic leukaemias and lymphomas are no longer considered to be different diseases. Rather, the essential feature of the definition is the tumour cells, and a neoplasm of a particular lymphoid cell type may present as either leukaemia or a solid tumour mass (lymphoma) in a given patient. This has a bearing on the assessment of associations with exposures in epidemiological studies, which previously considered leukaemias (all types combined, or specific categories such as acute lymphocytic leukaemia) separately from non-Hodgkin lymphomas. The WHO classification indicates that the previous practice is no longer appropriate and that lymphomas and leukaemias should be combined in tabulations of the incidence of disease, at least for leukaemias and lymphomas of the same cell type, e.g. chronic lymphocytic leukemia/small lymphocytic lymphoma. However, this reclassification is difficult or impossible to achieve in epidemiological studies that rely on death certificates issued many years ago.

References

IARC (1987) *IARC Monographs on the Evaluation of Carcinogenic Risks to Humans*, Suppl. 7, *Overall Evaluations of Carcinogenicity: An Updating of* IARC Monographs *Volumes 1 to 42*, Lyon, pp. 373–376

IARC (1994) *IARC Monographs on the Evaluation of Carcinogenic Risks to Humans*, Vol. 60, *Some Industrial Chemicals*, Lyon, pp. 73–159

IARC (1995) *IARC Monographs on the Evaluation of Carcinogenic Risks to Humans*, Vol. 63, *Dry Cleaning, Some Chlorinated Solvents and Other Industrial Chemicals*, Lyon, pp. 467–475

IARC (1999) *IARC Monographs on the Evaluation of Carcinogenic Risks to Humans*, Vol. 71, *Re-evaluation of Some Organic Chemicals, Hydrazine and Hydrogen Peroxide*, Lyon, pp. 109–225, 923–928

Jaffe, E.S., Harris, N.L., Stein, H. & Vardiman, J.W., eds (2001) *Pathology and Genetics of Tumours of Haematopoietic and Lymphoid Tissues*, Lyon, IARC

Kauppinen, T., Toikkanen, J., Pedersen, D., Young, R., Ahrens, W., Boffetta, P., Hansen, J., Kromhout, H., Maqueda Blasco, J., Mirabelli, D., de la Orden-Rivera, V., Pannett, B., Plato, N., Savela, A., Vincent, R. & Kogevinas, M. (2000) Occupational exposure to carcinogens in the European Union. *Occup. environ. Med.*, **57**, 10–18

NOES (1997) *National Occupational Exposure Survey 1981–83, Unpublished Data as of November 1997*, Cincinnati, OH, US Department of Health and Human Services, Public Health Service, National Institute for Occupational Safety and Health

Swerdlow, S.H., Campo, E., Harris, N.L., Jaffe, E.S., Pileri, S.A., Stein, H., Thiele, J. & Vardiman, J.W., eds (2008) *WHO Classification of Tumours of Haematopoietic and Lymphoid Tissues*, Lyon, IARC

WHO (1975) *International Classification of Diseases*, 9th rev., Geneva

THE MONOGRAPHS

1,3-BUTADIENE

This substance was considered by previous Working Groups in June 1985 (IARC, 1986; see also correction, IARC, 1987a), March 1987 (IARC, 1987b), October 1991 (IARC, 1992) and February 1998 (IARC, 1999). Since that time, new data have become available, and these have been incorporated into the monograph and taken into consideration in the present evaluation.

One of the metabolites of 1,3-butadiene, 1,2:3,4-diepoxybutane, was also evaluated previously by an IARC Working Group (IARC, 1976), and its re-evaluation by the present Working Group is included in this monograph.

1. Exposure Data

1.1 Chemical and physical data

Butadiene

1.1.1 *Nomenclature* (IARC, 1999; IPCS-CEC, 2000; O'Neil, 2006)

Chem. Abstr. Serv. Reg. No.: 106-99-0
Chem. Abstr. Name: 1,3-Butadiene
IUPAC Systematic Name: 1,3-Butadiene
RTECS No.: EI9275000
UN TDG No.: 1010 (stabilized)
EC No.: 601-013-00-X
Synonyms: Biethylene; bivinyl; butadiene; buta-1,3-diene; α,γ-butadiene; *trans*-butadiene; divinyl; erythrene; pyrrolylene; vinylethylene

1.1.2 *Structural and molecular formulae and relative molecular mass*

$$H_2C = CH - CH = CH_2$$

C_4H_6 Relative molecular mass: 54.09

1.1.3   *Chemical and physical properties of the pure substance*

From IARC (1999), IPCS-CEC (2000), Lide (2005) and O'Neil (2006) unless otherwise specified

(a)   *Description*: Colourless gas
(b)   *Boiling-point*: –4.4 °C
(c)   *Melting-point*: –108.9 °C
(d)   *Density*: d_4^{20} 0.6149
(e)   *Spectroscopy data*: Ultraviolet (Grasselli & Ritchey, 1975), infrared (Sadtler Research Laboratories, 1995; prism [893a], grating [36758]), nuclear magnetic resonance and mass spectral data (NIH/EPA Chemical Information System, 1983) have been reported.
(f)   *Solubility*: Slightly soluble in water (1 g/L at 20 °C); soluble in ethanol, diethyl ether, benzene and organic solvents; very soluble in acetone (see also Verschueren, 1996)
(g)   *Vapour pressure*: 120 kPa at 0 °C; 273 kPa at 25 °C (Grub & Löser, 2005)
(h)   *Relative vapour density (air = 1)*: 1.87 (Verschueren, 1996)
(i)   *Stability*: As a result of flow and agitation, electrostatic charges can be generated. The vapours are uninhibited and may form polymers in vents or flame arresters of storage tanks, and result in the blockage of vents. On exposure to air, the substance can form peroxides and initiate explosive polymerization. It may also polymerize due to warming by fire or an explosion. It decomposes explosively on rapid heating under pressure and may react vigorously with oxidants and many other substances, causing fire and explosion hazards (IPCS-CEC, 2000).
(j)   *Flash-point*: –76 °C (IPCS-CEC, 2000)
(k)   *Auto-ignition temperature*: 414 °C (IPCS-CEC, 2000)
(l)   *Explosive limits*: Lower, 1.1%; upper, 12.3% (IPCS-CEC, 2000)
(m)   *Octanol/water partition coefficient*: log P_{ow}, 1.99 (IPCS-CEC, 2000)
(n)   *Odour threshold*: 1–1.6 ppm [2.2–3.5 mg/m^3] (recognition) (ACGIH, 2001)
(o)   *Henry's law constant (calculated at 25 °C and 101.325 kPa)*: 7460 Pa × m^3/mol (Health Canada, 1999)
(p)   *Organic carbon partition coefficient*: log K_{oc}, 1.86–2.36 (Health Canada, 1999)
(q)   *Conversion factor*: mg/m^3 = 2.21 × ppm[1]

Diepoxybutane

Diepoxybutane is the racemic mixture of four different isomers, with the following Chem. Abstr. Serv. Reg. Nos: 1464-53-5, diepoxybutane; 298-18-0, (±)-diepoxybutane;

---

[1] Calculated from: mg/m^3 = (molecular weight/24.47) × ppm, assuming normal temperature (25 °C) and pressure (101.3 kPa)

564-00-1, *meso*-diepoxybutane; 30419-67-1, D-diepoxybutane; 30031-64-2, L-diepoxy-butane.

1.1.1   Nomenclature

Chem. Abstr. Name: 2,2′-Bioxirane
IUPAC Systematic Name: 1,2:3,4-Diepoxybutane
Synonyms: Butadiene dioxide (diepoxybutane); 1,3-butadiene diepoxide ((±)-di-epoxybutane); D-1,2:3,4-diepoxybutane (D-diepoxybutane): L-1,2:3,4-diepoxybutane; (5,5)-1,2:3,4-diepoxybutane (L-diepoxybutane)

1.1.2   Structural and molecular formulae and relative molecular mass

$$\underset{H}{\overset{O}{\underset{|}{\overset{/\backslash}{H_2C-C}}}}\underset{O}{\overset{H}{\underset{\backslash/}{-C-CH_2}}}$$

$C_4H_6O_2$ Relative molecular mass: 86.10

1.1.3   Chemical and physical properties

From O'Neil (2006)
(a)   *Description*: Colourless liquid
(b)   *Boiling-point*: 138 °C
(c)   *Melting-point*: –19 °C
(d)   *Solubility*: Miscible with water (hydrolyses)
(e)   *Vapour pressure:* 918 Pa at 25 °C

1.1.4   Technical products and impurities

In the production of polymers such as styrene–butadiene copolymer resins, the polymerization catalysts used are sensitive to some impurities such as oxygen and moisture. Butadiene that is used for polymerization is 99.9% pure. Up to 22 different volatile components of light molecular mass were detected as impurities with the ASTM method D2593-93 (reapproved in 2004; ASTM, 2004).

1.1.5   Analysis

Selected methods for the analysis of butadiene in various matrices are listed in Table 1. Those for the analysis of butadiene in air have been evaluated; there appears to be no single preferred method, but more recent ones give a higher performance. Thermal desorption provides high levels of accuracy and precision (Bianchi *et al.*, 1997).

Several gas detector tubes are used in conjunction with common colorimetric reactions to detect butadiene. The reactions include the reduction of chromate or dichromate to chromous ion and the reduction of ammonium molybdate and palladium sulfate to molybdenum blue (Saltzman & Harman, 1989).

Passive dosimeters that use different techniques (thermal desorption and gas chromatography, colorimetric reactions) are also available for the detection of butadiene.

Table 1. Selected methods for the analysis of butadiene in various matrices

Sample matrix	Sample preparation	Assay procedure	Limit of detection	Reference
Air	Adsorb (charcoal); extract (carbon disulfide)	GC/FID	200 µg/m³	Occupational Safety and Health Administration (1990a)
	Adsorb (charcoal); extract (dichloromethane)	GC/FID	0.2 µg/sample	Eller (1994)
	Adsorb on Perkin-Elmer ATD 400 packed with polymeric or synthetic adsorbent material; thermal desorption	GC/FID	200 µg/m³	Health and Safety Executive (1992)
	3M passive monitoring	GC/FID	0.029 mg/m³ for a 20.5-L sample	Anttinen-Klemetti et al. (2004)
Foods and plastic food-packaging material	Dissolve (N,N-dimethylacetamide) or melt; inject headspace sample	GC/MS–SIM	~1 µg/kg	Startin & Gilbert (1984)
Plastics, liquid foods	Dissolve in ortho-dichlorobenzene; inject headspace sample	GC/FID	2–20 µg/kg	Food and Drug Administration (1987)
Solid foods	Cut or mash; inject headspace sample	GC/FID	2–20 µg/kg	Food and Drug Administration (1987)

GC/FID, gas chromatography/flame ionization detection; GC/MS–SIM, gas chromatography/mass spectrometry with single-ion monitoring

1.2   Production and use

1.2.1   *Production*

Butadiene was first produced in the late nineteenth century by pyrolysis of various organic materials. Commercial production began in the 1930s (Sun & Wristers, 2002).

(a)   *Manufacturing processes*

(i)   *Ethylene co-production*

Butadiene is manufactured primarily as a co-product of the steam cracking of hydro-carbon streams to produce ethylene. This process accounts for over 95% of global buta-diene production (White, 2007).

Steam cracking is a complex, highly endothermic pyrolysis reaction, during which a hydrocarbon feedstock is heated to approximately 800 °C and 34 kPa for less than 1 sec and the carbon–carbon and carbon–hydrogen bonds are broken. As a result, a mixture of olefins, aromatic compounds, tar and gases is formed. These products are cooled and separated into specific boiling-range cuts of C_1, C_2, C_3 and C_4 compounds. The C_4 fraction contains butadiene, isobutylene, 1-butene, 2-butene and some other minor hydrocarbons. The overall yields of butadiene during the process depend on both the parameters of the process and the composition of feedstocks. Generally, heavier steam-cracking feedstocks produce greater amounts of butadiene. Separation and purification of butadiene from other components is carried out mainly by an extractive distillation process. The most commonly used solvents are acetonitrile and dimethylformamide; dimethylacetamide, furfural and *N*-methyl-2-pyrrolidinone have also been used to this end (Sun & Wristers, 2002; Walther, 2003).

(ii)   *Dehydrogenation*

The intentional dehydrogenation of *n*-butane or *n*-butenes also yields butadiene. This is achieved by the Houdry process for dehydrogenation of *n*-butane or by oxidative dehydrogenation of *n*-butenes (Walther, 2003).

(iii)   *Ethanol-based production*

A plant in India produces butadiene in a two-step process from ethanol. Initial de-hydrogenation is achieved through a copper catalyst, and the resulting mixture is then dehydrated at atmospheric pressure in the presence of a zirconium oxide or tantalum oxide–silica gel catalyst at 300–350 °C. Overall yields of butadiene in the second reaction are about 70%. This process is very similar to the adol condensation of acetaldehyde (Walther, 2003).

(b)   *Butadiene extraction processes*

Regardless of the production process, final purification of butadiene requires removal of any butane, butene or acetylene impurities. Currently, seven different commercial processes exist for the extraction of butadiene that employ different extraction solvents. The processes, identified by the licencer and type of solvent, are: BASF Aktiengesellshaft — *N*-methylpyrrolidone; Lyondell Petrochemical Company — acetonitrile; Zeon Corporation — dimethylformamide; ConocoPhillips — furfural; Shell Chemical Company — acetonitrile; Solutia — β-methoxyproprionitrile with 15% furfural; Dow (formerly Union Carbide Corporation) — dimethylacetamide; and (no licencer) — cuprous ammonium acetate solution (Walther, 2003).

(c)   Production volume

An estimated 9.3 million tonnes of butadiene were produced worldwide in 2005 (CMAI, 2006). Production volumes for different regions for the years 2004 and 2006 are given in Table 2.

World capacity grew by 3.5% per year between 1997 and 2002. During that period, most of the increase in capacity occurred in Asia, South America and the Middle East. Asia is now the largest producer of butadiene, and accounts for one-third of the world capacity (Walther, 2003).

Diepoxybutane is not believed to be produced commercially except in small quantities for research purposes (National Library of Medicine, 2008).

Table 2. Butadiene production (in tonnes) by world region from 1981 to 2006

Region	1981	1990	1996	2004	2006
North America	1480	1593	1956	2862	2878
South America	–	–	–	377	377
Western Europe	636[a]	1256	1017[b]	1902	2232
Eastern Europe	–	–	–	1170	736
Middle East/Africa	–	–	–	180	340
Asia/Pacific	518[c]	1253	1755[d]	3104	4405

From IARC (1999), CMAI (2004, 2006)
[a] No data available for Germany
[b] No data available for the United Kingdom or Italy
[c] Value for Japan only
[d] No data available for China

1.2.2   Use

Butadiene is used primarily in the production of synthetic rubbers and polymers. These polymers are used in a wide variety of industrial and consumer products, to improve their functionality, performance and safety and lower their costs. Butadiene-based products are important components of automobiles, construction materials, appliance parts, computers and telecommunications equipment, clothing, protective clothing, pack-aging and household articles (White, 2007).

The synthetic rubbers that are produced from butadiene include styrene–butadiene rubber, polybutadiene rubber, styrene–butadiene latex, chloroprene rubber and nitrile rubber. Important plastics that contain butadiene as a monomeric component are shock-resistant polystyrene, a two-phase system that consists of polystyrene and polybutadiene; polymers that consist of acrylonitrile, butadiene and styrene; and a copolymer of methyl methacrylate, butadiene and styrene, which is used as a modifier for poly(vinyl)chloride. Butadiene is also used as an intermediate in the production of chloroprene, adiponitrile and other basic petrochemicals (White, 2007).

Diepoxybutane has been proposed for use in curing polymers and cross-linking textile fibres (National Library of Medicine, 2008).

1.3   Occurrence

1.3.1   *Natural occurrence*

Butadiene is not known to occur as a natural product.

1.3.2   *Occupational exposure*

According to the 1990–93 CAREX database (see General Remarks) for 15 countries of the European Union (Kauppinen *et al.*, 2000) and the 1981–83 US National Occupational Exposure Survey (NOES, 1997), approximately 31 500 workers in Europe and 50 000 workers in the USA were potentially exposed to butadiene.

Based on data from CAREX, the major categories of industrial exposure to butadiene in 15 European countries are the manufacture of industrial chemicals (8000 persons), rubber products (7000 persons), plastic products (7000 persons), petroleum refining (2200 persons) and building construction (1600 persons) (Kauppinen *et al.*, 2000).

In the studies presented below, the accuracy of the levels of exposure to butadiene measured with the methods used until the mid-1980s may have been affected by the inability to distinguish between butadiene and other C_4 compounds, low desorption efficiency at low concentrations, possible sample breakthrough in charcoal tubes and possible loss during storage (Lunsford *et al.*, 1990; Bianchi *et al.*, 1997).

(a)   *Petroleum refining and butadiene monomer production*

Detailed industrial hygiene surveys were conducted in the USA by the National Institute for Occupational Safety and Health in 1985 in four of 10 facilities where butadiene was produced by solvent extraction of C_4 fractions that originated from ethylene co-product streams (Krishnan *et al.*, 1987). Levels of butadiene to which workers in various job categories were exposed are summarized in Table 3. Jobs that required workers to handle or transport containers, such as emptying sample cylinders or loading and unloading tank trucks or rail cars, presented the greatest potential exposure. Geometric means of full-shift exposure levels for other job categories were below 1 ppm [2.2 mg/m³]. Short-term samples showed that activities such as open-loop sampling and emptying cylinders were associated with peak exposures of 100 ppm [220 mg/m³]. Full-shift area samples indicated that ambient concentrations of butadiene were greatest in the rail car terminals (geometric mean, 1.8 ppm [3.9 mg/m³]) and in the tank storage farm (2.1 ppm [4.7 mg/m³]).

Table 3. Eight-hour time-weighted average exposure levels in personal breathing zone samples at four butadiene monomer production facilities in the USA, 1985

Job category	No. of samples	Exposure level (ppm [mg/m³])		
		Arithmetic mean	Geometric mean	Range
Process technician				
Control room	10	0.45 [1.0]	0.09 [0.2]	< 0.02–1.87 [< 0.04–4.1]
Process area	28	2.23 [4.9]	0.64 [1.4]	< 0.08–34.9 [< 0.18–77]
Loading area				
Rail car	9	14.6 [32.4]	1.00 [2.2]	0.12–124 [0.27–273]
Tank truck	3	2.65 [5.9]	1.02 [2.3]	0.08–5.46 [0.18–12.1]
Tank farm	5	0.44 [0.97]	0.20 [0.44]	< 0.04–1.53 [< 0.09–3.4]
Laboratory technician				
Analysis	29	1.06 [2.3]	0.40 [0.88]	0.03–6.31 [0.07–14.0]
Cylinder emptying	3	126 [277]	7.46 [16.5]	0.42–374 [0.93–826]

From Krishnan *et al.* (1987)

Monitoring in a plant in Finland generally indicated ambient air levels of butadiene of less than 10 ppm [22 mg/m³] at different sites (33 samples; mean sampling time, 5.3 h). In personal samples for 16 process workers, the concentrations ranged from < 0.1 to 477 ppm [< 0.22–1050 mg/m³] (mean, 11.5 ppm [25 mg/m³]; median, < 0.1 ppm [< 0.22 mg/m³]; 46 samples; mean sampling time, 2.5 h). The highest concentrations were measured during the collection of samples, for which protective clothing and respirators were used (Work Environment Fund, 1991).

A study of biological monitoring for the mutagenic effects of exposure to butadiene reported estimated average exposures of 1 ppm [2.2 mg/m³] for workers in a butadiene monomer plant. Ambient air concentrations in production areas averaged 3.5 ppm [7.7 mg/m³], while average concentrations of 0.03 ppm [0.07 mg/m³] were reported for the control area (Ward, J.B. *et al.*, 1996).

Levels of exposure to butadiene of workers in various job groups in the production and distribution of gasoline (see IARC, 1989) are shown in Table 4. Table 5 shows exposures in 1984–87 of workers in different areas of petroleum refineries and

Table 4. Personal exposures to butadiene associated with gasoline in 1984–85 in 13 European countries[a] (540 measurements)

Activity	Exposure level (mg/m^3)		
	Arithmetic mean	Range	Duration (TWA)
Production on-site (refining)	0.3	ND–11.4	8 h
Production off-site (refining)	0.1	ND–1.6	8 h
Loading ships (closed system)	6.4	ND–21.0	8 h
Loading ships (open system)	1.1	ND–4.2	8 h
Loading barges	2.6	ND–15.2	8 h
Jetty man	2.6	ND–15.9	8 h
Bulk loading road tankers			
Top loading < 1 h	1.4	ND–32.3	< 1 h
Top loading > 1 h	0.4	ND–4.7	8 h
Bottom loading < 1 h	0.2	ND–3.0	< 1 h
Bottom loading > 1 h	0.4	ND–14.1	8 h
Road tanker delivery (bulk plant to service station)	ND		
Rail car top loading	0.6	ND–6.2	8 h
Drumming	ND		
Service station attendant (dispensing fuel)	0.3	ND–1.1	8 h
Self-service station (filling tank)	1.6	ND–10.6	2 min

From CONCAWE (1987)
ND, not detected; TWA, time-weighted average
[a] Countries included not reported

Table 5. Eight-hour time-weighted average concentrations of butadiene to which workers in different jobs in petroleum refineries and petrochemical facilities were exposed in the USA, 1984–87

Job area	No. of facilities	Arithmetic mean[a]		Range	
		ppm	mg/m^3	ppm	mg/m^3
Production	7	0.24	0.53	0.008–2.0	0.02–4.4
Maintenance	6	0.11	0.24	0.02–0.37	0.04–0.82
Distribution	1	2.90	6.41	–	–
Laboratory	4	0.18	0.40	0.07–0.4	0.16–0.88

From Heiden Associates (1987)
[a] Weighted by number of exposed workers

petrochemical facilities where crude butadiene was produced (usually a C_4 stream obtained as a by-product of ethylene production). Table 6 shows more recent data on crackers at butadiene production plants for the years 1986–93 (ECETOC, 1997).

Exposure data from 15 monomer extraction sites for the years 1984–93 showed that less than 10% of the measured concentrations exceeded 5 ppm [11 mg/m³] (Table 7); in 1995 (Table 8), personal exposure levels in general were below 5 ppm [11 mg/m³] (ECETOC, 1997).

In 1998, personal exposure to butadiene was measured for 24 workers in a monomer production facility in the Czech Republic. The mean (± standard deviation [SD]) concentration of butadiene, calculated from 217 individual time-weighted average (TWA) measurements, was 0.6 ± 2.1 mg/m³ [0.27 ± 0.95 ppm]. The personal TWA measurements from all monomer production workers ranged from undetectable to 19.9 mg/m³. The mean concentration for the control group was 0.03 ± 0.03 mg/m³ [0.01 ± 0.01 ppm], calculated from 28 personal TWA exposure measurements (Albertini et al., 2003a).

Personal exposure to butadiene of 10 workers who held different jobs in a petrochemical plant in Finland was assessed using passive monitors shortly after the threshold limit value (TLV) of 1 ppm had come into force. A total of 119 personal breathing zone samples were taken and 117 were analysed. Of these, 32 (27%) samples were under the limit of quantification (0.029 mg/m³ [0.013 ppm] in a 20.5-L sample), 81 samples (69%) were between the limit of quantification and 1 ppm [2.2 mg/m³] and four samples (3%) were over the Finnish occupational exposure limit of 1 ppm. The mean value of all samples was 0.17 ppm [0.38 mg/m³] and the mean value of the samples that exceeded the Finnish occupational exposure limit was 1.75 ppm [3.87 mg/m³]. The mean level of exposure varied significantly ($p = 0.03$) between the 10 workers. Smoking did not significantly affect the values, but the seasonal effect was significant ($p = 0.02$) (Anttinen-Klemetti et al., 2004).

The occupational exposure of 42 workers in a petrochemical plant in Italy where butadiene was produced and used to prepare polymers was assessed by biomonitoring. The control group originated from the same industrial complex and included 43 workers who had no significant occupational exposure to butadiene. Active sampling from the breathing zone of the workers was performed during a full shift. Each exposed worker was assessed three to four times over a period of 6 weeks during different shifts. The mean exposure level of the control group was 0.9 μg/m³ [0.4 ppb] (SD, 1.0) and the lowest and highest values were < 0.1 and 3.8 μg/m³ [< 0.05 and 1.7 ppb], respectively. The mean exposure level of the exposed group was 11.5 μg/m³ [5.2 ppb] (SD, 35.8) and the lowest and highest values were < 0.1 and 220.6 μg/m³ [< 0.04 and 99.8 ppb], respectively (Fustinoni et al., 2004).

An exposure assessment was carried out in southern Taiwan, China, on a 120-acre [486 000 m²] petrochemical complex that comprised 11 different manufacturing plants. Butadiene was produced in two of the plants, which had an annual production of about 156 000 tonnes per year. Using the Fourier transform infrared spectroscopy technique, data were collected on 77 days during the period 1997–99. The relative number of samples that

Table 6. Personal exposures to butadiene of crackers in butadiene production plants in the European Union

Job category	Year of measurement	No. of workers	No. of samples	Exposure level (ppm)							
				<1	1–2	2–3	3–4	4–5	5–10	10–25	≥25
Unloading, loading, storage	1986–92	210	92	82	3	3	2	0	0	1	0
Distillation (hot)	1986–93	394	92	382	0	3	1	2	0	2	2
Laboratory, sampling	1986–93	132	184	178	2	1	2	1	0	0	0
Maintenance	1986–92	282	371	364	5	0	1	0	0	1	0
Other	1990–92	467	509	487	18	2	1	1	ND	0	0
Total	1986–93	1485	1548	1493	28	9	8	4	0	4	2

From ECETOC (1997)

ND, not detected [limit of detection not stated]

Table 7. Personal exposures to butadiene in extraction units[a] of butadiene production plants in the European Union

Job category	Year of measurement	No. of workers	No. of samples	Exposure level (ppm)							
				<1	1–2	2–3	3–4	4–5	5–10	10–25	≥25
Unloading, loading, storage	1986–93	392	224	178	9	8	7	2	11	22	7
Distillation (hot)	1985–93	256	626	535	20	19	6	11	8	12	15
Laboratory, sampling	1985–93	45	48	29	4	2	2	2	3	5	1
Maintenance	1986–93	248	127	93	14	3	2	1	3	4	7
Other	1984–92	45	10	8	2	0	0	0	0	0	0
Total	1984–93	986	1035	843	49	32	17	16	25	23	30

From ECETOC (1997)

[a] Isolation of butadiene from C_4 stream

Table 8. Personal exposures to butadiene at 15 monomer extraction sites in the European Union in 1995

Job category	Exposure level (ppm)	
	Time-weighted averages	Range of values
Production		
Extraction	< 0.01–2	0–14
Derivation[a]	1.4–3.4	0.07–60
Storage and filling	< 0.02–5	0–18.1
Transport	< 0.1–0.7	0.02–1.2
Laboratory	0.03–1	0–13.1

From ECETOC (1997)
[a] Integrated monomer extraction and styrene–butadiene production on same site

were above the detection limit was 15.2% and the mean value of the measurements was 10.5 ± 36.7 ppb [23.2 ± 81.1 μg/m^3]. The maximum concentration measured was 3.1 ppm [6.8 mg/m^3] (Chan *et al.*, 2006). [Measurements were area samples and may underestimate exposure of the workers.]

In the monomer industry, potential exposure to compounds other than butadiene includes exposure to extraction solvents and components of the C$_4$ feedstock. Extraction solvents differ between facilities: common solvents include dimethylformamide, dimethylacetamide, acetonitrile, β-methoxypropionitrile (Fajen, 1985a), furfural and aqueous cuprous ammonium acetate (Occupational Safety and Health Administration, 1990b). Stabilizers are commonly used to prevent the formation of peroxides in air and during polymerization. No information was available on these exposures or on exposure to chemicals other than butadiene that are produced in some facilities such as butylenes, ethylene, propylene, polyethylene and polypropylene resins, methyl-*tert*-butyl ether and aromatic hydrocarbons (Fajen, 1985b,c).

(b)   Production of polymers and derivatives

In samples taken at a styrene–butadiene rubber plant in the USA in 1976 (Table 9), levels of butadiene above 100 ppm [220 mg/m^3] were encountered by technical services personnel (115 ppm [253 mg/m^3]) and an instrument man (174 ppm [385 mg/m^3]; Meinhardt *et al.*, 1978). At another styrene–butadiene rubber manufacturing plant in the USA in 1979, the only two departments in which levels were greater than 10 ppm [22 mg/m^3] were the tank farm (53.4 ppm [118 mg/m^3]) and maintenance (20.7 ppm [46 mg/m^3]; Checkoway & Williams, 1982). Overall mean 8-h TWA exposure levels differed

Table 9. Eight-hour time-weighted average exposure levels of butadiene measured in two styrene–butadiene rubber manufacturing plants in the USA

Reference	Year of sampling	Job classification or department	No. of samples	Exposure level	
				ppm	mg/m^3
Meinhardt	1976	Instrument man	3	58.6	130
et al. (1978)		Technical services personnel	12	19.9	43.9
		Head production operator	5	15.5	34.3
		Carpenter	4	7.80	17.2
		Production operator	24	3.30	7.29
		Maintenance mechanic	17	3.15	6.96
		Common labourer	17	1.52	3.36
		Production foreman	1	1.16	2.56
		Operator helper	3	0.79	1.75
		Pipe fitter	8	0.74	1.64
		Electrician	5	0.22	0.49
Checkoway &	1979	Tank farm	8	20.0	44.3
Williams (1982)		Maintenance	52	0.97	2.1
		Reactor recovery	28	0.77	1.7
		Solution	12	0.59	1.3
		Factory service	56	0.37	0.82
		Shipping and receiving	2	0.08	0.18
		Storeroom	1	0.08	0.18

considerably between the two plants: 13.5 ppm [30 mg/m^3] and 1.24 ppm [2.7mg/m^3], respectively (Meinhardt et al., 1982).

Detailed industrial hygiene surveys were conducted in 1986 in five of 17 facilities in the USA where butadiene was used to produce styrene–butadiene rubber, nitrile–butadiene rubber, polybutadiene rubber, neoprene and adiponitrile (Fajen, 1988). Levels of butadiene to which workers in various job categories were exposed are summarized in Table 10. Process technicians in unloading, in the tank farm and in the purification, polymerization and reaction areas, laboratory technicians and maintenance technicians were exposed to the highest levels. Short-term sampling showed that activities such as sampling a barge and laboratory work were associated with peak exposures of more than 100 ppm [220 mg/m^3]. Full-shift area sampling indicated that geometric mean ambient concentrations of butadiene were less than 0.5 ppm [1.1 mg/m^3] and usually less than 0.1 ppm [0.22 mg/m^3] in all locations measured at the five plants.

A biological monitoring study that used personal sampling reported average levels of butadiene of 0.30, 0.21 and 0.12 ppm [0.66, 0.46 and 0.27 mg/m^3] for the high-, inter-mediate- and low-exposure groups, respectively, in a styrene–butadiene rubber plant in Texas, USA (Ward, J.B. et al., 1996).

Table 10. Eight-hour time-weighted average exposure levels in personal breathing zone samples at five plants that produced butadiene-based polymers and derivatives in the USA, 1986

Job category	No. of samples	Exposure level (ppm [mg/m³])		
		Arithmetic mean	Geometric mean	Range
Process technician				
Unloading area	2	14.6 [32.27]	4.69 [10.37]	0.770–28.5 [1.7–63.0]
Tank farm	31	2.08 [4.60]	0.270 [0.60]	< 0.006–23.7 [< 0.01–2.4]
Purification	18	7.80 [17.24]	6.10 [13.48]	1.33–24.1 [3.0–53.3]
Polymerization or reaction	81	0.414 [0.92]	0.062 [0.14]	< 0.006–11.3 [< 0.01–5.0]
Solutions and coagulation	33	0.048 [0.11]	0.029 [0.06]	< 0.005–0.169 [< 0.01–4]
Crumbing and drying	35	0.033 [0.07]	0.023 [0.05]	< 0.005–0.116 [< 0.01–0.26]
Packaging	79	0.036 [0.08]	0.022 [0.05]	< 0.005–0.154 [< 0.01–0.34]
Warehouse	20	0.020 [0.04]	0.010 [0.02]	< 0.005–0.068 [< 0.01–0.15]
Control room	6	0.030 [0.07]	0.019 [0.04]	< 0.012–0.070 [< 0.03–0.16]
Laboratory technician	54	2.27 [5.02]	0.213 [0.47]	< 0.006–37.4 [< 0.01–82.65]
Maintenance technician	72	1.37 [3.02]	0.122 [0.27]	< 0.006–43.2 [< 0.01–95.47]
Utilities operator	6	0.118 [0.26]	0.054 [0.12]	< 0.006–0.304 [< 0.01–0.67]

From Fajen (1988)

In 13 of 27 European sites where styrene–butadiene rubber and styrene–butadiene latex were produced, less than 10% of the concentrations measured exceeded 5 ppm (Table 11; ECETOC, 1997).

Data from the Netherlands are available from 1976 onwards, but the measurement methods used in the early surveys are unknown (Kwekkeboom, 1996; Dubbeld, 1998). No clear trend can be seen for the years 1990–97, but average exposures were relatively low (arithmetic mean < 3 ppm [6.6 mg/m³]) (Table 12).

Exposure of 38 workers was measured in a butadiene polymer production facility in China. Personal full-shift measurements established that workers in butadiene operations were exposed to a median level of 2.0 ppm [4.4 mg/m³]. Short-term breathing zone measurements of butadiene showed great extremes in exposure; DMF [dimethyl-formamide] analysts had a median exposure of 54 ppm [119 mg/m³] (range, below detection to 3090 ppm [6829 mg/m³]; 50 samples), polymer analysts had a median exposure of 6.5 ppm [14.4 mg/m³] (range, below detection to 1078 ppm [2382 mg/m³]; 41 samples) and maintenance-recovery workers had a median exposure of 7.0 ppm [15.5 mg/m³] (range, below detection to > 12 000 ppm [> 26 520 mg/m³]; 24 samples) (Hayes *et al.*, 2001).

A biomonitoring study carried out in a styrene–butadiene rubber plant in Southeast Texas, in which 37 workers were monitored during their entire work shift using passive samplers, demonstrated that levels in the tank area exceeded the current Occupational

Table 11. Eight-hour time-weighted average personal exposures to butadiene in styrene–butadiene rubber plants in the European Union (1984–93)

Job category	No. of workers	No. of samples	Exposure level (ppm)								
			< 0.5	0.51–1	1.01–2	2.01–3	3.01–4	4.01–5	5.01–10	10.01–25	≥ 25
Unloading, loading and storage	132	77	47	1	8	6	3	0	5	5	2
Polymerization	324	147	61	23	25	18	6	4	7	3	0
Recovery	103	165	113	9	9	14	7	4	5	4	0
Finishing	247	120	90	16	3	4	5	1	1	0	0
Laboratory sampling	115	113	68	13	12	6	4	2	3	5	0
Maintenance	141	39	28	1	2	1	1	2	1	2	1
Total	1062	661	407	63	59	49	26	13	22	19	3

From ECETOC (1997)

Table 12. Eight-hour time-weighted average exposure levels of butadiene in personal breathing zone samples at a plant that produced styrene–butadiene polymer in the Netherlands, 1990–97

Year	No. of samples	Exposure level (mg/m^3 [ppm])		
		Arithmetic mean	Range	Method[a]
1990	27	5.45 [2.47]	0.35–69.06 [0.16–31.24]	3M 3500
1991	19	1.11 [0.50]	0.09–2.88 [0.04–1.30]	NIOSH 1024
1992	23	2.79 [1.26]	0.13–11.78 [0.06–5.33]	3M 3520
1993	38	2.87 [1.30]	0.15–13.13 [0.07–5.94]	3M 3520/ NIOSH 1024
1996/97 process operators	20	2.77 [1.25]	0.13–46.62 [0.06–21.10]	3M 3520
1996/97 maintenance workers	14	0.54 [0.24]	0.12–9.89 [0.05–4.48]	3M 3520

From Kwekkeboom (1996); Dubbeld (1998)
[a] Analytical methods used are described by Bianchi et al. (1997). Methods 3M 3500 and 3M 3520 involve absorption onto butadiene-specific activated charcoal, followed by desorption with carbon disulfide or with dichloromethane, respectively, and analysis by direct-injection gas chromatography with flame ionization detection.

Safety and Health Administation permissible exposure limit for butadiene. However, the workers wore protective equipment on this particular job. TWA values in various work areas are summarized in Table 13 (Ward et al., 2001).

In 1998, 319 personal workshift TWA measurements of exposure to butadiene were obtained for 34 workers in a polymer production plant in the Czech Republic. The mean ($\pm$ SD) concentration of butadiene was 1.8 ± 4.7 mg/m^3 [0.8 ± 2.1 ppm]. The individual TWA measurements from all polymer production workers ranged from 0.002 to 39.0 mg/m^3 [0.001–17.6 ppm]. The level of exposure of the control group was 0.03 ± 0.03 mg/m^3 [0.01 ± 0.01 ppm], calculated from 28 personal TWA measurements (Albertini et al., 2003a).

A Finnish study assessed personal exposure to butadiene in three plants that manufactured styrene–butadiene latex. Full-shift air samples were collected from the breathing zone of 28 workers using passive samplers over 4 months. A total of 885 samples were collected and the number of samples per participant ranged from 19 to 39. Samples were collected at the same time in all three plants. The data showed that 624 (70.5%) of the samples were below the limit of quantification; 240 (27.1%) samples were between the limit of quantification and 1 ppm [2.2 mg/m^3] and 21 (2.4%) were over the Finnish occupational exposure limit of 1 ppm [2.2 mg/m^3]. Mean butadiene concentrations in the three plants were 0.068, 0.125 and 0.302 ppm [0.15, 0.28 and 0.67 mg/m^3], respectively.

Table 13. Time-weighted average exposures to butadiene in a styrene–butadiene rubber plant in the USA, 1998

Work area	Subjects	Detectable samples	Samples below the LOD[a]	Exposure level (mean ± SD) (ppm [mg/m³])
Tank farm	6	17	0	4.04 ± 3.45 [8.9 ± 7.6]
Recovery	6	17	0	1.09 ± 2.35 [2.41 ± 5.19]
Reactor	9	17	3	0.64 ± 1.26 [1.41 ± 2.78]
Low areas[b]	14	22	19	0.05 ± 0.06 [0.11 ± 0.13]
Laboratory	1	2	0	0.29 ± 0.33 [0.64 ± 0.73]
Blending	1	3	0	0.49 ± 0.24 [1.08 ± 0.53]

From Ward et al. (2001)

LOD, limit of detection; SD, standard deviation

[a] Half of the 0.002 ppm detection limit was used to calculate exposure to butadiene for the samples

[b] Coagulation, baling, packing, water paint, shipping, warehouse and control room

Statistical analysis of the data did not indicate any significant difference between the plants when all results were considered (Anttinen-Klemetti et al., 2006).

In a Czech study that included 26 female control workers, 23 female butadiene-exposed workers, 25 male control workers and 30 male butadiene-exposed workers, 10 personal full-shift (8-h) measurements per worker over a 4-month period showed mean 8-h TWA exposure levels of 0.008 mg/m³ and 0.4 mg/m³ [0.004 and 0.18 ppm] for control and exposed women, respectively. The highest single 8-h TWA value among exposed women was 9.8 mg/m³ [4.5 ppm]. Mean 8-h TWA exposure levels were 0.007 mg/m³ and 0.8 mg/m³ [0.003 and 0.36 ppm] for control and exposed men, respectively; personal single 8-h TWA values of up to 12.6 mg/m³ [5.7 ppm] were measured in the exposed group. The concentrations for butadiene-exposed workers were significantly higher than those for the controls for both men and women; the concentrations for butadiene-exposed workers were significantly higher for men than for women (Albertini et al., 2007). [The difference in exposure levels may be due to differences in tasks performed by men and women.]

Data from a Canadian styrene–butadiene rubber plant indicate a clear decrease in exposure from 1977 to 1991 (Sathiakumar & Delzell, 2007; Table 14). The data were used to validate the estimates of historical exposure to butadiene (Macaluso et al., 1996, 2004; Sathiakumar et al., 2007).

The manufacture of butadiene-based polymers and butadiene derivatives implies potential exposure to a number of other chemical agents that vary according to product and process and include other monomers (styrene, acrylonitrile, chloroprene), solvents, additives (e.g. activators, antioxidants, modifiers), catalysts, mineral oils, carbon black, chlorine, inorganic acids and caustic solutions (Fajen, 1986a,b; Roberts, 1986). Styrene, benzene and toluene levels were measured in 1979 in various departments of a plant that manufactured styrene–butadiene rubber in the USA: mean 8-h TWA levels of styrene were below 2 ppm [8.4 mg/m^3], except for tank-farm workers (13.7 ppm [57.5 mg/m^3], eight samples); mean benzene levels did not exceed 0.1 ppm [0.3 mg/m^3], and those of toluene did not exceed 0.9 ppm [3.4 mg/m^3] (Checkoway & Williams, 1982). Meinhardt *et al.* (1982) reported that the mean 8-h TWA levels of styrene in two styrene–butadiene rubber manufacturing plants were 0.94 ppm [3.9 mg/m^3] (55 samples) and 1.99 ppm [8.4 mg/m^3] (35 samples) in 1977; the average level of benzene measured in one of the plants was 0.1 ppm [0.3 mg/m^3] (three samples). Average levels of styrene, toluene, benzene, vinyl cyclohexene and cyclooctadiene were reported to be below 1 ppm in another styrene–butadiene rubber plant in 1977 (Burroughs, 1977). Dimethyldithiocarbamate has been used in some plants and dermal exposure to this compound potentially exists (Delzell *et al.*, 2001).

Table 14. Exposure levels of butadiene in a styrene–butadiene rubber plant in Canada

Year	No. of jobs monitored	No. of measurements	Exposure level (mean[a] ± SD) (ppm [mg/m^3])
1977	3	56	24.8 ± 69.9 [54.8 ± 154.5]
1978	11	527	16.0 ± 166.6 [35.4 ± 368.2]
1979	13	274	10.6 ± 153.2 [23.4 ± 338.6]
1980	13	301	14.5 ± 137.8 [32.0 ± 304.5]
1981	15	307	4.8 ± 38.4 [10.6 ± 84.9]
1982	21	406	3.8 ± 28.2 [8.4 ± 62.3]
1983	13	113	3.9 ± 19.4 [8.6 ± 42.9]
1984	27	658	2.5 ± 20.3 [5.5 ± 44.9]
1985	27	482	2.6 ± 18.4 [5.7 ± 40.7]
1986	30	504	2.3 ± 16.2 [5.08 ± 35.8]
1987	26	310	0.85 ± 6.3 [1.9 ± 13.9]
1988	28	417	1.0 ± 5.2 [2.2 ± 11.5]
1989	27	238	1.5 ± 5.5 [3.3 ± 12.2]
1990	27	223	0.63 ± 3.3 [1.4 ± 7.3]
1991	25	162	0.34 ± 0.61 [0.75 ± 1.35]

From Sathiakumar *et al.* (2007)
SD, standard deviation
[a] Weighted by the number of measurements for job/year combinations in a year

(c) Manufacture of rubber and plastics products

In a tyre and tube manufacturing plant in the USA in 1975, a cutter man/Banbury operator was reported to have been exposed to 2.1 ppm [4.6 mg/m^3] butadiene (personal 6-h sample) (Ropert, 1976).

Personal 8-h TWA measurements taken in 1978 and 1979 in companies where acrylonitrile–butadiene–styrene moulding operations were conducted showed levels of

< 0.05–1.9 mg/m^3 [< 0.11–4.2 ppm] (Burroughs, 1979; Belanger & Elesh, 1980; Ruhe & Jannerfeldt, 1980).

In a polybutadiene rubber warehouse, levels of 0.003 ppm [0.007 mg/m^3] butadiene were found in area samples; area and personal samples taken in tyre plants revealed levels of 0.007–0.05 ppm [0.016–0.11 mg/m^3] butadiene (Rubber Manufacturers' Association, 1984).

Unreacted butadiene was detected as a trace (0.04–0.2 mg/kg) in 15 of 37 bulk samples of polymers and other chemicals synthesized from butadiene and analysed in 1985–86. Only two samples contained measurable amounts of butadiene: tetrahydro-phthalic anhydride (53 mg/kg) and vinylpyridine latex (16.5 mg/kg) (JACA Corp., 1987).

Detailed industrial hygiene surveys were conducted in 1984–87 in the USA at a rubber tyre plant and an industrial hose plant where styrene–butadiene rubber, poly-butadiene and acrylonitrile–butadiene rubber were processed. No butadiene was detected in any of 124 personal full-shift samples from workers in the following job categories that were identified as involving potential exposure to butadiene: Banbury operators, mill operators, extruder operators, curing operators, conveyer operators, calendering operators, wire winders, tube machine operators, tyre builders and tyre repair and buffer workers (Fajen et al., 1990).

Occupational exposures to many other agents in the rubber goods manufacturing industry have been reviewed previously (IARC, 1982).

(d)   Comparison of exposure levels in monomer and styrene–butadiene rubber production facilities

Exposures measured in monomer production facilities in the USA demonstrated overall mean levels of 3.5 ppm [7.7 mg/m^3] (measured in 1979–92; number not reported; stationary sampling; Cowles et al., 1994) and 7.1 ppm [15.7 mg/m^3] (measured in 1985; 87 samples; personal sampling; Krishnan et al., 1987). Recently reported values from the Czech Republic and Finland were 0.64 ppm [1.41 mg/m^3] (measured in 1998; 217 samples; personal sampling) and 0.17 ppm [0.38 mg/m^3] (measured in 2002; 117 samples; personal sampling) (Albertini et al., 2003a; Anttinen-Klemetti et al., 2004).

Measurement of butadiene concentrations in a styrene–butadiene rubber plant in Canada demonstrated a decrease in exposure during the 14 years of monitoring. The levels dropped from 24.8 ppm in 1977 [54.8 mg/m^3] to 0.34 ppm [0.75 mg/m^3] in 1991 (Table 14) (Sathiakumar et al., 2007).

The decreasing trend of exposure was apparent in both monomer and styrene–butadiene rubber production; however, the lack of data from the 1940s to the 1970s does not allow comparison between the two processes.

1.3.3   Environmental occurrence

According to the Environmental Protection Agency Toxic Chemical Release Inventory in the USA, industrial releases of butadiene to the atmosphere from industrial facilities in the USA were 4425 tonnes in 1987, 2360 tonnes in 1990 and 1385 tonnes in 1995. According to the same database, fugitive air emissions were 157 973 kg and point source air emissions were 450 926 kg in 2005 (Environmental Protection Agency Toxic Release Inventory, 2005; National Library of Medicine, 2008).

Under laboratory conditions, non-catalyst vehicles emitted butadiene at a rate of 20.7 ± 9.2 mg/kg. Vehicles that had a functioning catalyst–emission control device had an average emission rate of 2.1 ± 1.5 mg/km. Based on these numbers, the authors concluded that vehicle emissions of butadiene have been substantially underestimated (Ye *et al.*, 1997). Based on an average of 20 000 km per year per car and approximately 243 million registered cars in the USA in 2004, and considering the average emission rates estimated by Ye *et al.* (1997), emissions of butadiene from automobile exhausts can be estimated to amount to approximately 106 770 tonnes per year.

Butadiene is also released to the atmosphere from the smoke of bush fires, the thermal breakdown or burning of plastics and by volatization from gasoline (Agency for Toxic Substances and Disease Registry, 1992; see IARC, 1992).

Kim *et al.* (2001, 2002) measured the concentrations of 15 volatile organic compounds, including butadiene, in a wide range of urban micro-environments in the United Kingdom (Table 15) and estimated the personal exposure of 12 urban dwellers directly and indirectly via static monitoring combined with a personal activities diary (Table 16).

Table 15. Mean concentrations of butadiene in micro-environments in the United Kingdom

Environment	No. of samples	Concentration (mean ± SD) (μg/m^3)
Home	64	1.1 ± 1.9
Office	12	0.3 ± 0.2
Restaurant	6	1.5 ± 0.8
Public house	6	3.0 ± 2.0
Department store	8	0.6 ± 0.4
Cinema	6	0.6 ± 0.3
Perfume store	3	0.9 ± 0.1
Library	6	0.4 ± 0.2
Laboratory	8	0.2 ± 0.1
Train station	12	2.2 ± 1.7
Coach station	12	0.9 ± 0.7
Road with traffic	12	1.8 ± 0.9
Car	35	7.9 ± 4.7
Train	18	1.0 ± 0.6
Bus	18	1.7 ± 0.9
Smoking home	32	1.7 ± 2.5
Nonsmoking home	32	0.5 ± 0.3

From Kim *et al.* (2001)
SD, standard deviation

Table 16. Daytime and night-time concentrations (μg/m^3) of butadiene recorded during personal exposure monitoring in the United Kingdom, 1999–2000

Period	No. of samples	Mean	Standard deviation	Minimum	Maximum
Daytime	473	1.1	0.4	ND	26.3
Night-time	99	0.8	0.4	ND	7.9

From Kim *et al.* (2002)
ND, not detected

Environmental exposure to emissions, including butadiene, was compared between bus and cycling commuters on a route in Dublin. Samples were collected during both morning and afternoon rush-hour periods using continuous sampling. The average concentrations experienced by the cyclist and the bus passenger for all journeys were 0.47 ppb [103 μg/m^3] (SD, 0.19; min., 0.24; max., 0.81) and 0.78 ppb [1.7 μg/m^3] (SD, 0.34; min., 0.34; max., 1.49), respectively (O'Donoghue *et al.*, 2007).

In the United Kingdom, the estimated emission of butadiene in 1996 was 10.6 thousand tonnes. Road vehicle exhaust emissions dominated and comprised 68% of the total emissions, while emissions from off-road vehicles and machinery accounted for 14%. The remaining emissions arose from the chemical industry, during the manufacture of butadiene and its use in the production of various rubber compounds. These two processes accounted for 8 and 10%, respectively, of total emissions in the United Kingdom in 1996 (Dollard *et al.*, 2001).

Municipal structural fires are a source of butadiene, and the mean level of butadiene from nine fires ranged from 0.03 to 4.84 ppm [0.07–9.9 mg/m^3] (Austin *et al.*, 2001). Domestic wood burning also has an impact on levels of butadiene in homes. Wood burners had a significantly higher personal exposure to butadiene (median, 0.18 μg/m^3) than the reference group. Similarly, significantly higher indoor levels were reported (median, 0.23 μg/m^3) in homes of wood burners than in the homes of the reference group (Gustafson *et al.*, 2007).

The intake of butadiene that results from exposure to environmental tobacco smoke for a person who lives with one or more smokers in homes where smoking is permitted was estimated to be in the range of 16–37 μg per day (Nazaroff & Singer, 2004). The levels of butadiene in public houses in Dublin were assessed before and after the smoking ban in 2004. The average level before the ban was 4.15 μg/m^3 [1.87 ppb]. The levels of butadiene recorded in the same establishments when cigarettes were no longer being smoked dropped significantly to 0.22 μg/m^3 [0.1 ppb], which is still higher than the average ambient level (0.12 μg/m^3 [0.05 ppb]) (McNabola *et al.*, 2006).

In the metropolitan area of Mexico City, three persons who were simultaneously monitored for butadiene inside the home and outdoors had median levels of 2.1 μg/m^3 [1 ppb] (max., 11.5 μg/m^3 [5.2 ppb]), 2.0 μg/m^3 [0.9 ppb] (max., 8.3 μg/m^3 [3.7 ppb]) and

0.8 µg/m^3 [0.4 ppb] (max., 4.6 µg/m^3 [2.1 ppb]) for personal, indoor and outdoor exposure, respectively (Serrano-Trespalacios *et al.*, 2004).

Ambient concentrations of butadiene were measured in Japan during the years 1997–2003 at general environmental stations, roadside stations and industrial vicinity stations. The mean levels in 1998 were 0.28, 0.56 and 0.37 µg/m^3 [0.13, 0.25 and 0.17 ppb] for the general environment, roadside and industrial vicinity, respectively. The overall level was 0.36 µg/m^3 [0.16 ppb]. In 2003, corresponding levels were 0.22, 0.42 and 0.31 µg/m^3 [0.10, 0.19 and 0.14 ppb], with an overall level of 0.29 µg/m^3 [0.13 ppb] (Higashino *et al.*, 2006).

Mainstream and sidestream cigarette smoke contain approximately 20–40 µg and 80–130 µg butadiene per cigarette, respectively; levels of butadiene in smoky indoor environments are typically 10–20 µg/m^3 [5–9 ppb] (IARC, 2004).

Based on its physical and chemical properties, butadiene is unlikely to be detected in water or in soil (Agency for Toxic Substances and Disease Registry, 1992).

1.4   Regulations and guidelines

Occupational exposure limits and guidelines for butadiene in several countries, regions or organizations are given in Table 17.

The government of the United Kingdom has imposed an air quality standard for butadiene of 2.25 µg/m^3 [1.00 ppb] to be achieved by December 2003 (running annual mean) (AEA Energy & Environment, 2002).

Table 17. Occupational exposure limits and guidelines for butadiene in several countries/regions or organizations

Country/region or organization	TWA (ppm)[a]	STEL (ppm)[a]	Carcinogenicity[b]	Notes
Belgium	2		Ca	
Brazil	780			
Canada				
Alberta	2			Schedule 2
British Columbia	2	2		K2
Ontario	5			
Quebec	2		A2	
China (mg/m^3)	5	12.5		STEL based on the 'ultra limit coefficient'
China, Hong Kong SAR	2		A2	
Czech Republic (mg/m^3)	10	20		
Finland	1			
Germany-MAK			1	
Ireland	1		Ca2	
Japan-JSOH			1	
Malaysia	2			

Table 17 (contd)

Country/region or organization	TWA (ppm)[a]	STEL (ppm)[a]	Carcinogenicity[b]	Notes
Mexico	1000	1250	A2	
Netherlands	21		Ca	
New Zealand	10		A2	
Norway	1		Ca	
Poland-MAC (mg/m³)	10	40		
South Africa-DOL CL	10			
Spain	2		Ca1	
Sweden	0.5	5	Ca	
United Kingdom	10		R45	
USA				
ACGIH (TLV)	2		A2	Cancer
NIOSH IDLH (ceiling)		2000	Ca	
OSHA PEL	1	5		

From ACGIH® Worldwide (2005)
ACGIH, American Conference of Governmental Industrial Hygienists; DOL CL, Department of Labour – ceiling limits; IDLH, immediately dangerous to life or health; JSOH, Japanese Society of Occupational Health; MAC, maximum acceptable concentration; MAK, maximum allowed concentration; NIOSH, National Institute for Occupational Safety and Health; OSHA, Occupational Safety and Health Administration; PEL, permissible exposure limit; STEL, short-term exposure limit; TLV, threshold limit value; TWA, time-weighted average
[a] Unless otherwise specified
[b] Ca (Belgium, Netherlands, Sweden, NIOSH), carcinogen/substance is carcinogenic; Ca (Norway), potential cancer-causing agent; 2, considered to be carcinogenic to humans; A2, suspected human carcinogen/carcinogenicity suspected in humans; 1, substance which causes cancer in man/carcinogenic to humans; Ca2, suspected human carcinogen; Ca1, known or presumed human carcinogen; R45, may cause cancer

2.   Studies of Cancer in Humans

2.1   Background

Over the last 30 years, the relationship between exposure to butadiene and cancer in human populations has been investigated in numerous studies. The most relevant investigations focused on working populations who were employed in butadiene monomer and styrene–butadiene rubber production.

Three independent cohorts of monomer production workers in the USA have been studied: at two Union Carbide plants in West Virginia (Ward et al., 1995), at a Texaco plant in Texas (Divine & Hartman, 2001) and at a Shell plant in Texas (Tsai et al., 2001).

Two independent groups of styrene–butadiene rubber production workers have been studied. One was studied by the National Institute of Occupational Safety and Health (NIOSH) in a two-plant complex in Ohio, USA (McMichael *et al.*, 1974, 1976; Meinhardt *et al.*, 1982), and the other comprised workers from eight facilities in the USA and Canada who were studied by researchers from the Johns Hopkins' University (Matanoski & Schwartz, 1987; Matanoski *et al.*, 1990, 1993).

Subsequently, researchers from the University of Alabama at Birmingham (Delzell *et al.* 1996) studied the two-plant complex originally investigated by NIOSH plus seven of the eight plants studied by the Johns Hopkins' University. The Johns Hopkins' researchers also conducted nested case–control studies within this working population (Santos-Burgoa *et al.*, 1992; Matanoski *et al.*, 1997). The University of Alabama at Birmingham group recently updated the follow-up of the cohort and revised and refined their assessment of exposures both to butadiene and to possible confounding co-exposures (Macaluso *et al.*, 2004). A number of largely overlapping publications from these groups have been reviewed. The most recent results were published by Graff *et al.* (2005), Sathiakumar *et al.* (2005), and Cheng *et al.* (2007).

In addition to industry-based studies, a population-based case–control study in Canada (Parent *et al.*, 2000) and a cohort study of students at a high school adjacent to a styrene–butadiene rubber production plant in the USA (Loughlin *et al.*, 1999) are also reviewed here.

Overall, the available studies focused consistently on a possible increased risk for neoplasms of the lymphatic and haematopoietic system from exposure to butadiene.

Epidemiological studies of cancer and exposure to butadiene are summarized in Table 18.

2.2   Industry-based studies

2.2.1   *Monomer production*

A cohort mortality study included men who were assigned to any of three butadiene production units located within several chemical plants in the Kanawha Valley of West Virginia, USA. Of the 364 men included in the study, 277 (76%) were employed in a 'Rubber Reserve' plant that operated during the Second World War (Ward *et al.*, 1995). The plants produced butadiene from ethanol or from olefin cracking. The butadiene production units included in this study were selected from an index of chemical departments that was developed by the Union Carbide Corporation and included only departments where butadiene was a primary product and neither benzene nor ethylene oxide was present. The cohort studied was part of a large cohort of 29 139 chemical workers whose mortality experience had been reported earlier, although without regard to specific exposures (Rinsky *et al.*, 1988). Three subjects were lost to follow-up (0.8%). Mortality from all cancers was not increased (48 deaths; standardized mortality ratio [SMR], 1.1; 95% confidence interval [CI], 0. 8–1.4). Seven deaths from lymphatic and

Table 18. Epidemiological studies of exposure to 1,3-butadiene and the risk for lympho-haematopoietic neoplasms

Butadiene monomer production

Reference, location	Cohort description	Exposure assessment	Organ site (ICD code)	Exposure categories	No. of cases/ deaths	Relative risk (95% CI)	Adjustment for potential confounders	Comments
Ward, E.H. *et al.* (1995, 1996), USA	364 male workers in three units	Employment in butadiene departments; no benzene or ethylene oxide present	All (140–208)		48	**SMR** 1.1 (0.8–1.4)	Age, time period; county reference rates	All 4 cases of lympho/reticulo-sarcomas had been employed ≥ 2 years (SMR, 8.3; 95% CI, 1.6–14.8), as had those of stomach cancer (SMR, 6.6; 95% CI, 2.1–15.3); all occurred in the rubber reserve plant.
			Lymphatic and haematopoietic		7	1.8 (0.7–3.6)		
			Lymphosarcoma and reticulosarcoma (200)		4	5.8 (1.6–14.8)		
			Leukaemia (204–208)		2	1.2 (0.2–4.4)		
Divine & Hartman (2001), USA	2800 male workers employed ≥ 6 months in 1943–96	Industrial hygiene sampling data	All cancers (140–209)	Employed	333	**SMR** 0.9 (0.8–1.0)	Age, time period, age at hire	No increasing trend by duration of employment; no increasing trend by exposure group; lymphatic haematopoietic cancers and lymphosarcoma significantly increased in the highest exposure category; elevations were found in workers employed < 1950, and were highest in short-term workers.
				< 5 years	170	1.0 (0.8–1.1)		
				5–19 years	55	0.8 (0.6–1.1)		
				≥ 20 years	108	0.8 (0.7–1.0)		
			Lymphohaematopoietic (200–209)	Employed	50	1.4 (1.1–1.9)		
				< 5 years	26	1.6 (1.0–2.3)		
				5–19 years	8	1.2 (0.5–2.4)		
				≥ 20 years	16	1.3 (0.8–2.2)		
				High exposure				
				< 5 years	20	1.8 (1.1–2.8)		
				≥ 5 years	14	1.5 (0.8–2.5)		
				First employed				
				1942–49	46	1.5 (1.1–2.1)		
				≥ 1950	4	0.7 (0.2–1.8)		

Table 18 (contd)

Reference, location	Cohort description	Exposure assessment	Organ site (ICD code)	Exposure categories	No. of cases/ deaths	Relative risk (95% CI)	Adjustment for potential confounders	Comments
Divine & Hartman (2001) (contd)			Non-Hodgkin lymphoma (200, 202)	Employed	19	1.5 (0.9–2.3)		
				< 5 years	12	1.3 (0.3–3.7)		
				5–19 years	3	0.9 (0.3–2.3)		
				≥ 20 years	4	2.0 (0.9–3.9)		
				High exposure				
				< 5 years	8	1.1 (0.3–2.9)		
				≥ 5 years	4	1.6 (0.9–2.6)		
				First employed				
				1942–49	17	1.6 (0.9–2.6)		
				≥ 1950	2	0.9 (0.1–3.2)		
			Leukaemia (204–207)	Employed	18	1.3 (0.8–2.0)		
				< 5 years	9	1.4 (0.6–2.6)		
				5–19 years	2	0.7 (0.1–2.6)		
				≥ 20 years	7	1.5 (0.6–3.1)		
				High exposure				
				< 5 years	8	1.9 (0.8–3.7)		
				≥ 5 years	5	1.4 (0.4–3.2)		
				First employed				
				1942–49	18	1.5 (0.9–2.4)		
				≥ 1950	0	0 (0–178)		
Tsai et al. (2001), USA	614 male workers	Employed ≥ 5 years in butadiene production; most 8-h TWAs for butadiene < 10 ppm	All cancers		16	**SMR** 0.6 (0.3–0.9)	Age, race, calendar year; reference county-specific rates	A concurrent morbidity study failed to show differences in haematological values between butadiene-exposed and unexposed workers within the complex.
			Lymphatic and haemopoietic (200–209)		3	1.1 (0.3–1.5)		

Table 18 (contd)

Styrene–butadiene rubber (SBR) production

Reference, location	Cohort description	Exposure assessment	Organ site (ICD code)	Exposure categories	No. of cases/ deaths	Relative risk (95% CI)	Adjustment for potential confounders	Comments
McMichael et al. (1976), USA	Case–cohort of 6678 male rubber workers	Employment for > 2 years in SBR production based on work histories	All lymphatic and haematopoietic (200–9)	≥ 5 years in synthetic plant	51	6.2 (4.1–12.5)[a]	Age	No information on exposure to specific agents
			Lymphatic leukaemia (204)		14	3.9 (2.6–8.0)[a]		
Meinhardt et al. (1982), USA (overlapping with Delzell et al., 1996)	2756 white men employed for at least 6 months (Plant A, 1662 men; Plant B, 1094 men)	Duration and time of employment	Lymphatic and haematopoietic (200–5)	Plant A	9	**SMR** 1.6	Age, time period, race	
			Lymphosarcoma and reticulosarcoma	Plant A, total	3	1.8		
				Plant A, working 1943–45	3	2.1		
				Plant B, total	1	1.3		
			Leukaemia (204)	Plant A, total	5	2.0		
				Plant A, working 1943–45	5	2.8		
				Plant B, total	1	1.0		

Table 18 (contd)

Reference, location	Cohort description	Exposure assessment	Organ site (ICD code)	Exposure categories	No. of cases/ deaths	Relative risk (95% CI)	Adjustment for potential confounders	Comments
Delzell et al. (1996), USA and Canada (includes data from Meinhardt et al. (1982); Matanoski & Schwartz, 1987; Lemen et al., 1990; Matanoski et al., 1990; Santos-Burgoa et al., 1992; Matanoski et al., 1993, 1997)	15 649 workers employed for at least 1 year in eight production plants in 1943–91	8281 unique combinations of work area/job title, grouped in 308 work areas with similar exposure	All cancers (140–208) Lymphosarcoma (200) Other lymphopoietic (202) Leukaemia (204–208)	Five main process groups and seven sub-groups Polymerization Maintenance Labour Laboratories	950 11 42 48 15 13 10	0.93 (0.87–0.99) 0.8 (0.4–1.4) 1.0 (0.7–1.5) 1.3 (1.0–1.7) 2.5 (1.4–4.1) 2.7 (1.4–4.5) 4.3 (2.1–7.9)	Age, race, calendar time	Among 'ever hourly paid' workers, 45 leukaemia deaths (SMR, 1.4; 95% CI, 1.0–1.9); SMR for hourly workers having worked for > 10 years and hired ≥ 20 years ago, 2.2 (95% CI, 1.5–3.2) based on 28 leukaemia deaths
Macaluso et al. (1996), USA and Canada (overlapping with Delzell et al., 1996)	12 412 subjects	Retrospective quantitative estimates of exposure to butadiene, styrene and benzene by work area	Leukaemia (204–208)	*ppm–years* 0 < 1 1–19 20–79 ≥ 80 *p*-trend	8 4 12 16 18	**SMR** 0.8 (0.3–1.5) 0.4 (0.4–1.1) 1.3 (0.7–2.3) 1.7 (1.0–2.7) 2.6 (1.6–4.1) = 0.01	Age, race, co-exposure to styrene and benzene; Mantel-Haenszel rate ratios adjusted by race, cumulative exposure to styrene	Including 7 decedents for whom leukaemia was listed as contributory cause of death
				0 < 1 1–19 20–79 ≥ 80 *p*-trend		**Mantel-Haenszel** 1.0 2.0 (NR) 2.1 (NR) 2.4 (NR) 4.5 (NR) 0.01		

Table 18 (contd)

Reference, location	Cohort description	Exposure assessment	Organ site (ICD code)	Exposure categories	No. of cases/ deaths	Relative risk (95% CI)	Adjustment for potential confounders	Comments
Matanoski et al. (1997), USA and Canada (overlapping with Delzell et al., 1996)	Nested case–control study from a cohort of 12 113 employees at SBR plant	Estimated cumulative exposure and average intensity of exposure to butadiene	Hodgkin lymphoma (201) Leukaemia	Average intensity of exposure to butadiene, 1 ppm compared with 0 ppm	8 26	1.7 (0.99–3.0) 1.5 (1.1–2.1)	Birth year, age at hire before 1950, race, length of employment	Additional results from the same cohort are presented in the text (Matanoski & Schwartz, 1987; Matanoski et al., 1990; Santos-Burgoa et al., 1992); non-Hodgkin lymphoma and multiple myeloma were not associated with exposure to butadiene.
Sathiakumar et al. (1998), USA and Canada (same as Delzell et al., 1996)	12 412 subjects	See Macaluso et al. (1996)	Non-Hodgkin lymphoma (202)	Hourly workers ≥ 10 years worked and ≥ 20 years since hire	15	**SMR** 1.4 (0.8–2.3)	Age, race, calendar time	No pattern by duration of employment, time since hire, period of hire or process group

Table 18 (contd)

Reference, location	Cohort description	Exposure assessment	Organ site (ICD code)	Exposure categories	No. of cases/ deaths	Relative risk (95% CI)	Adjustment for potential confounders	Comments
Delzell et al. (2001), USA and Canada	13 130 men employed for at least 1 year during 1943–91 at 6 SBR plants	Quantitative estimates	Leukaemia (204–208)	*Butadiene ppm–years*		**Poisson regression**	Age, years since hire	The association of risk for leukaemia with butadiene was stronger for ppm–years due to exposure intensities > 100 ppm.
				0	7	1.0		
				> 0–< 86.3	17	1.2 (0.5–3.0)		
				86.3–< 362.2	18	2.0 (0.8–4.8)		
				≥ 362.2	17	3.8 (1.6–9.1)		
				p-trend		< 0.001		
				Butadiene ppm–years			Age, years since hire, co-exposure to other agents	
				0	7	1.0		
				> 0–< 86.3	17	1.3 (0.4–4.3)		
				86.3–< 362.2	18	1.3 (0.4–4.6)		
				≥ 362.2	17	2.3 (0.6–8.3)		
				p-trend		= 0.250		
				Butadiene ppm–years exposure intensity < 100 ppm			Age, years since hire	
				0	7	1.0		
				> 0–< 37.8	17	1.1 (0.5-2.7)		
				37.8–< 96.3	17	2.8 (1.2-6.8)		
				≥ 96.3	18	3.0 (1.2-7.1)		
				p-trend		= 0.25		
				Butadiene ppm–years exposure intensity > 100 ppm			Age, years since hire	
				0	7	1.0		
				> 0–< 46.5	17	2.1 (0.9–5.1)		
				46.5–< 234.3	17	2.8 (1.2–6.7)		
				≥ 234.3	18	5.8 (2.4–13.8)		
				p-trend		= 0.01		

Table 18 (contd)

Reference, location	Cohort description	Exposure assessment	Organ site (ICD code)	Exposure categories	No. of cases/ deaths	Relative risk (95% CI)	Adjustment for potential confounders	Comments
Graff et al. (2005), USA and Canada	16 579 men working at 6 plants ≥ 1 year by 1991 and followed up through to 1998	Same as Delzell et al. (2001); cumulative exposure estimates for butadiene, styrene and DMDTC	Leukaemia (204–208)	*Butadiene ppm–years*		**Poisson regression**	Age, years since hire	SMR analyses with external reference rates (national and state-specific) also conducted and results for leukaemia consistent with those of internal analysis using Poisson regression models.
				0	10	1.0		
				> 0–< 33.7	7	1.4 (0.7–3.1)		
				33.7–< 184.7	18	1.2 (0.6–2.7)		
				184.7–< 425.0	18	2.9 (1.4–6.4)		
				≥ 425.0	18	3.7 (1.7–8.0)		
				p-trend		< 0.001		
			Leukaemia (204–208)	*Butadiene ppm–years*			Age, years since hire, other agents	
				0	10	1.0		
				> 0–< 33.7	17	1.4 (0.5–3.9)		
				33.7–< 184.7	18	0.9 (0.3–2.6)		
				184.7–< 425.0	18	2.1 (0.7–6.2)		
				≥ 425.0	18	3.0 (1.0–9.2)		
				p-trend		= 0.028		
			Chronic lymphocytic leukaemia (204.1)	< 33.7	7	1.0		
				33.7–< 425.0	11	1.5 (0.6–4.0)		
				≥ 425.0	7	3.9 (1.3–11.0)		
				p-trend		= 0.014		
			Chronic myelogenous leukaemia (205.1)	< 33.7	3	1.0		
				33.7–< 425.0	8	2.7 (0.7–10.4)		
				≥ 425.0	5	7.2 (1.7–30.5)		
				p-trend		= 0.007		
			Other leukaemia	< 33.7	5	1.0		
				33.7–< 425.0	5	1.1 (0.3–3.9)		
				≥ 425.0	4	4.0 (0.3–15.0)		
				p-trend		= 0.060		

Table 18 (contd)

Reference, location	Cohort description	Exposure assessment	Organ site (ICD code)	Exposure categories	No. of cases/ deaths	Relative risk (95% CI)	Adjustment for potential confounders	Comments
Sathiakumar et al. (2005), USA and Canada	17 924 male workers employed ≥ 1 year before 1992 followed through to 1998	Same as Delzell et al. (1996)	Non-Hodgkin lymphoma (200, 202)	All workers	53	**SMR** 1.0 (0.8–1.3)	Age, race, calendar period	Leukaemia excesses in production mainly due to chronic lymphatic leukaemia: polymerization (8 cases; SMR, 4.97; 95% CI, 2.15–9.80), coagulation (5 cases; SMR, 6.07; 95% CI, 1.97–14.17) and finishing (7 cases; SMR, 3.44; 95% CI, 1.38–7.09); myelogenous leukaemia particularly high in maintenance labour (acute, 5 cases; SMR, 2.95; 95% CI, 0.96–6.88) and laboratory (total, 6 cases; SMR, 3.31; 95% CI, 1.22–7.20; chronic, 3 cases; SMR, 5.22; 95% CI, 1.08–15.26)
				Hourly workers	49	1.1 (0.8–1.5)		
			All cancer		1608	0.92 (0.88–0.97)		
			Lymphohaematopoietic (200–208)		162	1.06 (0.9–1.2)		
			Hodgkin lymphoma		12	1.1 (0.6–2.0)		
			Multiple myeloma (203)		26	0.95 (0.62–1.4)		
			Leukaemia (204–208)	All workers	71	1.2 (0.9–1.5)		
				Hourly workers	63	1.2 (0.9–1.6)		
				Hourly workers ≥ 20 years since hire –10 years worked	19	2.6 (1.6–4.0)		
				Production Polymerization	18	2.0 (1.2–3.2)		
				Coagulation	10	2.3 (1.1–4.3)		
				Finishing	19	1.6 (0.9–2.4)		
				Labour maintenance	15	2.0 (1.1–3.4)		
				Laboratories	14	3.3 (1.8–5.5)		
			Chronic lymphocytic leukaemia (204.1)	All workers	16	1.5 (0.9–2.5)		
				Hourly workers	15	1.7 (0.96–2.8)		

Table 18 (contd)

Reference, location	Cohort description	Exposure assessment	Organ site (ICD code)	Exposure categories	No. of cases'/deaths	Relative risk (95% CI)	Adjustment for potential confounders	Comments
Delzell et al. (2006), USA and Canada				*Butadiene ppm–years*			Age, years since hire, other agents	
			Non-Hodgkin lymphoma (200, 202)	0	11	1.0		
				>0–<33.7	16	1.0 (0.4–2.6)		
				33.7–<184.7	10	0.4 (0.1–1.2)		
				184.7–<425.0	12	0.9 (0.3–2.7)		
				≥425.0	9	0.7 (0.2–2.3)		
			Non-Hodgkin lymphoma and chronic lymphocytic leukaemia combined (200, 202, 204.1)	0	12	1.0		
				>0–<33.7	18	0.9 (0.4–2.1)		
				33.7–<184.7	14	0.4 (0.2–1.1)		
				184.7–<425.0	17	1.0 (0.4–2.7)		
				≥425.0	14	0.9 (0.3–2.7)		
			Lymphoid neoplasms (200–204)	0	24	1.0		
				>0–<33.7	28	0.9 (0.5–2.0)		
				33.7–<184.7	25	0.7 (0.3–1.6)		
				184.7–<425.0	21	1.3 (0.6–3.1)		
				≥425.0	22	1.5 (0.6–3.8)		
			Myeloid neoplasms (205, 206), (erythroleukaemia, myelofibrosis, myelosdysplasia, polycythemia vera, myeloproliferative disease)	<33.7	19	1.0		
				33.7–<184.7	15	0.8 (0.3–1.7)		
				184.7–<425.0	11	1.6 (0.6–4.1)		
				≥425.0	11	2.4 (0.9–6.8)		

Table 18 (contd)

Reference, location	Cohort description	Exposure assessment	Organ site (ICD code)	Exposure categories	No. of cases/ deaths	Relative risk (95% CI)	Adjustment for potential confounders	Comments
Cheng *et al.* (2007), USA and Canada	Same as Sathiakumar *et al.* (2005)	Same as Delzell *et al.* (2001)	Leukaemia (204–208)	*Cumulative ppm–years*	81	**Cox regression coefficient (β) for exposure–response SE, *p*-value**	Age, year of birth, race, plant, years since hire, DMDTC	Lymphoid neoplasms associated with butadiene ppm–years and myeloid neoplasms with butadiene peaks; neither trend significant after adjusting for covariates; DMDTC as a continuous variable not associated with leukaemia; risk estimates for quartiles of exposure to DMDTC significantly increased without monotonic trend.
				Continuous		$\beta = 3.0*10^{-4}$ SE $1.4*10^{-4}$, $p = 0.04$ $(0.1*10^{-4} – 5.8*10^{-4})$		
				Mean scored deciles		$\beta = 5.8*10^{-4}$ SE $2.7*10^{-4}$, $p = 0.03$ $(0.5*10^{-4} – 11.1*10^{-4})$		
				Total number of peaks Continuous		$\beta = 5.6*10^{-5}$ SE $2.4*10^{-5}$, $p = 0.02$ $(0.8*10^{-5} – 10.4*10^{-5})$		
				Mean scored deciles		$\beta = 7.5*10^{-5}$ SE $3.7*10^{-5}$, $p = 0.04$ $(0.3*10^{-5} – 14.7*10^{-5})$		
				Average intensity Continuous		$\beta = 3.6*10^{-3}$ SE $2.1*10^{-3}$, $p = 0.09$ $(-0.5*10^{-3} – 7.7*10^{-3})$		
				Mean scored deciles		$\beta = 3.8*10^{-3}$ SE $3.7*10^{-3}$, $p = 0.40$ $(-3.5*10^{-3} – 11.0*10^{-3})$		

CI, confidence interval; DMDTC, dimethyldithiocarbamate; ICD, International Classification of Diseases; NR, not reported; SE, standard error; SMR, standardized mortality ratio; TWA, time-weighted average

[a] 99.9% confidence interval

haematopoietic cancers occurred (SMR, 1.8; 95% CI, 0.7–3.6), including four cases of lymphosarcoma and reticulosarcoma (SMR, 5.8; 95% CI, 1.6–14.8). Three cases had a duration of employment of 2 years or more (SMR, 8.3; $p < 0.05$). Two cases of leukaemia (SMR, 1.2; 95% CI, 0.2–4.4) also occurred. A non-significant excess of mortality from stomach cancer was observed (SMR, 2.4; 95% CI, 0.8–5.7). All five cases of stomach cancer occurred among the subset of workers who had been employed in the 'Rubber Reserve' plant for 2 years or more (SMR, 6.6; 95% CI, 2.1–15.3).

The mortality of a cohort of workers who manufactured butadiene monomer in Texas, USA (Downs *et al.*, 1987), has been investigated repeatedly with updated and extended follow-up (Divine, 1990; Divine *et al.*, 1993; Divine & Hartman, 1996). The latest available update, that included 5 additional years of follow-up up to 31 December 1999, was reported by Divine and Hartman (2001). The cohort at that time included 2800 male workers (of whom 216 were non-white and 10 were of unknown race) who had been employed for at least 6 months between 1943 and 1996. Exposure assessment was based on job history and industrial hygiene sampling data for the years after 1981. Each job was assigned a score for exposure to butadiene that took into account calendar period and type of operation. No information was reported on exposure to chemicals other than butadiene. The number of workers lost to follow-up was 192 (6.7%), all but 17 (< 1%) of whom were known to be alive at the end of 1998. A total of 1422 deaths were identified through to 1999, and death certificates were obtained for all but 19 (1.3%) of the deaths. SMRs were calculated using mortality rates for the US population as the reference. The SMR for all causes of death was 0.9 (95% CI, 0.8–0.9) and that for all cancers (333 deaths) was 0.9 (95% CI, 0.8–1.0). Fifty deaths from lymphatic and haematopoietic cancers (International Classification of Diseases [ICD]-8, 200–209; SMR, 1.4; 95% CI, 1.1–1.9), nine deaths from lymphosarcoma and reticulosarcoma (ICD-8, 200; SMR, 2.0; 95% CI, 0.9–3.9), 19 deaths from non-Hodgkin lymphoma (ICD-8, 200, 202; SMR, 1.5; 95% CI, 0.9–2.3), four deaths from Hodgkin lymphoma (ICD-8, 201; SMR, 1.6; 95% CI, 0.4–4.1), 18 deaths from leukaemia (ICD-8, 204–207; SMR, 1.3; 95% CI, 0.8–2.0), seven deaths from multiple myeloma (ICD-8, 203; SMR, 1.3; 95% CI, 0.5–2.6) and 18 deaths from cancer of other lymphatic tissue (ICD-8, 202, 203, 208; SMR, 1.3; 95% CI, 0.8–2.1) were observed. However, the latter category overlapped with non-Hodgkin lymphoma and multiple myeloma. The SMRs for the lymphatic and haematopoietic cancers did not increase with length of employment. Analysis by date of employment showed an increased risk for lymphatic and haematopoietic cancers among those first employed between 1942 and 1949. A separate mortality analysis for non-whites showed lower than expected mortality for all malignant neoplasms (17 observed, 19 expected) and a single death from lymphatic and haematopoietic cancer. Subcohort analyses were made for groups that were classified as having background, low and varied exposure. The background-exposure group included persons in offices, transportation, utilities and warehouses; the low-exposure group had spent some time in operating units; and the varied-exposure group included those with greatest potential exposure in operating units, laboratories and maintenance. In the background-exposure group, four deaths from lymphatic and haematopoietic cancers

(ICD-8, 200–209) were observed among those employed for < 5 years (SMR, 1.9; 95% CI, 0.5–4.7) and four among those exposed for > 5 years (SMR, 1.7; 95% CI, 0.5–4.3). Eleven deaths from lymphatic and haematopoietic cancers (ICD-8, 200–209) were observed in the low-exposure group, seven of which were among those with < 5 years of employment (SMR, 0.9; 95% CI, 0.4–1.9) and four among those employed for > 5 years (SMR, 0.6; 95% CI, 0.2–1.6). In the varied-exposure group, with the highest potential for exposure to butadiene, 34 deaths from lymphatic and haematopoietic cancers (ICD-8, 200–209) were observed, 20 of which were among those employed for < 5 years (SMR, 1.8; 95% CI, 1.1–2.8) and 14 among those exposed for > 5 years (SMR, 1.5; 95% CI, 0.8–2.5). In all groups, the SMRs for lymphatic and haematopoietic cancer decreased with duration of employment. For lymphosarcoma and reticulosarcoma, two deaths occurred in the low-exposure group (one among those employed < 5 years and one among those employed > 5 years) and seven deaths were observed in the varied-exposure group, five of which were among those employed for < 5 years (SMR, 3.7; 95% CI, 1.2–8.7) and two among those employed for > 5 years (SMR, 1.87; 95% CI, 0.23–6.76). Three deaths from leukaemia occurred (SMR, 0.7; 95% CI, 0.1–2.0) in the low-exposure subgroup and 13 cases were observed in the varied-exposure group, eight of which were among those employed for < 5 years (SMR, 1.9; 95% CI, 0.8–3.7) and five among those employed > 5 years (SMR, 1.4; 95% CI, 0.4–3.2). Six deaths from non-Hodgkin lymphoma were observed in the low-exposure group, four among short-term employees (SMR, 1.5; 95% CI, 0.4–3.8) and two among those employed for > 5 years (SMR, 0.9; 95% CI, 0.1–3.2), and 12 deaths occurred in the varied-exposure group, eight of which were among those employed for < 5 years (SMR, 2.0; 95% CI, 0.9–3.9) and four among long-term employees (SMR, 1.1; 95% CI, 0.3–2.9). The 'varied-exposure' group with high potential for exposure to butadiene showed elevated SMR estimates for all subcategories of lymphatic and haematopoietic cancers, but the increase was statistically significant only for lympho/reticulosarcoma among those employed for < 5 years. Slightly elevated SMRs were also found in the low-exposure group for cancer of the kidney (three cases; SMR, 1.6; 95% CI, 0.3–4.6; and three cases; SMR, 1.9; 95% CI, 0.4–5.4; among short- and long-term employees, respectively). In the varied-exposure group, a suggestive excess incidence of kidney cancer was only present among those employed for > 5 years (four cases; SMR, 1.65; 95% CI, 0.45–4.22). Survival analysis by Cox regression was carried out using a cumulative exposure score as a time-dependent explanatory variable for all lymphohaematopoietic neoplasms, non-Hodgkin lymphoma and leukaemia. None of these cancers was significantly associated with the cumulative exposure score. The elevated risk for all the lymphohaematopoietic cancers and their subcategories occurred among persons who were first employed before 1950. [The Working Group noted that although there was no evidence of an exposure–response relationship, it is probable that many workers during the years of the Second World War would have had short but relatively intense exposures, and thus duration of exposure may not be the most relevant dose metric.]

Another relatively small retrospective mortality study, together with a prospective morbidity survey, was performed on male employees at the Shell Deer Park Manufacturing Complex in the USA (Cowles *et al.*, 1994) and was updated with a 9-year extension of the follow-up (Tsai *et al.*, 2001). Butadiene monomer production took place in the facility between 1941 and 1948 and from 1970 onwards. The cohort comprised 614 eligible male employees who had worked for 5 years or more in jobs that entailed potential exposure to butadiene. Also eligible were employees who had worked for at least half of their total duration of employment during 1948–89 in a job that entailed potential exposure to butadiene (with a minimum 3-month period in such jobs). Female employees were excluded because of the small number (35) who met the eligibility criteria. Industrial hygiene data from 1979 to 1992 showed that few exposures to butadiene exceeded 10 ppm [22 mg/m^3] as an 8-h TWA and that most were below 1 ppm [2.2 mg/m^3]; the arithmetic mean exposure was 3.5 ppm [7.7 mg/m^3]. Only one study member had unknown vital status at the end of the follow-up. Person–years were accrued after 1 April 1948 from the time that a person first met the eligibility criteria. Death certificates were obtained for all known decedents. SMRs adjusted for age, race and calendar year were calculated using county-specific mortality rates as the reference. Six hundred and fourteen cohort members contributed a total of 12 391 person–years during the expanded study period, during which 61 deaths were identified. The SMR for all causes of death was 0.55 (95% CI, 0.42–0.70) and that for all malignant neoplasms was 0.6 (16 deaths; 95% CI, 0.3–0.9). Eight deaths were due to lung cancer (SMR, 0.7; 95% CI, 0.2–3.1) and three to cancer of the lymphatic and haematopoietic tissues (SMR, 1.1; 95% CI, 0.3–1.5). No deaths from leukaemia were observed, whereas one death was expected. The morbidity study included 289 of the 614 cohort members who were actively employed at some time between 1 January 1992 and 31 December 1998. The morbidity experience of this group was compared with that of an internal comparison group of 1386 active employees during the same period who had had no exposure to butadiene. A morbidity event was defined as an absence from work of > 5 days during 1992–98 that resulted from a specific diagnosed disorder. No meaningful differences in morbidity events between the butadiene-exposed and unexposed employees in the rest of the Shell Deer Park Manufacturing Complex were observed. [The Working Group noted that one criteria for inclusion in the cohort (at least half of total employment during 1948–89 in a potentially exposed job) was a potential source of bias, and that the SMR for all causes was unusually low.]

2.2.2 *Styrene–butadiene rubber production*

The 9-year mortality experience of a cohort of 6678 male rubber workers from a single, large tyre manufacturing plant in Ohio, USA, approximately 4% of whom worked in the manufacture of synthetic rubber, was investigated during 1964–72 (McMichael *et al.*, 1974, 1976). Death rates from various specific causes were increased and included lymphatic and haematopoietic cancers in general (43 observed deaths; SMR, 1.36), lymphosarcoma and Hodgkin lymphoma (15 observed; SMR, 1.64) and leukaemia (17 observed; SMR, 1.26). A case–cohort study was nested within the cohort to investigate the association of excesses of mortality with specific jobs within the rubber industry to compare workers who died from cancers in the 10-year period 1964–73 with a sample of members of the whole cohort and to elucidate differences in work histories (McMichael *et al.*, 1976). A 6.2-fold increase in risk for lymphatic and haematopoietic cancers (99.9% CI, 4.1–12.5) and a 3.9-fold increase in risk for lymphatic leukaemia (99.9% CI, 2.6–8.0) were found in association with more than 5 years of work in manufacturing units that produced mainly styrene–butadiene rubber during 1940–60. [The Working Group noted that no information was provided on exposure to specific substances including potentially confounding chemicals such as benzene.]

Meinhardt *et al.* (1982) studied the mortality experience of white male workers who had been employed for at least 6 months in a two-plant complex styrene–butadiene rubber facility in the USA. A total of 1662 workers employed in Plant A between 1943 and 1976 and 1094 workers employed in Plant B between 1950 and 1976 were followed up through to 31 March 1976. Nine deaths from cancer of the lymphatic and haematopoietic tissues (ICD-7, 200–205) were seen in workers in Plant A (SMR, 1.6). The SMR among those from Plant A who were first employed between January 1943 and December 1945 was 2.1. Five deaths from leukaemia (ICD-7, 204) were observed in Plant A among workers employed between 1943 and 1945 (SMR, 2.8). In Plant B, two deaths from lymphatic and haematopoietic neoplasms (one lymphosarcoma/reticulosarcoma and one leukaemia) were observed.

Matanoski *et al.* (1990) investigated mortality patterns from 1943 (synthetic rubber production began in 1942) through to 1982 among 12 113 employees at styrene–butadiene rubber plants in Canada and the USA who had previously been followed up through to 1979 by Matanoski and Schwartz (1987). Overall, there were no increases in mortality from lymphatic and haematopoietic cancers. When employees were classified according to their longest-held job, production workers (presumed by the authors to be those with highest exposures to butadiene) had a significant excess of 'other lymphatic cancer' (nine deaths; SMR, 2.60; 95% CI, 1.19–4.94). When mortality among production workers was examined by race, a significant excess for leukaemia was seen in blacks (three deaths; SMR, 6.56; 95% CI, 1.35–19.06). Of 92 deaths among black production workers, six were from all lymphohaemopoietic cancers (SMR, 5.07; 95% CI, 1.87–11.07).

Nested case–control studies were conducted within the styrene–butadiene rubber cohort in the USA and Canada (Santos-Burgoa *et al.*, 1992; Matanoski *et al.*, 1997). In the study by Santos-Burgoa *et al.* (1992), 59 cases of lymphatic and haematopoietic cancer in male workers (1943–82) were matched to 193 controls by plant, age, year of hire, duration of employment and survival to time of death of the case. Each job was assigned an estimated rank of exposure to butadiene and styrene, and cumulated exposure for each worker was calculated using employment histories. A strong association was identified for both butadiene (odds ratio, 9.4; 95% CI, 2.1–22.9) and styrene (odds ratio, 3.1; 95% CI, 0.8–11.2). After controlling for the other exposure, the odds ratio for exposure to butadiene remained high and significant (odds ratio, 7.4; 95% CI, 1.3–41.3) whereas the relative risk estimate for styrene was approximately unity (odds ratio, 1.1; 95% CI, 0.23–4.95).

Matanoski *et al.* (1997) conducted a second case–control study that was nested in the styrene–butadiene cohort and included as cases most of the same lymphatic and haemato-poietic cancer decedents studied by Santos-Burgoa *et al.* (1992). In this study, hospital records obtained for 55 of the 59 cases studied by Santos-Burgoa *et al.* (1992) were re-viewed to confirm death certificate reports of lymphatic and haematopoietic cancer. The review confirmed all leukaemias, eliminated two cases and added one case of non-Hodgkin lymphoma and confirmed all cases of Hodgkin lymphoma and multiple myeloma. The final case groups included 58 total lymphatic and haematopoietic cancers, 12 non-Hodgkin lymphomas (seven lymphosarcomas and five other non-Hodgkin lymphomas), eight Hodgkin lymphomas, 26 leukaemias and 10 multiple myelomas. Controls were 1242 employees who were chosen to reflect the distribution of the cohort by plant and age, who had to have lived at least as long as cases and who represented approximately 1% of the cohort, but were not matched individually to cases. Quantitative exposure estimates for butadiene and styrene were developed by using exposure measurements for work areas and jobs, when available, and a modelling procedure to obtain estimates for jobs that had no measurements. Plant- and work area-specific exposure estimates were linked to work histories to obtain indices of cumulative exposure (ppm–months) and average intensity of exposure (ppm). Odds ratios for an average intensity of exposure of 1 ppm compared with 0 ppm and for ppm–months as a con-tinuous variable were estimated using logarithmically transformed exposure data in unconditional logistic regression models that controlled for year of birth, period of hire, age at hire, race and length of employment. Leukaemia and Hodgkin lymphoma were associated positively with average intensity of exposure to butadiene (odds ratio at 1 ppm: leukaemia, 1.50; 95% CI, 1.07–2.10; Hodgkin lymphoma, 1.7; 95% CI, 0.99–3.02) and with ppm–months of exposure to butadiene. Non-Hodgkin lymphoma and multiple myeloma were associated positively with average intensity of exposure and cumulative exposure to styrene but not with indices of exposure to butadiene. Further analyses indicated that, in models that included both average intensity of exposure to butadiene and an indicator for longest employment in service, labour and laboratory work areas, both variables were statistically significantly, positively associated with leukaemia. Separate analyses of lymphoid leukaemia (10 cases) and myeloid leukaemia (15 cases) found that the average intensity of exposure to butadiene, but not work area, was significantly associated with lymphoid leukaemia. Average intensity of exposure to butadiene and work area were both associated positively with myeloid leukaemia, but the association was significant only for work area. Matanoski *et al.* (1997) suggested that misclassi-fication of quantitative indices of exposure to butadiene could explain the latter results.

Delzell *et al.* (1996) and Sathiakumar *et al.* (1998) evaluated the mortality experience of 15 649 men (87% white and 13% black) who had been employed for at least 1 year at any of eight styrene–butadiene rubber plants in the USA and Canada and who had worked in styrene–butadiene rubber-related operations in these plants. Seven of the plants had been studied previously by Matanoski and Schwartz (1987), Matanoski *et al.* (1990), Santos-Burgoa *et al.* (1992) and Matanoski *et al.*(1993, 1997); the two-plant complex studied earlier by Meinhardt *et al.* (1982) and Lemen *et al.* (1990) was also included. Complete work histories were available for 97% of the subjects: about 75% was exposed to butadiene and 83% was exposed to styrene. A list was developed to identify every combination of work area and job title, for a total of 8281 unique combinations. Using information from the plant on processes and operations and on jobs and tasks within each type of operation, 308 groups of work area were specified, and comprised processes and jobs that were considered to be similar. For analysis, these were further classified into five main process groups and seven process subgroups. During 1943–91, the cohort had a total of 386 172 person–years of follow-up and 734 individuals were lost to follow-up (5%). A total of 3976 deaths were observed compared with 4553 deaths expected on the basis of general population mortality rates for the USA or (for the Canadian subcohort) Ontario (SMR, 0.87; 95% CI, 0.85–0.90). Mortality from cancer was slightly lower than expected (950 deaths; SMR, 0.93; 95% CI, 0.87–0.99). Eleven lymphosarcomas were observed (SMR, 0.80; 95% CI, 0.40–1.40) and 42 'other lymphopoietic cancers' (SMR, 0.97; 95% CI, 0.70–1.52) which included 17 non-Hodgkin lymphomas, eight Hodgkin lymphomas, 14 multiple myelomas, one polycythaemia vera and two myelofibroses. In addition, 48 deaths from leukaemia were observed in the full cohort (SMR, 1.31; 95% CI, 0.97–1.74), including 45 among 'ever hourly paid' (86% of the cohort) subjects (SMR, 1.43; 95% CI, 1.04–1.91). The excess was fairly consistent across plants and was concentrated among 'ever hourly paid' subjects with 10 or more years of employment and 20 or more years since hire (28 deaths; SMR, 2.24; 95% CI, 1.49–3.23) and among polymerization workers (15 deaths; SMR, 2.51; 95% CI, 1.40–4.14), maintenance labourers (13 deaths; SMR, 2.65; 95% CI, 1.41–4.53) and laboratory workers (10 deaths; SMR, 4.31; 95% CI, 2.07–7.93). Polymerization workers and maintenance labourers had potentially high exposure to butadiene but only low-to-moderate exposure to styrene. Sathiakumar *et al.* (1998) reported that, among subjects with ≥ 10 years of employment and ≥ 20 years since hire, moderately non-significantly increased mortality from non-Hodgkin lymphoma was also apparent (15 deaths; SMR, 1.37; 95% CI, 0.77–2.26), but without any consistent pattern by duration of employment, time since hire, period of hire or process group. Mortality from other types/sites of cancer was not significantly elevated in this cohort.

Macaluso *et al.* (1996) reported an additional analysis, with more detailed exposure assessment, of mortality from leukaemia among 16 610 subjects (12 412 exposed to butadiene) employed at six of the eight North American styrene–butadiene rubber manu-facturing plants investigated by Delzell *et al.* (1996) [14 295 workers were included but a further 2350 workers from the same plants who were not employed in styrene–butadiene rubber operations at those plants were not included in Delzell *et al.* (1996)]. A total of 418 846 person–years of follow-up through 1991 and 58 leukaemia deaths, seven of which were reported to be the contributory ('underlying') cause of death, were included only in analyses that used internal comparisons. Retrospective quantitative estimates of exposure to butadiene, styrene and benzene were developed and the estimation procedure identified work areas within each manufacturing process, historical changes in exposure potential and specific tasks that involved exposure. Mathematical models were then used to calculate job- and time period-specific average exposures. The resulting estimates were linked with work histories to obtain cumulative exposure estimates that were employed in stratified and Poisson regression analyses of mortality rates. Mantel-Haenszel rate ratios adjusted by race, age and cumulative exposure to styrene increased with cumulative exposure to butadiene from 1.0 in the unexposed category through to 2.0, 2.1, 2.4 and 4.5 in the estimated exposure categories $0, < 1, 1–19, 20–79$ and ≥ 80 ppm–years, respectively (p for trend $= 0.01$). The trend of increasing risk with exposure to butadiene was still significant after exclusion of the unexposed category ($p = 0.03$). The risk pattern was less clear and statistically non-significant for exposure to styrene (rate ratios, 0.9, 5.4, 3.4 and 2.7 in the estimated exposure categories of $< 5, 5–9, 10–39$ and ≥ 40 ppm–years, respectively; p for trend $= 0.14$) and the association with benzene disappeared after controlling for exposure to butadiene and styrene.

Irons and Pyatt (1998) suggested that apparently different patterns of risk for leukaemia between workers employed in butadiene monomer production and those involved in styrene–butadiene rubber production might be linked to a class of chemicals with haematotoxic and immunotoxic potential (dithiocarbamates) that were present in styrene–butadiene rubber but not butadiene monomer production. In particular, they suggested that dimethyldithiocarbamate, which was used between the early 1950s and 1965 in the majority of styrene–butadiene rubber plants as a stopping agent in the cold polymerization reaction, might confound an association between butadiene and leukaemia in exposed workers.

A further analysis was then conducted among the North American synthetic rubber industry workers to evaluate the relative relevance of butadiene, styrene and dimethyl-dithiocarbamate in the statistically significantly increased risk for mortality from leukaemia (Delzell *et al.*, 2001). The analysis included 13 130 men who had been employed for at least 1 year during 1943–91 at any of six synthetic rubber plants (of the eight previously studied by Delzell *et al.* (1996) and Sathiakumar *et al.* (1998)) that had sufficient information for quantitative exposure estimation. Revised exposure estimates for butadiene and styrene and new quantitative estimates for dimethyldithiocarbamate were developed (Macaluso *et al.*, 2004). Quantitative estimates of cumulative exposure were obtained by (*a*) identifying work area/job groups ('jobs') that consisted of homo-geneous work activities; (*b*) identifying the tasks that comprised each job; (*c*) identifying historical changes in exposure potential for each task; (*d*) computing time period-specific average exposure concentrations in parts per million for tasks and jobs; (*e*) compiling the job-specific estimates into a job–exposure matrix for each plant; and (*f*) linking the resulting job–exposure matrices with work histories to obtain cumulative exposure estimates. The job–exposure matrix contained plant-specific estimates of 8-h TWA exposure concentrations for butadiene and other chemicals for each job and for each year from 1943 through to 1991. Mathematical models were used to calculate plant-, task-, work area/job group- and time period-specific average exposures. The revised TWA exposure estimates, compared with the original estimates, were about four to six times higher for butadiene and two times higher for styrene. Estimates of the annual number of peaks of exposure in each job (i.e. for each job, the number of component tasks in which intensity exceeded 100 ppm for butadiene and 50 ppm for styrene) were also computed. Vital status at the end of 1991 was known for over 99% of subjects. A total of 234 416 person–years of observation (average, 18 person–years per subject) were accrued during the follow-up period and included in the analysis. Information from death certificates was available for 3813 (98%) of 3892 decedents; the death certificates of 58 decedents mentioned leukaemia as the underlying or contributing cause of death. For 48 of these, medical records confirmed that they had had leukaemia; for 10, medical records were not available and these were retained in the case group. An additional decedent had medical records that indicated leukaemia but the death certificate mentioned myelodysplasia: he was added to the case group (total, 59 decedents). Poisson regression analysis was used to estimate relative rates of mortality from leukaemia and their 95% CIs for a particular agent/exposure category compared with the category of workers who were unexposed or had low exposure; regression models for each agent took into account the level of exposure, age, years since hire and, in some models, co-exposure to one or both of the other chemicals. In some analyses, exposure was lagged under the assumption that exposures that occurred within 5 or 10 years before death were etiologically irrelevant. Mortality from leukaemia showed a consistently positive association with increasing exposure to butadiene (relative rate, 1.0; 1.2; 95% CI, 0.5–3.0; 2.0; 95% CI 0.8–4.8; and 3.8; 95% CI, 1.6–9.1; for exposure to 0, 0–86.3, 86.3–362.2 and ≥ 362.2 ppm–years, respectively) [p for trend < 0.001] and to styrene (relative rate, 1.0; 1.2; 95% CI, 0.5–3.3; 2.3; 95% CI, 0.9–6.2; and 3.2; 95% CI, 1.2–8.8; for exposure to 0, 0–20.6, 20.6–60.4 and ≥ 60.4 ppm–years, respectively) [p for trend $= 0.001$]. Exposure to dimethyldithio-carbamate also showed consistently increased relative rates, but with no monotonic trend. After controlling for exposure to styrene and dimethyldithiocarbamate as well as for age and years since hire, exposure to butadiene remained consistently but not statistically significantly associated with increasing mortality from leukaemia (relative rate, 1.0; 1.3; 95% CI, 0.4–4.3; 1.3; 95% CI, 0.4–4.6; and 2.3; 95% CI, 0.6–8.3) [p for trend $= 0.250$].

When exposure to total peaks (> 100 ppm for butadiene and > 50 ppm for styrene) was used in the analysis, a positive association of exposure to butadiene and styrene with mortality from leukaemia was again apparent; adjustments for other agents made the associations irregular and imprecise. Lagging for a 5- or 10-year exposure period did not alter the results materially. Models were also run to estimate relative rates for leukaemia for exposures to butadiene calculated at intensities of < 100 ppm and > 100 ppm. In the former analysis, a statistically non-significant trend of increasing relative rate with increasing number of butadiene ppm–years was found (relative rate, 1.0; 1.1; 95% CI, 0.5–2.7; 2.8; 95% CI, 1.2–6.8; and 3.0; 95% CI, 1.2–7.1; for exposure to 0, 0–37.8, 37.8–96.3 and ≥ 96.3 ppm–years, respectively; p for trend $= 0.25$), whereas the trend for exposure to > 100 ppm was statistically significant (relative rate, 1.0; 2.1; 95% CI, 0.9–

5.1; 2.8; 95% CI, 1.2–6.7; and 5.8; 95% CI, 2.4–13.8; for exposure to 0, 0–46.5, 46.5–234.3 and ≥ 234.3 ppm–years, respectively; p for trend = 0.01). Analyses based on quartiles or quintiles of exposure yielded patterns of results similar to those seen in the analyses based on tertiles shown above. Exposure to butadiene and dimethyldithio-carbamate was further categorized to study interaction, but no clear interaction between the two agents was apparent. The analysis confirmed a significant, although weaker, association with exposure to butadiene even after controlling for dimethyldithio-carbamate: the relative rate for leukaemia for exposure to 0–38.7, 38.7–287.3 and ≥ 287.3 ppm–years of butadiene was, respectively, 1.0, 1.5 (95% CI, 0.8–2.9) and 3.4 (95% CI, 1.8–6.4) when unadjusted for exposure to dimethyldithiocarbamate (p for trend = 0.0001) and 1.0, 1.0 (95% CI, 0.5–2.1) and 2.0 (95% CI, 0.9–4.3) when adjusted for exposure to dimethyldithiocarbamate (p for trend = 0.007). Dimethyldithiocarbamate was associated with a non-monotonically increasing risk and the trend was statistically non-significant after controlling for butadiene. The relative rate for exposure to 0–342.4, 342.4–1222.6 and ≥ 1222.6 mg–years/cm of dimethyldithiocarbamate was, respectively, 1.0, 3.6 (95% CI, 1.9–6.7) and 2.9 (95% CI, 1.5–5.3) when unadjusted for exposure to butadiene (p for trend = 0.003) and 1.0, 3.2 (95% CI, 1.6–6.3) and 2.1 (95% CI, 1.0–4.4) when adjusted for exposure to butadiene (p for trend = 0.196). A similar analysis was conducted for co-exposure to butadiene and styrene. The marginal trend was consistent and statistically significant for exposure to butadiene adjusted for styrene (p for trend = 0.006), but not for styrene adjusted for butadiene (p for trend = 0.763). Analyses by specific subgroups of leukaemia were conducted but sparse data rendered the results largely uninformative. [The Working Group noted the difficulties in estimating exposures to dimethyldithiocarbamate, which are primarily dermal, and that substantial mis-classification of exposure to this chemical was possible. Furthermore, the assessment of exposure to dimethyldithiocarbamate was performed with the knowledge of which departments had excess mortality from leukaemia and could conceivably have been biased by this knowledge.]

Mortality from lymphatic and haematopoietic cancer in the updated North American cohort was studied in relation to exposure to butadiene, styrene and dimethyldithiocarbamate (Graff et al., 2005). Two of the US plants were not included in this analysis because information on work area/job group was not sufficient for quantitative exposure estimation for all substances. Included were 16 579 men who had worked at any of the six study plants for at least 1 year by the end of 1991 and who were followed up between 1944 and 1998. All work histories and exposure data came from the previous study of Delzell et al. (2001), and exposure estimation procedures were those described by Macaluso et al. (2004). Information on vital status through to 1998 was established for 97% of the study group. Cause of death was ascertained through death certificates, the national death index and a search of medical records. Most analyses used Poisson regression models to obtain maximum likelihood estimates of the relative rate for the contrast between categories of one agent, adjusting for other agents and for additional potential confounders. SMR analyses by level of exposure to the agent were also made using state-specific US and Canadian male mortality rates as the comparison group and data from death certificates and the national death index only to determine causes of death. During the observation period, 500 174 person–years were accrued. Based on a review of medical records where possible, 81 deaths from leukaemia, 58 from non-Hodgkin lymphoma, 27 from multiple myeloma and 13 from Hodgkin disease were ascertained. Single-agent analyses, adjusting for age and years since hire, indicated a positive association between exposure to butadiene and leukaemia (relative risk, 1.0; 1.4; 95% CI, 0.7–3.1; 1.2; 95% CI, 0.6–2.7; 2.9; 95% CI, 1.4–6.4; and 3.7; 95% CI, 1.7–8.0; for exposure to 0, 0–33.7, 33.7–184.7, 184.7–425.0 and ≥ 425.0 ppm–years, respectively) [p for trend < 0.001] and between exposure to styrene and leukaemia (relative risk, 1.0, 1.3; 95% CI, 0.6–3.2; 1.6; 95% CI, 0.7–3.9; 3.0; 95% CI, 1.2–7.1; and 2.7; 95% CI, 1.1–6.4; for exposure to 0, 0–8.3, 8.3–31.8, 31.8–61.1 and ≥ 61.1 ppm–years, respectively) [p for trend = 0.001]. Exposure to dimethyldithiocarbamate was also positively associated, but with no monotonic increase (relative risk, 1.0; 2.5; 95% CI, 1.2–5.0; 3.0; 95% CI, 1.5–5.9; 4.9; 95% CI, 2.5–9.7; and 2.7; 95% CI, 1.4–5.4; for exposure to 0, 0–185.3, 185.3–739.4, 739.4–1610.3 and ≥ 1610.3 mg–years/cm, respectively) [p for trend = 0.001]. Similar results were obtained for butadiene and styrene when total peaks were used as exposure metrics. Exposures to butadiene, styrene and dimethyldithiocarbamate were found to be highly correlated. In the models that also controlled for other agents, the estimated relative rates for the increasing categories of butadiene ppm–years were 1.0, 1.4 (95% CI, 0.5–3.9), 0.9 (95% CI, 0.3–2.6), 2.1 (95% CI, 0.7–6.2) and 3.0 (95% CI, 1.0–9.2) [p for trend = 0.028]; for styrene, the association appeared to be negative [p for trend = 0.639]; and for dimethyldithiocarbamate, a positive association was still apparent with no monotonic exposure–response pattern (relative risk, 1.0, 2.6; 95% CI, 1.2–5.8; 3.1; 95% CI, 1.4–7.1; 4.4; 95% CI, 1.9–10.2; and 2.0; 95% CI, 0.8–4.8) [p for trend = 0.066]. Individual adjustment for one or both of the other main exposure factors yielded similar results: the positive increasing association between exposure to butadiene and leukaemia was slightly reduced; no association remained for styrene; dimethyldithiocarbamate still exhibited a positive association with leukaemia but with no dose–response. Leukaemia was positively associated with butadiene ppm–years accrued at exposure intensities > 100 ppm and < 100 ppm. There was no evidence of an interaction between butadiene and dimethyldithiocarbamate or between butadiene and styrene. Analyses by histological type clearly showed an association of butadiene ppm–years with chronic lymphocytic leukaemia (relative risk, 1.0; 1.5; 95% CI, 0.6–4.0; 3.9; 95% CI, 1.3–11.0) [p for trend = 0.014], chronic myelogenous leukaemia (relative risk, 1.0; 2.7; 95% CI, 0.7–10.4; 7.2; 95% CI, 1.7–30.5) [p for trend = 0.007] and other leukaemia (relative risk, 1.0; 1.1; 95% CI, 0.3–3.9; 4.0; 95% CI, 1.0–15.0) [p for trend = 0.060] for exposures to 0–33.7, 33.7–425.0 and ≥ 425.0 ppm–years, respectively. No associations were found for non-Hodgkin lymphoma, multiple myeloma or acute myelogenous leukaemia. Results for a case series comprised of chronic lymphocytic leukaemia and non-Hodgkin lymphoma combined were similar to those for non-Hodgkin lymphoma alone (Delzell et al., 2006). External analyses that compared mortality rates of workers in each cumulative exposure category to the rate in the general population and controlled for age, race and calendar year provided consistent results.

The mortality follow-up of North American synthetic rubber industry workers who had been employed for at least 1 year before 1 January 1992 at any of seven US and one Canadian styrene–butadiene rubber plants was later extended for a further 7 years from 1991 through to the end of 1998 (Sathiakumar et al., 2005) and included 17 924 subjects (15 583 white and 2341 non-white). Work histories provided information on each job held, a description of the work area and job and payroll classification. Analyses of data by work area were restricted to 15 612 subjects who had been employed in styrene–butadiene rubber-related operations in the eight plants and classified into five major work areas: production, maintenance, labour, laboratories and other operations. For six of the eight plants (a total of 14 273 subjects), work histories were sufficiently detailed to permit further specification of three subgroups of work area in production, two in maintenance and two in labour. Vital status was updated through to 1998 and ascertained for 97% of the study group. In total, 570 (3%) subjects were lost to follow-up. A total of 540 586 person–years of observation were accrued. SMRs were calculated using mortality rates of the male population in Ontario (Canada) and in the three US states where the plants were located. The update added 83 401 person–years (18% increase), 1578 deaths (34%), 492 deaths from cancer (44%) and 20 deaths from leukaemia (39%) to those of the previous study. Mortality from all causes was lower than that expected (6237 deaths; SMR, 0.86; 95% CI, 0.84–0.88) as was mortality from all cancers (1608 deaths; SMR, 0.92; 95% CI, 0.88–0.97). Mortality from lymphatic and haematopoietic cancer was slightly elevated (162 deaths; SMR, 1.06; 95% CI, 0.90–1.23); 12 deaths from Hodgkin lymphoma yielded an SMR of 1.11 (95% CI, 0.58–1.95) and 71 deaths from leukaemia represented a modest excess above expectation (SMR, 1.16; 95% CI, 0.91–1.47). Mortality from non-Hodgkin lymphoma was as expected (53 deaths; SMR, 1.00; 95% CI, 0.75–1.30) and that from multiple myeloma was lower than expected (26 deaths; SMR, 0.95; 95% CI, 0.62–1.40). No consistent patterns were observed when mortality was analysed by ever/never hourly paid, by years since hire or by years worked. In the overall study group, the excess mortality from leukaemia was concentrated among men who had been hired in the 1950s (31 deaths; SMR, 1.50; 95% CI, 1.01–2.11). The excess mortality from all leukaemias was highest among hourly paid workers (63 deaths; SMR, 1.23; 95% CI, 0.94–1.57), especially among those who had 20–29 years since hire and ≥ 10 years worked (19 deaths; SMR, 2.58; 95% CI, 1.56–4.03). Analysis by specific histological type was possible for 65 of the 71 leukaemias and for the 1968–98 time period only. For all subjects included in this analysis, the SMR for all forms of leukaemia (65 deaths) was 1.26 (95% CI, 0.97–1.61), that for lymphocytic leukaemia (19 deaths) was 1.28 (95% CI, 0.77–2.00) and that for myelogenous leukaemia (28 deaths) was 1.27 (95% CI, 0.84–1.83). In the SMR analysis restricted to 1968–98, hourly paid workers had an overall SMR for leukaemia (65 deaths) of 1.35 (95% CI, 1.03–1.75), and the excess mortality was particularly marked among those who had 20–29 years since hire and ≥ 10 years worked (SMR, 2.84; 95% CI, 1.68–4.49); a non-significant increase was seen for lymphocytic leukaemia (four deaths; SMR, 2.33; 95% CI, 0.65–5.97), whereas the excess for myelogenous leukaemia was significant (nine deaths; SMR, 3.20; 95% CI, 1.46–6.07) and was stronger for the chronic myelogenous form (six deaths; SMR, 6.55; 95% CI, 2.40–14.26). Analysis by production work areas in the whole cohort, with follow-up between 1944 and 1998, showed an association between mortality from leukaemia and working in the following areas: polymerization (18 deaths; SMR, 2.04; 95% CI, 1.21–3.22), coagulation (10 deaths; SMR, 2.31; 95% CI, 1.11–4.25) and finishing (19 deaths; SMR, 1.56; 95% CI, 0.94–2.44); in maintenance labour (15 deaths; SMR, 2.03; 95% CI, 1.14–3.35); and in laboratories (14 deaths; SMR, 3.26; 95% CI, 1.78–5.46). The excesses of mortality in production were mainly due to chronic lymphatic leukaemia: polymerization (eight deaths; SMR, 4.97; 95% CI, 2.15–9.80), coagulation (five deaths; SMR, 6.07; 95% CI, 1.97–14.17) and finishing (seven deaths; SMR, 3.44; 95% CI, 1.38–7.09), whereas mortality from myelogenous leukaemia was particularly high in maintenance labour (acute, five deaths; SMR, 2.95; 95% CI, 0.96–6.88) and in laboratory workers (total, six deaths; SMR, 3.31; 95% CI, 1.22–7.20; chronic, three deaths; SMR, 5.22; 95% CI, 1.08–15.26).

Cheng *et al.* (2007) used Cox proportional hazard models on the set of data analysed by Graff *et al.* (2005) to examine further the exposure–response relations between several butadiene exposure indices and leukaemia (81 decedents), and to assess exposure–response relations between butadiene and all lymphoid neoplasms (120 decedents from lymphatic leukaemia, non-Hodgkin lymphoma, Hodgkin lymphoma and multiple myeloma) and all myeloid neoplasms (56 decedents from myeloid and monocytic leukaemia, myelofibrosis, myelodysplasia, myeloproliferative disorders and polycythemia vera). Cox regression techniques were considered to permit estimation of the exposure–response relations throughout the exposure range, to provide optimal control of confounding by age and to be less affected by intercorrelations among exposure variables. A subset of 488 subjects was excluded because they dropped out from follow-up at ages below that of the youngest leukaemia decedent. Potential confounders for which the analyses controlled included dimethyldithiocarbamate, race, plant, years since hire and year of birth. The butadiene exposure indices used in these analyses were: cumulative exposure in ppm–years, total number of exposures to peaks (> 100 ppm) and average intensities of exposure in parts per million. All three exposure indices were associated positively with the risk for leukaemia. Penalized spline regression indicated that the natural logarithm of the hazard ratio for leukaemia increased in a fairly linear fashion in the exposure range below the 95th percentile for all three indices. Analysis by decile of exposure to butadiene showed an irregular pattern of estimated rate ratios. After controlling for all co-variates, estimated relative rates by decile range of values exhibited a non-monotonic trend that was of borderline statistical significance for ppm–years [p for trend = 0.049], but not for exposure to peaks [p for trend = 0.071] or average intensity of exposure [p for trend = 0.433]. Models that used continuous exposure variables indicated that, for butadiene ppm–years, the exposure–response relation with leukaemia was positive and statistically significant in all but two of the eight models evaluated. After adjustment for all co-variates, the regression coefficient β that estimated the slope of the exposure–response relation was 3.0×10^{-4} (95% CI, 0.1×10^{-4}–5.8×10^{-4}; $p = 0.04$) in models that used continuous, untransformed ppm–years, 5.8×10^{-4} (95% CI, 0.5×10^{-4}–11.1×10^{-4}; $p = 0.03$) in models that used mean scored deciles and 6.1×10^{-4} ($p = 0.04$) in models that used mean scored quintiles. The exposure–response trend for butadiene peaks and leukaemia was positive and statistically significant in all eight models. The regression coefficient β was 5.6×10^{-5} (95% CI, 0.8×10^{-5}–10.4×10^{-5}; $p = 0.02$) in models that used continuous, untransformed butadiene peaks and 7.5×10^{-5} (95% CI, 0.3×10^{-5}–14.7×10^{-5}; $p = 0.04$) in models that used mean scored deciles of butadiene peaks, after controlling for all covariates. The association of average intensity of exposure to butadiene with leukaemia was statistically significant only in the model that used the square-root transformation of parts per million butadiene. Lagging of exposure had a small impact on the value of the coefficients for the three exposure variables. Lymphoid neoplasms were associated with the ppm–years exposure index and myeloid neoplasms with exposure to peaks. However, neither of the relations was statistically significant after control for covariates. Cumulative exposure to dimethyldithiocarbamate, when treated as a continuous variable, was not associated with leukaemia in any of the models. The risk estimates for each quartile of cumulative exposure to dimethyldithiocarbamate were significantly increased, even after adjustment for cumulative exposure to butadiene, without, however, a monotonic trend. Relative rate estimates were, respectively, 2.4 (95% CI, 1.2–5.0), 2.9 (95% CI, 1.4–5.8), 4.5 (95% CI, 2.2–8.9) and 2.1 (95% CI, 1.0–4.4) [p for trend = 0.458].

[The Working Group noted that, given the strong correlation between original and revised estimates (Spearman's $r = 0.9$) reported, the validation of the exposure estimates in one plant during 1977–91 (Sathiakumar & Delzell, 2007) showed that estimates from the most recent measurements were in general very close to measured exposures, especially for the styrene–butadiene rubber-related job titles. The ranking of jobs had hardly changed from the first estimates (Macaluso et al., 1996) to the adjusted estimates (Macaluso et al., 2004). However, it is uncertain to what extent this validation can be extrapolated to the other plants.]

2.2.3   Other rubber production

Bond et al. (1992) reported a mortality study of 2904 male workers engaged in the development and manufacture of styrene-based products, including styrene–butadiene latex, who were potentially exposed to styrene and related chemicals [including butadiene] for at least 1 year between 1937 and 1971. The number of person–years of follow-up during 1970–86 for workers in this production was 11 754. In comparison with USA mortality rates, the SMR for all causes of death among styrene–butadiene latex workers was 0.9, based on 82 deaths. A total of 13 cancers were observed (22.0 expected; SMR, 0.6), and no site had an SMR that exceeded unity. One death from lymphatic and haematopoietic cancers occurred, which was due to leukaemia (ICD-8 204–207) versus

0.9 expected. [The Working Group noted the limited information relating to exposure to butadiene.]

2.3   Population-based studies

The risk for lymphatic and haematopoietic cancers was evaluated among students of a high school in eastern Texas, USA, that was bound at the rear by facilities that had produced synthetic styrene–butadiene rubber since 1943 (Loughlin *et al.*, 1999). A cohort of 15 043 students who had attended the school for at least 3 consecutive months during a school year between 1963 and 1993 was constructed. In total, 338 graduates (241 men and 97 women) had died during the follow-up period of 1963–95, which were fewer than expected. The SMR for all lymphatic and haematopoietic cancer was 0.84 (95% CI, 0.74–0.85) for men (12 observed deaths) and 0.47 (95% CI, 0.06–1.70) for women (two observed deaths). The SMR was higher for 1530 men who had attended the school for ≤ 2 years than for the 6352 who had attended for ≥ 2 years. For the former group, the SMR for all lymphatic and haematopoietic cancer was 3.20 (95% CI, 0.87–8.20).

A population-based case–control study in the Montréal area, Canada (Parent *et al.*, 2000), assessed the association between renal-cell carcinoma and a large number of occupational exposures among men aged 35–70 years between 1979 and 1985. Cases were identified at all large hospitals in the area and were histologically confirmed; case ascertainment was 95% complete. Comparison was carried out with two sets of controls: subjects with other types of cancer and people selected from the general population. Questionnaires on cancer risk factors that included lifetime occupational history were administered. Relative risks were estimated by odds ratios from unconditional logistic regression models. In the analysis, 142 cases, 533 population controls and 1900 other cancer controls were available. The odds ratio for exposure to 'styrene–butadiene rubber' was 2.1 (10 exposed cases; 95% CI, 1.1–4.2) after controlling for age, family income, tobacco smoke and body mass index and 1.8 (95% CI, 0.9–3.7) after controlling for other occupational exposures. [The Working Group noted that it was unclear what was meant by exposure to styrene–butadiene rubber.]

3.   Studies of Cancer in Experimental Animals

3.1   Inhalation exposure

3.1.1   *Mouse*

Groups of 50 male and 50 female B6C3F$_1$ mice, 8–9 weeks of age, were exposed by whole-body inhalation to 625 or 1250 ppm [1380 or 2760 mg/m^3] butadiene (minimum purity, > 98.9%) for 6 h per day on 5 days per week for 60 weeks (males) or 61 weeks (females). Equal numbers of animals were sham-exposed and served as controls. The study was terminated after 61 weeks because of a high incidence of lethal neoplasms in the exposed animals. Deaths were mainly due to malignant lymphomas. The numbers of survivors at 61 weeks were: males — 49/50 control, 11/50 low-dose and 7/50 high-dose; females — 46/50 control, 15/50 low-dose and 30/50 high-dose. As shown in Table 19, butadiene induced haemangiosarcomas that originated in the heart and metastasized to various organs. The incidence of haemangiosarcomas of the heart in historical controls was extremely low (1/2372 males, 1/2443 females). Other types of neoplasm for which the incidence was significantly increased (Fisher's exact test) in animals of each sex were malignant lymphomas, alveolar/bronchiolar adenomas or carcinomas of the lung and papillomas or carcinomas of the forestomach. Tumours that occurred with significantly increased incidence in females only included hepatocellular adenoma or carcinoma of the liver: 0/50 control, 2/47 ($p = 0.232$) low-dose and 5/49 ($p = 0.027$) high-dose; acinar-cell carcinoma of the mammary gland: 0/50 control, 2/49 low-dose and 6/49 ($p = 0.012$) high-dose; and granulosa-cell tumours of the ovary: 0/49 control, 6/45 ($p = 0.01$) low-dose and 12/48 ($p < 0.001$) high-dose. Gliomas were observed in the brain of one male mouse exposed to 1250 ppm and in two male mice exposed to 625 ppm butadiene (National Toxicology Program, 1984; Huff et al., 1985).

Table 19. Incidence of tumours in B6C3F$_1$ mice exposed to butadiene by inhalation at 625 and 1250 ppm for 61 weeks

	Male			Female		
	0	625 ppm	1250 ppm	0	625 ppm	1250 ppm
Haemangiosarcoma of heart (with metastases)	0/50	16/49 ($p < 0.001$)[a]	7/49 ($p = 0.006$)	0/50	11/48 ($p < 0.001$)	18/49 ($p < 0.001$)
Malignant lymphoma	0/50	23/50 ($p < 0.001$)	29/50 ($p < 0.001$)	1/50	10/49 ($p = 0.003$)	10/49 ($p = 0.003$)
Lung alveolar/bronchiolar adenoma or carcinoma	2/50	14/49 ($p < 0.001$)	15/49 ($p < 0.001$)	3/49	12/48 ($p = 0.01$)	23/49 ($p < 0.001$)
Forestomach papilloma or carcinoma	0/49	7/40 ($p = 0.003$)	1/44 ($p = 0.47$)	0/49	5/42 ($p = 0.018$)	10/49 ($p < 0.001$)

From National Toxicology Program (1984); Huff et al. (1985)
[a] p values from Fisher's exact test

    Because of the reduced survival of mice in the initial study, further studies were conducted at lower exposure concentrations. In one study, groups of 70–90 male and 70–90 female B6C3F$_1$ mice, 6.5 weeks of age, were exposed by whole-body inhalation to 0, 6.25, 20, 62.5, 200 or 625 ppm [0, 14, 44, 138, 440 or 1380 mg/m^3] butadiene (purity, > 99%) for 6 h per day on 5 days per week for up to 2 years. Up to 10 animals per group were killed and evaluated after 40 and 65 weeks of exposure. Survival was significantly reduced ($p < 0.05$) in all groups of mice exposed to 20 ppm or higher; terminal survivors were: males — 35/70 control, 39/70 at 6.25 ppm, 24/70 at 20 ppm, 22/70 at 62.5 ppm, 3/70 at 200 ppm and 0/90 at 625 ppm; females — 37/70 control, 33/70 at 6.25 ppm, 24/70 at 20 ppm, 11/70 at 62.5 ppm, 0/70 at 200 ppm and 0/90 at 625 ppm. As shown in Table 20, exposure to butadiene produced increases in both sexes in the incidence of lymphomas, heart haemangiosarcomas, lung alveolar/bronchiolar adenomas and carcinomas, forestomach papillomas and carcinomas, Harderian gland adenomas and adenocarcinomas and hepatocellular adenomas and carcinomas. The incidence of mammary gland adenocarcinomas and benign and malignant ovarian granulosa-cell tumours was increased in females. Lymphocytic lymphomas were seen as early as after 23 weeks of exposure and were the principal cause of death in male and female mice exposed to 625 ppm butadiene (Melnick *et al.*, 1990; National Toxicology Program, 1993).

In the same study, a stop-exposure experiment was conducted in which groups of 50 male B6C3F$_1$ mice, 6.5 weeks of age, were exposed to butadiene (purity, > 99%) by whole-body inhalation for 6 h per day on 5 days per week at concentrations of 200 ppm [440 mg/m^3] for 40 weeks, 312 ppm [690 mg/m^3] for 52 weeks, 625 ppm [1380 mg/m^3] for 13 weeks or 625 ppm [1380 mg/m^3] for 26 weeks. The multiple of the exposure concentration and duration of exposure (ppm–weeks) was approximately 8000 ppm–weeks or 16 000 ppm–weeks for the exposure groups. After the exposures were terminated, the animals were placed in control chambers for up to 104 weeks after the beginning of treatment. A group of 70 males served as chamber controls (0 ppm). [The Working Group noted that this was the same control group as that used in the experiment described in the above paragraph.] Survival was reduced ($p < 0.05$) in all exposed groups; the numbers of survivors at the end of the study were 35 controls, nine exposed to 200 ppm, one exposed to 312 ppm, five exposed to 625 ppm for 13 weeks and none exposed to 625 ppm for 26 weeks. As shown in Table 21, exposure to butadiene produced increases in the incidence of lymphomas, heart haemangiosarcomas, lung alveolar/bronchiolar adenomas and carcinomas, forestomach papillomas and carcinomas, Harderian gland adenomas and adenocarcinomas, preputial gland carcinomas and kidney tubular adenomas. This exposure protocol revealed additional tumour sites in males (preputial gland and renal cortex). The incidence of lymphocytic lymphoma was greater after exposure to higher concentrations of butadiene for a short time than after exposure to lower concentrations for an extended period (Melnick *et al.*, 1990; National Toxicology Program, 1993). Brain neoplasms including two neuroblastomas and three gliomas were observed in mice exposed to 625 ppm for 13 or 26 weeks in the stop-exposure study (National Toxicology Program, 1993). Brain neoplasms are rare and had never been seen in historical National Toxicology Program controls at the time of the study. [The Working Group noted that brain tumours are rare in mice and were observed, although at a low incidence, in both National Toxicology Program bioassays (National Toxicology Program, 1984, 1993).]

Follow-up studies were completed to test the hypothesis that the high incidence of lymphocytic lymphomas in mice exposed to concentrations of 200 ppm butadiene or higher was at least partially dependent on the activation of an endogenous retrovirus in

Table 20. Survival and incidence of tumours in mice exposed to butadiene by inhalation for up to 2 years

	Exposure concentration (ppm)					
	0	6.25	20	62.5	200	625
Males						
Initial number[a]	70	70	70	70	70	90
Number of survivors	35	39	24	22	3	0
Lymphoma	4 (8%)[b]	3 (6%)	8 (19%)	11 (25%)[c]	9 (27%)[c]	69 (97%)[c]
Heart haemangiosarcoma	0 (0%)	0 (0%)	1 (2%)	5 (13%)[c]	20 (57%)[c]	6 (53%)[c]
Lung alveolar/bronchiolar adenoma and carcinoma	22 (46%)	23 (48%)	20 (45%)	33 (72%)[c]	42 (87%)[c]	12 (73%)[c]
Forestomach papilloma and carcinoma	1 (2%)	0 (0%)	1 (2%)	5 (13%)	12 (36%)[c]	13 (75%)[c]
Harderian gland adenoma and adenocarcinoma	6 (13%)	7 (15%)	11 (25%)	24 (53%)[c]	33 (77%)[c]	7 (58%)[c]
Hepatocellular adenoma and carcinoma	31 (55%)	27 (54%)	35 (68%)	32 (69%)	40 (87%)[c]	12 (75%)
Preputial gland adenoma or carcinoma	0 (0%)	0 (0%)	0 (0%)	0 (0%)	5 (17%)[c]	0 (0%)
Females						
Initial number[a]	70	70	70	70	70	90
Number of survivors	37	33	24	11	0	0
Lymphoma	10 (20%)	14 (30%)	18 (4_%)[c]	10 (26%)	19 (58%)[c]	43 (89%)[c]
Heart haemangiosarcoma	0 (0%)	0 (0%)	0 (0%)	1 (3%)	20 (64%)[c]	26 (84%)[c]
Lung alveolar/bronchiolar adenoma and carcinoma	4 (8%)	15 (32%)[c]	19 (4_%)[c]	27 (61%)[c]	32 (81%)[c]	25 (83%)[c]
Forestomach papilloma and carcinoma	2 (4%)	2 (4%)	3 (8%)	4 (12%)	7 (31%)[c]	28 (85%)[c]
Harderian gland adenoma and adenocarcinoma	9 (18%)	10 (21%)	7 (17%)	16 (40%)[c]	22 (67%)[c]	7 (48%)[c]
Hepatocellular adenoma and carcinoma	17 (35%)	20 (41%)	23 (5_%)[c]	24 (60%)[c]	20 (68%)[c]	3 (28%)
Mammary gland adenocarcinoma	0 (0%)	2 (4%)	2 (5%)	6 (16%)[c]	13 (47%)[c]	13 (66%)[c]
Ovarian benign and malignant granulosa-cell tumour	1 (2%)	0 (0%)	0 (0%)	9 (24%)[c]	11 (44%)[c]	6 (44%)

From Melnick et al. (1990); National Toxicology Program (1993)

[a] Initial numbers include animals removed from the study for interim sacrifices at 40 and 65 weeks of exposure.

[b] Mortality-adjusted tumour rates are given in parentheses.

[c] $p < 0.05$, based on logistic regression analysis with adjustment for intercurrent mortality

Table 21. Survival and incidence of tumours in male mice exposed to butadiene in stop-exposure studies[a]

	Exposure				
	0 ppm	200 ppm, 40 weeks	312 ppm, 52 weeks	625 ppm, 13 weeks	625 ppm, 26 weeks
Initial number	70	50	50	50	50
Number of survivors	35	9	1	5	0
Lymphoma	4 (8%)[b]	12 (35%)[c]	15 (55%)[c]	24 (61%)[c]	37 (90%)[c]
Heart haemangiosarcoma	0 (0%)	15 (47%)[c]	33 (87%)[c]	7 (31%)[c]	13 (76%)[c]
Lung alveolar/bronchiolar adenoma and carcinoma	22 (46%)	35 (88%)[c]	32 (88%)[c]	27 (87%)[c]	18 (89%)[c]
Forestomach squamous-cell papilloma and carcinoma	1 (2%)	6 (20%)[c]	13 (52%)[c]	8 (33%)[c]	11 (63%)[c]
Harderian gland adenoma and adenocarcinoma	6 (13%)	27 (72%)[c]	28 (86%)[c]	23 (82%)[c]	11 (70%)[c]
Preputial gland adenoma and carcinoma	0 (0%)	1 (3%)	4 (21%)[c]	5 (21%)[c]	3 (31%)[c]
Renal tubular adenoma	0 (0%)	5 (16%)[c]	3 (15%)[c]	1 (5%)	1 (11%)

From Melnick et al. (1990); National Toxicology Program (1993)

[a] After exposures were terminated, animals were placed in control chambers until the end of the study at 104 weeks.

[b] Mortality-adjusted tumour rates are given in parentheses.

[c] $p < 0.05$, based on logistic regression analysis with adjustment for intercurrent mortality

the strain of mouse used in the study. Groups of 60 male B6C3F₁ and 60 male NIH Swiss mice, 4–6 weeks of age, were exposed to 0 or 1250 ppm [2760 mg/m³] butadiene (> 99.5% pure) by whole-body inhalation for 6 h per day on 5 days per week for 52 weeks. An additional group of 50 male B6C3F₁ mice was exposed similarly to butadiene for 12 weeks and held until termination of the experiment at 52 weeks. The incidence of thymic lymphomas was 1/60 control, 10/48 exposed for 12 weeks and 34/60 exposed for 52 weeks in B6C3F₁ mice and 8/57 in NIH Swiss mice exposed for 52 weeks. Haemangiosarcomas of the heart were observed in 5/60 B6C3F₁ mice and 1/57 NIH Swiss mice exposed for 52 weeks. Exposure of B6C3F₁ mice to 1250 ppm of butadiene for 6 h per day on 5 days per week for 3–21 weeks greatly increased the quantity of ecotropic retrovirus recovered from bone marrow, thymus and spleen. This was not the case for NIH Swiss mice in which proviral ecotropic sequences are truncated and the virus is not expressed. The authors suggested that the lack of retroviruses provides resistance to the induction of the lymphomas by butadiene (Irons *et al.*, 1987a, 1989; Irons, 1990). [The Working Group noted that Swiss mice are less sensitive to the induction of haemangiosarcomas of the heart and lymphomas and that genetic factors may contribute to the development of these tumours.]

One study addressed the question of whether a single, high level of exposure to butadiene was sufficient to induce neoplasia. Groups of 60 male and 60 female B6C3F₁ mice, 8–10 weeks of age, were exposed by whole-body inhalation for a single 2-h period to 0, 1000, 5000 or 10 000 ppm [0, 2200, 11 000 or 22 000 mg/m³] butadiene [purity unspecified]. The mice were then held for 2 years, at which time all survivors were killed and tissues and organs were examined histopathologically. Survival, weight gains and tumour incidence in exposed mice were not affected by exposure to butadiene (survival: males — 28/60 control, 34/60 low-dose, 44/60 mid-dose and 34/60 high-dose; females — 45/60, 36/60, 38/60 and 48/60, respectively) (Bucher *et al.*, 1993).

3.1.2   *Rat*

Groups of 100 male and 100 female Sprague-Dawley rats, 4–5 weeks of age, were exposed by whole-body inhalation to 0, 1000 or 8000 ppm [0, 2200 or 17 600 mg/m³] butadiene (minimal purity, 99.2%) for 6 h per day on 5 days per week for 111 weeks (males) or 105 weeks (females). Survival was reduced in low- ($p < 0.05$) and high-dose ($p < 0.01$) females and in high-dose males ($p < 0.05$); the numbers of survivors were: males — 45 control, 50 low-dose and 32 high-dose; females — 46 control, 32 low-dose and 24 high-dose. Tumours that occurred at a significantly increased incidence in males were pancreatic exocrine adenomas (control, 3/100; low-dose, 1/100; and high-dose, 10/100, $p \leq 0.001$) and interstitial-cell tumours of the testis (control, 0/100; low-dose, 3/100; and high-dose, 8/100; p for trend ≤ 0.001). Those that occurred at a significantly increased incidence in females were follicular-cell adenomas of the thyroid gland (control, 0/100; low-dose, 2/100; and high-dose, 10/100; p for trend ≤ 0.01), sarcomas of the uterus (control, 1/100; low-dose, 4/100; and high-dose, 5/100; p for trend ≤ 0.05), carcinomas of the Zymbal gland (control, 0/100; low-dose, 0/100; and high-dose, 4/100; p for trend ≤ 0.01) and benign and malignant mammary tumours (control, 50/100; low-dose, 79/100; and high-dose, 81/100; p for trend ≤ 0.001). Mammary adenocarcinomas were found in 18/100 control, 15/100 low-dose and 26/100 high-dose female rats (Owen *et al.*, 1987; Owen & Glaister, 1990).

3.2   Carcinogenicity of metabolites

3.2.1   *1,2-Epoxy-3-butene (epoxybutene)*

Mouse

A group of 30 male Swiss mice, 8 weeks of age, received dermal applications of 100 mg undiluted epoxybutene, the initial monoepoxide metabolite of butadiene, three times per week for life. The median survival time was 237 days; three skin papillomas and one squamous-cell carcinoma were observed (Van Duuren *et al.*, 1963). [The Working Group noted that this incidence was similar to that in control groups that were left untreated.]

3.2.2   *1,2:3,4-Diepoxybutane (diepoxybutane)*

(a)   *Mouse*

Two groups of 30 male Swiss mice, 8 weeks of age, received dermal applications of 100 mg D,L-diepoxybutane (10% in acetone) or 100 mg *meso*-diepoxybutane (10% in acetone) three times a week for life. The median survival times were 78 and 154 weeks, respectively. Two skin papillomas and one squamous-cell carcinoma were observed following treatment with D,L-diepoxybutane and six skin papillomas and four squamous-cell carcinomas were observed following treatment with *meso*-diepoxybutane. Eight skin papillomas and no carcinomas were observed in 120 acetone-treated controls (Van Duuren *et al.*, 1963).

D,L-Diepoxybutane induced one skin papilloma or 10 skin papillomas and six squamous-cell carcinomas when applied to the skin of two groups of 30 female Swiss mice, 8 weeks of age, at respective doses of 10 or 3 mg in 100 mg acetone three times per week for life. *meso*-Diepoxybutane induced five skin papillomas and four squamous-cell carcinomas or one skin papilloma when applied to the skin of two groups of 30 female Swiss mice at respective doses of 10 or 3 mg in 100 mg acetone three times per week for life. No tumours were observed in 60 acetone-treated control mice (Van Duuren *et al.*, 1965).

Groups of 15 male and 15 female strain A mice, 4–6 weeks of age, received 12 thrice weekly intraperitoneal injections of L-diepoxybutane at total doses ranging from 1.7 to 192 mg/kg bw (35–2200 µmol/kg bw) in water or tricaprylin. The experiment was terminated 39 weeks after the first injection. L-Diepoxybutane slightly increased the incidence (40–78% versus 27–37% in controls) and multiplicity (0.5–1.5 tumour/mouse versus 0.29–0.48 tumours/mouse in controls) of lung tumours (Shimkin *et al.*, 1966).

Groups of male Swiss mice, 6 weeks of age, received subcutaneous injections of 0.1 or 1.1 mg D,L-diepoxybutane in 0.05 mL tricaprylin once a week for 401–589 days. Five local fibrosarcomas and two adenocarcinomas of breast origin were observed in a group of 50 mice (0.1-mg dose) and five local sarcomas in a group of 30 mice (1.1-mg dose). No tumours were observed in three tricaprylin-treated control groups (total of 110 animals) (Van Duuren *et al.*, 1966).

Groups of 56 female B6C3F$_1$ mice [it is unclear whether the animals were 6 or 10–11 weeks of age] were exposed by inhalation to 0, 2.5 or 5.0 ppm D,L-diepoxybutane for 6 h per day on 5 days per week for 6 weeks. Eight animals per group were examined for acute toxicity at the end of the exposures and most of the 48 remaining animals in each group were held for 18 months to observe tumour development (four animals were actually held for 6 months and four others for 12 months). The exposures resulted in nasal lesions that led to reduced survival. At the end of the experiment, neoplastic lesions were observed in the nasal mucosa, reproductive organs, lymph nodes, bone, liver, Harderian gland, pancreas and lung, but the only statistically significant increase was in the incidence of Harderian gland lesions. The incidence of total Harderian gland tumours was 0/40 control, 2/42 low-dose and 5/36 high-dose animals ($p < 0.05$, χ^2 test) (Henderson *et al.*, 1999, 2000).

(b)   Rat

Subcutaneous injection of 1 mg D,L-diepoxybutane in 0.1 mL tricaprylin once a week for 550 days induced nine local fibrosarcomas and one adenocarcinoma of breast origin in 50 female Sprague-Dawley rats that were 6 weeks of age at the beginning of the experiment. One adenocarcinoma of breast origin was observed in 50 control animals (Van Duuren *et al.*, 1966).

A 5-mg/mL dose of diepoxybutane dissolved in 0.5 mL tricaprylin was administered once a week by a gastric feeding tube to five female Sprague-Dawley rats, 6 weeks of age, for 363 days. No gastric tumours were observed (Van Duuren *et al.*, 1966).

Groups of 56 female Sprague-Dawley rats [it is unclear whether the animals were 6 or 10–11 weeks of age] were exposed by inhalation to 0, 2.5 or 5.0 ppm D,L-diepoxybutane for 6 h per day on 5 days per week for 6 weeks. Eight animals per group were examined for acute toxicity at the end of the exposures and most of the 48 remaining animals in each group were held for 18 months to observe tumour development (four animals were actually held for 6 months and four others for 12 months). The exposures resulted in nasal lesions that led to reduced survival. At the end of the experiment, the only significant increase was in the incidence of neoplasms of the nasal mucosa. The incidence of these tumours, principally squamous-cell carcinomas, was 0/47 control, 12/48 low-dose and 24/48 high-dose animals. Three high-dose rats had multiple tumours (Henderson *et al.*, 1999, 2000).

4.   Mechanistic and Other Relevant Data

The toxicokinetics and toxicology of butadiene have been comprehensively reviewed (IARC, 1999). No measured data on the pharmacokinetics of butadiene in exposed humans were available at that time. Data on a limited number of metabolites and haemoglobin adducts of butadiene in exposed humans and data on butadiene and its metabolites in experimental systems using human tissues were included. However, considerably more information is currently available regarding the metabolic pathways of butadiene and its major metabolites (see Figure 1).

Figure 1. Metabolic pathways of butadiene deduced from findings in mammals *in vitro* and *in vivo*

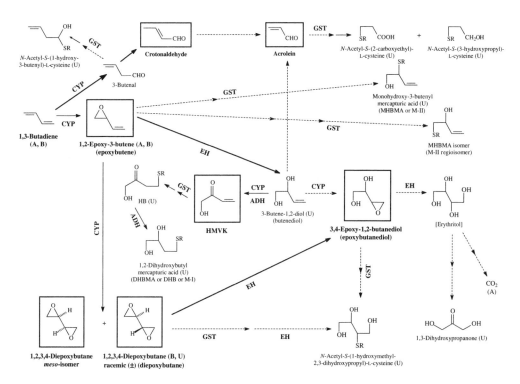

A, B, U, metabolites in exhaled air, blood, urine, respectively; ADH, alcohol dehydrogenase; CYP, cyto-chrome P450; DHB, 4-(N-acetyl-L-cystein-S-yl)-1,2-dihydroxybutane; EH, epoxide hydrolase; GST, gluta-thione-S-transferase; HB, 4-(N-acetyl-L-cystein-S-yl)-1-hydroxy-2-butanone; HMVK, hydroxymethylvinyl ketone
Solid frame, electrophilic metabolites that can form DNA or haemoglobin adducts; dashed lines, assumed pathways

4.1   Absorption, distribution, metabolism and excretion

4.1.1   *Humans*

(a)   *Butadiene*

Perbellini *et al.* (2003) determined the concentrations of butadiene in alveolar air, blood and urine in humans after non-occupational exposure. Breath, blood and urine samples were taken from 61 men who lived in small mountain villages of Northeast Italy. The mean age of the subjects was 44.5 years (range, 26–64 years); 15 were smokers and 46 were nonsmokers (11 of these were exposed to secondhand tobacco smoke). Samples were collected after overnight rest and analysed by headspace and GC–MS methods. The median concentrations of butadiene were 1.2 ng/L (range, < 0.8–13.2 ng/L) in alveolar air, 2.2 ng/L (range, < 0.5–50.2 ng) in blood and 1.1 ng/L (range, < 1–8.9 ng/L) in urine. Concentrations were significantly higher (two to three times) in smokers compared with nonsmokers in all biological media. The ratio of the median butadiene concentration in blood to alveolar air was 1.8, which is consistent with published values for measured blood:air partition coefficients.

Lin *et al.* (2001) conducted an inhalation study to identify influential physiological factors in the respiratory uptake of butadiene in humans. Healthy volunteers (71 men and 62 women) were exposed to 2 ppm [4.42 mg/m³] butadiene for 20 min followed by purified air for 40 min. Exhaled breath samples were collected during exposure to determine the uptake of butadiene (micrograms per kilogram of body weight (bw) butadiene absorbed), which varied from 0.6 to 4.9 µg/kg bw. The blood:air partition coefficient and alveolar ventilation were most significant in determining uptake. Women had a slightly higher uptake than men; increasing age and cigarette smoking resulted in decreased uptake. The mean percentage of total inhaled butadiene that was absorbed was 45.6% for men and 43.4% for women.

Lin *et al.* (2002) developed an automated exposure system to study the toxicokinetics of inhaled gases in humans. Butadiene was used for system validation at three levels (0.08, 0.4 and 2.0 ppm [0.18, 0.88 and 4.42 mg/m³]) and the system was tested in three subjects who were exposed to 2.0 ppm butadiene for 20 min. Steady-state levels of butadiene in alveolar air were obtained before the end of the 20-min exposure. Levels ranged between approximately 1 and 1.9 ppm. By the end of the 40-min post-exposure period, levels of butadiene in alveolar air had fallen by at least 10-fold.

Smith *et al.* (2001) assessed genetic and dietary factors that affect human metabolism of butadiene by monitoring exhaled breath during and after a 20-min exposure of 71 male and 62 female volunteers to 2 ppm [4.42 mg/m³] butadiene. Chlorzoxazone was administered following exposure and urine was collected to measure the cytochrome P450 (CYP) 2E1 phenotype. A physiologically based pharmacokinetic model was fit to the exhaled breath measurements of each volunteer to estimate model parameters, including metabolic rate. No correlation was found between total butadiene uptake and any of the parameters (metabolic rate, oxidation rate and CYP2E1 phenotype or genotype).

Gordon *et al.* (2002) used real-time breath measurement methods to investigate the suitability of volatile organic compounds, including butadiene, as breath biomarkers for active and passive smoking. Five adult smoker/nonsmoker pairs were recruited into the study. During cigarette smoking, smokers exhaled into the breath analyser throughout a 2–2.5-h smoking period. After smoking, the long-term decay in the breath of the smokers was recorded continuously for 15 min. Exhaled breath in nonsmokers, who were in the room with the smokers, was also monitored. The maximum breath concentration of butadiene was relatively constant among smokers and averaged 373 $\mu g/m^3$ [169 ppm]. Following cessation of smoking, the mean residence time was 0.47 min. The average room air concentration of butadiene was 18.9 $\mu g/m^3$ [42 ppm]. Many of the post-exposure measurements of the breath of nonsmokers were below the limit of quantitation. The average increase in breath concentration of butadiene in nonsmokers and smokers, respectively, was 14.4 and 353 $\mu g/m^3$ [6.5 and 160 ppm].

(b) Metabolites

Several investigators have quantified the presence of metabolites derived from butadiene in the urine of humans in controlled laboratory, environmental or workplace settings. A scheme that describes metabolic pathways of butadiene deduced from in-vitro and in-vivo findings in mammals is presented in Figure 1. Two urinary metabolites have been identified: 1,2-dihydroxybutyl mercapturic acid (DHBMA; also referred to as DHB, MI, M-I or M1) and monohydroxy-3-butenyl mercapturic acid (MHBMA; also referred to as MII, M-II or M2). Both metabolites are mercapturic acids and are derived from the glutathione (GSH) conjugates of electrophilic butadiene metabolites (Figure 1). MHBMA results from the enzyme-mediated reaction of 1,2-epoxy-3-butene (epoxybutene) with GSH. Two isomeric forms of MHBMA have been quantified in the urine of rats and mice (Elfarra *et al.*, 1995). It should be noted, however, that some of the early studies may have not quantified both of these isomers. DHBMA results from the hydrolysis of epoxybutene by epoxide hydrolase (EH) followed by further enzymatic reaction by CYP or alcohol dehydrogenase (ADH) to yield hydroxymethylvinyl ketone (HMVK) before eventual conjugation with GSH (Sprague & Elfarra, 2004). The relative proportions of these metabolites that were measured depended on the species. Due to the higher concentrations of DHBMA in control subjects, DHBMA appears to be a less specific biomarker for exposure than MHBMA, for which background levels are relatively low. However, both metabolites appear to be elevated in humans exposed to butadiene compared with unexposed controls.

Sapkota *et al.* (2006) collected personal air and urine samples from individuals in traffic-dense environments in order to characterize exposure to butadiene in this setting. Urine samples were analysed for MHBMA and DHBMA. Exposure to butadiene differed among the groups; median values were 2.38, 1.62 and 0.88 $\mu g/m^3$ [5, 3.6 and 1.9 ppm] for toll collectors (nine individuals), urban–weekday (seven individuals) and suburban–weekend (seven individuals) groups, respectively. These groups represented high, medium and low levels of exposure intensity. All individuals were nonsmokers in non-smoking households. For the three groups, mean levels of MHBMA were 9.7, 6.0 and 6.8 ng/mL and those of DHBMA were 378, 258, and 306 ng/mL, respectively.

Urban *et al.* (2003) applied a tandem liquid chromatography (LC)–MS method to determine levels of MHBMA and DHBMA in the urine of humans. Exposure to tobacco smoke had a significant effect on the urinary excretion of MHBMA and the metabolite ratio DHBMA/(DHBMA + MHBMA). Urine samples were collected over a 24-h period from 10 smokers and 10 nonsmokers. Mean MHBMA levels were 12.5 and 86.4 µg/24 h for nonsmokers and smokers, respectively. Mean DHBMA levels were 459 and 644 µg/24 h for nonsmokers and smokers, respectively. The metabolic ratio was 0.970 and 0.859 for the two groups, respectively.

Fustinoni *et al.* (2004) assessed exposure to butadiene in two groups who worked in a butadiene plant: 42 occupationally exposed workers and 43 unexposed controls. Personal exposure to butadiene was assessed by collecting air samples during the 8-h workshift (three to four times over a period of 6 weeks for the exposed and once for the control group). Urine and exhaled air samples were collected at the beginning and end of the workshift and blood samples were taken at the end of the workshift for the exposed; all samples were collected at the end of the workshift for the controls. Concentrations of DHBMA and MHBMA were determined in the urine samples. Mean airborne butadiene concentrations were 11.5 and 0.9 µg/m^3 [5.2 and 0.4 ppm] for exposed and control groups, respectively. Mean concentrations of butadiene metabolites in blood and urine were higher in exposed workers: 8.3 ng/L and 5.9 ng/L in blood and 4.3 ng/L and 3.1 ng/L in urine of exposed and control groups before the workshift, respectively. Concentrations of butadiene metabolites in urine at the end of the workshift were 605 µg/L and 602 µg/L DHBMA and 10.5 µg/L and 7.5 µg/L MHBMA in exposed and controls, respectively.

(c)   *Haemoglobin adducts*

While haemoglobin adducts are not causally related to mutagenic events, they provide an effective measure of exposure to reactive intermediates of chemicals. Haemoglobin adducts accumulate during the life of red cells which is approximately 120 days in humans. The butadiene metabolite, epoxybutene, has been shown to react with haemo-globin to form *N*-(2-hydroxy-3-butenyl)valine (MHbVal) adducts. Another haemoglobin adduct of butadiene is *N*-(2,3,4-trihydroxybutyl)valine (THbVal), which can be formed in humans by the reaction of 3,4-epoxy-1,2-butanediol (epoxybutanediol) with haemoglobin or by the reaction of 1,2:3,4-diepoxybutane (diepoxybutane) with haemoglobin followed by hydrolysis of the haemoglobin adduct (Swenberg *et al.*, 2000a). Swenberg *et al.* (2001) reviewed data on various biomarkers for butadiene and noted that those on both DNA and haemoglobin adducts strongly support the conclusion that epoxybutanediol is the major electrophile that binds to these macromolecules.

Boogaard (2002) reviewed the use of haemoglobin adducts to monitor exposure and drew several important conclusions. In theory, the removal of haemoglobin adducts is a zero-order process and is only determined by the life-span of the erythrocyte. Poor correlations were found between concentrations of adducts in a spot blood sample and air concentrations on a limited number of days (i.e. 1–3 days during the shift). In contrast, good correlations were found when very frequent air monitoring was carried out, such as 10 full-day shift measurements over a 2-month period. Good correlations were also found between an increase in adduct concentration over a short period of time and the cumulative exposure during this time, which was determined by continuous monitoring. The author noted that, when specific adducts are determined, information is also obtained regarding the chemical nature of the reactive intermediates. Butadiene forms at least two other reactive intermediates other than epoxybutene: diepoxybutane and epoxybutanediol, both of which form the same THbVal adducts. One of the major data gaps in the assessment of exposure to butadiene is a sensitive biomarker that is specific for diepoxybutane. One potential biomarker is the cyclic adduct, N,N-(2,3-dihydroxy-1,4-butadiyl)valine (PyrVal), which has recently been quantified in rats and mice exposed to levels as low as 1 ppm [2.21 mg/m^3] butadiene for 10 days, but its presence has yet to be quantified in human haemoglobin samples (Boysen et al., 2004; Swenberg et al., 2007).

The utility of haemoglobin adducts as biomarkers for human exposure to butadiene has been investigated in several molecular epidemiological studies that often included the measurement of urinary metabolites and personal air monitoring of butadiene, as well as genotoxicity end-points and metabolic phenotypes.

Van Sittert et al. (2000) and Boogaard et al. (2001a) reported on the assessment of urinary metabolites and haemoglobin adducts. One study involved 44 male workers in a butadiene monomer production facility in the Netherlands who were exposed to low levels of butadiene and 28 male administrative workers with no occupational exposure to butadiene. A second study conducted in a butadiene monomer and styrene–butadiene rubber production facility in Prague, Czech Republic, involved 24 male workers from the monomer unit, 34 from the polymer unit and 25 administrative workers. This study is described in detail by Albertini et al. (2001, 2003a). In the two studies, airborne levels of butadiene, MHBMA, DHBMA and MHbVal were determined. MHBMA was more sensitive than DHBMA for monitoring recent exposures and could be detected at an 8-h TWA exposure as low as 0.13 ppm [0.29 mg/m^3]. The sensitivity of DHBMA was restricted by high background levels, of which the origin is unknown. This study confirmed the higher hydrolytic activity in humans compared with rodents, as shown in other studies, which was reflected in the much higher ratio of DHBMA/(MHBMA + DHBMA).

In the study in the Netherlands, airborne levels of butadiene ranged from 0.2 to 9.5 ppm [0.09–4.3 mg/m^3] (8-h TWA) and levels of MHbVal ranged from 0.6 to 3.8 pmol/g haemoglobin in exposed workers and from 0.1 to 1.2 pmol/g haemoglobin in controls. In the study in Prague, airborne levels of butadiene ranged from 0 to 0.038 ppm [0–0.02 mg/m^3] for the controls, 0.02 to 1.6 ppm [0.009–0.72 mg/m^3] for the monomer workers and 0.02 to 4.2 ppm [0.009–1.9 mg/m^3] for the polymer workers. There was a strong correlation between the 60-day average airborne concentration of butadiene and

MHbVal, which the authors concluded was a sensitive method for monitoring cumulative exposures to butadiene above 0.35 ppm [0.16 mg/m^3]. In controls, urinary levels of MHBMA ranged from 0.1 to 7.3 µg/L and those of DHBMA from 197 to 747 µg/L. In the monomer and polymer workers, levels of MHBMA ranged from < 0.1 to 44 µg/L and from 1.7 to 962 µg/L, respectively, in end-of-shift urine samples. Levels of DHBMA ranged from 52 to 3522 µg/L in the monomer and from 190 to 26 207 µg/L in the polymer workers. For each metabolite there was a strong correlation between the urinary concentration and 8-h TWA levels of airborne butadiene.

Albertini *et al.* (2001, 2003a) conducted a molecular epidemiological study of humans exposed to butadiene in an occupational setting in Prague, Czech Republic (24 butadiene monomer production workers, 34 polymerization workers and 25 controls). Personal 8-h TWA measurements of exposure to butadiene were made on several occasions over a 60-day period, and biological samples were obtained for the measurement of biomarkers of butadiene metabolism: urinary metabolites of butadiene, MHBMA and DHBMA and the haemoglobin adducts, MHbVal and THbVal. Mean 8-h TWA levels of exposure to butadiene were 0.642 mg/m^3 [1.42 ppm] for the monomer workers, 1.794 mg/m^3 [3.96 ppm] for the polymerization workers and 0.023 mg/m^3 [0.05 ppm] for the controls. All four biomarkers were significantly correlated with levels of exposure to butadiene; the haemoglobin adducts were the most highly correlated. After a workshift, mean concentrations of DHBMA were 764, 4647 and 353 µg/L for the monomer production, polymerization and administration workers, respectively, and mean concentrations of MHBMA were 9.44, 120.17 and 1.70 µg/L, respectively. The proportion of MHBMA to the total urinary metabolites (MHBMA + DHBMA) was analysed relative to the glutathione-*S*-transferase (GST) genotypes, *GSTM1* and *GSTT1*, for all three exposure groups. The mean ratios for workers with the homozygous null genotypes in all groups were always lower than those for workers with positive genotypes. Thus, although MHBMA represents a minor pathway in butadiene metabolism, there is a decrease in the proportion of this metabolite formed by GST-null individuals. Concentrations of MHbVal were 0.47, 2.23 and 0.22 pmol/g haemoglobin for the monomer production, polymerization and administration workers, respectively. The group means were correlated with the measured mean levels of exposure to butadiene. Mean concentrations of the THbVal adduct were 178.73, 716.70 and 94.77 pmol/g haemoglobin for the three groups, respectively. Thus, the THbVal adduct is present at concentrations that are increased approximately fivefold over background. There was no effect of *GSTT1* or *GSTM1* genotype on the formation of haemoglobin adducts.

Albertini *et al.* (2007) reported a second study in Czech workers that included both men and women: 23 female workers exposed to butadiene, 26 female control workers, 30 male workers exposed to butadiene and 25 male control workers. Multiple external exposure measurements were made over a 4-month period before biological samples were collected. Mean 8-h TWA exposure levels were 0.008 mg/m^3 [0.0035 ppm] and 0.397 mg/m^3 [0.180 ppm] for female controls and exposed workers, respectively. Exposure levels for men were 0.007 mg/m^3 [0.0032 ppm] and 0.808 mg/m^3 [0.370 ppm] for controls and exposed, respectively. Urinary concentrations of MHBMA and DHBMA were elevated in exposed male and female workers compared with controls. Mean levels of DHBMA were 331.6 μg/L and 508.1 μg /L for control and exposed women, respectively, and 512.8 μg/L and 854.1 μg/L for control and exposed men, respectively. Mean levels of MHBMA were 8.3 μg/L and 19.2 μg /L for control and exposed women, respectively, and 14.9 μg/L and 47.9 μg/L for control and exposed men, respectively. As part of this study, assays were conducted to determine the presence of the haemoglobin adduct, PyrVal. This adduct is specific for the highly genotoxic metabolite of butadiene, diepoxybutane. All samples were below the limit of quantitation for the assay (0.3 pmol/g haemoglobin).

Swenberg et al. (2007) quantified PyrVal in the blood of mice and rats exposed to 1 ppm [2.21 mg/m^3] butadiene. For these comparative studies, 50 mg haemoglobin from workers, rats and mice were analysed by the method of Boysen et al. (2007). Whereas all rat and mouse samples had quantifiable amounts of PyrVal, none of the human samples did. The authors reported that, although the TWA exposures to butadiene in the Czech study were below 1 ppm [2.21 mg/m^3] for both men and women, the duration of exposure was much greater for humans than for rodents, which made the cumulative exposures comparable. Since haemoglobin adducts form over the lifespan of the erythrocyte (humans, 120 days; rats, 63 days; and mice, 43 days), human haemoglobin had a cumulative exposure similar to that of both rats and mice (women: 0.18 ppm butadiene × 17.1 weeks = 3.1 ppm–weeks; men: 0.37 ppm butadiene × 17.1 weeks = 6.3 ppm–weeks; rodents: 1 ppm butadiene × 4 weeks = 4.0 ppm–weeks). They also reported that the analytical peaks in samples from rats exposed to 1 ppm [2.21 mg/m^3] butadiene were sufficiently large that quantitative measurements could have been made with one-third of the haemoglobin, which suggests that humans form at least three times less PyrVal than similarly exposed rats and 100 times less than similarly exposed mice.

Fustinoni et al. (2002) investigated the role of genetic polymorphisms in the metabolism of butadiene in 40 Italian subjects. Thirty were occupationally exposed during butadiene monomer production or polymerization processes and 10 were unexposed administrative clerks. Air samples were collected from butadiene-exposed workers during the workshift using personal samplers. Personal exposure to airborne butadiene ranged from 4 to 201 μg/m^3 [1.8–90.5 ppm]. At the end of the workshift, blood and urine samples were collected from all subjects. Concentrations of the urinary metabolite DHBMA and the haemoglobin adduct THbVal were assessed. Median urinary DHBMA concentrations were 17.1 mg/g creatinine in exposed workers and 1.42 mg/g creatinine in unexposed workers; THBVal levels were 37 pmol/g haemoglobin and 35.3 pmol/g haemoglobin in exposed and unexposed groups, respectively. Smoking influenced the formation of haemoglobin adducts and higher THbVal levels were found in subjects with GSTM1 null and GSTT1 null genotypes.

Hayes et al. (2001) examined a spectrum of outcomes in 41 butadiene polymer production workers and 38 controls in China. Smokers accounted for 86.7% of the exposed group and 78.6% of the controls. Median butadiene concentrations (6-h TWA) were 2 ppm [0.90 mg/m^3] for the exposed group and 0 ppm for the controls, as determined during a 6-h workshift using personal samplers. A post-shift blood sample and during-shift urine samples were also collected. Median urinary concentrations of DHBMA were 1.3 µg/mg creatinine in the exposed group and 0.6 µg/mg creatinine in the controls. THbVal haemoglobin adducts were significantly more common [numerical data not provided] in exposed workers than in the unexposed ($p < 0.0001$) and correlated well with air measurement (Spearman's $\rho = 0.40$, $p = 0.03$) and weakly with urinary butadiene (Spearman's $\rho = 0.37$, $p = 0.24$).

(d)   Physiologically based toxicokinetic models

Physiologically based models founded on informative prior distributions for population parameters as well as previously published data on exhaled breath concentrations of butadiene in exposed humans have been designed to facilitate a global sensitivity analysis of the kinetics of butadiene and its metabolites in humans; the most recent was published by Brochot *et al.* (2007) and its purpose was to guide the design of new human experiments intended to collect critically useful kinetic data on butadiene and its metabolites.

4.1.2   Experimental systems

At the beginning of each of the following sections, brief highlights on the disposition of butadiene that were summarized previously (IARC, 1999) are presented. The reader should refer to that monograph for citations and more complete descriptions of the relevant studies. These highlights are followed by information that has been published since that time. For this and other sections, diepoxybutane refers to the (±) racemic mixture of diastereomers, unless otherwise specified.

(a)   Butadiene

Inhalation pharmacokinetic studies conducted in Sprague-Dawley rats and B6C3F$_1$ mice demonstrated linear metabolic elimination kinetics at exposures of up to about 1000 ppm [2200 mg/m^3]; maximal rates of butadiene metabolism were higher in mice (400 µmol/h/kg) than in rats (220 µmol/h/kg) (IARC, 1999). In the linear range, metabolism is limited by the uptake of this gas. At equivalent, non-saturating exposure levels, steady-state blood concentrations of butadiene are about twofold higher in mice than in rats. Numerous metabolites have been identified in the urine of rats and mice exposed to butadiene (Figure 1); the major urinary metabolites are mercapturic acids (DHBMA and MHBMA) that result from conjugation of epoxybutene or HMVK, a metabolite of butenediol, with GSH.

Exhaled epoxybutene was measured in chamber atmospheres in which male B6C3F$_1$ mice or Sprague-Dawley rats were exposed for up to 8 h to constant concentrations of butadiene that ranged from 1 ppm to 6000 ppm [2.21–13 260 mg/m^3] (mice) or 10 000 ppm [22 100 mg/m^3] (rats) (Filser *et al.*, 2007). In additional experiments, blood levels of diepoxybutane, butenediol and epoxybutanediol were measured at the end of 6-h exposures that ranged from 60 ppm [132.6 mg/m^3] up to about 1200 ppm [2652 mg/m^3]. Epoxybutanediol is formed by partial hydrolysis of diepoxybutane or by oxidation of butenediol (Figure 1). Blood concentrations of epoxybutene were estimated from the product of its atmospheric concentration at steady state and its blood:air partition coefficient. Mouse:rat ratios of blood concentrations of epoxybutene were 2.0–2.6 at concentrations of butadiene below 10 ppm [22.1 mg/m^3], 3.8 at 100 ppm [221 mg/m^3], 4.9 at 625 ppm [1381 mg/m^3] and 8.0 at 1250 ppm [2762.5 mg/m^3]. Blood concentrations of diepoxybutane in mice were 0.30, 2.2 and 3.2 μmol/L at 67, 630 and 1270 ppm [148, 1392.3 and 2806.7 mg/m^3] butadiene, respectively. Diepoxybutane was not detected in the blood of rats exposed to up to 900 ppm [1989 mg/m^3] butadiene (detection limit, 10 nmol/L) (Filser et al., 2007). However, previous studies (IARC, 1999) reported diepoxybutane levels of 2.4–5 nmol/L in male and 11 nmol/L in female Sprague-Dawley rats exposed to 62.5 ppm [138 mg/m^3] butadiene. Butenediol levels reached 60 μmol/L in both species exposed to 1200 ppm [2652 mg/m^3] butadiene, whereas maximum blood levels of epoxybutanediol were 42 μmol/L in mice exposed to 300 ppm [663 mg/m^3] butadiene and 9.5 μmol/L in rats exposed to 150 ppm [331.5 mg/m^3] butadiene. The limited epoxybutanediol formation was suggested to be due to competition by butadiene for the CYP-mediated oxidation of epoxybutene to diepoxybutane and of butenediol to epoxybutanediol. In rats, the total blood concentrations of epoxybutene and epoxybutanediol were greater after exposure to 200 ppm [442 mg/m^3] butadiene than after exposure to 1000 or 8000 ppm [2210 or 17 680 mg/m^3]; the latter values are the concentrations of butadiene that were used in a rat carcinogenicity study.

First-pass metabolism of butadiene to epoxybutene, diepoxybutane, butenediol, epoxybutanediol and crotonaldehyde was quantified in the livers of male Sprague-Dawley rats and B6C3F$_1$ mice perfused in a gas-tight all-glass system (Filser et al., 2001). Concentrations of butadiene in the perfusate and perfusion rates were 330 nmol/mL at 3–4 mL/min for mouse liver and 240 nmol/mL at 17–20 mL/min for rat liver. Concentrations of butadiene and its metabolites in the perfusate that entered and left the liver were measured during 100-min perfusions. The perfusate consisted of Krebs-Henseleit buffer that contained bovine erythrocytes, bovine serum albumin and a constant concentration of butadiene. The rate of single-pass butadiene metabolism was estimated to be 0.014 and 0.055 mmol/h per liver of mouse and rat, respectively. The mean concentration of epoxybutene was 1.1 nmol/mL in the rat liver effluent and 9.4 nmol/mL in the mouse liver effluent. Butenediol concentrations in the perfusates that left the liver were similar in rats and mice (approximately 7 and 8 nmol/mL, respectively). Levels of diepoxybutane and epoxybutanediol were below the limit of detection in the effluent from the rat liver and low in the mouse liver effluent (approximately 0.06 and 0.07 nmol/mL, respectively). Concentrations of crotonaldehyde were below the limit of detection (60 nmol/L) in both rat and mouse liver.

Filser et al. (2001) also studied butadiene metabolism in perfused livers obtained from rats that were depleted of GSH by pretreatment with diethylmaleate. Under these conditions, the rate of metabolism was not altered; however, concentrations of epoxybutene and butenediol were increased 25- and 10-fold, respectively, and concentrations of diepoxybutane and crotonaldehyde in the effluent perfusates were quantifiable (0.15 and 0.10 nmol/mL, respectively). The authors concluded that GST activity is important in controlling the production of diepoxybutane and crotonaldehyde in rats.

    (b)   Metabolites in vitro (see Figure 1)

    Butadiene is oxidized initially to epoxybutene by nicotinamide adenine dinucleotide phosphate (NADPH)-dependent metabolism that primarily involves CYP2E1 and CYP2A6. This metabolic pathway has been measured in microsomal fractions obtained from the livers and lungs of mice, rats and humans and from the kidney and testis of rats and mice (IARC, 1999). At low concentrations of butadiene, metabolism via CYP2E1 predominates. Liver microsomes from mice, rats and humans can also oxidize epoxybutene to diepoxybutane. Kinetic parameters (maximum velocity [V_{max}] and Michaelis-Menten constant [K_m]) indicated faster rates of oxidative metabolism of butadiene and epoxybutene in microsomes from mice than in those from rats, while human liver microsomes showed a wide range of activites (Csanady *et al.*, 1992; Duescher & Elfarra, 1994), but only a small number of human liver and lung samples were analysed. Mouse, rat and human microsomes can convert epoxybutene to both (±)-diepoxybutane and *meso*-diepoxybutane. The latter isomer is preferentially hydrolysed in rat and human liver microsomes (Krause & Elfarra, 1997). Epoxybutene and diepoxybutane are eliminated by microsomal EH (mEH) and by cytosolic GST activities. In-vitro kinetics of EH- and GST-catalysed metabolism of epoxybutene and diepoxybutane in microsomal and cytosolic fractions from livers and lungs of mice, rats and humans have also been reported (IARC, 1999). GST activities were highest in mouse and lowest in human cytosol; EH activities were highest in human and lowest in mouse microsomes. Bone-marrow cells of mice and humans can also oxidize butadiene to epoxybutene by a myeloperoxidase-catalysed reaction. A third epoxide intermediate of butadiene metabolism, epoxybutanediol, can be formed by the oxidation of butenediol (the product of epoxybutene hydrolysis) or by partial hydrolysis of diepoxybutane.

    Hepatocytes isolated from male B6C3F$_1$ mice and Sprague-Dawley rats were incubated with epoxybutene and evaluated for the formation of diepoxybutane, butenediol and GSH conjugates at 5-min intervals during incubations of up to 45 min (Kemper *et al.*, 2001). The results are shown in Table 22. Cumulative levels of combined racemic and *meso*-diepoxybutane (oxidation of epoxybutene) were higher in mouse than in rat hepatocyte cultures, whereas the cumulative levels of butenediol (hydrolysis of epoxybutene) were higher in the rat hepatocyte cultures. GSH conjugates were present at similar levels in both rat and mouse hepatocyte cultures.

    Hepatic microsomes pooled from cynomolgus monkeys or humans exposed to butadiene (monkey microsomes: 46 ppm, 290 ppm or 28 000 ppm [102, 641 or 61 880 mg/m^3]; human microsomes: 45 ppm, 450 ppm or 36 000 ppm [99, 995 or

79 560 mg/m^3]) produced epoxybutene at similar rates (Dahl & Henderson, 2000). Oxidation of epoxybutene to diepoxybutane, which is competitively inhibited by butadiene, was slightly faster in monkey than in human microsomes.

Table 22. Area under the concentration versus time curve (nmol·min/10^6 cells) for epoxybutene-derived metabolites in isolated mouse and rat hepatocytes during 45-min incubations with epoxybutene

Concentration of epoxybutene (μM)	Diepoxybutane	Butenediol	GSH conjugates
Mouse hepatocytes			
5	63 ± 23	9 ± 1	22 ± 14
25	197 ± 28	133 ± 24	117 ± 32
250	616 ± 53	908 ± 172	1101 ± 322
Rat hepatocytes			
5	5 ± 1	78 ± 20	27 ± 1
25	13 ± 3	435 ± 98	153 ± 9
250	80 ± 3	3403 ± 755	1552 ± 206

From Kemper *et al.* (2001)
GSH, glutathione

(c)   *Metabolites* in vivo (see Figure 1)

The identification of epoxybutene in exhaled breath, blood and multiple organs of rats or mice exposed to butadiene indicates the systemic availability of this metabolic intermediate. At equivalent exposure concentrations of butadiene, tissue levels of epoxybutene and diepoxybutane were higher in mice than in rats (IARC, 1999).

[14]C-Labelled epoxybutene was administered as a single intraperitoneal injection to male Sprague-Dawley rats and B6C3F$_1$ mice at doses of 1, 5, 20 and 50 mg/kg bw; urine and faeces were collected up to 48 h after treatment (Richardson *et al.*, 1998). Approximately 50% of the administered radioactivity was excreted in the urine and 2–5% in the faeces. Urinary metabolites identified in this study are listed in Table 23. Because the percentage of urinary radioactivity recovered for each metabolite did not differ in relation to the administered dose, mean values across the dose groups are shown. Both species preferentially metabolized epoxybutene by direct conjugation with GSH. In rats, 48–64% of the urinary radioactivity was derived from the direct reaction of epoxybutene with GSH and 14–25% was derived from hydrolysis of epoxybutene. In mice, 60–72% of the urinary radioactivity was derived from the direct reaction of epoxybutene with GSH and 6–10% was derived from hydrolysis of epoxybutene. No metabolites of diepoxybutane were detected in the urine of either species.

Table 23. Urinary metabolites in rats and mice given a single intraperitoneal injection of 1, 5, 20 or 50 mg/kg bw [4-^{14}C]epoxybutene

Metabolite[a]	% of recovered urinary radioactivity	
	Rat	Mouse
Polar fraction[b]	22 ± 2	23 ± 1
4-(N-Acetyl-L-cystein-S-yl)-1,2-dihydroxybutane and 4-(N-acetyl-L-cystein-S-yl)-2-hydroxybutanoic acid	14 ± 3	10 ± 2
3-(N-Acetyl-L-cystein-S-yl)propan-1-ol and 3-(N-acetyl-L-cystein-S-yl)propanoic acid	6 ± 2	–
(R)-2-(N-Acetyl-L-cystein-S-yl)-1-hydroxybut-3-ene	13 ± 1	11 ± 1
1-(N-Acetyl-L-cystein-S-yl)-2-(S)-hydroxybut-3-ene and 1-(N-acetyl-L-cystein-S-yl)-2-(R)-hydroxybut-3-ene	19 ± 5	26 ± 6
(S)-2-(N-Acetyl-L-cystein-S-yl)-1-hydroxybut-3-ene	25 ± 2	11 ± 2
4-(N-Acetyl-L-cystein-S-yl)-1-hydroxybut-2-ene	1 ± 0.4	–
S-(1-Hydroxybut-3-en-2-yl)mercaptoacetic acid	–	10 ± 2
S-(2-Hydroxybut-3-en-1-yl)mercaptoacetic acid	–	10 ± 2

From Richardson *et al.* (1998)
[a] Italicized metabolites are produced subsequent to hydrolysis of epoxybutene; the other metabolites listed are produced by direct reaction of epoxybutene with glutathione.
[b] Individual metabolites in the polar fraction were less than 1% of the recovered urinary radioactivity.

Male Sprague-Dawley rats and B6C3F$_1$ mice were exposed by nose-only inhalation to 200 ppm [442 mg/m^3] [2,3-^{14}C]butadiene for 6 h; radioactivity in urine, faeces, exhaled volatiles and [^{14}C]carbon dioxide was measured during and up to 42 h after exposure (Richardson *et al.*, 1999). Total uptake of butadiene was 0.19 mmol/kg bw (10.3 mg/kg) in rats and 0.38 mmol/kg bw (20.5 mg/kg) in mice. In rats, 40% of the recovered radioactivity was exhaled as [^{14}C]carbon dioxide, 42% was excreted in urine, 8% was excreted in faeces and 9% remained in the carcass. In mice, 6% of the recovered radioactivity was exhaled as [^{14}C]carbon dioxide, 71% was excreted in urine, 11% was excreted in faeces and 13% remained in the carcass. Because the position of the radiolabel in this study was on carbons 2 and 3, the formation of [^{14}C]carbon dioxide is a result of the loss of two carbon atoms from butadiene. Urinary metabolites identified in this study are listed in Table 24. Metabolites arising from the direct reaction of epoxybutene with GSH accounted for 8% of the metabolized dose in rats and 16% of the metabolized dose in mice. In contrast to the study of epoxybutene metabolism (Richardson *et al.*, 1998), the study on butadiene metabolism identified trihydroxybutyl mercapturic acids in the urine of exposed rats and mice.

Table 24. Urinary metabolites in rats and mice exposed to 200 ppm [^{14}C]butadiene for 6 h

Metabolite[a]	% of total radioactivity recovered	
	Rat	Mouse
Polar fraction	16.6 ± 0.6	33.0 ± 0.6
4-(N-Acetyl-L-cystein-S-yl)-1,2,3-trihydroxybutane and 3-(N-acetyl- L-cystein-S-yl)-1,2,4-trihydroxybutane	4.1 ± 0.2	6.7 ± 0.3
4-(N-Acetyl-L-cystein-S-yl)-1,2-dihydroxybutane	7.3 ± 1.2	7.1 ± 0.3
4-(N-Acetyl-L-cystein-S-yl)-2-hydroxybutanoic acid	1.1 ± 0.1	–
3-(N-Acetyl-L-cystein-S-yl)propan-1-ol and 3-(N-acetyl-L-cystein-S-yl)propanoic acid	0.4 ± 0.1	–
(R)-2-(N-Acetyl-L-cystein-S-yl-1-hydroxybut-3-ene	1.7 ± 0.3	1.9 ± 0.4
1-(N-Acetyl-L-cystein-S-yl)-2-(S)-hydroxybut-3-ene	0.2 ± 0.1	1.3 ± 0.2
1-(N-Acetyl-L-cystein-S-yl)-2-(R)-hydroxybut-3-ene	1.6 ± 0.4	6.1 ± 0.2
(S)-2-(N-Acetyl-L-cystein-S-yl)-1-hydroxybut-3-ene	4.2 ± 0.6	2.5 ± 0.1
4-(N-Acetyl-L-cystein-S-yl)-1-hydroxybut-2-ene	–	0.1 ± 0.1
S-(1-Hydroxybut-3-en-2-yl)mercaptoacetic acid	–	1.6 ± 0.4
S-(2-Hydroxybut-3-en-1-yl)mercaptoacetic acid	–	2.3 ± 0.1
Unknown	3.9 ± 0.8	–

From Richardson *et al.* (1999)
[a] Italicized metabolites are produced subsequent to hydrolysis of epoxybutene; the other metabolites listed are produced by direct reaction of epoxybutene with glutathione.

Urinary metabolites were also identified in male Sprague-Dawley rats and B6C3F$_1$ mice exposed by nose-only inhalation to 1, 5 or 20 ppm [2.21, 11 or 44 mg/m^3] [2,3-^{14}C]butadiene for 6 h (Booth *et al.*, 2004a). This study did not include measurements of radioactivity in faeces, exhaled volatiles, carbon dioxide or the carcass. Urine was collected over an 18-h period after exposure but not during exposure. The profiles of urinary metabolites were somewhat similar to those reported by Richardson *et al.* (1999).

Four mercapturic acids derived from HMVK were identified in the urine from male B6C3F$_1$ mice and Sprague-Dawley rats given a single intraperitoneal injection of 25, 62.5, 125 or 200 mg/kg bw butanediol (Sprague & Elfarra, 2004). The metabolites were N-acetyl-L-cystein-S-yl conjugates of 1,2-dihydroxybutane, 1-hydroxy-2-butanone, propanol and propionic acid. HMVK may be formed by ADH- or CYP-mediated oxidation of butenediol. These four HMVK-derived metabolites accounted for 7 and 11% of the total radioactivity recovered from rats and mice exposed to butadiene, respectively (Richardson *et al.*, 1999).

Trace amounts of 1-hydroxy-2-butanone, crotonic acid, propionic acid and 2-ketobutyric acid were detected in the urine of male B6C3F$_1$ mice and Sprague-Dawley rats administered butanediol by intraperitoneal injection (mice: 125 or 250 mg/kg bw; rats: 62.5, 125, 200 or 250 mg/kg bw) (Sprague & Elfarra, 2003). The combined concentration of these metabolites was less than 1% of the administered dose of butenediol; these low levels may be due to further metabolism of the carboxylic acids prior to their excretion in the urine. The detection of these metabolites suggests the possibility that toxic intermediary metabolites, such as crotonaldehyde, may be formed from butenediol.

(d)   Haemoglobin adducts

Epoxybutene can form two diastomeric pairs of adducts at the N-terminal valine of hacmoglobin termed MHbVal: N-(2-hydroxy-3-buten-1-yl)valine and N-(1-hydroxy-3-buten-2-yl)valine (IARC, 1999). Levels of these adducts formed in rats and mice are dependent on exposure concentrations of butadiene, duration of exposure and the turnover rates of red blood cells.

Much work has been carried out on the use of haemoglobin adducts as biomarkers of internal levels of the epoxide intermediates of butadiene metabolism. Epoxybutene, diepoxybutane and epoxybutanediol can react with the N-terminal valine to form MHbVal, PyrVal and THbVal adducts, respectively (Boysen et al., 2007). In addition, THbVal may also be formed by the reaction of haemoglobin with diepoxybutane and subsequent hydrolysis of the remaining epoxide group.

THbVal adduct levels in haemoglobin isolated from erythrocytes of male Sprague-Dawley rats and B6C3F$_1$ mice exposed by nose-only inhalation to 1, 5 or 20 ppm [2.2, 11 or 44 mg/m^3] [2,3-^{14}C]butadiene for 6 h per day for 5 days were 80, 179 and 512 pmol/g haemoglobin for rats, respectively, and 143, 351 and 1100 pmol/g haemoglobin for mice, respectively (Booth et al., 2004a). However, the level of radioactivity was approximately 1.3-fold higher in rat than in mouse haemoglobin. The measured levels of THbVal adduct represented only about 1–2% of the total radioactive adducts in the haemoglobin, which indicates that multiple alkylation sites within haemoglobin may be modified by butadiene metabolites. After incubation of epoxybutane with erythrocytes, Moll et al. (2000) detected 10 epoxybutane adducts on each of the α- and β-globin chains.

A specific ring-closed adduct, the pyrolidine adduct PyrVal, can be formed by the reaction of haemoglobin with diepoxybutane (Fred et al., 2004). This adduct has been measured after in-vitro reactions of rat and mouse erythrocyte haemolysates with diepoxybutane and after intraperitoneal injections of diepoxybutane into Fischer 344 rats and C57/BL mice. The levels of PyrVal adduct per administered dose were similar in rat and mouse haemoglobin after in-vitro or in-vivo exposure to diepoxybutane. In addition, THbVal adducts were measured in rats and mice given intraperitoneal injections of diepoxybutane or epoxybutanediol. Levels of this adduct were similar in mice and rats dosed with epoxybutanediol; however, after treatment with diepoxybutane, levels of THbVal adducts were three to four times higher in rats.

Several haemoglobin adducts were measured in rats and mice after inhalation exposure to butadiene (Boysen *et al.*, 2004, 2007). Female B6C3F$_1$ mice were exposed to 3, 62.5 or 1250 ppm [6.6, 138 or 3453 mg/m^3] butadiene for 6 h per day for 2 weeks, while female Fischer 344 rats were exposed to 3 or 62.5 ppm [6.6 or 138 mg/m^3] for 10 days. At equivalent butadiene exposures, the levels of MHbVal and PyrVal were higher in mice than in rats, while levels of THbVal were similar in these species (Table 25). The formation of each of these adducts in mice and rats was more efficient (pmol adduct/g haemoglobin per ppm butadiene) at 3 ppm butadiene than at higher exposure concentrations. The major adduct formed in mice and rats is THbVal. In rats, formation of THbVal reaches a plateau at exposures to butadiene above 62.5 ppm (Boysen *et al.*, 2007).

Table 25. *N*-Terminal haemoglobin adducts (pmol/g haemoglobin and adducts/ ppm butadiene) in mice and rats exposed to butadiene (BD) for 10 days

	Exposure (ppm)	MHbVal		PyrVal		THbVal	
		pmol/g	/ppm BD	pmol/g	/ppm BD	pmol/g	/ppm BD
Mice	0	0.91 ± 0.9				54 ± 8	
	3	38 ± 6	12.7	49 ± 3	16.2	339 ± 41	112.8
	62.5	145 ± 21	2.3	130 ± 64	2.1	3202 ± 302	51.2
	1250	7386 ± 227	5.9	2487 ± 426	2.0	14 838 ± 975	11.9
Rats	0	2.6 ± 0.6				60 ± 2	
	3	1.3 ± 0.7	4.3	4 ± 1	1.3	397 ± 12	132
	62.5	86 ± 1.2	1.4	38 ± 1	0.6	2937 ± 39	47
	1250	1682 ± 58	1.4			5555 ± 469	4.4

From Boysen *et al.* (2007)
MHbVal, *N*-(2-hydroxy-3-butenyl)valine; PyrVal, *N,N*-(2,3-dihydroxy-1,4-butadiyl)valine; THbVal, *N*-(2,3,4-trihydroxybutyl)valine

The levels of THbVal adducts in female B6C3F$_1$ mice exposed by inhalation to 6, 18 or 36 ppm butanediol for 6 h per day on 5 days per week for 4 weeks were approximately twofold higher than those in female Fischer 344 rats exposed to the same concentrations of this metabolite. The similarity in the shape of the dose–response curves for the formation of these adducts and the induction of hypoxanthine–guanine phosphoribosyl transferase gene (*Hprt*) mutant frequency in splenic T cells from mice and rats exposed to butenediol suggests that epoxybutanediol (the product of butenediol epoxidation) may play a significant role in the mutagenicity of butadiene (Powley *et al.*, 2005).

(e)   Physiological toxicokinetic models of butadiene disposition

Several physiologically based toxicokinetic models have been developed to characterize the disposition of butadiene and epoxybutene in rats and mice (IARC, 1999).

These models were based on species-specific physiological parameters, in-vitro metabolic parameters, and blood:air, tissue:air and tissue:blood partition coefficients. Adjustable parameters were estimated by fitting the models to data on butadiene and epoxybutene uptake in rats and mice exposed separately to these gases in closed chambers. Although each model was fairly effective in reproducing butadiene uptake in rats and mice, they overpredicted blood levels of epoxybutene measured subsequently in rats and mice exposed to butadiene. This discrepancy was reduced by assuming that epoxybutene formed from butadiene is partially sequestered in an intrahepatic compartment that allows first-pass metabolism of epoxybutene by EH or by assuming that only a small fraction of butadiene (19–24%) is oxidized to epoxybutene. None of the models included the formation or elimination of epoxybutanediol.

Predictions of human blood levels of diepoxybutane are sensitive to parameters that affect the metabolism of butadiene to epoxybutene, the rate at which epoxybutene is oxidized to diepoxybutane and the rates of hydrolysis of epoxybutene and diepoxybutane.

To address the finding that physiological models of butadiene disposition that reproduced the uptake of this gas and epoxybutene from closed chambers but overpredicted blood concentrations of epoxybutene measured subsequently in rats and mice exposed to butadiene, a modified model was proposed in which epoxybutene formed from butadiene has privileged access to EH (Kohn & Melnick, 2000; based on work of Oesch & Daly, 1972). This was then expanded to include equations for the production and metabolism of butenediol and epoxybutanediol (Kohn & Melnick, 2001). The model predicts higher concentrations of epoxybutanediol than either epoxybutene or diepoxybutane in all metabolizing tissues of rats and mice at all butadiene exposures examined.

4.2   Genetic and related effects

The genetic toxicology of butadiene and its major metabolites, epoxybutene and diepoxybutane, has been reviewed (IARC, 1999; Henderson, 2001).

4.2.1   *Humans*

The *HPRT* variant frequency in lymphocytes as well as the concentration of the urinary metabolite of butadiene, DHBMA, was examined in 49 workers in a styrene–butadiene rubber production facility in Texas, USA (Ammenheuser *et al.*, 2001). The study included 24 subjects who had high exposure and 25 who had low exposure for *HPRT* variant frequency analysis, 22 subjects who had high exposure and 24 who had low exposure for dosimeter measurements and 24 who had high exposure and 23 who had low exposure for urine analyses. The mean value of exposure to butadiene was 1.48 ± 0.37 ppm [3.27 ± 0.82 mg/m^3] (mean ± standard error [SE]) for the high-exposure group and 0.15 ± 0.02 ppm [0.33 ± 0.04 mg/m^3] for the low-exposure group. The frequency of *HPRT* variants was $6.66 \pm 1.4 \times 10^{-6}$ (mean ± SE) for the high-exposure group and $2.10 \pm$

0.2×10^{-6} for the low-exposure group ($p < 0.0002$). When smoking status was considered, the frequency of *HPRT* variants was $6.8 \pm 1.2 \times 10^{-6}$ for 19 nonsmokers in the high-exposure group and $1.8 \pm 0.2 \times 10^{-6}$ for 20 nonsmokers in the low-exposure group ($p < 0.0005$). The concentration of DHBMA was 2046 ± 348 ng/mg creatinine in the urine of the high-exposure group compared with 585 ± 98 ng/mg creatinine in the urine of the low-exposure group ($p < 0.0005$).

Another study was conducted in the same styrene–butadiene facility in 1998 (Ward *et al.*, 2001). The frequency of *HPRT* variants in lymphocytes as well as the concentration of the urinary metabolite of butadiene, DHBMA, were examined in 37 workers (22 who had high exposure and 15 who had low exposure). The mean value of exposure to butadiene was 1.71 ± 0.54 ppm [3.78 ± 1.2 mg/m^3] (mean $\pm$ SE) for the high-exposure group and 0.07 ± 0.03 ppm [0.15 ± 0.07 mg/m^3] for the low-exposure group. The frequency of *HPRT* variants was $10.67 \pm 1.51 \times 10^{-6}$ (mean $\pm$ SE) for the high-exposure group and $3.54 \pm 0.61 \times 10^{-6}$ for the low-exposure group ($p < 0.001$). The concentration of the metabolite was 378 ± 53 ng/mg creatinine in the urine of the high-exposure group compared with 271 ± 50 ng/mg creatinine in the urine of the low-exposure group. Unlike the previous study, this difference was not significant ($p > 0.05$).

A subset of the workers from the Texas facility was analysed for their frequency of *HPRT* mutants (Ma *et al.*, 2000). *HPRT* mutants were analysed by a multiplex polymerase chain reaction (PCR) and the frequency of large deletions in butadiene-exposed workers (17.5%; 25/143) was significantly higher than that in control subjects (9.7%; 21/217; $p < 0.05$). This increase in large deletions was due primarily to an increase in multiple exon deletions ($p < 0.05$). When the *HPRT* mutants were analysed for cDNA sequence mutations, the majority of the mutations observed in both exposure groups were single-base substitutions. However, the overall distribution of the types of mutation was significantly different between the two groups ($p < 0.05$). A non-significant increase in mutations at AT sites was observed in butadiene-exposed workers (46%) compared with the control group (39%), and the proportion of A:T→T:A transversions was also increased in the butadiene-exposed group (16%) compared with the control group (8%; $p = 0.25$). Three new mutable sites were identified at positions 116, 370 and 410. The frequency of -1 frame shift mutations was significantly higher (11%; $p < 0.05$) in exposed workers than in the controls (2%). Polymorphisms in the *mEH* gene may play a significant role in the sensitivity of humans to the genotoxic effects of butadiene. In workers exposed to > 150 ppb [331.5 µg/m^3] butadiene, individuals who had at least one polymorphic *mEH His* allele had a significant ($p < 0.001$) threefold increase in the frequency of *HPRT* variant (mutant) lymphocytes compared with individuals who had the *Tyr/Tyr* genotype (Abdel-Rahman *et al.*, 2001).

Blood samples from 19 exposed (butadiene monomer production unit) and 19 control (heat production unit) workers at a petrochemical company in the Czech Republic were analysed for chromosomal aberrations and sister chromatid exchange (Šrám *et al.*, 1998). The median exposure concentration of butadiene was 0.53 mg/m^3 [0.24 ppm] for the exposed group and 0.013 mg/m^3 [0.006 ppm] for the control group. A significant increase in the percentage of aberrant cells was observed in the exposed group (3.11 ± 1.33 versus $2.03 \pm 1.01\%$; $p < 0.01$). When smoking status was considered in the exposed group, no difference in the percentage of aberrant cells was observed between smokers (3.11 ± 1.50) and nonsmokers (3.10 ± 1.24), although nonsmokers were exposed to nearly three times more butadiene (1.73 mg/m^3) than smokers (0.53 mg/m^3). There was also a significant increase in the frequencies of sister chromatid exchange per cell in the exposed compared with the control groups (6.96 ± 1.51 and 4.87 ± 1.11 [mean $\pm$ SD], respectively; $p < 0.001$).

A comparison of conventional cytogenetic analyses and fluorescence in-situ hybridization (FISH) was conducted among 82 workers in a chemical plant in the Czech Republic (Šrám et al., 2004). Twenty-three subjects worked in monomer production and were exposed to 0.642 mg/m^3 [0.3 ppm] butadiene, 34 worked in polymer production (1.794 mg/m^3 [0.812 ppm] butadiene) and 25 matched controls (0.023 mg/m^3 [0.01 ppm] butadiene) worked in administration. Using both methods, no significant differences in chromosomal aberration frequency were detected between any of the groups. When subjects with suspected clonality were excluded, re-analysis of the data by FISH found a significant difference between the polymer production workers (2.73 ± 1.51 genomic frequencies of stable chromosomal exchanges) and the monomer production and control groups (1.72 ± 1.14 and 2.06 ± 1.31 genomic frequencies of stable chromosomal exchanges, respectively).

A study that used several different biomarkers to determine the effects of exposure to butadiene on workers was undertaken in the Czech Republic (Albertini et al., 2001). Eighty-three workers from the same industrial site were divided into three groups: controls (25 from administration), and monomer (24) and polymer (34) workers. Polymer workers typically had levels of exposure (1.76 ± 4.69 mg/m^3 [0.8 ppm]) that were significantly higher than those of the monomer workers (0.64 ± 2.06 mg/m^3 [0.29 ppm]) and controls (0.3 ± 0.03 mg/m^3 [0.14 ppm]). Analysis by autoradiography of *HPRT* mutations in 49 workers showed a significant difference between the control ($10.75 \pm 6.11 \times 10^{-6}$) and the monomer ($5.73 \pm 4.72 \times 10^{-6}$) and the polymer workers ($6.48 \pm 4.77 \times 10^{-6}$). This trend contradicts that expected. Analysis by a cloning assay of *HPRT* mutations in 75 workers showed no significant differences between the groups (controls, $13.00 \pm 8.1 \times 10^{-6}$; monomer workers, $10.69 \pm 5.4 \times 10^{-6}$; polymer workers, $18.83 \pm 17.41 \times 10^{-6}$). Assays for sister chromatid exchange were completed for 73 study subjects. No significant differences were observed between the groups. Chromosomal aberrations were analysed by traditional methods in 82 workers. The mean percentages of cells with aberrations were 1.56, 1.52 and 1.54% for the control, monomer and polymer groups, respectively. The mean number of chromosomal breaks per cell was also similar between the groups. Chromosomal changes analysed by FISH also showed no significant differences. [The Working Group noted the very high levels of butadiene-derived metabolites in the urine of controls.]

A Health Effects Institute Report summarized the study of workers in the Czech Republic (Albertini et al., 2003a). The conclusions on the genotoxicity studies were that 'none of these measures showed positive responses at exposure levels encountered in this study'. *HPRT* mutations analysed by cloning or autoradiographic techniques showed no effect of butadiene, and mutation spectra were not significantly different between exposed and unexposed workers. *HPRT* mutation frequencies were also unrelated to the metabolic genotypes examined. When smoking status was considered, there was no significant effect of smoking and no significant exposure group-by-smoking interaction on *HPRT* mutation frequencies. Chromosomal aberrations analysed by traditional or FISH methods and sister chromatid exchange were also unaffected by exposure to butadiene. The results of the study by Šrám *et al.* (1998) were in conflict with these conclusions and showed increased chromosomal aberrations.

Further molecular epidemiological analysis of butadiene-exposed workers in the Czech Republic was conducted to determine whether any gender differences in the response to butadiene existed (Albertini *et al.*, 2007). The average level of exposure to butadiene (mg/m^3) was 0.397 ± 0.502 (mean ± SD) [0.18 ppm] for the 23 women and 0.808 ± 1.646 [0.37 ppm] for the 30 men. Thus, exposed male workers had a significantly higher level of exposure than female workers in this study. It should be noted that exposed male workers also had higher levels of exposure to styrene than female workers and that exposed female workers had higher levels of exposure to toluene and benzene than the exposed male workers. Although urinary concentrations of the mercapturic acid metabolites of butadiene, DHBMA and MHBMA, were higher in butadiene-exposed women than in female controls, the differences were not significant. The levels of both DHBMA and MHBMA (μg/L) were significantly increased in male butadiene-exposed subjects (854.1 ± 567.0 and 47.9 ± 44.3, respectively) compared with male controls (512.8 ± 272.1 and 14.9 ± 10.3, respectively; $p < 0.05$). Thus, significantly higher concentrations of metabolites occurred in men than in women in both the control and exposed groups. *HPRT* mutations measured by the T-cell assay did not differ significantly between exposed and control groups of either sex. No significant associations between exposure to butadiene and sister chromatid exchange or chromosomal aberrations were detected in either sex. Effects of genotype were also examined. In this study, *GSTT1*-null workers showed a significantly slower rise in the rate of MHBMA excretion ($p < 0.05$). In addition, individuals with the EH genotype that specifies low activity showed a significantly higher rise in urinary MHBMA/(DHBMA + MHBMA) ratios with increasing exposure to butadiene.

Zhang *et al.* (2004) measured chromosomal changes in the peripheral blood lymphocytes of 39 butadiene polymer production workers and 38 unexposed controls in Yanshan, China. The median exposure level for the butadiene-exposed workers as a 6-h TWA was 2 ppm [4.42 mg/m^3] whereas the control group had a median level of 0 ppm. Tobacco use was controlled for by including a similar percentage of smokers with similar pack–years of smoking in both the control and exposed groups. No significant numerical or structural chromosomal changes were detected using FISH with probes for chromosomes 1, 7, 8 or 12. *GSTT1* and *GSTM1* genotypes had no significant effect on the frequency of hyperdiploidy of the above chromosomes or on the frequency of structural changes of chromosomes 8 and 12 in the butadiene-exposed group. The EH *EPHX1* Y113H polymorphism had no effect on chromosomal damage or *HPRT* mutant frequency in either the exposed or control workers. However, workers with the histidine arginine HR or RR allele of the *EPHX1* H139R polymorphism had increased levels of hyperdiploidy of chromosomes 1, 7 and 8. Overall, predicted EPHX1 activity did not influence genetic damage at low occupational exposures to butadiene. Further analysis at this plant of 41 workers exposed to the same median levels of butadiene (2 ppm) and 38 controls was undertaken (Hayes *et al.*, 2001). No differences were observed in the Glycophorin A assay between the exposed workers and the controls. The mutation frequency of *HPRT* measured with the T-cell cloning assay was also not significantly different and no significant increase was detected in sister chromatid exchange frequency.

Another study at a tyre plant in the Slovak Republic examined 110 workers, who were exposed to several xenobiotics of which butadiene was the most prominent, for markers of genotoxicity in relation to several polymorphisms (Vodicka *et al.*, 2004). The workers were divided into three groups: high exposure (butadiene concentration, 2.6 ± 0.2 mg/m^3 [1.18 ppm]), low exposure (butadiene concentration, 2.3 ± 2.2 mg/m^3 [1.04 ppm]) and no exposure (trace amounts). The frequencies of total chromosomal aberrations were significantly lower (1.3 ± 1.3; $p < 0.01$) in the low-exposure group compared with the high- and no-exposure groups (2.2 ± 1.4 and 2.3 ± 1.1, respectively). No significant differences were observed in DNA single-strand breaks or in single-strand break endo III-sensitive site frequencies. A non-significant twofold higher rate of DNA repair was found in the high-exposure group (0.6 ± 0.6 single-strand breaks/10^9 daltons) compared with the low- and no-exposure groups (0.3 ± 0.3 and 0.3 ± 0.4 single-strand breaks/10^9 daltons, respectively). A weak but non-significant association was found between CYP2E1 expression in peripheral blood lymphocytes and the frequency of chromosomal aberrations ($r = 0.298$; $p = 0.097$). In all individuals, assessment of several genetic polymorphisms suggested that individuals who had low *EPHX1*-activity genotypes had the highest level of chromosomal aberrations. Significantly lower frequencies of chromosomal aberration ($p = 0.024$) were detected in individuals who had the variant CC genotype associated with the XPD exon 23.

A study of 27 healthy male Caucasian workers exposed to butadiene and 26 matched controls from an Italian petrochemical plant analysed genotoxic effects (Lovreglio *et al.*, 2006). The mean exposure to butadiene was 6.4 ± 14.0 µg/m^3 [0.003 ppm] for the butadiene-exposed workers which was significantly different from that of the controls (0.8 ± 1.1 µg/m^3 [0.0004 ppm]; $p < 0.001$). No significant differences were observed in sister chromatid exchange, the percentage of cells with a high frequency of sister chromatid exchange, chromosomal aberrations or proliferation index in the peripheral blood lymphocytes of these two groups. When subjects were classified according to smoking status, a significant increase was observed in the mean frequency of sister chromatid exchange in smokers (6.6 ± 1.2) compared with nonsmokers (5.5 ± 0.8; $p = 0.001$). Exposure to butadiene was also higher in smokers than in nonsmokers but this was not statistically significant ($p = 0.3$).

4.2.2   *Experimental systems*

(a)   *Butadiene* (see Table 26 for details and references)

The genotoxicity of butadiene has been reviewed previously (IARC, 1999).

The frequency of DNA single-strand breaks was increased in NMRI mice exposed to butadiene *in vivo*.

Decreases in cloning efficiency of T cells and a significant increase in *Hprt* mutation frequency was observed in female B6C3F$_1$ mice exposed to 3 ppm [6.63 mg/m^3] butadiene for 2 weeks and in rats exposed to 62.5 ppm [138.1 mg/m^3] butadiene for 2 weeks; these are the currently reported lowest-observed-effect levels for butadiene that induced *Hprt* mutations in mice and rats, respectively. The *Hprt* mutation frequency was also increased in *Ephx*-1 null and *Xpc* (DNA repair enzyme) null mice exposed to butadiene for 4 weeks compared with normal mice.

Characterization of *Hprt* mutations in cDNA and genomic DNA from splenic T-cell mutants was carried out in male B6C3F$_1$ mice and Fischer 344 rats. The mean *Hprt* mutant frequency in mice was $9.20 \pm 3.25 \times 10^{-6}$ in the butadiene-exposed animals compared with $1.48 \pm 0.84 \times 10^{-6}$ ($p < 0.001$) in the controls. In rats, the mean *Hprt* mutant frequency in the exposed animals was $8.08 \pm 2.82 \times 10^{-6}$ compared with $3.07 \pm 0.98 \times 10^{-6}$ ($p < 0.001$) in the controls. In mice, real time PCR and cDNA sequencing showed a statistically significant difference in the overall proportion of mutation types detected in control versus butadiene-exposed mice ($p = 0.042$), while multiplex PCR of genomic DNA showed that deletion mutations were significantly increased in butadiene-exposed mice ($p = 0.031$). Analysis of the individual mutation types that occurred in both treated and control mice showed that exposure to butadiene significantly increased the frequencies of each type of base substitution, except for A:T→G:C transitions, and frameshifts and deletions. In male rats, no difference in the overall mutational spectra was detected using cDNA sequencing alone or when combined with multiplex PCR. Statistical analyses of the individual mutation types showed that exposure to butadiene significantly increased base substitution at A:T→T:A transversions in both mice and rats, and single-base insertions, deletion mutations and complex mutations as well as G:C→C:G transversions in mice.

In the bone marrow of B6C3F$_1$ *LacI* transgenic mice exposed to butadiene, a significant increase in point mutations was observed at A:T base pairs compared with air-exposed mice. In the spleen of the exposed mice, a significant increase in base substitution mutations (GC→AT transitions and GC→TA transversions at non-CpG sites) was detected, and a significant increase in A:T base pairs occurred, similar to that observed in the bone marrow.

Micronucleus formation was increased in NMRI mice and male and female B6C3F$_1$/CrBR mice exposed to butadiene. Male B6C3F$_1$ mice were exposed to butadiene and the bone marrow was harvested 24 h after onset of exposure (Jackson *et al.*, 2000). The frequencies of micronucleated polychromatic erythrocytes were significantly increased ($28.2 \pm 3.1/100$ cells; $p < 0.05$) compared with controls ($9.87 \pm 2.1/100$ cells) as

Table 26. Genetic and related effects of butadiene

Test system	Result[a] Without exogenous metabolic system	Result[a] With exogenous metabolic system	Dose[b] (LED or HID)	Reference
Salmonella typhimurium TA100, reverse mutation	–	+	1080 ppm	Araki *et al.* (1994)
Salmonella typhimurium TA1530, reverse mutation	–	+	86 ppm	de Meester *et al.* (1980)
Salmonella typhimurium TA1535, reverse mutation	–	+	216 ppm	Araki *et al.* (1994)
Salmonella typhimurium TA1537, TA98, reverse mutation	–	–	1080 ppm	Araki *et al.* (1994)
Escherichia coli WP2 *uvrA*, reverse mutation	–	–	1080 ppm	Araki *et al.* (1994)
Drosophila melanogaster, somatic mutation or recombination	–		10 000 ppm inh	Victorin *et al.* (1990)
Drosophila melanogaster, sex-linked recessive lethal mutation	–		500 ppm inh	Foureman *et al.* (1994)
DNA single-strand breaks, NMRI mouse alveolar macrophages *in vitro*	–	NT	40 ppm	Walles *et al.* (1995)
Gene mutation, mouse lymphoma L5178Y cells, *Tk* locus *in vitro*	–	–	650 ppm	McGregor *et al.* (1991)
Sister chromatid exchange, Chinese hamster ovary cells *in vitro*	–	(+)	1.35	Sasiadek *et al.* (1991a)
Sister chromatid exchange, human lymphocytes *in vitro*	+	+	108	Sasiadek *et al.* (1991b)
Binucleated cells, human bronchial epithelial cells *in vitro*	+	NT	25 µg as soot/mL medium	Catallo *et al.* (2001)
DNA cross-links, B6C3F₁ mouse liver *in vivo*	+		450 ppm inh 7 h	Jelitto *et al.* (1989)
DNA cross-links, B6C3F₁ mouse liver *in vivo*	–		2070 ppm inh 8 h/d, 7 d	Ristau *et al.* (1990)
DNA cross-links, B6C3F₁ mouse lung and liver *in vivo*	+		250 ppm inh 7 h	Vangala *et al.* (1993)
DNA single-strand breaks, B6C3F₁ mouse liver *in vivo*	+		2000 ppm inh 7 h/d, 7 d	Vangala *et al.* (1993)
DNA single-strand breaks, NMRI mouse lung and liver *in vivo*	+		200 ppm inh 16 h	Walles *et al.* (1995)
DNA strand breaks, CD-1 mouse liver, bone marrow or testis *in vivo*	–		130 ppm inh 6 h/d, 4 wk	Anderson *et al.* (1997)
DNA damage, CD-1 mouse testicular cells *in vivo*	+		125 ppm inh 6 h	Brinkworth *et al.* (1998)
DNA single-strand breaks and γ-irradiation-specific DNA repair activity, NMRI mice *in vivo*	+		500 mg/m³ 6 h/d, 28 d	Vodicka *et al.* (2006)
DNA cross-links, Sprague-Dawley rat liver *in vivo*	–		550 ppm inh 7 h	Jelitto *et al.* (1989)
DNA cross-links, Sprague-Dawley rat liver *in vivo*	–		1240 ppm inh 8 h/d, 7 d	Ristau *et al.* (1990)
DNA cross-links, Sprague-Dawley rat liver and lung *in vivo*	–		2000 ppm inh 7 h	Vangala *et al.* (1993)
DNA single-strand breaks, Sprague-Dawley rat liver *in vivo*	+		2000 ppm inh 7 h/d, 7 d	Vangala *et al.* (1993)

Table 26 (contd)

Test system	Result[a] Without exogenous metabolic system	Result[a] With exogenous metabolic system	Dose[b] (LED or HID)	Reference
Gene mutation, *lacZ* mouse bone marrow *in vivo*	+		625 ppm inh 6 h/d, 5 d/wk, 1 wk	Recio et al. (1992)
Gene mutation, B6C3F₁ mouse T lymphocytes, *Hprt* locus *in vivo*	+		625 ppm inh 6 h/d, 5 d/wk, 4 wk	Cochrane & Skopek (1993)
Gene mutation, B6C3F₁ mouse T lymphocytes, *Hprt* locus *in vivo*	+		625 ppm inh 6 h/d, 5 d/wk, 2 wk	Cochrane & Skopek (1994)
Gene mutation, *LacI* mice *in vivo*	+		62.5 ppm inh 6 h/d, 5 d/wk, 4 wk	Sisk et al. (1994)
Gene mutation, B6C3F₁ mouse T lymphocytes, *Hprt* locus *in vivo*	+		1300 ppm inh 6 h/d, 5 d/wk, 1 wk	Tates et al. (1994)
Gene mutation, *LacI* mice *in vivo*	+		1250 ppm inh 6 h/d, 5 d/wk, 4 wk	Recio & Meyer (1995)
Gene mutation, (102/E1 × C3H/E1)F₁ mouse splenocytes, *Hprt* locus *in vivo*	+		500 ppm inh 6 h/d, 5 d	Tates et al. (1998)
Gene mutation, CD-1 mouse splenocytes, *Hprt* locus *in vivo*	–		1300 ppm inh 6 h/d, 5 d/wk, 4 wk	Tates et al. (1998)
Gene mutation, female B6C3F₁ mice, *Hprt* locus *in vivo*	+		20 ppm 6 h/d, 5 d/wk, 2 wk	Meng et al. (1999a)
Gene mutation, female B6C3F₁ mouse thymic and splenic T cells, *Hprt* locus *in vivo*	+		20 ppm 6 h/d, 5 d/wk, 2 wk	Walker & Meng (2000)
Gene mutation, female Fischer 344 rats, *Hprt* locus *in vivo*	(+)		625 ppm 6 h/d, 5 d/wk, 4 wk	Walker & Meng (2000)
Gene mutation, female B6C3F₁ mice, *Hprt* locus *in vivo*	+		3 ppm 6 h/d, 5 d/wk, 2 wk	Meng et al. (2001)
Gene mutation, male B6C3F₁ mice and Fischer 344 rats, *Hprt* locus *in vivo*	+		1250 ppm 6 h/d, 5 d/wk, 2 wk	Meng et al. (2004)

Table 26 (contd)

Test system	Result[a]		Dose[b] (LED or HID)	Reference
	Without exogenous metabolic system	With exogenous metabolic system		
Gene mutation, B6C3F₁ *LacI* transgenic mice *in vivo*	+		625 ppm 6 h/d, 5 d/wk, 4 wk	Recio *et al.* (2001)
Gene mutation, B6C3F₁ mice, *Znfn1a1/Ikaros* gene *in vivo*	(+)		NG	Karlsson *et al.* (2002)
Gene mutation, *Ephx1*-plus mice, *Hprt* locus *in vivo*	(+)		20 ppm 7 h/d, 5 d/wk, 4 wk	Wickliffe *et al.* (2003, 2007)
Gene mutation, *Ephx1*-null mice, *Hprt* locus *in vivo*	+		20 ppm 7 h/d, 5 d/wk, 4 wk	Wickliffe *et al.* (2003, 2007)
Gene mutation, *Xpc*-plus mice, *Hprt* locus *in vivo*	(+)		20 ppm 7 h/d, 5 d/wk, 4 wk	Wickliffe *et al.* (2007)
Gene mutation, *Xpc*-null mice, *Hprt* locus *in vivo*	+		20 ppm 7 h/d, 5 d/wk, 4 wk	Wickliffe *et al.* (2007)
Gene mutation, male B6C3F₁ mice and female Fischer 344 rats, *Hprt* locus *in vivo*	+		1250 ppm 6 h/d, 5 d/wk, 2 wk	Meng *et al.* (2007a)
Gene mutation, female Fischer 344 rats, *Hprt* locus *in vivo*	(+)		62.5 ppm 6 h/d, 5 d/wk, 2 wk	Meng *et al.* (2007a)
Mouse spot test, female T-stock mice	+		500 ppm inh 6 h/d, 5 d/wk, 1 wk	Adler *et al.* (1994)
Sister chromatid exchange, B6C3F₁ mouse bone marrow *in vivo*	+		116 ppm inh 6 h	Cunningham *et al.* (1986)
Sister chromatid exchange, Sprague-Dawley rat bone marrow	−		4000 ppm inh 6 h	Cunningham *et al.* (1986)
Sister chromatid exchange, B6C3F₁ mouse bone marrow *in vivo*	+		7 ppm inh 6 h/d, 5 d/wk, 2 wk	Tice *et al.* (1987)
Micronucleus formation, B6C3F₁ mouse bone marrow *in vivo*	+		116 ppm inh 6 h	Cunningham *et al.* (1986)
Micronucleus formation, B6C3F₁ mouse peripheral blood *in vivo*	+		70 ppm inh 6 h/d, 5 d/wk, 2 wk	Tice *et al.* (1987)

Table 26 (contd)

Test system	Result[a]		Dose[b] (LED or HID)	Reference
	Without exogenous metabolic system	With exogenous metabolic system		
Micronucleus formation, B6C3F₁ mouse peripheral blood *in vivo*	+		7 ppm inh 6 h/d, 5 d/wk, 13 wk	Jauhar *et al.* (1988)
Micronucleus formation, NMRI mouse bone marrow *in vivo*	+		35 ppm inh 23 h	Victorin *et al.* (1990)
Micronucleus formation, (102/E1 × C3H/E1)F₁ and CB6F₁ mice *in vivo*	+		50 ppm inh 6 h/d, 5 d/wk	Adler *et al.* (1994); Autio *et al.* (1994)
Micronucleus formation, (102 × C3H) mice *in vivo*	+		200 ppm inh 6 h/d, 5 d/wk	Xiao & Tates (1995)
Micronucleus formation, (102/E1 × C3H/E1)F₁ mouse splenocytes *in vivo*	+		130 ppm inh 6 h/d, 5 d	Stephanou *et al.* (1998)
Micronucleus formation (102/E1 × C3H/E1)F₁ mouse spermatids *in vivo*	+		250 ppm inh 6 h/d, 5 d	Tommasi *et al.* (1998)
Micronucleus formation, male B6C3F₁ mice *in vivo*	+	NT	1100 ppm initial concentration 4 h	Jackson *et al.* (2000)
Micronucleus formation, male and female (102/E1 × C3H/EI)F₁ mouse primary lung fibroblasts *in vivo*	+	NT	500 ppm 6 h/d, 5 d	Ranaldi *et al.* (2001)
Micronucleus formation, male and female B6C3F₁/CrBR mice *in vivo*	+	NT	1000 ppm 6 h/d, 2 d	Bevan *et al.* (2001)
Micronucleus formation, NMRI mice *in vivo*	+	NT	500 mg/m³ 6 h/d, 28 d	Vodicka *et al.* (2006)
Micronucleus formation, Sprague-Dawley rat bone marrow *in vivo*	−		4000 ppm inh 6 h/d, 2 d	Cunningham *et al.* (1986)
Micronucleus formation, Sprague-Dawley rats *in vivo*	−		500 ppm 6 h/d, 5 d/wk	Autio *et al.* (1994)
Chromosomal aberrations, B6C3F₁, and NIH mouse bone marrow *in vivo*	+		1500 ppm inh 6 h	Irons *et al.* (1987b)
Chromosomal aberrations, B6C3F₁, mouse bone marrow *in vivo*	+		700 ppm inh 6 h/d, 5 d/wk, 2 wk	Tice *et al.* (1987)
Chromosomal aberrations, (102/E1 × C3H/E1)F₁ mouse embryos *in vivo*	+		130 ppm inh 6 h/d, 5 d	Pachierotti *et al.* (1998)
Aneuploidy, B6C3F₁ and NIH mouse bone marrow *in vivo*	−		1500 ppm inh 6 h	Irons *et al.* (1987b)

Table 26 (contd)

Test system	Result[a]		Dose[b] (LED or HID)	Reference
	Without exogenous metabolic system	With exogenous metabolic system		
Dominant lethal test, male CD-1 mice	+		233 ppm inh 6 h/d, 5 d/wk, 1 wk	Morrissey et al. (1990)
Dominant lethal test, CD-1 mice	+		1250 ppm inh 6 h/d, 5 d/wk, 10 wk	Anderson et al. (1993)
Dominant lethal test, CD-1 mice	–		6250 ppm inh 6 h	Anderson et al. (1993)
Dominant lethal test, (102/E1 × C3H/E1)F$_1$ mice	+		1300 ppm inh 6 h/d, 5 d/wk, 1 wk	Adler et al. (1994)
Dominant lethal test, (102/E1 × C3H/E1)F$_1$ mice	+		500 ppm inh 6 h/d, 5 d	Adler et al. (1998)
Dominant lethal test, CD-1 mice	+		65 ppm inh 6 h/d, 5 d/wk, 4 wk	Anderson et al. (1998)
Dominant lethal test, CD-1 mice	+		125 ppm inh 6 h/d, 5 d/wk, 10 wk	Brinkworth et al. (1998)
Dominant lethal test, Sprague-Dawley rats	–		1250 ppm inh 6 h/d, 5 d/wk, 10 wk	Anderson et al. (1998)
Mouse (C3H/E1) heritable translocation test	+		1300 ppm inh 6 h/d, 5 d/wk, 1 wk	Adler et al. (1995)
Mouse (102/E1 × C3H/E1)F$_1$ heritable translocation test	+		500 ppm inh 6 h/d, 5 d	Adler et al. (1998)
Binding to DNA, male B6C3F$_1$ mouse and male Wistar rat liver in vivo	+		13 ppm inh 4–6.6 h	Kreiling et al. (1986a)
Binding to DNA at N7 of guanine, male B6C3F$_1$ mouse liver in vivo	+		450 ppm inh 7 h	Jelitto et al. (1989)
Binding to DNA at N7 of guanine, male B6C3F$_1$ mouse liver in vivo	+		NG	Bolt & Jelitto (1996)
Binding to DNA at N^6 of adenine, mouse lung in vivo	+		200 ppm inh 6 h/d, 5 d/wk, 1 wk	Koivisto et al. (1996)

Table 26 (contd)

Test system	Result[a]		Dose[b] (LED or HID)	Reference
	Without exogenous metabolic system	With exogenous metabolic system		
Binding to DNA at N7 of guanine, mouse testis and lung *in vivo*	+		200 ppm 6 h/d, 5 d	Koivisto et al. (1998)
Binding to DNA at N7 of guanine, male Wistar rat liver *in vivo*	–		550 ppm inh 7 h	Jelitto et al. (1989)
Binding to DNA at N7 of guanine, male Wistar rat liver *in vivo*	–		NG	Bolt & Jelitto (1996)
Binding to DNA at N6 of adenine, rat lung *in vivo*	+		200 ppm inh 6 h/d, 5 d/wk, 1 wk	Koivisto et al. (1996)
Binding to DNA at N7 of guanine, male Sprague-Dawley rat liver *in vivo*	+		200 ppm inh 6 h/d, 5 d/wk, 1 wk	Koivisto et al. (1997)
Binding to protein, male B6C3F1 mouse and male Wistar rat liver *in vivo*	+		13 ppm inh 4–6.6 h	Kreiling et al. (1986a)
Sperm morphology, CD-1 mice *in vivo*	+		1165 ppm inh 6 h/d, 5 d/wk, 1 wk	Morrissey et al. (1990)

[a] +, positive; –, negative; (+), weakly positive; NT, not tested; NG, not given
[b] LED, lowest effective dose; HID, highest ineffective dose; d, day; inh, inhalation exposure; wk, week

determined by acridine orange staining. Two other methods to determine micronucleus frequency also showed similar results.

The contribution of CYP2E1 to the genotoxicity of butadiene was investigated by pretreating animals with 1,2-*trans*-dichloroethylene, a selective CYP2E1 inhibitor, and 1-aminobenzotriazole, an irreversible inhibitor of several CYPs, before exposure to butadiene (Jackson *et al.*, 2000). Pretreatment with 1,2-*trans*-dichloroethylene significantly lowered the micronucleus frequencies observed (19.8 ± 2.5) but the levels were still elevated over those in unexposed controls (11.5 ± 2.0). Pretreatment with 1-aminobenzotriazole caused the micronucleus frequency to fall to a level similar to that in unexposed animals. The frequency of kinetochore-negative micronuclei was also significantly increased in butadiene-exposed animals (21.3 ± 1.2) compared with controls (5.2 ± 1.7), indicating that butadiene is a clastogen.

(b)   Butadiene metabolites

(i)   *Epoxybutene* (see Table 27 for details and references)

Epoxybutene is mutagenic in *Salmonella typhimurium* in the presence and absence of a metabolic activation system.

The cII mutant frequency was increased only in Big Blue™ mice but not rat fibroblasts *in vitro*. The in-vitro mutational spectrum induced by epoxybutene (1 mM for 24 h) in Rat2 *LacI* cells was compared with a background spectrum. Significant increases in GC→AT transitions at non-CpG sites as well as GC→TA transversions (32% of the epoxybutene-induced mutations) were observed. At A:T base pairs, a significant increase was observed in AT→CG and AT→TA transversions.

Epoxybutene increased micronucleus formation in both Big Blue rat and mouse fibroblasts.

In a human B-lymphoblastoid cell line that does not express active CYP2E1, the mutational spectrum at *HPRT* induced by epoxybutene showed a significant increase in G:C→A:T and A:T→T:A mutations. The 2*S*-stereoisomer increased the *HPRT* mutation frequency in human lymphoblastoid TK6 cells whereas the 2*R*-isomer caused significant increases at higher doses only.

Mean frequencies of sister chromatid exchange were significantly increased in human whole blood lymphocyte cultures by epoxybutene in both the *GSTM1*-null ($p < 0.001$) and *GSTM1*-positive ($p = 0.03$) genotypes compared with unexposed controls.

The effect of *GSTM1* genotype as well as an adaptive dose of epoxybutene on the induction of sister chromatid exchange was examined. Without an adaptive dose, both genotypes showed a significant increase in sister chromatid exchange over controls. With the adaptive dose, the mean number of sister chromatid exchanges was significantly higher following exposure to epoxybutene in the *GSTM1*-null group (17.42 ± 2.43; $p = 0.01$) than in the control group (7.69 ± 1.00) or the *GSTM1*-positive group (14.07 ± 4.22). The results show an increased sensitivity of *GSTM1*-null subjects to the induction of sister chromatid exchange by epoxybutene.

Table 27. Genetic and related effects of epoxybutene

Test system	Result[a]		Dose[b] (LED or HID)	Reference
	Without exogenous metabolic system	With exogenous metabolic system		
Salmonella typhimurium TA100, TA1535, TA98, TA97a, reverse mutation	+	+	2–10 mM	Himmelstein *et al.* (2001)
Gene mutation, Big Blue™ mouse fibroblasts, cII locus *in vitro*	+		125 µM	Erexson & Tindall (2000a)
Gene mutation, Rat2 *LacI* transgenic fibroblasts, *LacI* locus *in vitro*	+		0.6 mM	Saranko *et al.* (1998); Recio *et al.* (2000)
Gene mutation, Big Blue™ rat fibroblasts, cII locus *in vitro*	(+)		500 µM	Erexson & Tindall (2000a)
Sister chromatid exchange, male CD-1 mouse and male CD rat splenic lymphocytes at G0 stage in the cell cycle *in vitro*	–		931 µM	Kligerman *et al.* (1999a,b)
Micronucleus formation, Big Blue™ mouse and rat fibroblasts *in vitro*	(+)		125 µM	Erexson & Tindall (2000a)
Micronuclei formation, Chinese hamster V79 cells *in vitro*	+		1 mM	Himmelstein *et al.* (2001)
Gene mutation, human lymphoblastoid TK6 cells, *HPRT* locus *in vitro*	+		400 µM for 24 h	Recio *et al.* (2000)
Gene mutation, human lymphoblastoid TK6 cells, *HPRT* and *TK* loci *in vitro*	+		400 µM 2S- or 2R-isomer for 24 h	Meng *et al.* (2007b)
Gene mutation, human lymphoblastoid TK6 cells, *HPRT* locus *in vitro*	+		400 µM 2R-isomer for 24 h	Meng *et al.* (2007b)
Gene mutation, human lymphoblastoid TK6 cells, *HPRT* locus *in vitro*	+		200 µM 2S-isomer for 24 h	Meng *et al.* (2007b)
Sister chromatid exchange, human whole blood at G0 stage in the cell cycle *in vitro*	–		931 µM	Kligerman *et al.* (1999a,b)
Sister chromatid exchange, human whole blood lymphocytes, *GSTM1*–, *GSTM1*+ *in vitro*	+		25 µM for 24 h	Sąsiadek *et al.* (1999)
Micronucleus formation, human lymphocytes *in vitro*	–		300 µM	Murg *et al.* (1999a)

Table 27 (contd)

Test system	Result[a] Without exogenous metabolic system	With exogenous metabolic system	Dose[b] (LED or HID)	Reference
Chromosomal aberrations, human peripheral blood lymphocytes treated with ara-C *in vitro*	+		931 μM	Kligerman *et al.* (1999b)
Hyperdiploidy and chromosomal breakage (1cen-q12 region), human lymphocytes *in vitro*	–		300 μM	Murg *et al.* (1999a)
Inhibition of IL-2 production, human CD4+ lymphocytes *in vitro*	–		10 μM	Irons *et al.* (2001)
Inhibition of clonogenic activity, human CD34+ bone marrow cells *in vitro*	–		1 mM	Irons *et al.* (2000)
Inhibition of clonogenic activity, human CD34+ bone marrow cells *in vitro*	–		100 μM	Irons *et al.* (2001)
Gene mutation, female B6C3F1 mouse splenic T cells, *Hprt* locus *in vivo*	+		2.5 ppm 6 h/d, 5 d/wk, 4 wk	Meng *et al.* (1999b)
Gene mutation, female Fischer 344 rats splenic T cells, *Hprt* locus *in vivo*	–		25 ppm 6 h/d, 5 d/wk, 4 wk	Meng *et al.* (1999b)
Gene mutation, female B6C3F1 *LacI* transgenic mouse spleen and bone marrow *in vivo*	–		29.9 ppm 6 h/d, 5 d/wk, 2 wk	Recio *et al.* (2000, 2001); Saranko *et al.* (2001)
Gene mutation, female B6C3F1 *LacI* transgenic mouse lung *in vivo*	(+)		29.9 ppm 6 h/d, 5 d/wk, 2 wk	Recio *et al.* (2000, 2001); Saranko *et al.* (2001)
Gene mutation, female Fischer 344 *LacI* transgenic rat spleen *in vivo*	–		29.9 ppm 6 h/d, 5 d/wk, 2 wk	Recio *et al.* (2000)
Gene mutation, female Fischer 344 *LacI* transgenic rat bone marrow *in vivo*	(+)		29.9 ppm 6 h/d, 5 d/wk, 2 wk	Recio *et al.* (2000)
Gene mutation, female B6C3F1 mouse splenic T cells, *Hprt* locus *in vivo*	+		2.5 ppm 6 h/d, 5 d/wk, 4 wk	Walker & Meng (2000)

Table 27 (contd)

Test system	Result[a]		Dose[b] (LED or HID)	Reference
	Without exogenous metabolic system	With exogenous metabolic system		
Gene mutation, female Fischer 344 rat splenic T cells, *Hprt* locus *in vivo*	–		2.5 ppm 6 h/d, 5 d/wk, 4 wk	Walker & Meng (2000)
Gene mutation, *Ephx1*-plus mice, *Hprt* locus *in vivo*	–		80 mg/kg/48 h × 3	Wickliffe *et al.* (2007)
Gene mutation, *Ephx1*-null mice, *Hprt* locus *in vivo*	+		80 mg/kg/48 h × 3	Wickliffe *et al.* (2007)
Gene mutation, *Xpc*-plus mice, *Hprt* locus *in vivo*	–		100 mg/kg/48 h × 3	Wickliffe *et al.* (2007)
Gene mutation, *Xpc*-null mice, *Hprt* locus *in vivo*	+		100 mg/kg/48 h × 3	Wickliffe *et al.* (2007)
Gene mutation, *Xpc* –/– mice, *Hprt* locus *in vivo*	+		150 mg/kg	Wickliffe *et al.* (2006)
Micronucleus formation, male C57/BL mouse polychromatic erythrocytes *in vivo*	+		250 µmol/kg	Fred *et al.* (2005)
Micronucleus formation, male Sprague-Dawley rat polychromatic erythrocytes *in vivo*	–		1125 µmol/kg	Fred *et al.* (2005)

IL, interleukin
[a] +, positive; –, negative; (+), weak positive; NT, not tested
[b] LED, lowest effective dose; HID, highest ineffective dose; d, day; wk, week

Epoxybutene did not induce sister chromatid exchange or chromosomal aberrations in human blood lymphocytes when added at the G_0 stage of the cell cycle. However, from further studies in which excision repair was inhibited, it is probable that epoxybutene induces chromosomal aberrations and DNA damage that is repaired by the excision process in G_0 lymphocytes (Kligerman *et al.*, 1999a,b).

In vivo, a significant increase in mutation frequency was observed at the *Hprt* locus in splenic T cells from female $B6C3F_1$ mice exposed to epoxybutene. Exposure to epoxy-butene by inhalation resulted in an approximately threefold increase in the frequency of *LacI* mutants in the lungs of female $B6C3F_1$ *LacI* transgenic mice ($8.3 \pm 3.0 \times 10^{-5}$ and $9.9 \pm 3.0 \times 10^{-5}$) compared with air-exposed controls ($3.1 \pm 0.7 \times 10^{-5}$ and $3.6 \pm 0.7 \times 10^{-5}$). Significant increases in GC→AT transitions at CpG sites ($p = 0.001$) were detected. A number of other alterations (insertions, deletions and tandem changes) were also increased in the lungs of exposed mice (10/54, 10%) compared with controls (2/59, 4%). When these alterations were considered separately, only the frequency of deletions was significantly increased ($p = 0.005$).

(ii)   *Epoxybutanediol* (see also Table 28 for details and references)

Epoxybutanediol has the least mutagenic potency of the butadiene epoxides in traditional mutagenic assays.

Epoxybutanediol increased cII mutant frequency in Big Blue™ mouse but not rat fibroblasts.

Mutational spectra of epoxybutanediol were obtained in the *Hprt* locus in Chinese hamster ovary-K1 cells. Of the 41 mutants analysed, 25 (61%) were base substitutions and 16 (39%) were deletions. The most common base substitutions were GC→AT and AT→GC transitions. Among the deletions, the majority of the mutants showed single exon loss.

Epoxybutanediol increased micronucleus formation in Big Blue™ rat fibroblasts *in vitro*. The same effect was seen in Big Blue™ mouse fibroblasts only at higher concentrations.

Epoxybutanediol weakly suppressed the haematopoietic progenitor clonogenic response in human $CD34^+$ bone-marrow cells.

(iii)   *Diepoxybutane* (see also Table 29 for details and references)

Diepoxybutane has been shown to be the most mutagenic of the butadiene epoxides in traditional mutagenicity assays.

Diepoxybutane is mutagenic in *S. typhimurium*, *Escherichia coli* and *Sulfolobus acidocaldarius* in the presence and absence of a metabolic activation system.

Thirty-nine diepoxybutane mutants were analysed in Chinese hamster ovary-K1 cells. Of these, 24 (62%) were base substitutions and 15 (38%) were deletions. The major base substitutions were GC→AT transitions (11/24) and AT→TA (5/24) and GC→CG (6/24) transversions. Among the deletions, the majority of the mutants showed single exon loss.

Table 28. Genetic and related effects of epoxybutanediol

Test system	Result[a]		Dose[b] (LED or HID)	Reference
	Without exogenous metabolic system	With exogenous metabolic system		
Gene mutation, Big Blue™ mouse fibroblasts, cII locus in vitro	+	NT	1000 μM	Erexson & Tindall (2000a)
Gene mutation, Big Blue™ rat fibroblasts, cII locus in vitro	–	NT	1000 μM	Erexson & Tindall (2000a)
Gene mutation, Chinese hamster ovary CHO-K1 cells, Hprt locus in vitro	+	NT	2 mM	Lee et al. (2002)
Micronucleus formation, Big Blue™ mouse fibroblasts in vitro	+	NT	500 μM	Erexson & Tindall (2000a)
Micronucleus formation, Big Blue™ rat fibroblasts in vitro	+	NT	250 μM	Erexson & Tindall (2000a)
Inhibition of IL-2 production, human CD4+ lymphocytes in vitro	–	NT	10 μM	Irons et al. (2001)
Inhibition of clonogenic activity, human CD34+ bone-marrow cells in vitro	–	NT	10^{-3} M	Irons et al. (2000)
Inhibition of clonogenic activity, human CD34+ bone-marrow cells in vitro	(+)	NT	100 μM	Irons et al. (2001)

IL, interleukin
[a] +, positive; –, negative; (+), weak positive; NT, not tested
[b] LED, lowest effective dose; HID, highest ineffective dose

Table 29. Genetic and related effects of diepoxybutane

Test system	Result[a]		Dose[b] (LED or HID)	Reference
	Without exogenous metabolic system	With exogenous metabolic system		
Escherichia coli TRG8, his+ revertants, + human O^6-alkylguanine-DNA alkyltransferase	+	NT	1 mM	Valadez *et al.* (2004)
Salmonella typhimurium YG7108, his+ revertants, + human O^6-alkylguanine-DNA alkyltransferase	+	NT	1 mM	Valadez *et al.* (2004)
Escherichia coli KL185, RC50, G1209, reverse mutation or genetic recombination	+	NT	5–300 µg/mL	Reilly & Grogan (2002)
Escherichia coli MBL50 cells, *supF* mutant frequency	+	NT	40 µM all isomers	Kim *et al.* (2007)
Salmonella typhimurium T100, TA97a, reverse mutation	–	–	10 mM	Himmelstein *et al.* (2001)
Salmonella typhimurium TA1535, TA98, reverse mutation	+	+	0.2 mM	Himmelstein *et al.* (2001)
Sulfolobus acidocaldarius DG29, DG38, DG64, reverse or forward mutation	+	NT	5–300 µg/mL	Reilly & Grogan (2002)
Gene mutation, Big Blue™ mouse and rat fibroblasts, cII locus *in vitro*	+	NT	2.5 µM	Erexson & Tindall (2000a)
Gene mutation, Chinese hamster ovary-K1 cells, *Hprt* locus *in vitro*	+	NT	20 µM	Lee *et al.* (2002)
Gene mutation, Rat2 transgenic fibroblasts, *LacI* locus *in vitro*	(+)	NT	10 µM	Recio *et al.* (2000)
Sister chromatid exchange, male CD rat and CD-1 mouse splenic lymphocytes, whole blood and isolated blood lymphocytes at G_0 stage in the cell cycle *in vitro*	+	NT	2.5 µM	Kligerman *et al.* (1999a)
Sister chromatid exchange, Big Blue™ mouse and rat fibroblasts *in vitro*	+	NT	2 µM	Erexson & Tindall (2000b)
Micronucleus formation, Big Blue™ mouse and rat fibroblasts *in vitro*	+	NT	2.5 µM	Erexson & Tindall (2000a)
Micronucleus formation, Rat2 *LacI* cells *in vitro*	+	NT	2 µM	Recio *et al.* (2000, 2001)
Micronucleus formation, Chinese hamster V79 cells *in vitro*	+	NT	12.5 µM	Himmelstein *et al.* (2001)

Table 29 (contd)

Test system	Result[a] Without exogenous metabolic system	With exogenous metabolic system	Dose[b] (LED or HID)	Reference
Gene mutation, human lymphoblastoid TK6 cells, *HPRT* locus *in vitro*	+	NT	4 μM for 24 h	Recio et al. (2000)
Gene mutation, human lymphoblastoid TK6 cells, *HPRT* locus *in vitro*	+	NT	2 μM all isomers for 24 h	Meng et al. (2007b)
Gene mutation, human lymphoblastoid TK6 cells, *TK* locus *in vitro*	+	NT	2 μM all isomers for 24 h	Meng et al. (2007b)
Sister chromatid exchange, human whole blood and isolated blood lymphocytes *in vitro*	+	NT	2.5 μM	Kligerman et al. (1999a)
Sister chromatid exchange, human whole blood lymphocytes *in vitro*	+	NT	5 μM	Schlade-Bartusiak et al. (2001, 2004)
Micronucleus formation, human lymphocytes *in vitro*	+	NT	2.5 μM	Murg et al. (1999a)
Chromosomal breakage (1cen-q12 region), AZH-1 cells from human lymphoblastoid TK6 cells	+	NT	5 μM	Murg et al. (1999b)
Chromosomal breakage (1 cen-q12 region), human lymphocytes *in vitro*	+	NT	2.5 μM	Murg et al. (1999a)
Hyperdiploidy (chromosome 1), AZH-1 cells from human lymphoblastoid TK6 cells	+	NT	10 μM	Murg et al. (1999b)
Hyperdiploidy, human lymphocytes *in vitro*	+	NT	10 μM	Murg et al. (1999a)
Inhibition of IL-2 production, human CD4[+] lymphocytes	–	NT	10 μM	Irons et al. (2001)
Inhibition of clonogenic activity, human CD34[+] bone-marrow cells	+	NT	2 μM *meso* or D,L	Irons et al. (2000, 2001)
Inhibition of clonogenic response, human CD34+ bone-marrow cells	+	NT	2 μM	Irons et al. (2001)
Cell cycle arrest in G_1/G_2, human embryonic lung fibroblasts	+	NT	100 μM for 1 h	Schmiederer et al. (2005)
Increased p53 and p21[cip1], human embryonic lung fibroblasts	+	NT	100 μM for 1 h	Schmiederer et al. (2005)

Table 29 (contd)

Test system	Result[a]		Dose[b] (LED or HID)	Reference
	Without exogenous metabolic system	With exogenous metabolic system		
Comet tail moments, *Ephx1*-plus mice *in vivo*	–	NT	15 mg/kg/24 h × 2	Wickliffe *et al.* (2003)
Comet tail moments, *Ephx1*-null mice *in vivo*	+	NT	1.5 mg/kg/24 h × 2	Wickliffe *et al.* (2003)
Gene mutation, female Fischer 344 rat and female B6C3F₁ mouse splenic T cells, *Hprt* locus *in vivo*	+	NT	2 ppm 6 h/d, 5 d/wk, 4 wk	Meng *et al.* (1999b); Walker & Meng (2000)
Gene mutation, female Fischer 344 *LacI* transgenic rat bone marrow *in vivo*	(+)	NT	3.8 ppm 6 h/d, 5 d/wk, 2 wk	Recio *et al.* (2000)
Gene mutation, female Fischer 344 *LacI* transgenic rat spleen and female B6C3F₁ *LacI* transgenic mouse bone marrow and spleen *in vivo*	–	NT	3.8 ppm 6 h/d, 5 d/wk, 2 wk	Recio *et al.* (2000)
Gene mutation, *Ephx1*-plus mice, *Hprt* locus *in vivo*	+	NT	15 mg/kg/24 h × 2	Wickliffe *et al.* (2003, 2007)
Gene mutation, *Ephx1*-null mice, *Hprt* locus *in vivo*	+	NT	15 mg/kg/24 h × 2	Wickliffe *et al.* (2003, 2007)

IL, interleukin

[a] +, positive; –, negative; (+), weak positive; NT, not tested

[b] LED, lowest effective dose; HID, highest ineffective dose; d, day; wk, week

At low concentrations of diepoxybutane, increases in the frequency of sister chromatid exchange were observed in Big Blue™ mouse and rat fibroblasts and of micronucleus formation in Rat2 *LacI* cells *in vitro* (Erexson & Tindall, 2000b; Recio *et al.*, 2000, 2001).

Increases in the *HPRT* and thymidine kinase (*TK*) mutation frequency in human lymphoblastoid TK6 cells were observed with all isomers (or the 2*R*,3*R*-, 2*S*,3*S*- and *meso*-stereoisomers) of diepoxybutane. The mutational spectrum of diepoxybutane at *HPRT* in human TK6 cells after exposure to racemic diepoxybutane was compared with background. Significant increases in A:T→T:A transversions and partial deletions were detected. Diepoxybutane increased the frequencies of sister chromatid exchange and micronucleus formation in human lymphocytes *in vitro*. Other genetic alterations such as chromosomal breakage and hyperdiploidy were observed as the concentration of diepoxybutane increased.

The effect of various polymorphisms on the frequency of sister chromatid exhange in whole blood lymphocytes from human volunteers after in-vitro exposure to diepoxybutane was examined. A significant difference in sister chromatid exchange was observed between the *GSTT1*-negative and *GSTT1*-positive individuals (79.28 ± 23.33 and 58.96 ± 17.44, respectively; $p < 0.01$). Individuals who were heterozygous for the C2 allele in CYP2E1 (C1/C2), which is associated with higher enzyme activity, had higher levels of sister chromatid exchange (70.83 ± 10.85) compared with C1/C1 individuals (56.83 ± 17.64; $p < 0.05$). The *RAD51* polymorphism as well as EH activity had no effect. In individuals with the *GSTT1*-null genotype, a significant difference was observed in individuals with very low or low expected EH activity (72.13 ± 12.41) and in individuals whose activity was expected to be high (102.73 ± 21.22). Similar results were observed in an earlier study in which *GSTT1*-null individuals had a sister chromatid exchange frequency of 84.8 ± 20.3 whereas individuals who were *GSTT1*-positive had a frequency of 67.9 ± 10.8 ($p < 0.001$). In this study, no effect was observed in individuals with different *GSTM1* genotypes (Schlade-Bartusiak *et al.*, 2000, 2004).

After in-vivo exposure of female B6C3F$_1$ mice and Fischer 344 rats to diepoxybutane, dose-related increases in mutation frequency at the *Hprt* locus were observed in the splenic T cells of both species. *LacI* transgenic mice and rats exposed to diepoxybutane showed no or a weak increase in *LacI* mutation frequency in the spleen and bone marrow.

4.2.3   *Mechanism of mutation induction*

(a)   DNA adducts

Many adducts with epoxybutene, epoxybutanediol and diepoxybutane have been identified in reactions with nucleosides and DNA *in vitro* (see Table 30 for details and references). The mutagenicity and mutation spectra of several of these adducts have been investigated (see Table 31 for details and references). Many of these adducts can also block replication by many polymerases or can cause misincorporation of proper nucleotides (see Table 32 for details and references). DNA adducts have been identified in humans exposed to butadiene and in animals exposed to butadiene and its metabolites.

Table 30. Reactivity of butadiene metabolites with DNA bases in vitro

Targets	Butadiene metabolite	Adducts formed	Kinetics	Analytical methods	Analytical methods
2′-Deoxyadenosine	EB	(R)-N6-(1-Hydroxy-3-buten-2-yl)deoxyadenosine; (S)-N6-(1-hydroxy-3-buten-2-yl)deoxyadenosine		NMR, MS, CD	Nechev et al. (2001)
2′-Deoxyguanosine	EB	(R)-N2-(1-Hydroxy-3-buten-2-yl)deoxyguanosine; (S)-N2-(1-hydroxy-3-buten-2-yl)deoxyguanosine		NMR, MS, CD spectra	Nechev et al. (2001)
2′-Deoxyguanosine	EB	N7-(2-Hydroxy-3-butenyl)guanine (G1) (equal amounts); N7-(1-(hydroxymethyl)-2-propenyl)guanine (G2) (equal amounts)	Neutral thermal hydrolysis	LC/MS, NMR	Boogaard et al. (2001b, 2004)
Single- and double-stranded calf thymus DNA	EB	N7-(2-Hydroxy-3-buten-1-yl)guanine (G1); N7-(1-hydroxy-3-buten-2-yl)guanine (G2); diastereomers of N3-(2-hydroxy-3-buten-1-yl)deoxyuridine; N6-(2-hydroxy-3-buten-1-yl)deoxyadenosine; N3-(2-hydroxy-3-buten-1-yl)adenine (A1); N3-(1-hydroxy-3-buten-2-yl)adenine (A2)	Enzymatic and neutral thermal hydrolysis, all adducts detected at EB ≥ 10 mM in ssDNA and ≥ 100 mM in dsDNA; I, II major adducts, III-V more prominent in ssDNA than dsDNA	HPLC, UV, FAB-MS	Selzer & Elfarra (1999); Elfarra et al. (2001)
Calf thymus DNA	EB	N7-(2-Hydroxy-3-butenyl)guanine (G1); N7-(1-(hydroxymethyl)-2-propenyl)guanine (G2); N3-(2-hydroxy-3-butenyl)adenine (A1); N3-(1-hydroxymethyl-2-propenyl)adenine (A2)	Neutral thermal hydrolysis, G1 ≥ G2 >> A2 > A1	HPLC, UV	Boogaard et al. (2004)
2′-Deoxyguanosine	EBD	N7-(1-(Hydroxymethyl)-2,3-dihydroxypropyl)guanine (major) (C3); N7-(2,3,4-trihydroxybut-1-yl)guanine (minor) (G4)	Neutral thermal hydrolysis	LC/MS, NMR	Boogaard et al. (2001b)
Deoxyadenosine 5′-monophosphate	EBD	N6-2,3,4-Trihydroxybutyladenine; N1-trihydroxybutyladenine	Base hydrolysis at 37 °C		Zhao et al. (1998)
2′-Deoxyguanosine-5′-phosphate, calf thymus DNA	EBD	N7-(2,3,4-Trihydroxybut-1-yl)guanine (G4)	Half-life, 30 ± 4 h	HPLC, UV	Koivisto et al. (1999)
Salmon testis DNA	DEB	N6-2,3,4-Trihydroxybutyladenine; N1-trihydroxybutyladenine	Base hydrolysis at 37 °C		Zhao et al. (1998)

Table 30 (contd)

Targets	Butadiene metabolite	Adducts formed	Kinetics	Analytical methods	Analytical methods
2′-Deoxyguanosine	DEB	Diastereomeric pairs of N-(2-hydroxy-1-oxiranylethyl)-2′-deoxyguanosine (P4-1 and P4-2); 7,8-dihydroxy-3-(2-deoxy-β-D-erythro-pentofuranosyl)-3,5,6,7,8,9-hexahydro-1,3-diazepino[1,2-a]purin-11(11H)one (P6); 1-(2-hydroxy-2-oxiranylethyl)-2′deoxyguanosine (P8 and P9); 1-[3-chloro-2-hydroxy-1-(hydroxymethyl)propyl]-2′-deoxyguanosine (1AP9 and 2AP9); 4,8-dihydroxy-1-(2-deoxy-β-D-erythro-pentofuranosyl)-9-hydroxymethyl-6,7,8,9-tetrahydro-1H-pyrimido[2,1-b] purinium ion (1BP4 and 2BP4); 6-oxo-2-amino-9-(2-deoxy-β-D-erythro-pentofuranosyl)-7-(2-hydroxy-2-oxiranylethyl)-6,9-dihydro-1H-purinium ion (P5 and P5′)	Product profile similar although much slower at DEB:dG ratio 10:1 compared to 80:1 at pH 7.4	HPLC, MS, NMR	Zhang & Elfarra (2003)
2′-Deoxyguanosine	DEB	7-Hydroxy-6-hydroxymethyl-5,6,7,8-tetrahydropyrimido[1,2-a]purin-10(1H)one (H2); 2-amino-1-(4-chloro-2,3-dihydroxybutyl)1,7-dihydro-6H-purine-6-one (H4); 2-amino-1-(2,3,4-trihydroxybutyl)-1,7-dihydro-6H-purin-6-one (H1′/H5′; 7,8-dihyroxy-1,5,6,7,8,9-hexahydro1,3-diazepino[1,2-a]purin-11(11H)one (H2′); 5-(3,4-dihydroxy-1-pyrrolidinyl)-2,6-diamino-4(3H)pyrimidinone (H3′); 2-amino-7-(3-chloro-2,4-dihydroxybutyl)-1,7-dihydro-6H-purin-6-one (H3); 2-amino-7-(2,3,4-trihydroxybutyl)-1,7-dihydro-6H-purin-6-one (H4′)	Acid hydrolysis H4′/H3 - hydrolysis products of P5/P5′; H2′- of P4-1, P4-2; H4, H1′/H5′, hydrolysis of P8/P9	HPLC, MS, NMR	Zhang & Elfarra (2004)
2′-Deoxyguanosine	DEB	Diastereomeric pairs of N-(2-hydroxy-1-oxiranylethyl)-2′-deoxyguanosine (P4-1 and P4-2; 7,8-dihydroxy-3-(2-deoxy-β-D-erythro-pentofuranosyl)-3,5,6,7,8,9-hexahydro-1,3-diazepino[1,2-a]purin-11(11H)one (P6); 1-(2-hydroxy-2-oxiranylethyl)-2′deoxyguanosine (P8 and P9); 6-oxo-2-amino-9-(2-deoxy-β-D-erythro-pentofuranosyl)-7-(2-hydroxy-2-oxiranylethyl)-6,9-dihydro-1H-purinium ion (P5 and P5′)	P5, P5′, P8, P9 half-lives of 2.6, 2.7, 16 and 16 h, respectively; P4-1, P4-2 and P6 are stable at physiological conditions (pH 7.4, 37 °C)	HPLC, UV, MS, NMR	Zhang & Elfarra (2005)

Table 30 (contd)

Targets	Butadiene metabolite	Adducts formed	Kinetics	Analytical methods	Analytical methods
2′-Deoxyguanosine	DEB	7,7′-(2,3-Dihydroxy-1,4-butanediyl)bis[2-amino-1,7-dihydro-6H-purin-6-one] (bis-N7G-BD); 2′-deoxy-1-[4-(2-amino-1,7-dihydro-6H-purin-6-on-7-yl)-2,3-dihydroxybutyl]-guanosine (N7G-N1dG-BD); 2-amino-9-hydroxymethyl-4-(4-acetyloxy-2,3-dihydroxybutyl)-8,5-dihydro-7H-[1,4]oxazepino[4,3,2-gh]purin-8-ol (PA1); 2-amino-9-hydroxymethyl-4-{4-[2-amino-9- or 7-(4-acetyloxy-2,3-dihydroxybutyl)-1,7-dihydro-6H-purin-6-on-7- or 9-yl]-2,3-dihydroxybutyl}-8,9-dihydro-7H-[1,4]-oxazepino[4,3,2-gh]purir-8-ol (PA2); 2-amino-7,9-bis(4-acetyloxy-2,3-dihydroxybutyl)-1,7-dihydro-6H-purin-6-one (PA3); 9,9′-bis(4-acetyloxy-2,3-dihydroxybutyl)-7,7′-(2,3-dihydroxy-1,4-butanediyl)bis[2-aminc-1,7-dihydro-6H-purin-6-one] (PA4)	PA1-PA4 formed in the reaction in acetic acid P5D +dG produces bis-N7G-BD P8, P9 + dG produces N7G-N1dG-BD	HPLC, UV, MS, NMR	Zhang & Elfarra (2006)
2′-Deoxyadenosine	DEB	(R,R)-N⁶-(2,3,4-Trihydroxybut-1-yl)deoxyadenosine; (S,S)-N⁶-(2,3,4-trihydroxybut-1-yl)deoxyadenosine		NMR, MS, CD	Nechev et al. (2001)
2′-Deoxyguanosine	DEB	(R,R)-N2-(2,3,4-Trihydroxybut-1-yl)deoxyguanosine; (S,S)-N2-(2,3,4-trihydroxybut-1-yl)deoxyguanosine		NMR, MS, CD spectra	Nechev et al. (2001)
2′-Deoxyguanosine	DEB	N7-(2,3,4-Trihydroxybutyl)guanine (G4) (major); N7-(1-(hydroxymethyl)-2,3-dihydroxypropyl)guanine (G3) (minor)	Neutral thermal hydrolysis	LC-MS, NMR	Boogaard et al. (2001b, 2004)
Guanosine	(±)-DEB	(±)-N7-(2,3,4-Trihydroxybutyl)guanine	Acid hydrolysis	LC-MS/MS	Oe et al. (1999)
Guanosine	meso-DEB	meso-N7-(2,3,4-Trihydroxybutyl)guanine (G4)	Acid hydrolysis	LC-MS/MS	Oe et al. (1999)
2′-Deoxyguanosine-5′-phosphate, calf thymus DNA	RR/SS DEB	N7-(2-Hydroxy-3,4-epoxy-1-yl)-5′dGMP	Half-life, 31 ± 3 h	HPLC, UV	Koivisto et al. (1999)

Table 30 (contd)

Targets	Butadiene metabolite	Adducts formed	Kinetics	Analytical methods	Analytical methods
Calf thymus DNA	Racemic DEB	1-(Aden-1-yl)-4-(guan-7-yl)-2,3-butanediol (N1A-N7G-BD; 1); 1-(aden-3-yl)-4-(guan-7-yl)-2,3-butanediol (N3A-N7G-BD; 2); 1-(aden-7-yl)-4-(guan-7-yl)-2,3-butanediol (N7A-N7G-BD; 3); 1-(aden-N^6-yl)-4-(guan-7-yl)-2,3-butanediol (N^6A-N7G-BD; 4)	Acid hydrolysis; half-lives in dsDNA: 2, 31 h; 3, 17 h; 1 and 4 not released	MS/MS, HPLC, UV	Park et al. (2004)
Guanosine; calf thymus DNA	DEB	1,4-bis-(Guan-7-yl)-2,3-butanediol (bis-N7G-BD); N7-(2′,3′,4′)trihydroxybutylguanine (N7-THBG)	Neutral thermal hydrolysis; half-life of bis-N7G-BD, 81.5 h; half-life of N7-THBG, 48.5 h	UV, MS, NMR	Park & Tretyakova (2004)
Guanosine	meso-DEB	meso-1,4-bis-(Guan-7-yl)-2,3-butanediol		UV, MS, NMR	Park et al. (2005)
2′-Deoxyguanosine; calf thymus DNA	HMVK	Diasteromeric pair of HMVK-derived 1,N^2-propanodeoxyguanosine C-6 adducts; as well as a diastereomeric pair of C-8 HMVK-derived 1,N^2-propanodeoxyguanosine adducts	2′-Deoxyguanosine reaction run at pH 11, calf thymus DNA experiment at pH 7.4	UV, MS, NMR	Powley et al. (2003)

BD, butadiene; CD, circular dichroism; DEB, diepoxybutane; dG, deoxyguanine; dGMP, desoxyguanosine monophosphate; dsDNA, double-stranded DNA; EB, epoxybutene; EBD, epoxybutane diol; FAB, positive ion fast atom bombardment; G, guanosine; HMVK, hydroxymethylvinyl ketone; HPLC, high-performance liquid chromatography; LC, liquid chromatography; LC–MS/MS, liquid chromatography in combination with tandem mass spectrometry; MS, mass spectrometry; NMR, nuclear magnetic resonance; ssDNA, single-stranded DNA; THBG, trihydroxybutylguanine; UV, ultraviolet

Table 31. Genetic and related effects of the DNA adducts of butadiene

Adduct	Test system	Result[a] (total mutation %)	Common mutations	References
R-EB-N^2-guanine	*E. coli* AB 2480	(±)	–	Carmical *et al.* (2000a)
S-EB-N^2-guanine	*E. coli* AB 2480	(+) (< 1)	G→T transversions (45%), G→A transitions (32%)	Carmical *et al.* (2000a)
R-EB-deoxyinosine	COS-7 cells	+ (59)	A→G (48%), A→C (7%)	Kanuri *et al.* (2002)
S-EB-deoxyinosine	COS-7 cells	+ (94.5)	A→G (79%), A→C (10%)	Kanuri *et al.* (2002)
R-EB-deoxyinosine	*E. coli* AB 2480	+ (53)	A→G (43%)	Kanuri *et al.* (2002)
S-EB-deoxyinosine	*E. coli* AB 2480	+ (96.5)	A→G (87%)	Kanuri *et al.* (2002)
R-EB-deoxyinosine	*E. coli* AB 2480	+ (90)	A→G (65%), A→T (29%)	Rodriguez *et al.* (2001)
S-EB-deoxyinosine	*E. coli* AB 2480	+ (91)	A→G (63%), A→C (32%)	Rodriguez *et al.* (2001)
R-EB-N^6-adenine	*E. coli* AB 2480	–	–	Carmical *et al.* (2000b)
S-EB-N^6-adenine	*E. coli* AB 2480	–	–	Carmical *et al.* (2000b)
R,R-EBD-N^6-adenine	*E. coli* AB 2480	(+) (0.13)	A→G	Carmical *et al.* (2000b)
S,S-EBD-N^6-adenine	*E. coli* AB 2480	(+) (0.25)	A→C	Carmical *et al.* (2000b)
EB-$N3$-2'-deoxyuridine	COS-7 cells	+ (97)	C→T transitions (53.4%), C→A transversions (32.5%)	Fernandes *et al.* (2006)
R,R-EBD-N^2-guanine	*E. coli* AB 2480	(+) (< 1)	G→A, G→T, G→C (nearly equal)	Carmical *et al.* (2000a)
S,S-EBD-N^2-guanine	*E. coli* AB 2480	(+) (< 1)	G→A, G→T, G→C (nearly equal)	Carmical *et al.* (2000a)
R,R-DEB-N^2-N^2-guanine cross-link	*E. coli* AB 2480	+	G→T	Carmical *et al.* (2000c)
S,S-DEB-N^2-N^2-guanine cross-link	*E. coli* AB 2480	+	G→A	Carmical *et al.* (2000c)
R,R-DEB-N^6-N^6-deoxyadenosine cross-link	*E. coli* AB 2480	(+) (8)	A→G (7.5%)	Kanuri *et al.* (2002)

Table 31 (contd)

Adduct	Test system	Result[a] (total mutation %)	Common mutations	References
S,S-DEB-N^6-N^6-deoxyadenosine cross-link	E. coli AB 2480	(+) (2.8)	A→G (2.3%)	Kanuri et al. (2002)
R,R-DEB-N^6-N^6-deoxyadenosine cross-link	COS-7 cells	+ (54)	A→G transitions(40%) A→C transversions (9%)	Kanuri et al. (2002)
S,S-DEB-N^6-N^6-deoxyadenosine cross-link	COS-7 cells	(+) (19.4)	A→G (13%) A→T (5.6%)	Kanuri et al. (2002)

[a]+, positive; (+), weakly positive; −, negative
DEB, diepoxybutane; EB, epoxybutene; EBD, epoxybutanediol

Table 32. Effect of the butadiene-derived DNA adducts on replication/repair

Adduct[a]	Test system	Blockage[b]	Single nucleotide incorporation[c]	Comment	References
R-EB-N6-adenine	E. coli DNA polymerases Pol I, II and III	–			Carmical et al. (2000b)
S-EB-N6-adenine	E. coli DNA polymerases Pol I, II and III	–			Carmical et al. (2000b)
R-EB-N2-guanine	E. coli DNA polymerases Pol I, II and III	+			Carmical et al. (2000a)
S-EB-N2-guanine	E. coli DNA polymerases Pol I, II and III	+			Carmical et al. (2000a)
R-EB N2-guanine	Yeast DNA polymerase η	–	Mostly C		Minko et al. (2001)
S-EB N2-guanine	Yeast DNA polymerase η	–	C	More efficient than R-stereoisomer	Minko et al. (2001)
R-EB N2-guanine	E. coli DNA polymerase Pol I	+			Minko et al. (2001)
S-EB N2-guanine	E. coli DNA polymerase Pol I	+			Minko et al. (2001)
EB-N3-2'-deoxyuridine	Bacterial Klenow (Kf)	+			Fernandes et al. (2006)
EB-N3-2'-deoxyuridine	Mammalian polymerase δ	(+)			Fernandes et al. (2006)
EB-N3-2'-deoxyuridine	Yeast polymerase δ	+			Fernandes et al. (2006)
EB-N3-2'-deoxyuridine	Mammalian polymerase ε	+			Fernandes et al. (2006)
R,R-EBD-N2-guanine	Yeast DNA polymerase η	–	C		Minko et al. (2001)
S,S-EBD-N2-guanine	Yeast DNA polymerase η	–	C	More efficient than R-stereoisomer	Minko et al. (2001)
R,R-EBD-N2-guanine	E. coli DNA polymerase Pol I	+			Minko et al. (2001)
S,S-EBD-N2-guanine	E. coli DNA polymerase Pol I	+			Minko et al. (2001)
R,R-EBD-N6-adenine	E. coli DNA polymerases Pol I, II and III	–			Carmical et al. (2000b)

Table 32 (contd)

Adduct[a]	Test system	Blockage[b]	Single nucleotide incorporation[c]	Comment	References
S,S-EBD-N^6-adenine	E. coli DNA polymerases Pol I, II and III	–			Carmical et al. (2000b)
R,R-EBD-N^2-guanine	E. coli DNA polymerases Pol I, II and III	+			Carmical et al. (2000a)
S,S-EBD-N^2-guanine	E. coli DNA polymerases Pol I, II and III	+			Carmical et al. (2000a)
R,R-EBD-N^2-guanine	Bacteriophage T7' DNA polymerase	(+)	dTTP		Zang et al. (2005)
S,S-EBD-N^2-guanine	Bacteriophage T7' DNA polymerase	(+)	dTTP	Misinsertion frequency 40-fold higher than the R,R-isomer	Zang et al. (2005)
R,R-EBD-N^2-guanine	HIV-1 reverse transcriptase	+			Zang et al. (2005)
S,S-EBD-N^2-guanine	HIV-1 reverse transcriptase	+			Zang et al. (2005)
R,R-DEB-N^2-N^2-guanine cross-link	E. coli AB2840 plaque-forming efficiency in vivo	+			Carmical et al. (2000c)
S,S-DEB-N^2-N^2-guanine cross-link	E. coli AB2840 plaque-forming efficiency in vivo	+			Carmical et al. (2000c)
R,R-DEB-N^2-N^2-guanine cross-link	E. coli DNA polymerases Pol I, II and III	+			Carmical et al. (2000c)
S,S-DEB-N^2-N^2-guanine cross-link	E. coli DNA polymerases Pol I, II and III	+			Carmical et al. (2000c)
R,R-DEB-N^2-N^2-guanine cross-link	E. coli UvrABC nuclease	+			Carmical et al. (2000c)

Table 32 (contd)

Adduct[a]	Test system	Blockage[b]	Single nucleotide incorporation[c]	Comment	References
S,S-DEB-N^2-N^2-guanine cross-link	$E.\ coli$ UvrABC nuclease	+			Carmical $et\ al.$ (2000a)
R,R-DEB-N^2-guanine-N^2-guanine cross-link	Yeast DNA polymerase η	+			Minko $et\ al.$ (2001)
S,S-DEB-N^2-guanine-N^2-guanine cross-link	Yeast DNA polymerase η	+			Minko $et\ al.$ (2001)

DEB, diepoxybutane; EB, epoxybutene; EBD, epoxybutanediol; HIV, human immunodeficiency virus

[a] Most were tested in an oligonucleotide

[b] +, highly blocked; (+), partially blocked; −, no blockage

[c] C, cytidine; dTTP, deoxythymidine triphosphate

(i)   *Butadiene*

Humans

The levels of the DNA adduct, N-1-(2,3,4-trihydroxybutyl)adenine, was determined in 15 male butadiene-exposed (monomer unit) and 11 male control workers from a butadiene monomer production plant in the Czech Republic (Zhao *et al.*, 2000). The median exposure concentration of butadiene for the exposed group was 0.53 mg/m^3 [0.24 ppm] whereas that for the control group was 0.013 mg/m^3 [0.006 ppm]. Because of interfering background peaks, the N-1-adenine adducts were converted to N^6-adenine adducts. This adduct was detected in 14 of 15 exposed workers and five of 11 controls. The difference in the levels of adducts between the butadiene-exposed workers (4.5 ± 7.7 adducts/10^9 nucleotides) and the control workers (0.8 ± 1.2 adducts/10^9 nucleotides) was significant ($p = 0.038$). When controls were subdivided into smokers and nonsmokers, the adduct levels were 1.5 ± 1.7 adducts/10^9 nucleotides for four smokers and 0.3 ± 0.6 adducts/10^9 nucleotides for seven nonsmokers but the difference was not significant. A significant correlation between the levels of the N-1-(2,3,4-trihydroxybutyl)adenine adduct in lymphocyte DNA and individual exposures to butadiene was found in the exposed group ($r = 0.707$; $p = 0.005$), control ($r = 0.733$; $p = 0.01$) and both groups combined ($r = 0.723$; $p < 0.001$; Zhao *et al.*, 2001). However, no significant correlations were found with other genotoxic effects such as DNA single-strand breaks or micronucleus formation.

Experimental systems

1,4-Bis(guan-7-yl)-2,3-butanediol is the N7-guanine–N7-guanine crosslink formed from the reaction of DNA with diepoxybutane. This compound has been identified in the livers and lungs of C57BL/6 mice that were exposed to 625 ppm [1381 mg/m^3] butadiene by inhalation for 7 h per day for 5 days (Goggin *et al.*, 2007). The DNA from livers and lungs contained 3.2 ± 0.4 and 1.8 ± 0.5 adducts/10^6 guanines from racemic diepoxybutane but no adducts from *meso*-diepoxybutane were detected.

Male B6C3F$_1$ mice and Sprague-Dawley rats were exposed for 6 h to 200 ppm [442 mg/m^3] [2,3-^{14}C]butadiene by nose-only inhalation and were killed 48 h after treatment; the livers and lungs were analysed for DNA adducts (Boogaard *et al.*, 2001b). In the livers and lungs of both rats and mice, N7-(2,3,4-trihydroxybut-1-yl)guanine (G4) was the major adduct detected. Mice had 102 ± 4 and 80 ± 4 G4 adducts/10^8 nucleotides (means ± SE) and rats had 10 ± 2 and 13 ± 0.2 G4 adducts/10^8 nucleotides in the liver and lung, respectively. Smaller amounts of N7-(2-hydroxy-3-buten-1-yl)guanine (G1) and N7-(1-hydroxy-3-buten-2-yl)guanine (G2) were detected. Mouse liver and lung contained 21 ± 9 and 3.4 ± 1.3 adducts/10^8 nucleotides, respectively, and rat liver and lung contained 1.9 ± 0.2 and 3.6 ± 1.2 adducts/10^8 nucleotides, respectively. In rats, no N7-(1,3,4-trihydroxybut-2-yl)guanine (G3) was detected whereas mouse liver and lung contained 25 ± 2 and 4.3 ± 0.1 adducts/10^8 nucleotides, respectively. A similar profile was also obtained in animals that were killed immediately after cessation of exposure (Boogaard *et al.*, 2004).

In another study, male B6C3F$_1$ mice and Sprague-Dawley rats were exposed to 20 ppm [44.2 mg/m^3] [2,3-^{14}C]butadiene for either 6 h or for 6 h per day for 5 days by nose-only inhalation, and the livers, lungs and testes were analysed for DNA adducts (Booth *et al.*, 2004b). Following the single 20-ppm exposure, G4 was the major adduct detected in all tissues in rats and mice. Mice had 13.91 ± 3.64, 13.67 ± 0.97 and 6.04 ± 0.8 G4 adducts/10^8 nucleotides and rats had 5.75 ± 1.32, 3.31 ± 1.74 and 1.39 ± 0.50 G4 adducts/10^8 nucleotides in liver, lung and testis, respectively. Small amounts of G3 (the exact identity was not determined) were detected consistently in mouse liver and in only one rat liver sample and was not detected in any other tissue. Following the 20-ppm 5-day exposure, G4 was again the main adduct detected and levels in mouse tissues were higher than those in corresponding rat tissues. G1 and G2 were detected in the liver and lung of mice and rats but not in mouse testis; rats had detectable levels in the testis. G3 was detected in mouse tissues and in the liver of rats. The amounts of these other metabolites were much lower than that of G4.

Female Sprague Dawley rats were exposed to 1000 ppm [2210 mg/m^3] butadiene by inhalation for 6 h per day on 5 days per week for 13 weeks. DNA was isolated from the liver and was analysed for the presence of the α-regioisomer of HMVK-derived 1,N^2-propanodeoxyguanosine by LC–MS/MS (Powley *et al.*, 2007). No adducts were detected.

Female B6C3F$_1$ mice and Fischer 344 rats were exposed by inhalation to butadiene for 6 h per day on 5 days per week for 2 weeks (Oe *et al.*, 1999; Blair *et al.*, 2000). The mean daily concentration of butadiene was approximately 1250 ppm [2762.5 mg/m^3]. DNA was isolated and analysed for the presence of ($\pm$)-G4 and *meso*-G4. On exposure day 10, mouse liver had 3.9 and 2.2 ($\pm$)-G4 and *meso*-G4 adducts/10^6 normal bases, respectively. On the same exposure day, rat liver had 1.6 and 0.8 ($\pm$)-G4 and *meso*-G4 adducts/10^6 normal bases, respectively. The in-vivo half-lives were 4.1 and 5.5 days for ($\pm$)-G4 and *meso*-G4, respectively, in mouse liver DNA. Half-lives for ($\pm$)-G4 and *meso*-G4 in rat liver DNA were 3.6 and 4.0 days, respectively.

DNA adducts were measured in the livers, lungs and kidneys of Fischer 344 rats and B6C3F$_1$ mice after exposure to 0, 20, 62.5 or 625 ppm [0, 44.2, 138 or 1381 mg/m^3] butadiene for 6 h per day or 5 days per week for 4 weeks (Swenberg *et al.*, 2000b). Adducts corresponding to the *N*7-guanine adducts of epoxybutene (G1 and G2) and the 2,3,4-trihydroxybutane–guanine adduct (G4) that can be formed from either epoxybutanediol or diepoxybutane were analysed. More G4 was detected in mice and rats than G1 and G2. In rats, adduct levels in the different tissues were similar. In general, mouse tissues contained higher levels of DNA adducts.

DNA adducts were measured in the livers, lungs and kidneys of Fischer 344 rats and B6C3F$_1$ mice after exposure to 0, 20, 62.5 or 625 ppm [0, 44.2, 138 or 1381 mg/m^3] butadiene for 6 h per day on 5 days per week for 4 weeks (Koc *et al.*, 1999). Both racemic and *meso*-G4 and G1 and G2 were analysed by LC–MS/MS. At 625 ppm [1381 mg/m^3] butadiene, mouse liver had 31.9 ± 6.5, 32.2 ± 4.2, 3.0 ± 0.1 and 2.4 ± 0.3 racemic G4, *meso-* G4, G1 and G2 adducts/10^6guanine bases, respectively. At 625 ppm butadiene, rat liver had 7.7 ± 4.5, 4.2 ± 2.5, 1.2 ± 0.5 and 0.9 ± 0.5 racemic G4, *meso-* G4, G1 and G2 adducts/10^6guanine bases, respectively. The number of adducts for both G4 and G1 and G2 was similar for all three tissues at all doses examined in both rats and mice. Mice had significantly higher amounts of G4 adducts than rats in all three tissues after exposure to 625 ppm. This difference was also significant in lung and kidney at 62.5 ppm but not at 20 ppm. Overall, the amounts of G1 and G2 adducts were lower than those of G4 adducts in both species.

In the lungs of mice exposed to 500 ppm [1105 mg/m^3] butadiene for 6 h per day for 5 days, *N*7-guanine DNA adducts arising from epoxybutene and epoxybutanediol were analysed (Koivisto & Peltonen, 2001). All four epoxybutene-derived adducts were detected, most of which arose from *S*-epoxybutene. For epoxybutanediol, 75% of the total adducts originated from the 2*R*-diol-3*S*-epoxybutene isomer and the reaction occurred almost exclusively at the terminal carbon.

Rats were exposed to 300 ppm [663 mg/m^3] butadiene for 6 h per day for 5 days and their liver DNA was analysed for the N^6-(2,3,4-trihydroxy-but-1-yl)adenine adduct (Zhao *et al.*, 1998). The average level of adduct detected in treated rats was 4.5 adducts/10^9 nucleotides whereas none was detected in control rat liver.

(ii)   *Butadiene metabolites in experimental systems*

Epoxybutene

Male B6C3F$_1$ mice and Sprague-Dawley rats received a single intraperitoneal injection of 1–50 mg/kg bw [^{14}C]epoxybutene and were killed 48 h later (Boogaard *et al.*, 2004). DNA was isolated from liver and lung and analysed for the presence of adducts. No adducts were detected in the lungs in either rats or mice. Adduct levels in the liver were below the limit of detection in rats treated with 1 mg/kg bw and in mice treated with 1 and 5 mg/kg bw epoxybutene. Overall, the adduct profiles were similar in rats and mice but rats had much higher levels of adducts than mice. In mice treated with 21 mg/kg bw epoxybutene, the average concentrations of G1 and G2, G3 and G4 were 368, 28 and 50 adducts/10^8 nucleotides, respectively. In rats treated with 18 mg/kg bw epoxybutene, the concentrations of G1 and G2, G3 and G4 were 857 ± 291, 21 ± 12 and 101 ± 25 adducts/10^8 nucleotides, respectively.

The livers and lungs of male B6C3F$_1$ mice and Sprague-Dawley rats that received an intraperitoneal injection of 20 mg/kg bw [4-^{14}C]epoxybutene and were killed 48 h later were analysed for DNA adducts. In rats, 857 G1 and G2 adducts/10^8 nucleotides and 101 G4 adducts/10^8 nucleotides were detected whereas 368 G1 and G2 adducts/10^8 nucleotides and 50 G4 adducts/10^8 nucleotides were detected in mice (Boogaard *et al.*, 2001b). No DNA adducts were detected in the lung.

Butanediol

Female B6C3F$_1$ mice and Fischer 344 rats were exposed by inhalation to 0–36 ppm [0–129.6 mg/m^3] butanediol. DNA was isolated from liver and lung and analysed for the presence of G4 (Powley *et al.*, 2005). Both racemic and *meso*-isomers of this compound can be formed and values were reported as total G4. Mice had significantly greater amounts of adduct than rats in both liver and lung at 6 and 18 ppm [21.6 and 64.8 mg/m^3] but there was little difference between the tissue levels. At 6 ppm, mice had 6030 ± 1740 and 5570 ± 540 fmol adducts/mg DNA whereas rats had 2560 ± 180 and 2320 ± 640 fmol adducts/mg DNA in the liver and lung, respectively. Similarily shaped dose–response curves were observed for G4 and the *Hprt* mutant frequency in splenic T cells in rodents exposed to butanediol.

However, when female Fischer 344 or Sprague-Dawley rats were exposed to higher concentrations of butanediol (36 ppm or 1000 ppm, respectively, for 6 h per day on 5 days per week for 4 weeks), no adducts were detectable in the DNA of the liver of these animals (Powley *et al.*, 2007).

Diepoxybutane

Diepoxybutane induces the formation of DNA–protein cross-links with the DNA repair protein, O^6-alkylguanine–DNA alkyltransferase (AGT) (Loeber *et al.*, 2006). The product of initial DNA alkylation by diepoxybutane, $N7$-(2'-hydroxy-3',4'-epoxybut-1'-yl)–deoxyguanosine, was incubated with recombinant human AGT and analysed by HPLC–electrospray ionization MS. Analysis of the whole protein showed the presence of a monoalkylated protein and a protein that contained two butanediol cross-links. Peptide mapping revealed that the DNA–AGT cross-link involved the sulfhydryls of Cys^{145} or Cys^{150} within the human AGT active site and the $N7$ position of guanine in duplex DNA. No cross-linking was detected with Cys^5, Cys^{24} or Cys^{62}. The resulting structure was 1-(*S*-cysteinyl)-4-(guan-7-yl)-2,3-butanediol.

The effect of the stereochemistry of the isomers of diepoxybutane and their abilities to form cross-links with calf thymus DNA was investigated (Park *et al.*, 2005). Comparable amounts of total 1,4-bis-(guan-7-yl)-2,3-butanediol (bis-$N7$-guanine–butadiene) cross-links and G4 adducts were observed. However, the types of cross-link (either interstrand or intrastrand) varied depending on the stereoisomer used. *S,S*-Diepoxybutane produced the highest amount of 1,3 interstrand cross-links (96%) followed closely by racemic diepoxybutane (90%). *meso*-Diepoxybutane produced almost equal amounts of 1,3 interstrand (49%) and 1,2 intrastrand cross-links (51%). *R,R*-Diepoxybutane produced 19% 1,2 intrastrand cross-links and 68% 1,3 interstrand cross-links but also produced a large quantity of 1,2 interstrand cross-links (13%) that were not detected with the other stereoisomers.

N^6-(2-Hydroxy-3,4-epoxybut-1-yl)adenine can potentially be produced from the reaction of diepoxybutane with DNA. This compound as well as its corresponding DNA oligomer have been synthesized (Antsypovich *et al.*, 2007). Yields of the compounds were lower than expected and both readily cyclized to an unidentified exocyclic diepoxybutane–deoxyadenosine side-product. Formation of cross-links by this compound was minimal. The half-life of N^6-(2-hydroxy-3,4-epoxybut-1-yl)adenine in single-stranded DNA was < 2 h at physiological conditions.

Calf thymus DNA incubated with a 40-fold molar excess of epoxybutene resulted in the detection of equimolar amounts of the two $N7$-guanine adducts of epoxybutene (G1 and G2) (Blair et al., 2000); when diepoxybutane was used, the (±)-G4 adduct was detected as the major product. When human TK6 cells were exposed to 400 μM epoxybutene for 24 h, the concentration of G1 and G2 adducts was 4.3 ± 0.9 and 4.1 ± 1.0 adducts/10^6normal cells, respectively. Urine samples from Fischer 344 rats and B6C3F$_1$ mice exposed to 1250 ppm [3453 mg/m^3] butadiene were analysed for the presence of $N7$-guanine adducts. For all 3 days on which the adducts were analysed, rats excreted significantly more G1 and G2 and (±)-G4; G1 was the major adduct excreted. In mice, a small amount of meso-G4 was detected but none was found in rat urine.

DNA adducts were analysed in MCF-7 cells after a 6-h exposure to epoxybutanediol and diepoxybutane at concentrations of 100–1000 μmol/mg DNA (Koivisto et al., 1999). At all concentrations tested, more diepoxybutane–$N7$-guanine adducts were detected. In the lungs of mice exposed to 50–1300 ppm [110.5–2873 mg/m^3] butadiene for 6 h per day for 5 days, large amounts of epoxybutanediol–$N7$-guanine (G4) adducts were detected. A small peak for the adduct between diepoxybutane and guanine at $N7$ was detected; however, this peak also elutes closely with an epoxybutene-derived adduct.

(b)   Structural effects of the adducts on DNA

The $(2R,3R)$-N^6-(2,3,4-trihydroxybutyl)-2'-deoxyadenosyl (BDT) DNA adduct of epoxybutanediol causes low levels of A→G mutations and the $(2S,3S)$-BDT DNA adduct causes low levels of A→C mutations. These adducts were incorporated at the X^6 position in the ras61 oligodeoxynucleotide that was then used to examine structural perturbations in duplex DNA (Merritt et al., 2004; Scholdberg et al., 2004). Both adducts were oriented in the major groove of the DNA, which resulted in minimal structural perturbation and allowed the Watson-Crick binding to remain intact. However, the major difference between the two stereoisomers was the orientation of the BDT moiety in the major groove. For the R,R-BDT adduct, the BDT moiety was orientated in plane with the modified base-pair X^6.T^{17} whereas the S,S-BDT adduct was tilted out of the base-pairing plane. This difference is due to differential interactions of $T^{17}O^4$ with the hydroxyl groups of the BDT moieties. To determine if a structural basis existed for the low levels of A→C mutations observed with the $(2S,3S)$-BDT DNA adduct, it was incorporated site-specifically into the ras61 oligodeoxynucleotide opposite a mismatched deoxyguanine in the complementary strand opposite the adducted deoxyadenine (Scholdberg et al., 2005a). Nuclear magnetic resonance studies revealed two conformations of the adducted mismatched duplex. In the major conformation, the presence of the trihydroxy adduct allowed formation of an A·G mismatched base pair in which the adduct was in the major groove of DNA and both mismatched bases were intrahelical. Thus, if this adduct is not repaired, the subsequent mismatch would result in the observed A→C mutations.

$N1$-[1-Hydroxy-3-buten-2(R)-yl]-2'-deoxyinosine, a DNA adduct of epoxybutene, is highly mutagenic in several systems and causes a large portion of A→G mutations. By incorporating this adduct into the *ras61* oligodeoxynucleotide at the second position of codon 61, positioning of the adduct in DNA could be determined (Merritt *et al.*, 2005a). This adduct caused a significant structural perturbation and showed the rotation of the adduct into a syn conformation, which placed the butadiene moiety into the major groove of the DNA duplex. This positioning disrupted Watson-Crick hydrogen bonding and some altered base stacking was observed. This syn conformation may also facilitate incorporation of desoxy cytosine triphosphate via Hoogsteen-type templating with deoxyinosine and result in A→G mutations.

*N*1-[1-Hydroxy-3-buten-2(*S*)-yl]-2′-deoxyinosine has been synthesized into an oligonucleotide that contained the epoxybutene adduct at the second position of codon 61 of the human N-*ras* proto-oncogene (Scholdberg *et al.*, 2005b). The adducted deoxyinosine was rotated into a high syn conformation, which allowed the adduct to be accommodated into the major groove of the DNA. This conformation positions the adduct to form the protonated Hoogsteen-pairing interaction with desoxy cytosine triphosphate during DNA replication thus generating A→G mutations. Some base–base stacking interactions were also perturbed.

The effect of the 1,4-bis(2′-deoxyadenosin-N^6-yl)-2*R*,3*R*-butanediol cross link in an oligonucleotide that contains the cross-link between the second and third adenines of codon 61 in the human N-*ras* proto-oncogene in duplex DNA was studied (Merritt *et al.*, 2005b). The adduct was orientated in the DNA major groove. Watson-Crick base-pairing was disrupted at $X^6 \cdot T^{17}$. At the cross-link site, an opening of base-pair $X^6 \cdot T^{17}$ altered base stacking patterns and caused slight unwinding of the DNA duplex.

Examination of the effect of the 1,4-bis(2'-deoxyadenosin-N^6-yl)-2*S*,3*S*-butanediol cross-link was also undertaken in a manner similar to that for the *R*,*R* isomer (Xu *et al.*, 2007). The adduct orientation was similar to that of the *R*,*R* adduct and it also disrupted Watson-Crick hydrogen bonding at the same base pair. The largest difference between the *S*,*S* and *R*,*R* adducts was in the conformation of the butadiene chain. Because of the anti-conformation of the two hydroxyl groups on the *S*,*S* adduct, a greater structural perturbation to the DNA duplex occurred, and resulted in a 10° bending of the cross-linked duplex.

Biochemical data suggest that both stereoisomers of N^6,N^6-deoxyadenosine intrastrand cross-linked adducts are by-passed by a variety of DNA polymerases, yet can be significantly mutagenic and lead to A→G transitions (Kanuri *et al.*, 2002).

4.2.4   *Alterations in oncogenes and suppressor genes in tumours*

A specific codon 13 mutation in K-*ras* has been described previously (see IARC, 1999).

Lymphomas induced in B6C3F₁ mice by exposure to butadiene were analysed for gross structural alterations and point mutations in several proto-oncogenes that are implicated in the *ras*, *p53* or *pRb* pathways (Zhuang & Söderkvist, 2000). Using southern blotting, no structural alterations or amplifications were detected in *Raf1*, *Mdm2*, *c-Myc*,

Cdc25a or *Cdc25b*. Ten tumours exhibited four identical silent base substitutions (GAC522AAC, GTG531GTC, TCG533TCC, GCT543ACT) and allelotypic analysis showed loss of heterozygosity of the *Raf1* locus in six of 31 butadiene-induced lymphomas. No changes were detected in lymphomas induced by long-term inhalation of 20–625 ppm [44.2–1381 mg/m^3] butadiene in B6C3F$_1$ mice that were analysed for genetic alterations in *Rb1*, *Ccnd1* and *Cdk4* genes. These results suggest that, if the inactivation of other tumour-suppressor genes may be involved in the development of a subset of butadiene-induced lymphomas, the genetic alterations in the above proto-oncogenes do not play an important role in the development of these tumours.

Studies using the *supF* gene and the three diepoxybutane isomers showed that *S,S*-diepoxybutane was the most potent mutagen followed by *R,R*-diepoxybutane and *meso*-diepoxybutane (Kim *et al.*, 2007). The major form of mutation was A:T→T:A transversion following treatment with all three stereoisomers. However, *S,S*-diepoxybutane induced larger numbers of G:C→A:T transitions while *R,R*-diepoxybutane resulted in a higher frequency of G:C→T:A transversions.

Rarely is the nervous system a target in chemical carcinogenesis but, in B6C3F$_1$ mice exposed to 625 ppm [1381 mg/m^3] butadiene, six malignant gliomas and two neuroblastomas were observed. Only one tumour has been reported in more than 500 historical control mice. Morphologically, the characteristics of the malignant gliomas and neuroblastomas were consistent with those reported for humans. Tumours were also evaluated for genetic alterations in *p53*, K- and H-*ras* genes (Kim *et al.*, 2005). One neuroblastoma had a mutation in codon 61 of the H-*ras* gene. Missense mutations in *p53* exons (exons 5–8) were detected in two neuroblastomas and three of six malignant gliomas and consisted mostly of G→A transitions (5/6). Three of five malignant gliomas and both neuroblastomas showed nuclear accumulation of p53 protein. Loss of heterozygosity at the *p53* gene locus was also observed in four of five malignant gliomas and both neuroblastomas. All of these tumours displayed loss of the C57 (B) allele at the *Ink4a/Arf* gene locus, which codes for the *p16^{Ink4a}* that may play a key role in the development of mouse brain tumours.

Male and female B6C3F$_1$ mice were exposed to a total of 8100 ppm [17 901 mg/m^3]–weeks and 16 200 ppm [35 802 mg/m^3]–weeks butadiene (Ton *et al.*, 2007). Of 51 lung tumours, 34 had a GGC→CGC transversion mutation in the codon 13 of the K-*ras* gene. A loss of heterozygosity on chromosome 6 was observed in 14 of 51 of the lung tumours and all were in the region of K-*ras*. There is mounting evidence that K-*ras*, which is a known oncogene, functions as a tumour-suppressor gene and its loss may play a major role in mouse lung carcinogenesis.

Point mutations in *ras* genes were analysed in forestomach tumours from male and female B6C3F$_1$ mice that had been exposed to 6.25–625 ppm [13.8–1381 mg/m^3] butadiene by inhalation for 6 h per day on 5 days per week for 1–2 years (Sills *et al.*, 2001). Among the butadiene-induced tumours, 20 of 24 contained *ras* gene mutations compared with four of 11 spontaneous forestomach neoplasms. In butadiene-induced forestomach tumours, the most common transversions were GGC→CGC in codon 13 in K-*ras*, and CAA→CTA in codon 61 in H-*ras*.

In male and female B6C3F$_1$ mice exposed to 6.25–625 ppm [13.8–1381 mg/m^3] butadiene by inhalation for 6 h per day on 5 days per week for 2 years, an increase in the incidence of cardiac haemangiosarcomas was observed. Eleven of these haemangio-sarcomas were analysed for alterations in the *p53* gene and *ras* proto-oncogenes (Hong *et al.*, 2000). Most of the butadiene-induced haemangiosarcomas (9/11) had K-*ras* muta-tions and all nine had G→C transversions in codon 13. Of the nine haemangiosarcomas with the K-*ras* mutations, five also had an H-*ras* codon 61 CGA mutation. Mutations in exons 5–8 of the *p53* gene were identified in five of 11 haemangiosarcomas.

Butadiene-induced mammary tumours (17) were collected from female B6C3F$_1$ mice that were exposed to 6.25–625 ppm [13.8–1381 mg/m^3] butadiene by inhalation for up to 2 years (Zhuang *et al.*, 2002). Genetic alterations in the *p53* gene were found in seven of 17 tumours. All of these tumours also showed loss of the wild-type *p53* allele. Missense mutations in codons 12, 13 or 61 of the H-*ras* gene were found in nine of 17 tumours. Seven of these nine H-*ras* mutations were G→C transversions in the first base of codon 13. Missense mutations in the β-catenin gene were identified in three of 17 tumours. No mutations were identified in the *Apc* or *Axin* genes.

4.3   Mechanistic considerations

The carcinogenicity of butadiene is most probably mediated by its metabolic intermediates. This view is based largely on the fact that butadiene-induced mutagenicity requires metabolic activation, and the DNA-reactive epoxides formed during butadiene biotransformation are direct-acting mutagens (IARC, 1999; Melnick & Kohn, 1995). The first step in butadiene metabolism primarily involves CYP-mediated oxidation to epoxybutene. At low concentrations of butadiene, metabolism via CYP2E1 predominates (IARC, 1999). Epoxybutene may be metabolized by conjugation with GSH via GST or by hydrolysis via EH. Epoxybutene may also be oxidized to multiple diastereomers of diepoxybutane (Krause & Elfarra, 1997), while dihydroxybutene formed by hydrolysis of epoxybutene may be oxidized to epoxybutanediol. The latter epoxides are also detoxified by GST or EH. Partial hydrolysis of diepoxybutane also produces epoxybutanediol. Each of these epoxide intermediates may contribute to the mutagenicity and carcinogenicity of butadiene. Factors that impact their relative contributions include tissues levels, reactivity with DNA and repair of covalent DNA adducts. For example, genetically modified mice that are deficient in mEH activity are more susceptible than wild-type mice to the mutagenic effects of butadiene and diepoxybutane (Wickliffe *et al.*, 2003). The detection of metabolites derived from HMVK and crotonaldehyde in the urine of rats or mice treated with butenediol suggests that these compounds may also be formed during the metabolism of butadiene (Sprague & Elfarra, 2003, 2004). The potential contributions of these DNA alkylating agents (crotonaldehyde and HMVK) to the mutagenicity and carcinogenicity of butadiene are not fully known.

The enzymes that regulate epoxide formation and elimination are polymorphic in human populations. While there are reports that indicate that genetic polymorphisms in GST and mEH affect the in-vitro mutagenicity of butadiene-derived epoxides or the mutagenicity of butadiene in occupationally exposed workers (Wiencke *et al.*, 1995; Abdel-Rahman *et al.*, 2003), the extent to which these enzyme variabilities impact the carcinogenicity of butadiene is not known. In addition, CYP is inducible by a variety of environmental and pharmaceutical agents. The reported range and distribution of butadiene or epoxybutene oxidation kinetics in human tissues *in vitro* is limited by the high interindividual variability in CYP, EH and GST activities and the fact that small numbers of human liver and lung samples have been analysed (Bolt *et al.*, 2003; Thier *et al.*, 2003; Norppa, 2004; Schlade-Bartusiak *et al.*, 2004).

The metabolism of butadiene in mice and rats demonstrates linear metabolic elimination kinetics at exposures of up to about 1000 ppm [2210 mg/m^3] (Kreiling *et al.*, 1986b). Toxicity studies conducted with much higher exposures add little additional information on the health effects of butadiene metabolites due to saturation of butadiene metabolism. Responses that increase proportionally with exposures above 1000 ppm butadiene probably represent effects of the parent compound. In the range of linear kinetics, mice metabolize butadiene at about twice the rate observed in rats. Species differences in metabolic clearance of butadiene at low exposure concentrations are largely due to differences in blood:air partition coefficients and physiological parameters that include alveolar ventilation rate, cardiac output and blood flow to metabolizing tissues (Kohn & Melnick, 1993; Sweeney *et al.*, 2001).

Although the formation of epoxybutene occurs primarily by CYP-mediated oxidation of butadiene, formation of this alkylating agent by a myeloperoxidase-catalysed reaction in bone-marrow cells (Maniglier-Poulet *et al.*, 1995) may be relevant to the induction of haematopoietic cancers in mice and humans.

Data on urinary metabolites indicate that the elimination of epoxybutene in mice occurs to a greater extent by conjugation with GSH than by hydrolysis (IARC, 1999). Although no studies have been reported that characterize the full profile of urinary metabolites for butadiene in humans, the high ratio of DHBMA to MHBMA in exposed workers indicates that epoxybutene is preferentially metabolized by hydrolysis before GSH conjugation in humans. In rats, metabolic elimination of epoxybutene formed from butadiene occurs to a similar extent by hydrolysis or GSH conjugation. In molecular epidemiological studies of occupational exposures to butadiene, the ratio of MHBMA to MHBMA + DHBMA was lower in workers who had homozygous null genotypes for *GSTM1* and *GSTT1* (Albertini *et al.*, 2001, 2003a).

The formation of epoxybutanediol or diepoxybutane requires a second oxidation step on either butenediol or epoxybutene, respectively. At increasing exposure concentrations of butadiene, competition between butadiene and butenediol or epoxybutene for CYP may limit the extent to which the second oxidation reaction may occur. Consequently, the blood concentration of epoxybutanediol is greater in rats exposed to 200 ppm [442 mg/m^3] butadiene than in those exposed to levels of 1000 ppm [2210 mg/m^3] or higher (Filser *et al.*, 2007). Competitive inhibition by butadiene of the second oxidation (Filser *et al.*, 2001) may account for the greater *Hprt* mutation efficiency in rats exposed to 62.5 ppm [138 mg/m^3] or mice exposed to 3 ppm [6.63 mg/m^3] compared with exposure of either species to 625 or 1250 ppm [1381 or 2762.5 mg/m^3] (Meng *et al.*, 2007a). Thus, high-dose studies of butadiene in animals ($\geq$ 625 ppm) may not adequately reveal the full carcinogenic potential of this gas at lower levels of exposure.

Haemoglobin adducts have been measured as biomarkers of internal levels of the epoxide intermediates of butadiene metabolism. Levels of MHbVal, PyrVal and THbVal adducts are reflective of blood concentrations of epoxybutene, diepoxybutane and epoxybutanediol, respectively. Each of these adducts has been measured in rats and mice exposed to butadiene at concentrations as low as 3 ppm [6.63 mg/m^3]. At equivalent exposures to butadiene, the levels of MHbVal and PyrVal were higher in mice than in rats, while levels of the major adduct, THbVal, were similar in these species (Boysen *et al.*, 2004, 2007). The formation of each of these adducts in mice and rats was more efficient at 3 ppm than at higher exposure concentrations of butadiene. MHbVal and THbVal have also been measured in workers exposed to butadiene (mean 8-h TWA exposures of 0.3–0.8 ppm [0.66–1.76 mg/m^3]), while levels of PyrVal in workers exposed to mean concentrations of 0.37 ppm [0.82 mg/m^3] were below the limit of detection (Albertini *et al.*, 2003a, 2007). Species differences in the levels of these haemoglobin adducts reflect differences in exposure to butadiene, blood levels of the epoxide intermediates, reactivity of the epoxide with the *N*-terminal valine and other reactive sites of haemoglobin and the half-life of red blood cells. When adduct levels are normalized per gram of haemoglobin per part per million of butadiene, the levels of MHbVal adducts in workers are slightly lower than those in rats exposed to 3 ppm [6.63 mg/m^3] butadiene, while the levels of THbVal adducts are higher in workers than in rats or mice exposed to 3 ppm butadiene. These data demonstrate the systemic availability of epoxybutene and epoxybutanediol in workers at occupational exposure levels of butadiene. In workers exposed to butadiene, THbVal levels are affected by the combined polymorphisms for *CYP2E1*, *GSTM1* and *GSTT1* genes (Fustinoni *et al.*, 2002).

The major DNA adducts formed in the liver, lung and kidney of rats and mice exposed to butadiene are at the *N7* position of guanine. G4 adducts are much more abundant than G1 and G2 adducts, which are derived from epoxybutene (Koc *et al.*, 1999). G4 adducts reach a plateau in rats at about 62 ppm [137 mg/m^3] butadiene, while G1 and G2 adducts increase nearly linearly with exposures to butadiene of up to 625 ppm [1381 mg/m^3]. The similarity in the shape of the dose–response curves for the formation of THbVal adducts, G4 adducts and the *Hprt* mutation frequency in splenic T cells from mice and rats exposed to butenediol suggests that epoxybutanediol may play a role in the mutagenicity and carcinogenicity of butadiene (Powley *et al.*, 2005). *N7*-Guanine adducts can undergo spontaneous depurination from DNA and create apurinic sites. Epoxide metabolites of butadiene can also react at base-pairing sites to form adducts at *N3*-cytosine, *N1*-adenine, *N^6*-adenine, *N1*-guanine and *N^2*-guanine (Selzer & Elfarra, 1996a,b, 1997; Zhao *et al.*, 1998; Zhang & Elfarra, 2004). An increase in *N1*-

trihydroxybutyladenine adducts was detected in lymphocytes of workers occupationally exposed to butadiene (Zhao *et al.*, 2000). Alkylation of *N*1-adenine by epoxybutene followed by hydrolytic deamination to form deoxyinosine has been shown to be highly mutagenic (Rodriguez *et al.*, 2001); this DNA lesion strongly codes for incorporation of cytosine during DNA replication which leads to the generation of A→G mutations. Diepoxybutane is a bifunctional alkylating agent that can form DNA–DNA crosslinks through binding at the *N*7 position of guanine of double-stranded DNA to produce bis-*N*7-guanine-2,3-butanediol (Park & Tretyakova, 2004). Depurination of these interstrand or intrastrand lesions can induce point mutations and large deletion mutations. However, when diepoxybutane alkylates an N^6-adenine in DNA, an exocyclic adenine adduct is formed preferentially to DNA–DNA cross-linked products (Antsypovich *et al.*, 2007).

Butadiene and its epoxide metabolites are genotoxic at multiple tissue sites in mice and rats and in a variety of other test systems. In-vitro studies demonstrate that diepoxybutane is more potent than epoxybutene or epoxybutanediol in the induction of micronuclei and gene mutations in mammalian cells. Epoxybutanediol, epoxybutene and diepoxybutane induced G→A transition mutations, adenine mutations (A→T and A→G) and deletions (Recio *et al.*, 2001; Lee *et al.*, 2002). The observed base substitution mutations induced by these alkylating agents are consistent with their DNA adduct profiles. A→T and G→C transversions are the most common mutations observed after in-vivo exposure to butadiene or in-vitro exposure to epoxybutene or diepoxybutane.

Markers of individual susceptibility can modulate the genotoxic effects of butadiene. In experimental studies, mice that lack a functional mEH gene were more susceptible than wild-type mice to the mutagenic effects of butadiene or diepoxybutane (Wickliffe *et al.*, 2003). EH activity varies considerably among individuals. Butadiene-exposed workers with the low EH activity genotype were reported to be more susceptible to butadiene-induced genotoxicity (lymphocyte *HPRT* mutant variant frequency) than individuals with the more common EH genotype (Abdel-Rahman *et al.*, 2001, 2003). In contrast, no significant effects were observed for induction of *HPRT* mutations or sister chromatid exchange in individuals with *GST* (M1 or T1) polymorphisms (Abdel-Rahman *et al.*, 2001). These differences in response are consistent with the known important role of EH in the detoxification of butadiene epoxides in tissues in which these intermediates are produced. Several other molecular epidemiological studies report no effect of butadiene on *HPRT* mutations or chromosomal changes at levels of occupational exposure and no significant associations with genotype (Zhang *et al.*, 2004; Albertini *et al.*, 2001, 2007). Discrepancies among these studies may be related to differences in workplace levels of exposure to butadiene, the impact of exposures to butadiene or other genotoxic agents from other sources (e.g. cigarette smoke, automobile exhaust), group size and the level of enzyme activity associated with a particular genotype.

The induction of sister chromatid exchange in human lymphocytes exposed *in vitro* to diepoxybutane was significantly higher in lymphocytes from *GSTT1*-null individuals than *GSTT1*-positive individuals (Wiencke *et al.*, 1995), which indicates that the GST pathway may be important in the detoxification of diepoxybutane released into whole blood.

Epoxybutene can induce sister chromatid exchange and chromosomal aberrations in human peripheral lymphocytes treated *in vitro*; the lack of induction of these effects in G_0 lymphocytes appears to be due to effective DNA excision repair (Kligerman *et al.*, 1999b). Other studies demonstrate the importance of DNA repair in the genotoxicity of butadiene-derived epoxides. For example, mice deficient in nucleotide excision repair activity are more susceptible than wild-type mice to the mutagenic effects of butadiene and diepoxybutane (Wickliffe *et al.*, 2007).

The mechanistic link between animal and human neoplasia induced by butadiene is supported by the identification in mice of genetic alterations in butadiene-induced tumours that are frequently involved in the development of a variety of human cancers. The K-*ras*, H-*ras*, *p53*, *p16/p15* and *β-catenin* mutations detected in tumours in mice probably occurred as a result of the DNA reactivity and genotoxic effects of butadiene-derived epoxides. A consistent pattern of K-*ras* mutations (G→C transversions at codon 13) was observed in butadiene-induced cardiac haemangiosarcomas, neoplasms of the lung and forestomach and lymphomas (Hong *et al.*, 2000; Sills *et al.*, 2001; Ton *et al.*, 2007). Alterations in the *p53* gene in mouse brain tumours were mostly G→A transition mutations (Kim *et al.*, 2005). Inactivation of the tumour-suppressor genes *p16* and *p15* may also be important in the development of butadiene-induced lymphomas (Zhuang *et al.*, 2000). Mammary gland adenocarcinomas induced by butadiene in mice had frequent mutations in the *p53*, H-*ras* and *β-catenin* genes (Zhuang *et al.*, 2002). These observations point to a genotoxic mechanism that underlies the development of butadiene-induced cancers. Although genotoxicity data indicate that diepoxybutane is the most genotoxic of the butadiene epoxides, the relative contribution of these metabolic intermediates to the mutagenicity and carcinogenicity of butadiene is not known.

A comparison of the degree of evidence on metabolism, haemoglobin adduct formation and genetic changes in rodents and humans exposed to butadiene is given in Table 33.

Table 33. Comparison of the degree of evidence on metabolism, haemoglobin adduct formation and genetic changes in rodents and humans exposed to butadiene

Parameter	Rats	Mice	Humans
In-vitro metabolism of butadiene to epoxybutene	Strong	Strong	Strong
In-vitro metabolism of epoxybutene to diepoxybutane	Strong	Strong	Strong
In-vivo measure of epoxybutene in blood	Strong	Strong	NI
In-vivo measure of diepoxybutane in blood	Strong	Strong	NI
N-(2,3,4-Trihydroxybutyl)valine haemoglobin adducts	Strong	Strong	Strong
N-(2-Hydroxy-3-butenyl)valine haemoglobin adducts	Strong	Strong	Strong

Table 33 (contd)

Parameter	Rats	Mice	Humans
N,N-(2,3-Dihydroxy-1,4-butadiyl)valine haemoglobin adduct	Strong	Strong	Weak[a]
Urinary excretion of butadiene-derived mercapturic acid metabolites	Strong	Strong	Strong
DNA adducts	Strong	Strong	Strong
Mutations in reporter genes in somatic cells	Strong	Strong	Inconsistent[b]
Chromosomal aberrations or micronuclei	No evidence	Strong	Weak[a]

NI, no information
[a] Possibly due to a lack of adequate studies
[b] Three negative and one positive studies

5.   Summary of Data Reported

5.1   Exposure data

1,3-Butadiene is a colourless gas that is produced by three different methods. More than 95% of global production is as a co-product from the industrial synthesis of ethylene. Regardless of the process, the production of butadiene monomer requires the removal of impurities. Butadiene is used primarily (85%) in the production of synthetic rubbers and polymers (polymer production).

The highest exposure to butadiene occurs in occupational settings. No measurements of exposure in butadiene monomer production before the 1970s are available, but levels of exposure have decreased from the late 1970s to the early 2000s from < 20 mg/m^3 to < 2 mg/m^3.

In styrene–butadiene polymer production, the estimated median levels of exposure to butadiene in earlier decades varied from 8 mg/m3 to 20 mg/m^3, while current measurements of exposure in modern facilities in North America and western Europe are generally below 2 mg/m^3. Levels reported in China are somewhat higher (~4 mg/m^3). Regardless of the type of factory, production process or country, some tasks are still characterized by very high exposures (~200 mg/m^3) that are typically short in duration.

Butadiene is a ubiquitous environmental contaminant and levels lower than those found in occupational settings have been reported in ambient air (< 0.02 mg/m^3); these mainly originate from combustion products (e.g. motor vehicle emissions and tobacco smoke).

The American Conference of Governmental Industrial Hygienists has reported occupational exposure limits for butadiene in various countries that range from 1 to 1000 ppm (2–2210 mg/m^3).

5.2   Cancer in humans

The Working Group reviewed studies of three cohorts of workers in the butadiene monomer industry and two cohorts of workers in the styrene–butadiene rubber industry. A study of styrene–butadiene rubber workers by researchers at the University of Alabama at Birmingham was considered by the Working Group to be the most informative. This study examined the mortality rates of approximately 17 000 workers from eight styrene–butadiene rubber facilities in the USA and Canada. Earlier studies of some of the facilities included in this study were carried out by researchers at the National Institute for Occupational Safety and Health and at Johns Hopkins' University.

A limiting factor in the present evaluation was that the diagnosis and classification of lymphatic and haematopoietic malignancies are extremely complex and have undergone several changes over the course of time (see General Remarks).

Although overall mortality from leukaemia was only slightly elevated in the most recent update of the University of Alabama at Birmingham cohort, larger excesses of mortality from leukaemia were seen in workers in the most highly exposed areas of the plants and among hourly paid workers, especially those who had been hired in the early years and had had longer employment (i.e. ≥ 10 years). These excesses were attributable to increased rates of mortality from both chronic lymphocytic and chronic myelogenous leukaemia. Furthermore, a significant exposure–response relationship between cumulative exposure to butadiene and mortality from leukaemia was observed in this study. Exposure–response relationships were apparent for both chronic lymphocytic and chronic myelogenous leukaemia. An exposure–response relationship between cumulative exposure to butadiene and leukaemia was also apparent in an earlier analysis conducted by the University of Alabama at Birmingham that used a different method for the assessment of exposure and in the previous Johns Hopkin's study. While concerns had been raised that these findings might have been due to confounding from exposure to other chemicals in the styrene–butadiene rubber industry, the most recent analyses indicated that the exposure–response relationship for butadiene and leukaemia was independent of exposures to benzene, styrene and dimethyldithiocarbamate.

A slight overall excess of mortality from leukaemia was also observed in two of the studies of the butadiene monomer industry, whereas a small deficit in mortality was observed in the third cohort study. The excess of mortality from leukaemia in one of the monomer industry cohorts was more pronounced among workers who had been exposed during the Second World War when exposures to butadiene had probably been higher. The excess of leukaemia in this cohort did not increase with duration of exposure or cumulative exposure.

The strongest evidence for an association between butadiene and non-Hodgkin lymphoma derives from the studies of workers in the monomer industry. Based on four cases (lymphosarcoma and reticulosarcoma), an approximately sixfold statistically significant excess risk was observed in one of the three studies. An approximately 50% non-significant excess of mortality from non-Hodgkin lymphoma was reported in another study of the monomer industry. Although the excess of mortality from non-Hodgkin lymphoma in this study did not increase with duration of exposure, it was more pronounced among workers who had been exposed during the Second World War when exposures had presumably been higher. The third study of the monomer industry reported only one case of non-Hodgkin lymphoma (0.2 expected). A non-significant twofold excess of mortality from lymphosarcoma and reticulosarcoma was reported in one of the two plants included in the earlier National Institute for Occupational Safety and Health study of styrene–butadiene rubber workers. No overall excess of mortality from non-Hodgkin lymphoma was observed in the University of Alabama at Birmingham study.

Overall, the epidemiological studies provide evidence that exposure to butadiene causes cancer in humans. This excess risk cannot be reasonably explained by confounding, bias or chance. This conclusion is primarily based on the evidence for a significant exposure–response relationship between exposure to butadiene and mortality from leukaemia in the University of Alabama in Birmingham study, which appears to be independent of other potentially confounding exposures. It is also supported by elevated relative risks for non-Hodgkin lymphoma in other studies, particularly in the butadiene monomer production industry. The Working Group was unable to determine the strength of the evidence for particular histological subtypes of lymphatic and haematopoietic neoplasms because of the changes in coding and diagnostic practices for these neoplasms that have occurred during the course of the epidemiological investigations. However, the Working Group considered that there was compelling evidence that exposure to butadiene is associated with an increased risk for leukaemias.

5.3   Cancer in experimental animals

Two bioassays of butadiene by inhalation exposure in mice showed increases in the incidence of lymphoma and neoplasms of the heart, lung, forestomach, liver, Harderian gland, preputial gland and kidney in males and increases in the incidence of lymphomas and neoplasms of the heart, lung, forestomach, liver, Harderian gland, ovary and mammary gland in females. The heart neoplasms were highly malignant and distinctive forms of haemangiosarcoma that were very rare in historical controls. The second bioassay was undertaken at much lower exposure levels than the first, but tumours developed at the same organ sites in both studies. The second study included exposure levels that were comparable with or even lower than historical levels of occupational exposure in humans.

In a single study of inhalation exposure in rats, butadiene caused increases in the incidence of pancreatic exocrine adenomas and carcinomas and interstitial-cell tumours of the testis in males. In females, increases in the incidence of thyroid follicular-cell tumours, uterine sarcomas, Zymbal gland carcinomas and benign and malignant mammary tumours were observed. This study was conducted at exposure levels that were much higher than those used in the inhalation bioassays in mice.

D,L-Diepoxybutane, a metabolite of butadiene, was tested for carcinogenicity in mice by repeated subcutaneous injection, by repeated intraperitoneal injection and by inhalation exposure. It caused fibrosarcomas at the site of subcutaneous injection and increased the incidence of Harderian gland tumours following inhalation exposure.

D,L-Diepoxybutane was tested for carcinogenicity in rats in one study by inhalation and caused squamous-cell carcinomas of the nasal mucosa. It also induced fibrosarcomas in rats at the site of repeated subcutaneous injection, but did not cause gastric tumours when administered by gavage.

meso-Diepoxybutane was tested for carcinogenicity by skin application in one study in male and one study in female mice in direct comparison with D,L-diepoxybutane. In both studies, *meso*-diepoxybutane caused an increased incidence of squamous-cell papillomas and carcinomas of the skin at the site of application while D,L-diepoxybutane gave negative results.

5.4   Mechanistic and other relevant data

The carcinogenicity of butadiene is most probably mediated by its metabolic intermediates. This assumption is based largely on the fact that butadiene-induced mutagenicity requires metabolic activation and that the DNA-reactive epoxides (stereoisomers of epoxybutene, epoxybutanediol and diepoxybutane) that are formed during the biotransformation of butadiene are direct-acting mutagens. Studies in humans indicate that butadiene is absorbed via inhalation and that the blood:air partition coefficient and alveolar ventilation are important parameters in the determination of uptake. Several studies have quantified the presence of metabolites derived from butadiene in the urine of humans exposed via inhalation in controlled laboratory, environmental or workplace settings. Two urinary metabolites have been identified in humans: 1,2-dihydroxybutyl mercapturic acid and monohydroxy-3-butenyl mercapturic acid, which are derived from the conjugation with glutathione of hydroxymethylvinyl ketone (a metabolite of butenediol) and epoxybutene, respectively.

Several molecular epidemiological studies have assessed the utility of haemoglobin adducts as biomarkers of human exposure to butadiene. The butadiene metabolite, epoxybutene, can react with the *N*-terminal valine of haemoglobin to form *N*-(2-hydroxy-3-butenyl)valine adducts, which have been observed in workers exposed to butadiene. The haemoglobin adduct, *N*-(2,3,4-trihydroxybutyl)valine, which is formed from epoxybutanediol or diepoxybutane, has also been observed in these workers. *N*,*N*-(2,3-Dihydroxy-1,4-butadiyl)valine, which is another adduct formed by the reaction of diepoxybutane with haemoglobin, has not been detected in butadiene-exposed workers. The presence of *N*-(2,3,4-trihydroxybutyl)valine and *N*-(2-hydroxy-3-butenyl)valine in workers exposed to butadiene demonstrates the systemic availability of the metabolites epoxybutene and epoxybutanediol at occupational exposure levels.

Several studies in humans have demonstrated the DNA-binding properties and clastogenic effects of butadiene. An increase in N1-(2,3,4-trihydroxybutyl)adenine adducts — derived from epoxybutanediol or diepoxybutane — was detected in the lymphocytes of workers occupationally exposed to butadiene. One study in workers exposed to butadiene found an increase in the frequency of chromosomal aberrations and sister chromatid exchange. Other studies found no significant increases in chromosomal alterations in workers, although the exposure concentrations were lower than those used in studies with mice.

The enzymes that regulate epoxide formation and elimination are polymorphic in human populations. The extent to which the variabilities of these enzymes modulate the carcinogenicity of butadiene is not known. Butadiene-exposed workers with the low epoxide hydrolase activity genotype were more susceptible to butadiene-induced geno-toxicity (frequency of human hypoxanthine–guanine phosphoribosyl transferase gene variants in lymphocytes).

More than 10 urinary metabolites, including the conjugation products monohydroxy-3-butenyl mercapturic acid and 1,2-dihydroxybutyl mercapturic acid, have been identified in butadiene-exposed rats and mice.

At equivalent exposures to butadiene, blood levels of the haemoglobin adducts N-(2-hydroxy-3-butenyl)valine and N,N-(2,3-dihydroxy-1,4-butadiyl)valine were higher in mice than in rats, while levels of the major adduct, N-(2,3,4-trihydroxybutyl)valine, were similar in these species. All of these adducts have been measured in rats and mice exposed to butadiene at concentrations as low as 3 ppm (6 mg/m^3).

Butadiene is clastogenic in mice and induces chromosomal aberrations, micronucleus formation and sister chromatid exchange. It has not been found to be clastogenic in rats.

The most abundant DNA adduct measured in rats and mice exposed to butadiene is N7-trihydroxybutylguanine, which is derived from either epoxybutanediol or diepoxy-butane. Epoxide metabolites of butadiene can also react at base-pairing sites to form adducts at N3-cytosine, N1-adenine, N^6-adenine, N1-guanine and N^2-guanine. Butadiene and its epoxide metabolites are genotoxic at multiple tissue sites in mice and rats and in a variety of other test systems.

Mutations in *ras* proto-oncogenes and the *p53* tumour-suppressor gene (genes that are involved in the development of a variety of cancers) were identified in several different types of tumour induced by butadiene in mice. A→T and G→C transversions are the most common mutations observed after in-vivo exposure to butadiene or in-vitro exposure to epoxybutene or diepoxybutane.

Although genotoxicity data indicate that diepoxybutane is the most genotoxic epoxide formed from butadiene, the relative contribution of all epoxide metabolites to the mutagenicity and carcinogenicity of butadiene is not known.

6.   Evaluation and Rationale

6.1   Carcinogenicity in humans

There is *sufficient evidence* in humans for the carcinogenicity of 1,3-butadiene.

6.2   Carcinogenicity in experimental animals

There is *sufficient evidence* in experimental animals for the carcinogenicity of 1,3-butadiene.

There is *sufficient evidence* in experimental animals for the carcinogenicity of D,L-diepoxybutane.

6.3   Overall evaluation

1,3-Butadiene is *carcinogenic to humans (Group 1)*.

7.   References

Abdel-Rahman, S.Z., Ammenheuser, M.M. & Ward, J.B., Jr (2001) Human sensitivity to 1,3-butadiene: Role of microsomal epoxide hydrolase polymorphisms. *Carcinogenesis*, **22**, 415–423

Abdel-Rahman, S.Z., El-Zein, R.A., Ammenheuser, M.M., Yang, Z., Stock, T.H., Morandi, M. & Ward, J.B., Jr (2003) Variability in human sensitivity to 1,3-butadiene: Influence of the allelic variants of the microsomal epoxide hydrolase gene. *Environ. mol. Mutag.*, **41**, 140–146

ACGIH (2001) *1,3-Butadiene. CD ROM*, Cincinnati, OH, American Conference of Government Industrial Hygienists

ACGIH® Worldwide (2005) *Documentation of the TLVs® and BEIs® with Other Worldwide Occupational Exposure Values — 2005 CD-ROM*, Cincinnati, OH, American Conference of Government Industrial Hygienists

Adler, I.-D., Cao, J., Filser, J.G., Gassner, P., Kessler, W., Kliesch, U., Neuhäuser-Klaus, A. & Nüsse, M. (1994) Mutagenicity of 1,3-butadiene inhalation in somatic and germinal cells of mice. *Mutat. Res.*, **309**, 307–314

Adler, I.-D., Filser, J.G., Gassner, P., Kessler, W., Schöneich, J. & Schriever-Schwemmer, G. (1995) Heritable translocations induced by inhalation exposure of male mice to 1,3-butadiene. *Mutat. Res.*, **347**, 121–127

Adler, I.D., Filser, J., Gonda, H., & Schriever-Schwemmer, G. (1998) Dose–response study for 1,3-butadiene-induced dominant lethal mutations and heritable translocations in germs cells of male mice. *Mutat. Res.*, **397**, 85–92

AEA Energy & Environment (2002) [http://www.airquality.co.uk/archive/standards.php; accessed 09.01.2008]

Agency for Toxic Substances and Disease Registry (1992) *Toxicological Profile for 1,3-Butadiene* (Report No. TR-91/07), Atlanta, GA

Albertini, R.J., Sram, R.J., Vacek, P.M., Lynch, J., Wright, M., Nicklas, J.A., Boogaard, P.J., Henderson, R.F., Swenberg, J.A., Tates, A.D. & Ward, J.B., Jr (2001) Biomarkers for assessing occupational exposures to 1,3-butadiene. *Chem.-biol. Interact.*, **135–136**, 429–453

Albertini, R.J., Sram, R.J., Vacek, P.M., Lynch, J., Nicklas, J.A., van Sittert, N.J., Boogaard, P.J., Henderson, R.F., Swenberg, J.A., Tates, A.D., Ward, J.B., Jr, Wright, M., Ammenheuser, M.M., Binkova, B., Blackwell, W., de Zwart, F.A., Krako, D., Krone, J., Megens, H., Musilova, P., Rajska, G., Ranasinghe, A., Rosenblatt, J.I., Rossner, P., Rubes, J., Sullivan, L., Upton, P. & Zwinderman, A.H. (2003) Biomarkers in Czech workers exposed to 1,3-butadiene: A transitional epidemiologic study. *Res. Rep. Health Eff. Inst.*, **116**, 1–141

Albertini, R.J., Sram, R.J., Vacek, P.M., Lynch, J., Rossner, P., Nicklas, J.A., McDonald, J.D., Boysen, G., Georgieva, N. & Swenberg, J.A. (2007) Molecular epidemiological studies in 1,3-butadiene exposed Czech workers: Female–male comparisons. *Chem.-biol. Interact.*, **166**, 63–77

Ammenheuser, M.M., Bechtold, W.E., Abdel-Rahman, S.Z., Rosenblatt, J.I., Hastings-Smith, D.A. & Ward, J.B., Jr (2001) Assessment of 1,3-butadiene exposure in polymer production workers using HPRT mutations in lymphocytes as a biomarker. *Environ. Health Perspect.*, **110**, 1249–1255

Anderson, D., Edwards, A.J. & Brinkworth, M.H. (1993) Male-mediated F_1 effects in mice exposed to 1,3-butadiene. In: Sorsa, M., Peltonen, K., Vainio, H. & Hemminki, K., eds, *Butadiene and Styrene: Assessment of Health Hazards* (IARC Scientific Publications No. 127), Lyon, IARC, pp. 171–181

Anderson, D., Dobrzynka, M.M., Jackson, L.I., Yu, T.W. & Brinkworth, M.H. (1997) Somatic and germ cell effects in rats and mice after treatment with 1,3-butadiene and its metabolites, 1,2-epoxybutene and 1,2,3,4-diepoxybutane. *Mutat. Res.*, **391**, 233–242

Anderson, D., Hughes, J.A., Edwards, A.J. & Brinkworth, M.H. (1998) A comparison of male-mediated effects in rats and mice exposed to 1,3-butadiene. *Mutat. Res.*, **397**, 77–84

Antsypovich, S., Quirk-Dorr, D., Pitts, C. & Tretyakova, N. (2007) Site specific N^6-(2-hydroxy-3,4-epoxybut-1-yl)adenine oligodeoxynucleotide adducts of 1,2,3,4-diepoxybutane: Synthesis and stability at physiological pH. *Chem. Res. Toxicol.*, **20**, 641–649

Anttinen-Klemetti, T., Vaaranrinta, R., Mutanen, P. & Peltonen, K. (2004) Personal exposure to 1,3-butadiene in a petrochemical plant, assessed by use of diffusive samplers. *Int. Arch. occup. environ. Health*, **77**, 288–292

Anttinen-Klemetti, T., Vaaranrinta, R., Mutanen, P. & Peltonen, K. (2006) Inhalation exposure to 1,3-butadiene and styrene in styrene–butadiene copolymer production. *Int. J. Hyg. environ. Health*, **209**, 151–158

Araki, A., Noguchi, T., Kato, F. & Matsushima, T. (1994) Improved method for mutagenicity testing of gaseous compounds by using a gas sampling bag. *Mutat. Res.*, **307**, 335–344

ASTM (2004) *ASTM D2593-93. Standard Test Method for Butadiene Purity and Hydrocarbon Impurities by Gas Chromatography*, West Conshohocken, PA, American Society for Testing and Materials

Austin, C.C., Wang, D., Ecobihon, D.J. & Dussault, G. (2001) Characterization of volatile organic compounds in smoke at municipal structural fires. *J. Toxicol. environ. Health*, **63**, 437–458

Autio, K., Renzi, L., Catalan, J., Albrecht, O.E. & Sorsa, M. (1994) Induction of micronuclei in peripheral blood and bone marrow erythrocytes of rats and mice exposed to 1,3-butadiene by inhalation. *Mutat. Res.*, **309**, 315–320

Belanger, P.L. & Elesh, E. (1980) *Health Hazard Evaluation Determination, Bell Helmets Inc., Norwalk, CA* (Report No. 79-36-646), Cincinnati, OH, National Institute for Occupational Safety and Health

Bevan, C., Keller, D.A., Panepinto, A.S. & Bentley, K.S. (2001) Effect of 4-vinylcyclohexene on micronucleus formation in the bone marrow of rats and mice. *Drug chem. Toxicol.*, **24**, 273–285

Bianchi, A., Boyle, B., Harrison, P., Lawrie, P., Le Lendu, T., Rocchi, P., Taalman, R. & Wieder, W. (1997) *A Review of Analytical Methods and their Significance to Subsequent Occupational Exposure Data Evaluation for 1,3-Butadiene* (Analytical Working Report), Brussels, European Chemical Industry Council

Blair, I.A., Oe, T., Kambouris, S. & Chaudhary, A.K. (2000) 1,3-Butadiene: Cancer, mutations, and adducts. Part IV: Molecular dosimetry of 1,3-butadiene. *Res. Rep. Health Eff. Inst.*, **92**, 151–190

Bolt, H.M. & Jelitto, B. (1996) Biological formation of the 1,3-butadiene DNA adducts 7-*N*-(2-hydroxy-3-buten-1-yl)guanine, 7-*N*-(1-hydroxy-3-buten-2-yl)guanine and 7-*N*-(2,3,4-trihydroxy-butyl)guanine. *Toxicology*, **113**, 328–330

Bolt, H.M., Roos, P.H. & Thier, R. (2003) The cytochrome P-450 isoenzyme CYP2E1 in the biological processing of industrial chemicals: Consequences for occupational and environmental medicine. *Int. Arch. occup. environ. Health*, **76**, 174–185

Bond, G.G., Bodner, K.M., Olsen, G.W. & Cook, R.R. (1992) Mortality among workers engaged in the development or manufacture of styrene-based products — An update. *Scand. J. Work Environ. Health*, **18**, 145–54

Boogaard, P.J. (2002) Use of haemoglobin adducts in exposure monitoring and risk assessment. *J. Chromatogr. B anal. Technol. biomed. Life Sci.*, **778**, 309–322

Boogaard, P.J., van Sittert, N.J. & Megens, H.J.J.J. (2001a) Urinary metabolites and haemoglobin adducts as biomarkers of exposure to 1,3-butadiene: A basis for 1,3-butadiene cancer risk assessment. *Chem.-biol. Interact.*, **135–136**, 695–701

Boogaard, P.J., van Sittert, N.J., Watson, W.P. & de Kloe, K.P. (2001b) A novel DNA adduct, originating from 1,2-epoxy-3,4-butanediol, is the major DNA adduct after exposure to [2,3-^{14}C]-1,3-butadiene, but not after exposure to [4-^{14}C]-1,2-epoxy-3-butene. *Chem.-biol. Interact.*, **135–136**, 687–693

Boogaard, P.J., de Kloe, K.P., Booth, E.D., & Watson, W.P. (2004) DNA adducts in rats and mice following exposure to [4-^{14}C]-1,2-epoxy-3-butene and to [2,3-^{14}C]-1,3-butadiene. *Chem.-biol. Interact.*, **148**, 69–92

Booth, E.D., Kilgour, J.D. & Watson, W.P. (2004a) Dose responses for the formation of hemoglobin adducts and urinary metabolites in rats and mice exposed by inhalation to low concentrations of 1,3-[2,3-^{14}C]-butadiene. *Chem.-biol. Interact.*, **147**, 213–232

Booth, E.D., Kilgour, J.D., Robinson, S.A. & Watson, W.P. (2004b) Dose responses for DNA adduct formation in tissues of rats and mice exposed by inhalation to low concentrations of 1,3-(2,3-[^{14}C])-butadiene. *Chem.-biol. Interact.*, **147**, 195–211

Boysen, G., Georgieva, N.I., Upton, P.B., Jayaraj, K., Li, Y., Walker, V.E. & Swenberg, J.A. (2004) Analysis of diepoxide-specific cyclic N-terminal globin adducts in mice and rats after inhalation exposure to 1,3-butadiene. *Cancer Res.*, **64**, 8517–8520

Boysen, G., Georgieva, N.I., Upton, P.B., Walker, V.E. & Swenberg, J.A. (2007) N-Terminal globin adducts as biomarkers for formation of butadiene derived epoxides. *Chem.-biol. Interact.*, **166**, 84–92

Brinkworth, M.H., Anderson, D., Hughes, J.A., Jackson, L.I., Yu, T.W. & Nieschlag, E. (1998) Genetic effects of 1,3-butadiene on the mouse testis. *Mutat. Res.*, **397**, 67–75

Brochot, C., Smith, T.J. & Bois, F.Y. (2007) Development of a physiologically based toxicokinetic model for butadiene and four major metabolites in humans: Global sensitivity analysis for experimental design issues. *Chem.-biol. Interact.*, **167**, 168–183

Bucher, J.R., Melnick, R.L. & Hildebrandt, P.K. (1993) Lack of carcinogenicity in mice exposed once to high concentrations of 1,3-butadiene. *J. natl Cancer Inst.*, **85**, 1866–1867

Burroughs, G.E. (1977) *Health Hazard Evaluation Determination, Firestone Synthetic Rubber Company, Akron, OH* (Report No. 77-1-426), Cincinnati, OH, National Institute for Occupational Safety and Health

Burroughs, G.E. (1979) *Health Hazard Evaluation Determination, Piper Aircraft Corporation, Vero Beach, FL* (Report No. 78-110-585), Cincinnati, OH, National Institute for Occupational Safety and Health

Carmical, J.R., Zhang, M., Nechev, L., Harris, C.M., Harris, T.M. & Lloyd, R.S. (2000a) Mutagenic potential of guanine N^2 adducts of butadiene mono- and diolepoxide. *Chem. Res. Toxicol.*, **13**, 18–25

Carmical, J.R., Nechev, L.V., Harris, C.M., Harris, T.M. & Lloyd, R.S. (2000b) Mutagenic potential of adenine N^6 adducts of monoepoxide and diolepoxide derivatives of butadiene. *Environ. mol. Mutag.*, **35**, 48–56

Carmical, J.R., Kowalczyk, A., Zou, Y., Van Houten, B., Nechev, L.V., Harris, C.M., Harris, T.M. & Lloyd, R.S. (2000c) Butadiene-induced intrastrand DNA cross-links: A possible role in deletion mutagenesis. *J. biol. Chem.*, **275**, 19482–19489

Catallo, W.J., Kennedy, C.H., Henk, W., Barker, S.A., Grace, S.C. & Penn, A. (2001) Combustion products of 1,3-butadiene are cytotoxic and genotoxic to human bronchial epithelial cells. *Environ. Health Perspect.*, **109**, 965–971

Chan, C.C., Shie, R.H., Chang, T.Y. & Tsai, D.H. (2006) Workers' exposures and potential health risks to air toxics in a petrochemical complex assessed by improved methodology. *Int. Arch. occup. environ. Health*, **79**, 135–142

Checkoway, H. & Williams, T.M. (1982) A hematology survey of workers at a styrene–butadiene synthetic rubber manufacturing plant. *Am. ind. Hyg. Assoc. J.*, **43**, 164–169

Cheng, H., Sathiakumar, N., Graff, J., Matthews, R. & Delzell, E. (2007) 1,3-Butadiene and leukemia among synthetic rubber industry workers: Exposure–response relationships. *Chem.-biol. Interact.*, **166**, 15–24

CMAI (Chemical Marketing Associates International) (2004) Product focus. Butadiene. *Chem. Week*, **February 11**, 26

CMAI (Chemical Marketing Associates International) (2006) Product focus. Butadiene. *Chem. Week*, **February 8**, 26

Cochrane, J.E. & Skopek, T.R. (1993) Mutagenicity of 1,3-butadiene and its epoxide metabolite in human TK6 cells and in splenic T cells isolated from exposed B6C3F1 mice. In: Sorsa, M., Peltonen, K., Vainio, H. & Hemminki, K., eds, *Butadiene and Styrene: Assessment of Health Hazards* (IARC Scientific Publications No. 127), Lyon, IARC, pp. 195–204

Cochrane, J.E. & Skopek, T.R. (1994) Mutagenicity of butadiene and its epoxide metabolites: II. Mutational spectra of butadiene, 1,2-epoxybutene and diepoxybutane at the *hprt* locus in splenic T cells from exposed B6C3F1 mice. *Carcinogenesis*, **15**, 719–723

CONCAWE (1987) *A Survey of Exposures to Gasoline Vapour* (Report No. 4/87), The Hague, Conservation of Clean Air and Water in Europe

Cowles, S.R., Tsai, S.P., Snyder, P.J. & Ross, C.E. (1994) Mortality, morbidity, and haematological results from a cohort of long-term workers involved in 1,3-butadiene monomer production. *Occup. environ. Med.*, **51**, 323–329

Csanady, G.A., Guengerich, F.P. & Bond, J.A. (1992) Comparison of the biotransformation of 1,3-butadiene and its metabolite, butadiene monoepoxide, by hepatic and pulmonary tissues from humans, rats and mice. *Carcinogenesis*, **13**, 1143–1153

Cunningham, M.J., Choy, W.N., Arce, G.T., Rickard, L.B., Vlachos, D.A., Kinney, L.A. & Sarrif, A.M. (1986) In vivo sister chromatid exchange and micronucleus induction studies with 1,3-butadiene in B6C3F1 mice and Sprague-Dawley rats. *Mutagenesis*, **1**, 449–452

Dahl, A.R. & Henderson, R.F. (2000) Comparative metabolism of low concentrations of butadiene and its monoepoxide in human and monkey hepatic microsomes. *Inhal. Toxicol.*, **12**, 439–451

Delzell, E., Sathiakumar, N., Hovinga, M., Macaluso, M., Julian, J., Larson, R., Cole, P. & Muir, D.C. (1996) A follow-up study of synthetic rubber workers. *Toxicology*, **113**, 182–189

Delzell, E., Macaluso, M., Sathiakumar, N. & Matthews, R. (2001) Leukemia and exposure to 1,3-butadiene, styrene and dimethyldithiocarbamate among workers in the synthetic rubber industry. *Chem.-biol. Interact.*, **135–136**, 515–534

Delzell, E., Sathiakumar, N., Graff, J., Macaluso, M., Maldonado, G. & Matthew, R. (2006) *An Updated Study of Mortality among North American Synthetic Rubber Industry Workers*, Boston, MA, Health Effects Institute

Divine, B.J. (1990) An update on mortality among workers at a 1,3-butadiene facility — Preliminary results. *Environ. Health Perspect.*, **86**, 119–128

Divine, B.J. & Hartman, C.M. (1996) Mortality update of butadiene production workers. *Toxicology*, **113**, 169–181

Divine, B.J. & Hartman, C.M. (2001) A cohort mortality study among workers at a 1,3-butadiene facility. *Chem.-biol. Interact.*, **135–136**, 535–553

Divine, B.J., Wendt, J.K. & Hartman, C.M. (1993) Cancer mortality among workers at a butadiene production facility. In: Sorsa, M., Peltonen, K., Vainio, H. & Hemminki, K., eds, *Butadiene and Styrene: Assessment of Health Hazards* (IARC Scientific Publications No. 127), Lyon, IARC, pp. 345–362

Dollard, G.J., Dore, C.J. & Jenkin, M.E. (2001) Ambient concentrations of 1,3-butadiene in the UK. *Chem.-biol. Interact.*, **135–136**, 177–206

Downs, T.D., Crane, M.M. & Kim, K.W. (1987) Mortality among workers at a butadiene facility. *Am. J. ind. Med.*, **12**, 311–329

Dubbeld, H. (1998) *Follow-up Study on a Model for Control of Health Hazards Resulting from Exposure to Toxic Substances* (Internal Report 1998-298), Wageningen, Wageningen Agricultural University, Environmental and Occupational Health Group

Duescher, R.J. & Elfarra, A.A. (1994) Human liver microsomes are efficient catalysts of 1,3-butadiene oxidation: Evidence for major roles by cytochromes P450 2A6 and 2E1. *Arch. Biochem. Biophys.*, **311**, 342–349

ECETOC (1997) *1,3-Butadiene OEL Criteria Document* (Special Report No. 12), Brussels, European Centre of Ecotoxicology and Toxicology of Chemicals

Elfarra, A.A., Sharer, J.E. & Duescher, R.J. (1995) Synthesis and characterization of *N*-acetyl-L-cysteine *S*-conjugates of butadiene monoxide and their detection and quantitation in urine of rats and mice given butadiene monoxide. *Chem. Res. Toxicol.*, **8**, 68–76

Elfarra, A.A., Moll, T.S., Krause, R.J., Kemper, R.A. & Selzer, R.R. (2001) Reactive metabolites of 1,3-butadiene: DNA and hemoglobin adduct formation and potential roles in carcinogenicity. *Adv. exp. Med. Biol.*, **500**, 93–103

Eller, P.M., ed. (1994) *NIOSH Manual of Analytical Methods* (DHHS (NIOSH) Publ. No. 94-113), 4th Ed., Cincinnati, OH, National Institute for Occupational Safety and Health [Method 1024]

Environmental Protection Agency Toxic Chemical Release Inventory (2005) [http://www.epa.gov]

Erexson, G.L. & Tindall, K.R. (2000a) Micronuclei and gene mutations in transgenic Big Blue® mouse and rat fibroblasts after exposure to the epoxide metabolites of 1,3-butadiene. *Mutat. Res.*, **472**, 105–117

Erexson, G.L. & Tindall, K.R. (2000b) Reduction of diepoxybutane-induced sister chromatid exchanges by glutathione peroxidase and erythrocytes in transgenic Big Blue® mouse and rat fibroblasts. *Mutat. Res.*, **447**, 267–274

Fajen, J.M. (1985a) *Industrial Hygiene Walk-through Survey Report of Texaco Company, Port Neches, TX* (Report No. 147.14), Cincinnati, OH, National Institute for Occupational Safety and Health

Fajen, J.M. (1985b) *Industrial Hygiene Walk-through Survey Report of Mobil Chemical Company, Beaumont, TX* (Report No. 147.11), Cincinnati, OH, National Institute for Occupational Safety and Health

Fajen, J.M. (1985c) *Industrial Hygiene Walk-through Survey Report of ARCO Chemical Company, Channelview, TX* (Report No. 147.12), Cincinnati, OH, National Institute for Occupational Safety and Health

Fajen, J.M. (1986a) *Industrial Hygiene Walk-through Survey Report of E.I. du Pont deNemours and Company, LaPlace, LA* (Report No. 147.31), Cincinnati, OH, National Institute for Occupational Safety and Health

Fajen, J.M. (1986b) *Industrial Hygiene Walk-through Survey Report of the Goodyear Tire and Rubber Company, Houston, TX* (Report No. 147.34), Cincinnati, OH, National Institute for Occupational Safety and Health

Fajen, J.M. (1988) *Extent of Exposure Study: 1,3-Butadiene Polymer Production Industry*, Cincinnati, OH, National Institute for Occupational Safety and Health

Fajen, J.M., Roberts, D.R., Ungers, L.J. & Krishnan, E.R. (1990) Occupational exposure of workers to 1,3-butadiene. *Environ. Health Perspect.*, **86**, 11–18

Fernandes, P.H., Hackfeld, L.C., Kozekov, I.D., Hodge, R.P. & Lloyd, R.S. (2006) Synthesis and mutagenesis of the butadiene-derived N3 2′-deoxyuridine adducts. *Chem. Res. Toxicol.*, **19**, 968–976

Filser, J.G., Faller, T.H., Bhowmik, S., Schuster, A., Kessler, W., Pütz, C. & Csanady, G.A. (2001) First-pass metabolism of 1,3-butadiene in once-through perfused livers of rats and mice. *Chem.-biol. Interact.*, **135–136**, 249–265

Filser, J.G., Hutzler, C., Meischner, V., Veereshwarayya, V. & Csanady, G.A. (2007) Metabolism of 1,3-butadiene to toxicologically relevant metabolites in single-exposed mice and rats. *Chem.-biol. Interact.*, **166**, 93–193

Food and Drug Administration (1987) 1,3-Butadiene. In: Fazio, T. & Sherma, J., eds, *Food Additives Analytical Manual*, Vol. II, *A Collection of Analytical Methods for Selected Food Additives*, Arlington, VA, Association of Official Analytical Chemists, pp. 58–68

Foureman, P., Mason, J.M., Valencia, R. & Zimmering, S. (1994) Chemical mutagenesis testing in *Drosophila*. IX. Results of 50 coded compounds tested for the National Toxicology Program. *Environ. mol. Mutag.*, **23**, 51–63

Fred, C., Kautiainen, A., Athanassiadis, I. & Tornqvist, M. (2004) Hemoglobin adduct levels in rat and mouse treated with 1,2:3,4-diepoxybutane. *Chem. Res. Toxicol.*, **17**, 785–794

Fred, C., Grawe, J. & Tornqvist, M. (2005) Hemoglobin adducts and micronuclei in rodents after treatment with isoprene monoxide or butadiene monoxide. *Mutat. Res.*, **585**, 21–32

Fustinoni, S., Soleo, L., Warholm, M., Begemann, P., Rannug, A., Neumann, H.G., Swenberg, J.A., Vimercati, L., Foa, V. & Colombi, A. (2002) Influence of metabolic genotypes on biomarkers of exposure to 1,3-butadiene in humans. *Cancer Epidemiol. Biomarkers Prev.*, **11**, 1082–1090

Fustinoni, S., Perbellini, L., Soleo, L., Manno, M. & Foa, V. (2004) Biological monitoring in occupational exposure to low levels of 1,3-butadiene. *Toxicol. Lett.*, **149**, 353–360

Goggin, M., Loeber, R., Park, S., Walker, V., Wickliffe, J. & Tretyakova, N. (2007) HPLC-ESI(+)-MS/MS analysis of N7-guanine–N7-guanine DNA cross-links in tissues of mice exposed to 1,3-butadiene. *Chem. Res. Toxicol.*, **20**, 839–847

Gordon, S.M., Wallace, L.A., Brinkman, M.C., Callahan, P.J. & Kenny, D.V. (2002) Volatile organic compounds as breath biomarkers for active and passive smoking. *Environ. Health Perspect.*, **110**, 689–698

Graff, J.J., Sathiakumar, N., Macaluso, M., Maldonado, G., Matthews, R. & Delzell, E. (2005) Chemical exposures in the synthetic rubber industry and lymphohematopoietic cancer mortality. *J. occup. environ. Med.*, **47**, 916–932

Grasselli, J.G. & Ritchey, W.M., eds (1975) *CRC Atlas of Spectral Data and Physical Constants for Organic Compounds*, Vol. 2, Cleveland, OH, CRC Press, p. 565

Grub, J. & Löser, E. (2005) Butadiene. In: *Ullmann's Encyclopedia of Industrial Chemistry*, 7th Ed., Weinheim, Wiley-VCH Publishers (on line)

Gustafson, P., Barregard, L., Strandberg, B. & Sällsten, G. (2007) The impact of domestic wood burning on personal, indoor and outdoor levels of 1,3-butadiene, benzene, formaldehyde and acetaldehyde. *J. environ. Monit.*, **9**, 23–32

Hayes, R.B., Zhang, L., Swenberg, J.A., Yin, S.N., Xi, L., Wiencke, J., Bechtold, W.E., Yao, M., Rothman, N., Haas, R., O'Neill, J.P., Wiemels, J., Dosemeci, M., Li, G. & Smith, M.T. (2001) Markers for carcinogenicity among butadiene-polymer workers in China. *Chem.-biol. Interact.*, **135–136**, 455–464

Health and Safety Executive (1992) *Methods for the Determination of Hazardous Substances (MDHS) 53—Pumped, Molecular Sieve*, London, Her Majesty's Stationery Office

Health Canada (1999) *Priority Substances List Assessment Report, 1-3 Butadiene*, Ottawa

Heiden Associates (1987) *Additional Industry Profile Data for Evaluating Compliance with Three Butadiene Workplace PEL Scenarios*, Washington DC

Henderson, R.F. (2001) Species differences in the metabolism of olefins: Implications for risk assessment. *Chem.-biol. Interact.*, **135–136**, 53–64

Henderson, R.F., Hahn, F.F., Barr, E.B., Belinsky, S.A., Ménache, M.G. & Benson, J.M. (1999) Carcinogenicity of inhaled butadiene diepoxide in female B6C3F1 mice and Sprague-Dawley rats. *Toxicol. Sci.*, **52**, 33–44

Henderson, R.F., Barr, E.B., Belinsky, S.A., Benson, J.M., Hahn, F.F. & Ménache, M.G. (2000) 1,3-Butadiene: Cancer, mutations, and adducts. Part I: Carcinogenicity of 1,2,3,4-diepoxy-butane. *Res. Rep. Health Eff. Inst.*, **92**, 11–43

Higashino, H., Mita, K., Yoshikado, H., Iwata, M. & Nakanishi, J. (2006) Exposure and risk assessment of 1,3-butadiene in Japan. *Chem.-biol. Interact.*, **1–3**, 52–62

Himmelstein, M.W., Gladnick, N.L., Donner, E.M., Snyder, R.D. & Valentine, R. (2001) In vitro genotoxicity testing of (1-chloroethenyl)oxirane, a metabolite of beta-chloroprene. *Chem.-biol. Interact.*, **135–136**, 703–713

Hong, H.H.L., Devereux, T.R., Melnick, R.L., Moomaw, C.R., Boorman, G.A. & Sills, R.C. (2000) Mutations of ras protooncogenes and p53 tumor suppressor gene in cardiac hemangiosarcomas from B6C3F1 mice exposed to 1,3-butadiene for 2 years. *Toxicol. Pathol.*, **28**, 529–534

Huff, J.E., Melnick, R.L., Solleveld, H.A., Haseman, J.K., Powers, M. & Miller, R.A. (1985) Multiple organ carcinogenicity of 1,3-butadiene in B6C3F$_1$ mice after 60 weeks of inhalation exposure. *Science*, **227**, 548–549

IARC (1976) *IARC Monographs on the Evaluation of Carcinogenic Risk of Chemicals to Man*, Vol. 11, *Cadmium, Nickel, some Epoxides, Miscellaneous Industrial Chemicals and General Considerations on Volatile Anaesthetics*, Lyon, pp. 115–123

IARC (1982) *IARC Monographs on the Evaluation of the Carcinogenic Risk of Chemicals to Humans*, Vol. 28, *The Rubber Industry*, Lyon

IARC (1986) *IARC Monographs on the Evaluation of the Carcinogenic Risk of Chemicals to Humans*, Vol. 39, *Some Chemicals Used in Plastics and Elastomers*, Lyon, pp. 155–179

IARC (1987a) *IARC Monographs on the Evaluation of the Carcinogenic Risk of Chemicals to Humans*, Vol. 42, *Silica and Some Silicates*, Lyon

IARC (1987b) *IARC Monographs on the Evaluation of Carcinogenic Risks to Humans*, Suppl. 7, *Overall Evaluations of Carcinogenicity: An Updating of* IARC Monographs *Volumes 1 to 42*, Lyon, pp. 136–137

IARC (1989) *IARC Monographs on the Evaluation of Carcinogenic Risks to Humans*, Vol. 45, *Occupational Exposures in Petroleum Refining; Crude Oil and Major Petroleum Fuels*, Lyon, pp. 169–174

IARC (1992) *IARC Monographs on the Evaluation of Carcinogenic Risks to Humans*, Vol. 54, *Occupational Exposures to Mists and Vapours from Strong Inorganic Acids; and Other Industrial Chemicals*, Lyon, pp. 237–285

IARC (1999) *IARC Monographs on the Evaluation of Carcinogenic Risks to Humans*, Vol. 71, *Re-evaluation of Some Organic Chemicals, Hydrazine and Hydrogen Peroxide*, Lyon, Part 1, pp. 109–225

IARC (2004) *IARC Monographs on the Evaluation of Carcinogenic Risks to Humans*, Vol. 83, *Tobacco Smoke and Involuntary Smoking*, Lyon

IPCS-CEC (2000) *International Chemical Safety Card 0017*, Geneva, World Health Organization

Irons, R.D. (1990) Studies on the mechanism of 1,3-butadiene-induced leukemogenesis: The potential role of endogenous murine leukemia virus. *Environ. Health Perspect.*, **86**, 49–55

Irons, R.D. & Pyatt, D.W. (1998) Dithiocarbamates as potential confounders in butadiene epidemiology. *Carcinogenesis*, **19**, 539–542

Irons, R.D., Stillman, W.S. & Cloyd, M.W. (1987a) Selective activation of endogenous ecotropic retrovirus in hematopoietic tissues of B6C3F1 mice during the preleukemic phase of 1,3-butadiene exposure. *Virology*, **161**, 457–462

Irons, R.D., Oshimura, M. & Barrett, J.C. (1987b) Chromosome aberrations in mouse bone marrow cells following in vivo exposure to 1,3-butadiene. *Carcinogenesis*, **8**, 1711–1714

Irons, R.D., Cathro, H.P., Stillman, W.S., Steinhagen, W.H. & Shah, R.S. (1989) Susceptibility to 1,3-butadiene-induced leukemogenesis correlates with endogenous ecotropic retroviral background in the mouse. *Toxicol. appl. Pharmacol.*, **101**, 170–176

Irons, R.D., Pyatt, D.W., Stillman, W.S., Som, D.B., Claffey, D.J. & Ruth, J.A. (2000) Comparative toxicity of known and putative metabolites of 1,3-butadiene in human CD34$^+$ bone marrow cells. *Toxicology*, **150**, 99–106

Irons, R.D., Stillman, W.S., Pyatt, D.W., Yang, Y., Le, A., Gustafson, D.L. & Zeng, J.H. (2001) Comparative toxicity of dithiocarbamates and butadiene metabolites in human lymphoid and bone marrow cells. *Chem.-biol. Interact.*, **135–136**, 615–625

JACA Corp. (1987) *Draft Final Report. Preliminary Economic Analysis of the Proposed Revision to the Standard for 1,3-Butadiene: Phase II*, Fort Washington, PA

Jackson, T.E., Lilly, P.D., Recio, L., Schlosser, P.M. & Medinsky, M.A. (2000) Inhibition of cytochrome P450 2E1 decreases, but does not eliminate, genotoxicity mediated by 1,3-butadiene. *Toxicol. Sci.*, **55**, 266–273

Jauhar, P.P., Henika, P.R., MacGregor, J.T., Wehr, C.M., Shelby, M.D., Murphy, S.A. & Margolin, B.H. (1988) 1,3-Butadiene: Induction of micronucleated erythrocytes in the peripheral blood of B6C3F1 mice exposed by inhalation for 13 weeks. *Mutat. Res.*, **209**, 171–176

Jelitto, B., Vangala, R.R. & Laib, R.J. (1989) Species differences in DNA damage by butadiene: Role of diepoxybutane. *Arch. Toxicol.*, **13** (Suppl.), 246–249

Kanuri, M., Nechev, L.V., Tamura, P.J., Harris, C.M., Harris, T.M. & Lloyd, R.S. (2002) Mutagenic spectrum of butadiene-derived N1-deoxyinosine adducts and N^6,N^6-deoxyadenosine intrastrand cross-links in mammalian cells. *Chem. Res. Toxicol.*, **15**, 1572–1580

Karlsson, A., Söderkvist, P. & Zhuang, S.M. (2002) Point mutations and deletions in the znfn1a1/ikaros gene in chemically induced murine lymphomas. *Cancer Res.*, **62**, 2650–2653

Kauppinen, T., Toikkanen, J., Pedersen, D., Young, R., Ahrens, W., Boffetta, P., Hansen, J., Kromhout, H., Maqueda Blasco, J., Mirabelli, D., de la Orden-Rivera, V., Pannett, B., Plato, N., Savela, A., Vincent, R. & Kogevinas, M. (2000) Occupational exposure to carcinogens in the European Union. *Occup. environ. Med.*, **57**, 10–18 [data partially available on the CAREX web site: http://www.ttl.fi/NR/rdonlyres/407B368B-26EF-475D-8F2B-DA0024B853E0/0/5 _exposures_by_agent_and_industry.pdf.]

Kemper, R.A., Krause, R.J. & Elfarra, A.A. (2001) Metabolism of butadiene monoxide by freshly isolated hepatocytes from mice and rats: Different partitioning between oxidative, hydrolytic, and conjugation pathways. *Drug Metab. Dispos.*, **29**, 830–836

Kim, Y.M., Harrad, S. & Harrison, R.M. (2001) Concentrations and sources of VOCs in urban domestic and public microenvironments. *Environ. Sci. Technol.*, **35**, 997–1004

Kim, Y.M., Harrad, S. & Harrison, R.M. (2002) Levels and sources of personal inhalation exposure to volatile organic compounds. *Environ. Sci. Technol.*, **36**, 5405–5410

Kim, Y., Hong, H.H., Lachat, Y., Clayton, N.P., Devereux, T.R., Melnick, R.L., Hegi, M.E., & Sills, R.C. (2005) Genetic alterations in brain tumors following 1,3-butadiene exposure in B6C3F1 mice. *Toxicol. Pathol.*, **33**, 307–312

Kim, M.Y., Tretyakova, N., & Wogan, G.N. (2007) Mutagenesis of the supF gene by stereo-isomers of 1,2,3,4-diepoxybutane. *Chem. Res. Toxicol.*, **20**, 790–797

Kligerman, A.D., DeMarini, D.M., Doerr, C.L., Hanley, N.M., Milholland, V.S. & Tennant, A.H. (1999a) Comparison of cytogenetic effects of 3,4-epoxy-1-butene and 1,2:3,4-diepoxybutane in mouse, rat and human lymphocytes following in vitro G_0 exposures. *Mutat. Res.*, **439**, 13–23

Kligerman, A.D., Doerr, C.L. & Tennant, A.H. (1999b) Cell cycle specificity of cytogenetic damage induced by 3,4-epoxy-1-butene. *Mutat. Res.*, **444**, 151–158

Koc, H., Tretyakova, N.Y., Walker, V.E., Henderson, R.F. & Swenberg, J.A. (1999) Molecular dosimetry of N-7 guanine adduct formation in mice and rats exposed to 1,3-butadiene. *Chem. Res. Toxicol.*, **12**, 566–574

Kohn, M.C. & Melnick, R.L. (1993) Species differences in the production and clearance of 1,3-butadiene metabolites: A mechanistic model indicates predominantly physiological, not bio-chemical, control. *Carcinogenesis*, **14**, 619–628

Kohn, M.C. & Melnick, R.L. (2000) The privileged access model of 1,3-butadiene disposition. *Environ. Health Perspect.*, **108**, 911–917

Kohn, M.C. & Melnick, R.L. (2001) Physiological modeling of butadiene disposition in mice and rats. *Chem.-biol. Interact.*, **135–136**, 285–301

Koivisto, P. & Peltonen, K. (2001) N7-Guanine adducts of the epoxy metabolites of 1,3-butadiene in mice lung. *Chem.-biol. Interact.*, **135–136**, 363–372

Koivisto, P., Adler, I.-D., Sorsa, M. & Peltonen, K. (1996) Inhalation exposure of rats and mice to 1,3-butadiene induces N6-adenine adducts of epoxybutene detected by ^{32}P-postlabeling and HPLC. *Environ. Health Perspect.*, **104** (Suppl. 3), 655–657

Koivisto, P., Sorsa, M., Pacchierotti, F. & Peltonen, K. (1997) ^{32}P-Postlabelling/HPLC assay reveals an enantioselective adduct formation in N7 guanine residues *in vivo* after 1,3-butadiene inhalation exposure. *Carcinogenesis*, **18**, 439–443

Koivisto, P., Adler, I.-D., Pacchierotti, F. & Peltonen, K. (1998) DNA adducts in mouse testis and lung after inhalation exposure to 1,3-butadiene. *Mutat. Res.*, **397**, 3–10

Koivisto, P., Kilpeläinen, I., Rasanen, I., Adler, I.-D., Pacchierotti, F. & Peltonen, K. (1999) Butadiene diolepoxide- and diepoxybutane-derived DNA adducts at N7-guanine: A high occurrence of diolepoxide-derived adducts in mouse lung after 1,3-butadiene exposure. *Carcinogenesis*, **20**, 1253–1259

Krause, R.J. & Elfarra, A.A. (1997) Oxidation of butadiene monoxide to *meso*- and (±)-diepoxybutane by cDNA-expressed human cytochrome P450s and by mouse, rat, and human liver microsomes: Evidence for preferential hydration of *meso*-diepoxybutane in rat and human liver microsomes. *Arch. Biochem. Biophys.*, **337**, 176–184

Kreiling, R., Laib, R.J. & Bolt, H.M. (1986a) Alkylation of nuclear proteins and DNA after exposure of rats and mice to [1,4-^{14}C]1,3-butadiene. *Toxicol. Lett.*, **30**, 131–136

Kreiling, R., Laib, R.J., Filser, J.G. & Bolt, H.M. (1986b) Species differences in butadiene metabolism between mice and rats evaluated by inhalation pharmacokinetics. *Arch. Toxicol.*, **58**, 235–238

Krishnan, E.R., Ungers, L.J., Morelli-Schroth, P.A. & Fajen, J.M. (1987) *Extent-of-exposure Study: 1,3-Butadiene Monomer Production Industry*, Cincinnati, OH, National Institute for Occupational Safety and Health

Kwekkeboom, J. (1996) [A Model for Control of Health Hazards Resulting from Exposure to Toxic Substances (Report V-415)], Wageningen, Wageningen Agricultural University, Department of Air Quality (in Dutch)

Lee, D.H., Kim, T.H., Lee, S.Y., Kim, H.J., Rhee, S.K., Yoon, B., Pfeifer, G.P. & Lee, C.S. (2002) Mutations induced by 1,3-butadiene metabolites, butadiene diolepoxide, and 1,2,3,4-diepoxy-butane at the Hprt locus in CHO-K1 cells. *Mol. Cells*, **14**, 411–419

Lemen, R.A., Meinhardt, T.J., Crandall, M.S., Fajen, J.M. & Brown, D.P. (1990) Environmental epidemiologic investigations in the styrene–butadiene rubber production industry. *Environ. Health Perspect.*, **86**, 103–106

Lide, D.R., ed. (2005) *CRC Handbook of Chemistry and Physics*, 86th Ed., Boca Raton, FL, CRC Press, pp. 3–72

Lin, Y.S., Smith, T.J., Kelsey, K.T. & Wypij, D. (2001) Human physiologic factors in respiratory uptake of 1,3-butadiene. *Environ. Health Perspect.*, **109**, 921–926

Lin, Y.S., Smith, T.J. & Wang, P.Y. (2002) An automated exposure system for human inhalation study. *Arch. environ. Health*, **57**, 215–223

Loeber, R., Rajesh, M., Fang, Q., Pegg, A.E., & Tretyakova, N. (2006) Cross-linking of the human DNA repair protein O6-alkylguanine DNA alkyltransferase to DNA in the presence of 1,2,3,4-diepoxybutane. *Chem. Res. Toxicol.*, **19**, 645–654

Loughlin, J.E., Rothman, K.J. & Dreyer, N.A. (1999) Lymphatic and haematopoietic cancer mortality in a population attending school adjacent to styrene–butadiene facilities, 1963–1993. *J. Epidemiol. Community Health*, **53**, 283–287

Lovreglio, P., Bukvic, N., Fustinoni, S., Ballini, A., Drago, I., Foa, V., Guanti, G. & Soleo, L. (2006) Lack of genotoxic effect in workers exposed to very low doses of 1,3-butadiene. *Arch. Toxicol.*, **80**, 378–381

Lunsford, R.A., Gagnon, Y.T., Palassis, J., Fajen, J.M., Roberts, D.R. & Eller, P.M. (1990) Determination of 1,3-butadiene down to sub-part-per-million levels in air by collection on charcoal and high resolution gas chromatography. *Appl. occup. environ. Hyg.*, **5**, 310–320

Ma, H., Wood, T.G., Ammenheuser, M.M., Rosenblatt, J.I. & Ward, J.B., Jr (2000) Molecular analysis of hprt mutant lymphocytes from 1, 3-butadiene-exposed workers. *Environ. mol. Mutag.*, **36**, 59–71

Macaluso, M., Larson, R., Delzell, E., Sathiakumar, N., Hovinga, M., Julian, J., Muir, D. & Cole, P. (1996) Leukemia and cumulative exposure to butadiene, styrene and benzene among workers in the synthetic rubber industry. *Toxicology*, **113**, 190–202

Macaluso, M., Larson, R., Lynch, J., Lipton, S. & Delzell, E. (2004) Historical estimation of exposure to 1,3-butadiene, styrene, and dimethyldithiocarbamate among synthetic rubber workers. *J. occup. environ. Hyg.*, **1**, 371–390

Maniglier-Poulet, C., Cheng, X., Ruth, J.A. & Ross, D. (1995) Metabolism of 1,3-butadiene to butadiene monoxide in mouse and human bone marrow cells. *Chem.-biol. Interact.*, **97**, 119–129

Matanoski, G.M. & Schwartz, L. (1987) Mortality of workers in styrene–butadiene polymer production. *J. occup. Med.*, **29**, 675–680

Matanoski, G.M., Santos-Burgoa, C. & Schwartz, L. (1990) Mortality of a cohort of workers in the styrene–butadiene polymer manufacturing industry (1943–1982). *Environ. Health Perspect.*, **86**, 107–117

Matanoski, G., Francis, M., Correa-Villasenor, A., Elliott, E., Santos-Burgoa, C. & Schwartz, L. (1993) Cancer epidemiology among styrene–butadiene rubber workers. In: Sorsa, M., Peltonen, K., Vainio, H. & Hemminki, K., eds, *Butadiene and Styrene: Assessment of Health Hazards* (IARC Scientific Publication No. 127), Lyon, IARC, pp. 363–374

Matanoski, G., Elliott, E., Tao, X., Francis, M., Correa-Villasenor, A. & Santos-Burgoa, C. (1997) Lymphohematopoietic cancers and butadiene and styrene exposure in synthetic rubber manufacture. *Ann. N.Y. Acad. Sci.*, **837**, 157–169

McGregor, D., Brown, A.G., Cattanach, P., Edwards, I., McBride, D., Riach, C., Shepherd, W. & Caspary, W.J. (1991) Responses of the L5178Y mouse lymphoma forward mutation assay: V. Gases and vapors. *Environ. mol. Mutag.*, **17**, 122–129

McMichael, A.J., Spirtas, R. & Kupper, L.L. (1974) An epidemiologic study of mortality within a cohort of rubber workers, 1964–72. *J. occup. Med.*, **16**, 458–464

McMichael, A.J., Spirtas, R., Gamble, J.F. & Tousey, P.M. (1976) Mortality among rubber workers: Relationship to specific jobs. *J. occup. Med.*, **18**, 178–185

McNabola, A., Broderick, B., Johnston, P. & Gill, L. (2006) Effects of the smoking ban on benzene and 1,3-butadiene levels in pubs in Dublin. *J. environ. Sci. Health*, **41**, 799–810

de Meester, C., Poncelet, F., Roberfroid, M. & Mercier, M. (1980) The mutagenicity of butadiene towards *Salmonella typhimurium*. *Toxicol. Lett.*, **6**, 125–130

Meinhardt, T.J., Young, R.J. & Hartle, R.W. (1978) Epidemiologic investigations of styrene–butadiene rubber production and reinforced plastics. *Scand. J. Work Environ. Health*, **4** (Suppl. 2), 240–246

Meinhardt, T.J., Lemen, R.A., Crandall, M.S. & Young, R.J. (1982) Environmental epidemiologic investigation of the styrene–butadiene rubber industry. Mortality patterns with discussion of the hematopoietic and lymphatic malignancies. *Scand. J. Work Environ. Health*, **8**, 250–259

Melnick, R.L. & Kohn, M.C. (1995) Mechanistic data indicate that 1,3-butadiene is a human carcinogen. *Carcinogenesis*, **16**, 157–163

Melnick, R.L., Huff, J., Chou, B.J. & Miller, R.A. (1990) Carcinogenicity of 1,3-butadiene in C57BL/6 × C3H F$_1$ mice at low exposure concentrations. *Cancer Res.*, **50**, 6592–6599

Meng, Q., Henderson, R.F., Chen, T., Heflich, R.H., Walker, D.M., Bauer, M.J., Reilly, A.A. & Walker, V.E. (1999a) Mutagenicity of 1,3-butadiene at the *Hprt* locus of T-lymphocytes following inhalation exposures of female mice and rats. *Mutat. Res.*, **429**, 107–125

Meng, Q., Henderson, R.F., Walker, D.M., Bauer, M.J., Reilly, A.A. & Walker, V.E. (1999b) Mutagenicity of the racemic mixtures of butadiene monoepoxide and butadiene diepoxide at the *Hprt* locus of T-lymphocytes following inhalation exposures of female mice and rats. *Mutat. Res.*, **429**, 127–140

Meng, Q., Henderson, R.F., Long, L., Blair, L., Walker, D.M., Upton, P.B., Swenberg, J.A. & Walker, V.E. (2001) Mutagenicity at the Hprt locus in T cells of female mice following inhalation exposures to low levels of 1,3-butadiene. *Chem.-biol. Interact.*, **135–136**, 343–361

Meng, Q., Walker, D.M., Scott, B.R., Seilkop, S.K., Aden, J.K., & Walker, V.E. (2004) Characterization of Hprt mutations in cDNA and genomic DNA of T-cell mutants from control and 1,3-butadiene-exposed male B6C3F1 mice and F344 rats. *Environ. mol. Mutag.*, **43**, 75–92

Meng, Q., Walker, D.M., McDonald, J.D., Henderson, R.F., Carter, M.M., Cook, D.L., Jr, McCash, C.L., Torres, S.M., Bauer, M.J., Seilkop, S.K., Upton, P.B., Georgieva, N.I., Boysen, G., Swenberg, J.A. & Walker, V.E. (2007a) Age-, gender-, and species-dependent mutagenicity in T cells of mice and rats exposed by inhalation to 1,3-butadiene. *Chem.-biol. Interact.*, **166**, 121–131

Meng, Q., Redetzke, D.L., Hackfeld, L.C., Hodge, R.P., Walker, D.M. & Walker, V.E. (2007b) Mutagenicity of stereochemical configurations of 1,2-epoxybutene and 1,2:3,4-diepoxybutane in human lymphoblastoid cells. *Chem.-biol. Interact.*, **166**, 207–218

Merritt, W.K., Scholdberg, T.A., Nechev, L.V., Harris, T.M., Harris, C.M., Lloyd, R.S. & Stone, M.P. (2004) Stereospecific structural perturbations arising from adenine N^6 butadiene triol adducts in duplex DNA. *Chem. Res. Toxicol.*, **17**, 1007–1019

Merritt, W.K., Kowalczyk, A., Scholdberg, T.A., Dean, S.M., Harris, T.M., Harris, C.M., Lloyd, R.S. & Stone, M.P. (2005a) Dual roles of glycosyl torsion angle conformation and stereochemical configuration in butadiene oxide-derived N1 beta-hydroxyalkyl deoxyinosine adducts: A structural perspective. *Chem. Res. Toxicol.*, **18**, 1098–1107

Merritt, W.K., Nechev, L.V., Scholdberg, T.A., Dean, S.M., Kiehna, S.E., Chang, J.C., Harris, T.M., Harris, C.M., Lloyd, R.S. & Stone, M.P. (2005b) Structure of the 1,4-bis(2'-deoxy-adenosin-N^6-yl)-2R,3R-butanediol cross-link arising from alkylation of the human N-ras codon 61 by butadiene diepoxide. *Biochemistry*, **44**, 10081–10092

Minko, I.G., Washington, M.T., Prakash, L., Prakash, S. & Lloyd, R.S. (2001) Translesion DNA synthesis by yeast DNA polymerase eta on templates containing N^2-guanine adducts of 1,3-butadiene metabolites. *J. biol. Chem.*, **276**, 2517–2522

Moll, T.S., Harms, A.C. & Elfarra, A.A. (2000) A comprehensive structural analysis of hemoglobin adducts formed after in-vitro exposure of erythrocytes to butadiene monoxide. *Chem. Res. Toxicol.*, **13**, 1103–1113

Morrissey, R.E., Schwetz, B.A., Hackett, P.L., Sikov, M.R., Hardin, B.D., McClanahan, B.J., Decker, J.R. & Mast, T.J. (1990) Overview of reproductive and developmental toxicity studies of 1,3-butadiene in rodents. *Environ. Health Perspect.*, **86**, 79–84

Murg, M.N., Schuler, M. & Eastmond, D.A. (1999a) Evaluation of micronuclei and chromosomal breakage in the 1cen-q12 region by the butadiene metabolites epoxybutene and diepoxybutane in cultured human lymphocytes. *Mutagenesis*, **14**, 541–546

Murg, M.N., Schuler, M. & Eastmond, D.A. (1999b) Persistence of chromosomal alterations affecting the 1cen-q12 region in a human lymphoblastoid cell line exposed to diepoxybutane and mitomycin C. *Mutat. Res.*, **446**, 193–203

National Library of Medicine (2008) *Toxic Chemical Release Inventory (TRI87, TRI90, TRI95, TRI05, TRI08) Databases*, Bethesda, MD [available at http://toxnet.nlm.nih.gov]

National Toxicology Program (1984) *Toxicology and Carcinogenesis Studies of 1,3-Butadiene (CAS No. 106-99-0) in B6C3F₁ Mice (Inhalation Studies)* (Tech. Rep. Ser. No. 288), Research Triangle Park, NC

National Toxicology Program (1993) *Toxicology and Carcinogenesis Studies of 1,3-Butadiene (CAS No. 106-99-0) in B6C3F₁ Mice (Inhalation Studies)* (Tech. Rep. Ser. No. 434), Research Triangle Park, NC

Nazaroff, W.W. & Singer, B.C. (2004) Inhalation of hazardous air pollutants from environmental tobacco smoke in US residents. *J. Expo. Anal. environ. Epidemiol.*, **14**, S71–S77

Nechev, L.V., Zhang, M., Tsarouhtsis, D., Tamura, P.J., Wilkinson, A.S., Harris, C.M. & Harris, T.M. (2001) Synthesis and characterization of nucleosides and oligonucleotides bearing adducts of butadiene epoxides on adenine N^6 and guanine N^2. *Chem. Res. Toxicol.*, **14**, 379–388

NIH/EPA Chemical Information System (1983) *Carbon-13 NMR Spectral Search System, Mass Spectral Search System, and Infrared Spectral Search System*, Arlington, VA, Information Consultants

NOES (1997) *National Occupational Exposure Survey 1981–83*, Unpublished data as of November 1997, Cincinnati, OH, US Department of Health and Human Services, Public Health Service, National Institute for Occupational Safety and Health

Norppa, H. (2004) Cytogenetic biomarkers and genetic polymorphisms. *Toxicol. Lett.*, **149**, 309–334

Occupational Safety and Health Administration (1990a) *OSHA Analytical Methods Manual*, Part 1: *Organic Substances*, Vol. 3, *Methods 55-80*, Salt Lake City, UT [Method 56]

Occupational Safety and Health Administration (1990b) Occupational exposure to 1,3-butadiene. *Fed. Regist.*, **55**, 32736–32826

O'Donoghue, R.T., Gill, L.W., McKevitt, R.J. & Broderick, B. (2007) Exposure to hydrocarbon concentrations while commuting or exercising in Dublin. *Environ. int.*, **33**, 1–8

Oe, T., Kambouris, S.J., Walker, V.E., Meng, Q., Recio, L., Wherli, S., Chaudhary, A.K., & Blair, I.A. (1999) Persistence of N7-(2,3,4-trihydroxybutyl)guanine adducts in the livers of mice and rats exposed to 1,3-butadiene. *Chem. Res. Toxicol.*, **12**, 247–257

Oesch, F. & Daly, J. (1972) Conversion of naphthalene to trans-naphthalene dihydrodiol: Evidence for the presence of a coupled aryl monooxygenase–epoxide hydrase system in hepatic microsomes. *Biochem. biophys. Res. Commun.*, **46**, 1713–1720

O'Neil, M.J., ed. (2006) *Merck Index*, 14th Ed., Whitehouse Station, NJ, Merck, p. 248

Owen, P.E. & Glaister, J.R. (1990) Inhalation toxicity and carcinogenicity of 1,3-butadiene in Sprague-Dawley rats. *Environ. Health Perspect.*, **86**, 19–25

Owen, P.E., Glaister, J.R., Gaunt, I.F. & Pullinger, D.H. (1987) Inhalation toxicity studies with 1,3-butadiene. 3. Two year toxicity/carcinogenicity study in rats. *Am. ind. Hyg. Assoc. J.*, **48**, 407–413

Pacchierotti, F., Adler, I.-D., Anderson, D., Brinkworth, M., Demopoulos, N.A., Lahdetie, J., Osterman-Golkar, S., Peltonen, K., Russo, A., Tates, A. & Waters, R. (1998) Genetic effects of 1,3-butadiene and associated risk for heritable damage. *Mutat. Res.*, **397**, 93–115

Parent, M.E., Hua, Y. & Siemiatycki, J. (2000) Occupational risk factors for renal cell carcinoma in Montreal. *Am. J. ind. Med.*, **38**, 609–618

Park, S. & Tretyakova, N. (2004) Structural characterization of the major DNA–DNA cross-link of 1,2,3,4-diepoxybutane. *Chem. Res. Toxicol.*, **17**, 129–136

Park, S., Hodge, J., Anderson, C. & Tretyakova, N. (2004) Guanine–adenine DNA cross-linking by 1,2,3,4-diepoxybutane: Potential basis for biological activity. *Chem. Res. Toxicol.*, **17**, 1638–1651

Park, S., Anderson, C., Loeber, R., Seetharaman, M., Jones, R. & Tretyakova, N. (2005) Interstrand and intrastrand DNA–DNA cross-linking by 1,2,3,4-diepoxybutane: Role of stereochemistry. *J. Am. chem. Soc.*, **127**, 14355–14365

Perbellini, L., Princivalle, A., Cerpelloni, M., Pasini, F. & Brugnone, F. (2003) Comparison of breath, blood and urine concentrations in the biomonitoring of environmental exposure to 1,3-butadiene, 2,5-dimethylfuran, and benzene. *Int. Arch. occup. environ. Health*, **76**, 461–466

Powley, M.W., Jayaraj, K., Gold, A., Ball, L.M. & Swenberg, J.A. (2003) 1,N^2-Propano-deoxyguanosine adducts of the 1,3-butadiene metabolite, hydroxymethylvinyl ketone. *Chem. Res. Toxicol.*, **16**, 1448–1454

Powley, M.W., Li, Y., Upton, P.B., Walker, V.E. & Swenberg, J.A. (2005) Quantification of DNA and hemoglobin adducts of 3,4-epoxy-1,2-butanediol in rodents exposed to 3-butene-1,2-diol. *Carcinogenesis*, **26**, 1573–1580

Powley, M.W., Walker, V.E., Li, Y., Upton, P.B., & Swenberg, J.A. (2007) The importance of 3,4-epoxy-1,2-butanediol and hydroxymethylvinyl ketone in 3-butene-1,2-diol associated mutagenicity. *Chem.-biol. Interact.*, **166**, 182–190

Ranaldi, R., Bassani, B. & Pacchierotti, F. (2001) Genotoxic effects of butadiene in mouse lung cells detected by an ex vivo micronucleus test. *Mutat. Res.*, **491**, 81–85

Recio, L. & Meyer, K.G. (1995) Increased frequency of mutations at A:T base pairs in the bone marrow of B6C3F1 *lacI* transgenic mice exposed to 1,3-butadiene. *Environ. mol. Mutag.*, **26**, 1–8

Recio, L., Osterman-Golkar, S., Csanady, G.A., Turner, M.J., Myhr, B., Moss, O. & Bond, J.A. (1992) Determination of mutagenicity in tissues of transgenic mice following exposure to 1,3-butadiene and N-ethyl-N-nitrosourea. *Toxicol. appl. Pharmacol.*, **117**, 58–64

Recio, L., Saranko, C.J. & Steen, A.M. (2000) 1,3-Butadiene: Cancer, mutations, and adducts. Part II: Roles of two metabolites of 1,3-butadiene in mediating its in vivo genotoxicity. *Res. Rep. Health Eff. Inst.*, **92**, 49–87

Recio, L., Steen, A.M., Pluta, L.J., Meyer, K.G. & Saranko, C.J. (2001) Mutational spectrum of 1,3-butadiene and metabolites 1,2-epoxybutene and 1,2,3,4-diepoxybutane to assess mutagenic mechanisms. *Chem.-biol. Interact.*, **135–136**, 325–341

Reilly, M.S. & Grogan, D.W. (2002) Biological effects of DNA damage in the hyperthermophilic archaeon Sulfolobus acidocaldarius. *FEMS Microbiol. Lett.*, **208**, 29–34

Richardson, K.A., Peters, M.M., Megens, R.H., van Elburg, P.A., Golding, B.T., Boogaard, P.J., Watson, W.P. & van Sittert, N.J. (1998) Identification of novel metabolites of butadiene mono-epoxide in rats and mice. *Chem. Res. Toxicol.*, **11**, 1543–1555

Richardson, K.A., Peters, M.M., Wong, B.A., Megens, R.H., van Elburg, P.A., Booth, E.D., Boogaard, P.J., Bond, J.A., Medinsky, M.A., Watson, W.P. & van Sittert, N.J. (1999) Quantitative and qualitative differences in the metabolism of ^{14}C-1,3-butadiene in rats and mice: Relevance to cancer susceptibility. *Toxicol. Sci.*, **49**, 186–201

Rinsky, R.A., Ott, G., Ward, E., Greenberg, H., Halperin, W. & Leet, T. (1988) Study of mortality among chemical workers in the Kanawha Valley of West Virginia. *Am. J. ind. Med.*, **13**, 429–438

Ristau, C., Deutschmann, S., Laib, R.J. & Ottenwalder, H. (1990) Detection of diepoxybutane-induced DNA–DNA crosslinks by cesium trifluoracetate (CsTFA) density-gradient centri-fugation. *Arch. Toxicol.*, **64**, 343–344

Roberts, D.R. (1986) *Industrial Hygiene Walk-through Survey Report of Copolymer Rubber and Chemical Corporation, Baton Rouge, LA* (Report No. 147.22), Cincinnati, OH, National Institute for Occupational Safety and Health

Rodriguez, D.A., Kowalczyk, A., Ward, J.B., Jr, Harris, C.M., Harris, T.M. & Lloyd, R.S. (2001) Point mutations induced by 1,2-epoxy-3-butene N1 deoxyinosine adducts. *Environ. mol. Mutag.*, **38**, 292–296

Ropert, C.P., Jr (1976) *Health Hazard Evaluation Determination, Goodyear Tire and Rubber Company, Gadsden, AL* (Report No. 74-120-260), Cincinnati, OH, National Institute for Occupational Safety and Health

Rubber Manufacturers' Association (1984) *Requests for Information Regarding 1,3-Butadiene, 49 Fed. Reg. 844 and 845 (Jan. 5 1984)*, Washington DC

Ruhe, R.L. & Jannerfeldt, E.R. (1980) *Health Hazard Evaluation, Metamora Products Corporation, Elkland, PA* (Report No. HE-80-188-797), Cincinnati, OH, National Institute for Occupational Safety and Health

Sadtler Research Laboratories (1995) *The Sadtler Standard Spectra, Cumulative Index,* Philadelphia, PA

Saltzman, B.E. & Harman, J.N. (1989) Direct reading colorimetric indicators. In: Lodge, J.P., Jr, ed., *Methods of Air Sampling and Analysis*, Chelsea, MI, Lewis Publishers, pp. 171–187

Santos-Burgoa, C., Matanoski, G.M., Zeger, S. & Schwartz, L. (1992) Lymphohematopoietic cancer in styrene–butadiene polymerization workers. *Am. J. Epidemiol.*, **136**, 843–854

Sapkota, A., Halden, R.U., Dominici, F., Groopman, J.D. & Buckley, T.J. (2006) Urinary biomarkers of 1,3-butadiene in environmental settings using liquid chromatography isotope dilution tandem mass spectrometry. *Chem.-biol. Interact.*, **160**, 70–79

Saranko, C.J., Pluta, L.J. & Recio, L. (1998) Molecular analysis of lacI mutants from transgenic fibroblasts exposed to 1,2-epoxybutene. *Carcinogenesis*, **19**, 1879–1887

Saranko, C.J., Meyer, K.G., Pluta, L.J., Henderson, R.F. & Recio, L. (2001) Lung-specific mutagenicity and mutational spectrum in B6C3F1 lacI transgenic mice following inhalation exposure to 1,2-epoxybutene. *Mutat. Res.*, **473**, 37–49

Sasiadek, M., Jarventaus, H. & Sorsa, M. (1991a) Sister-chromatid exchanges induced by 1,3-butadiene and its epoxides in CHO cells. *Mutat. Res.*, **263**, 47–50

Sasiadek, M., Norppa, H. & Sorsa, M. (1991b) 1,3-Butadiene and its epoxides induce sister-chromatid exchanges in human lymphocytes *in vitro*. *Mutat. Res.*, **261**, 117–121

Sasiadek, M., Hirvonen, A., Noga, L., Paprocka-Borowicz, M. & Norppa, H. (1999) Glutathione S-transferase M1 genotype influences sister chromatid exchange induction but not adaptive response in human lymphocytes treated with 1,2-epoxy-3-butene. *Mutat. Res.*, **439**, 207–212

Sathiakumar, N. & Delzell, E. (2007) A follow-up study of women in the synthetic rubber industry: Study methods. *Chem.-biol. Interact.*, **166**, 25–28

Sathiakumar, N., Delzell, E., Hovinga, M., Macaluso, M., Julian, J.A., Larson, R., Cole, P. & Muir, D.C. (1998) Mortality from cancer and other causes of death among synthetic rubber workers. *Occup. environ. Med.*, **55**, 230–235

Sathiakumar, N., Graff, J., Macaluso, M., Maldonado, G., Matthews, R. & Delzell, E. (2005) An updated study of mortality among North American synthetic rubber industry workers. *Occup. environ. Med.*, **62**, 822–829

Sathiakumar, N., Delzell, E., Cheng, H., Lynch, J., Sparks, W. & Macaluso, M. (2007) Validation of 1,3-butadiene exposure estimates for workers at a synthetic rubber plant. *Chem.-biol. Interact.*, **166**, 29–43

Schlade-Bartusiak, K., Sasiadek, M. & Kozlowska, J. (2000) The influence of GSTM1 and GSTT1 genotypes on the induction of sister chromatid exchanges and chromosome aberrations by 1,2:3,4-diepoxybutane. *Mutat. Res.*, **465**, 69–75

Schlade-Bartusiak, K., Rozik, K., Laczmanska, I., Ramsey, D. & Sasiadek, M. (2004) Influence of GSTT1, mEH, CYP2E1 and RAD51 polymorphisms on diepoxybutane-induced SCE frequency in cultured human lymphocytes. *Mutat. Res.*, **558**, 121–130

Schmiederer, M., Knutson, E., Muganda, P. & Albrecht, T. (2005) Acute exposure of human lung cells to 1,3-butadiene diepoxide results in G1 and G2 cell cycle arrest. *Environ. mol. Mutag.*, **45**, 354–364

Scholdberg, T.A., Nechev, L.V., Merritt, W.K., Harris, T.M., Harris, C.M., Lloyd, R.S. & Stone, M.P. (2004) Structure of a site specific major groove (2S,3S)-N^6-(2,3,4-trihydroxybutyl)-2′-deoxyadenosyl DNA adduct of butadiene diol epoxide. *Chem. Res. Toxicol.*, **17**, 717–730

Scholdberg, T.A., Nechev, L.V., Merritt, W.K., Harris, T.M., Harris, C.M., Lloyd, R.S. & Stone, M.P. (2005a) Mispairing of a site specific major groove (2S,3S)-N^6-(2,3,4-trihydroxybutyl)-2′-deoxyadenoxyl DNA adduct of butadiene diol epoxide with deoxyguanosine: Formation of a dA(anti).dG(anti) pairing intcraction. *Chem. Res. Toxicol.*, **18**, 145–153

Scholdberg, T.A., Merritt, W.K., Dean, S.M., Kowalcyzk, A., Harris, C.M., Harris, T.M., Rizzo, C.J., Lloyd, R.S. & Stone, M.P. (2005b) Structure of an oligodeoxynucleotide containing a butadiene oxide-derived N1 beta-hydroxyalkyl deoxyinosine adduct in the human N-ras codon 61 sequence. *Biochemistry*, **44**, 3327–3337

Selzer, R.R. & Elfarra, A.A. (1996a) Characterization of N1- and N6-adenosine adducts and N1-inosine adducts formed by the reaction of butadiene monoxide with adenosine: Evidence for the N1-adenosine adducts as major initial products. *Chem. Res. Toxicol.*, **9**, 875–881

Selzer, R.R. & Elfarra, A.A. (1996b) Synthesis and biochemical characterization of N1-, N2-, and N7-guanosine adducts of butadiene monoxide. *Chem. Res. Toxicol.*, **9**, 126–132

Selzer, R.R. & Elfarra, A.A. (1997) Chemical modification of deoxycytidine at different sites yields adducts of different stabilities: Characterization of N3- and O2-deoxycytidine and N3-deoxyuridine adducts of butadiene monoxide. *Arch. Biochem. Biophys.*, **343**, 63–72

Selzer, R.R. & Elfarra, A.A. (1999) In vitro reactions of butadiene monoxide with single- and double-stranded DNA: Characterization and quantitation of several purine and pyrimidine adducts. *Carcinogenesis*, **20**, 285–292

Serrano-Trespalacios, P.I., Ryan, L. & Spengler, J.D. (2004) Ambient, indoor and personal exposure relationships of volatile organic compounds in Mexico City Metropolitan Area. *J. Expo. Anal. environ. Epidemiol.*, **14**, S118–S132

Shimkin, M.B., Weisburger, J.H., Weisburger, E.K., Gubareff, N. & Suntzeff, V. (1966) Bioassay of 29 alkylating chemicals by the pulmonary-tumor response in strain A mice. *J. natl Cancer Inst.*, **36**, 915–935

Sills, R.C., Hong, H.L., Boorman, G.A., Devereux, T.R. & Melnick, R.L. (2001) Point mutations of K-ras and H-ras genes in forestomach neoplasms from control B6C3F1 mice and following exposure to 1,3-butadiene, isoprene or chloroprene for up to 2-years. *Chem.-biol. Interact.*, **135–136**, 373–386

Sisk, S.C., Pluta, L.J., Bond, J.A. & Recio, L. (1994) Molecular analysis of lacI mutants from bone marrow of B6C3F1 transgenic mice following inhalation exposure to 1,3-butadiene. *Carcinogenesis*, **15**, 471–477 van Sittert, N.J., Megens, H.J., Watson, W.P. & Boogaard, P.J. (2000) Biomarkers of exposure to 1,3-butadiene as a basis for cancer risk assessment. *Toxicol. Sci.*, **56**, 189–202

Smith, T.J., Lin, Y.S., Mezzetti, M., Bois, F.Y., Kelsey, K. & Ibrahim, J. (2001) Genetic and dietary factors affecting human metabolism of 1,3-butadiene. *Chem.-biol. Interact.*, **135–136**, 407–428

Sprague, C.L. & Elfarra, A.A. (2003) Detection of carboxylic acids and inhibition of hippuric acid formation in rats treated with 3-butene-1,2-diol, a major metabolite of 1,3-butadiene. *Drug Metab. Dispos.*, **31**, 986–992

Sprague, C.L. & Elfarra, A.A. (2004) Mercapturic acid urinary metabolites of 3-butene-1,2-diol as in vivo evidence for the formation of hydroxymethylvinyl ketone in mice and rats. *Chem. Res. Toxicol.*, **17**, 819–826

Šrám, R.J., Rössner, P., Peltonen, K., Podrazilova, K., Mrackova, G., Demopoulos, N.A., Stephanou, G., Vlachodimitropoulos, D., Darroudi, F. & Tates, A.D. (1998) Chromosomal aberrations, sister-chromatid exchanges, cells with high frequency of SCE, micronuclei and comet assay parameters in 1,3-butadiene-exposed workers. *Mutat. Res.*, **419**, 145–154

Šrám, R.J., Beskid, O., Binkova, B., Rossner, P. & Smerhovsky, Z. (2004) Cytogenetic analysis using fluorescence in situ hybridization (FISH) to evaluate occupational exposure to carcinogens. *Toxicol. Lett.*, **149**, 335–344

Startin, J.R. & Gilbert, J. (1984) Single ion monitoring of butadiene in plastics and foods by coupled mass-spectrometry–automatic headspace gas chromatography. *J. Chromatogr.*, **294**, 427–430

Stephanou, G., Russo, A., Vlastos, D., Andrianopoulos, C. & Demopoulos, N.A. (1998) Micronucleus induction in somatic cells of mice as evaluated after 1,3-butadiene inhalation. *Mutat. Res.*, **397**, 11–20

Sun, H.N. & Wristers, J.P. (2002) Butadiene. In: *Kirk-Othmer Encyclopedia of Chemical Technology*, Vol. 4, New York, J. Wiley & Sons, pp. 365–392 (on line)

Sweeney, L.M., Himmelstein, M.W. & Gargas, M.L. (2001) Development of a preliminary physiologically based toxicokinetic (PBTK) model for 1,3-butadiene risk assessment. *Chem.-biol. Interact.*, **135–136**, 303–322

Swenberg, J.A., Christova-Gueorguieva, N.I., Upton, P.B., Ranasinghe, A., Scheller, N., Wu, K.Y., Yen, T.Y. & Hayes, R. (2000a) 1,3-Butadiene: Cancer, mutations, and adducts. Part V: Hemoglobin adducts as biomarkers of 1,3-butadiene exposure and metabolism. *Res. Rep. Health Eff. Inst.*, **92**, 191–210

Swenberg, J.A., Ham, A., Koc, H., Morinello, E., Ranasinghe, A., Tretyakova, N., Upton, P.B. & Wu, K.Y. (2000b) DNA adducts: Effects of low exposure to ethylene oxide, vinyl chloride and butadiene. *Mutat. Res.*, **464**, 77–86

Swenberg, J.A., Koc, H., Upton, P.B., Georguieva, N., Ranasinghe, A., Walker, V.E. & Henderson, R. (2001) Using DNA and hemoglobin adducts to improve the risk assessment of butadiene. *Chem.-biol. Interact.*, **135–136**, 387–403

Swenberg, J.A., Boysen, G., Georgieva, N., Bird, M.G. & Lewis, R.J. (2007) Future directions in butadiene risk assessment and the role of cross-species internal dosimetry. *Chem.-biol. Interact.*, **166**, 78–83

Tates, A.D., van Dam, F.J., de Zwart, F.A., van Teylingen, C.M.M. & Natarajan, A.T. (1994) Development of a cloning assay with high cloning efficiency to detect induction of 6-thioguanine-resistant lymphocytes in spleen of adult mice following in vivo inhalation exposure to 1,3-butadiene. *Mutat. Res.*, **309**, 299–306

Tates, A.D., van Dam, F.J., van Teylingen, C.M., de Zwart, F.A. & Zwinderman, A.H. (1998) Comparison of induction of *hprt* mutations by 1,3-butadiene and/or its metabolites 1,2-epoxybutene and 1,2,3,4-diepoxybutane in lymphocytes from spleen of adult male mice and rats *in vivo. Mutat. Res.*, **397**, 21–36

Thier, R., Bruning, T., Roos, P.H., Rihs, H.P., Golka, K., Ko, Y. & Bolt, H.M. (2003) Markers of genetic susceptibility in human environmental hygiene and toxicology: The role of selected CYP, NAT and GST genes. *Int. J. Hyg. environ. Health*, **206**, 149–171

Tice, R.R., Boucher, R., Luke, C.A. & Shelby, M.D. (1987) Comparative cytogenetic analysis of bone marrow damage induced in male B6C3F1 mice by multiple exposures to gaseous 1,3-butadiene. *Environ. Mutag.*, **9**, 235–250

Tommasi, A.M., de Conti, S., Dobrzynska, M.M. & Russo, A. (1998) Evaluation and characterization of micronuclei in early spermatids of mice exposed to 1,3-butadiene. *Mutat. Res.*, **397**, 45–54

Ton, T.V., Hong, H.H., Devereux, T.R., Mclnick, R.L., Sills, R.C. & Kim, Y. (2007) Evaluation of genetic alterations in cancer-related genes in lung and brain tumors from B6C3F1 mice exposed to 1,3-butadiene or chloroprene. *Chem.-biol. Interact.*, **166**, 112–120

Tsai, S.P., Wendt, J.K. & Ransdell, J.D. (2001) A mortality, morbidity, and hematology study of petrochemical employees potentially exposed to 1,3-butadiene monomer. *Chem.-biol. Interact.*, **135–136**, 555–567

Urban, M., Gilch, G., Schepers, G., van Miert, E. & Scherer, G. (2003) Determination of the major mercapturic acids of 1,3-butadiene in human and rat urine using liquid chromatography with tandem mass spectrometry. *J. Chromatogr. B*, **796**, 131–140

Valadez, J.G., Liu, L., Loktionova, N.A., Pegg, A.E. & Guengerich, F.P. (2004) Activation of bis-electrophiles to mutagenic conjugates by human O^6-alkylguanine-DNA alkyltransferase. *Chem. Res. Toxicol.*, **17**, 972–982

Van Duuren, B.L., Nelson, N., Orris, L., Palmes, E.D. & Schmitt, F.L. (1963) Carcinogenicity of epoxides, lactones, and peroxy compounds. *J. natl Cancer Inst.*, **3**, 41–55

Van Duuren, B.L., Orris, L. & Nelson, N. (1965) Carcinogenicity of epoxides, lactones, and peroxy compounds. Part II. *J. natl Cancer Inst.*, **35**, 707–717

Van Duuren, B.L., Langseth, L., Orris, L., Teebor, G., Nelson, N. & Kuschner, M. (1966) Carcinogenity of epoxides, lactones, and peroxy compounds. IV. Tumor response in epithelial and connective tissue in mice and rats. *J. natl Cancer Inst.*, **37**, 825–838

Vangala, R.R., Laib, R.J. & Bolt, H.M. (1993) Evaluation of DNA damage by alkaline elution technique after inhalation exposure of rats and mice to 1,3-butadiene. *Arch. Toxicol.*, **67**, 34–38

Verschueren, K. (1996) *Handbook of Environmental Data on Organic Chemicals*, 3rd Ed., New York, Van Nostrand Reinhold, pp. 347–348

Victorin, K., Busk, L., Cederberg, H. & Magnusson, J. (1990) Genotoxic activity of 1,3-butadiene and nitrogen dioxide and their photochemical reaction products in *Drosophila* and in mouse bone marrow micronucleus assay. *Mutat. Res.*, **228**, 203–209

Vodicka, P., Kumar, R., Stetina, R., Musak, L., Soucek, P., Haufroid, V., Sasiadek, M., Vodickova, L., Naccarati, A., Sedikova, J., Sanyal, S., Kuricova, M., Brsiak, V., Norppa, H., Buchancova, J. & Hemminki, K. (2004) Markers of individual susceptibility and DNA repair rate in workers exposed to xenobiotics in a tire plant. *Environ. mol. Mutag.*, **44**, 283–292

Vodicka, P., Stetina, R., Smerak, P., Vodickova, L., Naccarati, A., Barta, I. & Hemminki, K. (2006) Micronuclei, DNA single-strand breaks and DNA-repair activity in mice exposed to 1,3-butadiene by inhalation. *Mutat. Res.*, **608**, 49–57

Walker, V.E. & Meng, Q. (2000) 1,3-Butadiene: Cancer, mutations, and adducts. Part III: In vivo mutation of the endogenous hprt genes of mice and rats by 1,3-butadiene and its metabolites. *Res. Rep. Health Eff. Inst.*, **92**, 89–139

Walles, S.A.S., Victorin, K. & Lundborg, M. (1995) DNA damage in lung cells *in vivo* and *in vitro* by 1,3-butadiene and nitrogen dioxide and their photochemical reaction products. *Mutat. Res.*, **328**, 11–19

Walther, M.W. (2003) *CEH Marketing Research Report – Butadiene*, Zürich, SRI Consulting

Ward, E.M., Fajen, J.M., Ruder, A.M., Rinsky, R.A., Halperin, W.E. & Fessler-Flesch, C.A. (1995) Mortality study of workers in 1,3-butadiene production units identified from a chemical workers cohort. *Environ. Health Perspect.*, **103**, 598–603

Ward, E.M., Fajen, J.M., Ruder, A.M., Rinsky, R.A., Halperin, W.E. & Fessler-Flesch, C.A. (1996) Mortality study of workers employed in 1,3-butadiene production units identified from a large chemical workers cohort. *Toxicology*, **113**, 157–168

Ward, J.B., Ammenheuser, M.M., Whorton, E.B., Jr, Bechtold, W.E., Kelsey, K.T. & Legator, M.S. (1996) Biological monitoring for mutagenic effects of occupational exposure to butadiene. *Toxicology*, **113**, 84–90

Ward, J.B., Jr, Abdel-Rahman, S.Z., Henderson, R.F., Stock, T.H., Morandi, M., Rosenblatt, J.I. & Ammenheuser, M.M. (2001) Assessment of butadiene exposure in synthetic rubber manufacturing workers in Texas using frequencies of hprt mutant lymphocytes as a biomarker. *Chem.-biol. Interact.*, **135–136**, 465–483

White, W.C. (2007) Butadiene production process overview. *Chem.-biol. Interact.*, **166**, 10–14

Wickliffe, J.K., Ammenheuser, M.M., Salazar, J.J., Abdel-Rahman, S.Z., Hastings-Smith, D.A., Postlethwait, E.M., Lloyd, R.S. & Ward, J.B., Jr (2003) A model of sensitivity: 1,3-Butadiene increases mutant frequencies and genomic damage in mice lacking a functional microsomal epoxide hydrolase gene. *Environ. mol. Mutag.*, **42**, 106–110

Wickliffe, J.K., Galbert, L.A., Ammenheuser, M.M., Herring, S.M., Xie, J., Masters, O.E., III, Friedberg, E.C., Lloyd, R.S. & Ward, J.B., Jr (2006) 3,4-Epoxy-1-butene, a reactive metabolite of 1,3-butadiene, induces somatic mutations in Xpc-null mice. *Environ. mol. Mutag.*, **47**, 67–70

Wickliffe, J.K., Herring, S.M., Hallberg, L.M., Galbert, L.A., Masters, O.E., III, Ammenheuser, M.M., Xie, J., Friedberg, E.C., Lloyd, R.S., Abdel-Rahman, S.Z. & Ward, J.B., Jr (2007) Detoxification of olefinic epoxides and nucleotide excision repair of epoxide-mediated DNA damage: Insights from animal models examining human sensitivity to 1,3-butadiene. *Chem.-biol. Interact.*, **166**, 226–231

Wiencke, J.K., Pemble, S., Ketterer, B. & Kelsey, K.T. (1995) Gene deletion of glutathione S-transferase theta: Correlation with induced genetic damage and potential role in endogenous mutagenesis. *Cancer Epidemiol. Biomarkers Prev.*, **4**, 253–259

Work Environment Fund (1991) *Development and Evaluation of Biological and Chemical Methods for Exposure Assessment of 1,3-Butadiene* (Contract No. 88-0147), Helsinki, Institute of Occupational Health

Xiao, Y. & Tates, A.D. (1995) Clastogenic effects of 1,3-butadiene and its metabolites 1,2-epoxybutene and 1,2,3,4-diepoxybutane in splenocytes and germ cells of rats and mice in vivo. *Environ. Health Perspect.*, **26**, 97–108

Xu, W., Merritt, W.K., Nechev, L.V., Harris, T.M., Harris, C.M., Lloyd, R.S. & Stone, M.P. (2007) Structure of the 1,4-bis(2′-deoxyadenosin-N⁶-yl)-2S,3S-butanediol intrastrand DNA cross-link arising from butadiene diepoxide in the human N-ras codon 61 sequence. *Chem. Res. Toxicol.*, **20**, 187–198

Ye, Y., Galbally, I.E. & Weeks, I.A. (1997) Emission of 1,3-butadiene from petrol-driven motor vehicle. *Atmos. Environ.*, **31**, 1157–1165

Zang, H., Harris, T.M. & Guengerich, F.P. (2005) Kinetics of nucleotide incorporation opposite DNA bulky guanine N^2 adducts by processive bacteriophage T7 DNA polymerase (exonuclease-) and HIV-1 reverse transcriptase. *J. biol. Chem.*, **280**, 1165–1178

Zhang, X.Y. & Elfarra, A.A. (2003) Identification and characterization of a series of nucleoside adducts formed by the reaction of 2′-deoxyguanosine and 1,2,3,4-diepoxybutane under physiological conditions. *Chem. Res. Toxicol.*, **16**, 1606–1615

Zhang, X.Y. & Elfarra, A.A. (2004) Characterization of the reaction products of 2′-deoxyguanosine and 1,2,3,4-diepoxybutane after acid hydrolysis: Formation of novel guanine and pyrimidine adducts. *Chem. Res. Toxicol.*, **17**, 521–528

Zhang, X.Y. & Elfarra, A.A. (2005) Reaction of 1,2,3,4-diepoxybutane with 2′-deoxyguanosine: Initial products and their stabilities and decomposition patterns under physiological conditions. *Chem. Res. Toxicol.*, **18**, 1316–1323

Zhang, X.Y. & Elfarra, A.A. (2006) Characterization of 1,2,3,4-diepoxybutane-2′-deoxyguanosine cross-linking products formed at physiological and nonphysiological conditions. *Chem. Res. Toxicol.*, **19**, 547–555

Zhang, L., Hayes, R.B., Guo, W., McHale, C.M., Yin, S., Wiencke, J.K., O'Neill, J.P., Rothman, N., Li, G.L. & Smith, M.T. (2004) Lack of increased genetic damage in 1,3-butadiene-exposed Chinese workers studied in relation to EPHX1 and GST genotypes. *Mutat. Res.*, **558**, 63–74

Zhao, C., Koskinen, M. & Hemminki, K. (1998) ³²P-Postlabelling of N⁶-adenine adducts of epoxybutanediol in vivo after 1,3-butadiene exposure. *Toxicol. Lett.*, **102–103**, 591–594

Zhao, C., Vodicka, P., Sram, R.J. & Hemminki, K. (2000) Human DNA adducts of 1,3-butadiene, an important environmental carcinogen. *Carcinogenesis*, **21**, 107–111

Zhao, C., Vodicka, P., Sram, R.J. & Hemminki, K. (2001) DNA adducts of 1,3-butadiene in humans: Relationships to exposure, GST genotypes, single-strand breaks, and cytogenetic end points. *Environ. mol. Mutag.*, **37**, 226–230

Zhuang, S.M. & Söderkvist, P. (2000) Genetic analysis of Raf1, Mdm2, c-Myc, Cdc25a and Cdc25b proto-oncogenes in 2′,3′-dideoxycytidine- and 1,3-butadiene-induced lymphomas in B6C3F1 mice. *Mutat. Res.*, **452**, 19–26

Zhuang, S.M., Wiseman, R.W. & Söderkvist, P. (2000) Mutation analysis of the pRb pathway in 2′,3′-dideoxycytidine- and 1,3-butadiene-induced mouse lymphomas. *Cancer Lett.*, **152**, 129–134

Zhuang, S.M., Wiseman, R.W. & Söderkvist, P. (2002) Frequent mutations of the Trp53, Hras1 and beta-catenin (Catnb) genes in 1,3-butadiene-induced mammary adenocarcinomas in B6C3F1 mice. *Oncogene*, **21**, 5643–5648

ETHYLENE OXIDE

This substance was considered by previous Working Groups in February 1976 (IARC, 1976), June 1984 (IARC, 1985), March 1987 (IARC, 1987) and February 1994 (IARC, 1994). Since that time, new data have become available, and these have been incorporated into the monograph and taken into consideration in the present evaluation.

1. Exposure Data

1.1 Chemical and physical data

1.1.1 *Nomenclature*

From IARC (1994) and IPCS-CEC (2001)
Chem. Abstr. Serv. Reg. No.: 75-21-8
Replaced CAS Reg. No.: 19034-08-3; 99932-75-9
Chem. Abstr. Name: Oxirane
IUPAC Systematic Name: Oxirane
RTECS No.: KX2450000
UN TDG No.: 1040
EC Index No.: 603-023-00-X
EINECS No.: 200-849-9
Synonyms: Dihydrooxirene; dimethylene oxide; EO ; 1,2-epoxyethane; epoxyethane; ethene oxide; EtO; ETO; oxacyclopropane; oxane; oxidoethane

1.1.2 *Structural and molecular formulae and relative molecular mass*

$$H_2C \overbrace{}^{} CH_2$$
$$O$$

C_2H_4O Relative molecular mass: 44.06

1.1.3 *Chemical and physical properties of the pure substance*

From IARC (1994), Dever *et al.* (2004), Lide (2005), Rebsdat and Mayer (2005) and O'Neil (2006), unless otherwise specified

(a) *Description*: Colourless gas
(b) *Boiling-point*: 13.2 °C at 746 mm Hg [99.4 kPa]; 10.4–10.8 °C at 760 mm Hg [101.3 kPa]
(c) *Freezing-point*: –111 °C
(d) *Density (liquid)*: 0.8824 at 10 °C/10 °C
(e) *Spectroscopy data*: Infrared [prism, 1109] and mass spectral data have been reported (Weast & Astle, 1985; Sadtler Research Laboratories, 1991).
(f) *Solubility*: Soluble in water, acetone, benzene, ethanol and diethyl ether
(g) *Vapour pressure*: 145.6 kPa at 20 °C (Hoechst Celanese Corp., 1992)
(h) *Relative vapour density (air = 1)*: 1.5 at 20 °C (IPCS-CEC, 2001)
(i) *Stability*: Reacts readily with acids; reactions proceed mainly via ring opening and are highly exothermic; explosive decomposition of vapour may occur at higher temperatures if dissipation of heat is inadequate.
(j) *Lower explosive limit*: 2.6–3.0% by volume in air
(k) *Octanol-water partition coefficient*: log P_{ow}, –0.30 (Sangster, 1989)
(l) *Flash-point*: Flammable gas (IPCS-CEC, 2001)
(m) *Inflammability limits in air*: 2.6–99.99% (V) (Shell Chemicals, 2005)
(n) *Autoignition temperature*: 428 °C (Shell Chemicals, 2005)
(o) *Dynamic viscosity*: 0.41 mPa at 0 °C (Shell Chemicals, 2005)
(p) *Conversion factor*: $mg/m^3 = 1.80 \times ppm$[1]

1.1.4 *Technical products and impurities*

Ethylene oxide for use as a fumigant and sterilizing agent used to be available in mixtures with nitrogen, carbon dioxide or dichlorodifluoromethane. Mixtures of 8.5–80% ethylene oxide/91.5–20% carbon dioxide (Allied Signal Chemicals, 1993) and 12% ethylene oxide in dichlorodifluoromethane were commonly used. As a result of concern about the role of chlorofluorocarbons in the depletion of stratospheric ozone and the phase-out of dichlorofluoromethane under the Montreal Protocol, the fluorocarbon materials now used to make blends of non-flammable ethylene oxide sterilants are hydrochlorofluorocarbons, hydrofluorocarbons and other flame-retardant diluent gases (Dever *et al.*, 2004).

---

[1] Calculated from: mg/m^3 = (relative molecular mass/24.45) × ppm, assuming normal temperature (25 °C) and pressure (101.3 kPa)

1.1.5   *Analysis*

Ethylene oxide in air can be determined by packed column gas chromatography (GC) with an electron capture detector (ECD) (NIOSH Method 1614), with an estimated limit of detection of 1 µg ethylene oxide per sample (National Institute for Occupational Safety and Health, 1987). A similar method is reported by the Occupational Safety and Health Administration in the USA (Tucker & Arnold, 1984; Cummins *et al.*, 1987). In a similar method reported by the Canadian Research Institute for Health and Safety at Work (IRSST Method 81-2), the sample is absorbed on an active charcoal tube (SKC ST-226-36), desorbed by benzylic alcohol and analysed by GC/flame ionization detection (FID) (IRSST, 2005).

In another technique (NIOSH Method 3702), a portable gas chromatograph is used with a photoionization detector or photoacoustic detector (IRSST 39-A). The sample is either drawn directly into a syringe or collected as a bag sample; it is then injected directly into the gas chromatograph for analysis. The estimated limit of detection of this method is 2.5 pg/mL injection (0.001 ppm [0.002 mg/m^3]) (National Institute for Occupational Safety and Health, 1998).

Passive methods use derivatization techniques that convert ethylene oxide to 2-bromoethanol followed by GC/ECD analysis or collect ethylene oxide in acidic solution (in which it is converted to ethylene glycol) or on a selective membrane followed by colorimetric analysis (Kring *et al.*, 1984; Puskar & Hecker, 1989; Puskar *et al.*, 1990, 1991; Szopinski *et al.*, 1991).

Methods for the analysis and quantification of ethylene oxide in emissions from production plants and commercial sterilizers by GC/FID have been reviewed (Steger, 1989; Margeson *et al.*, 1990).

Ethylene oxide has been measured in alveolar air and blood (Brugnone *et al.*, 1986). Several methods have been reported for the determination of *N*-(2-hydroxyethyl) adducts with cysteine, valine and histidine in haemoglobin: a radioimmunological technique, a modified Edman degradation procedure with GC/mass spectrometry (MS), a GC method with selective ion monitoring MS and a GC/ECD method (Farmer *et al.*, 1986; Bailey *et al.*, 1987; Bolt *et al.*, 1988; Föst *et al.*, 1991; Hagmar *et al.*, 1991; Kautiainen & Törnqvist, 1991; Sarto *et al.*, 1991; van Sittert *et al.*, 1993; Schettgen *et al.*, 2002).

Methods have been reported for the detection of residues of ethylene oxide used as a sterilant: headspace GC (Marlowe *et al.*, 1987) and GC (Wojcik-O'Neill & Ello, 1991) for the analysis of medical devices; capillary GC for the analysis of drugs and plastics (Danielson *et al.*, 1990); and headspace GC for the analysis of packaging materials and ethylene oxide in ethoxylated surfactants and demulsifiers (Dahlgran & Shingleton, 1987). Methods have also been developed for the determination of ethylene oxide residues in processed food products. In one such method, ethylene oxide is converted to ethylene iodohydrin and analysed by GC/ECD (Jensen, 1988).

1.2   Production and use

1.2.1   *Production*

Production of ethylene oxide began in 1914 by the chlorohydrin process, the main method used until 1937, in which ethylene chlorohydrin is converted to ethylene oxide by reaction with calcium oxide. The production of ethylene chlorohydrin resulted in the formation of two main organochlorine by-products, 1,2-dichloroethane and bis(2-chloroethyl)ether (see IARC, 1999a). Ethylene chlorohydrin was produced in either the same or a separate unit and was pumped over to the ethylene oxide production sector. The chlorohydrin process for the production of ethylene oxide was inefficient, because most of the chlorine that was used was lost as calcium chloride. Since 1931, that process has gradually been replaced by the direct vapour-phase oxidation process, in which ethylene is oxidized to ethylene oxide with air or oxygen and a silver catalyst at 10–30 atm (1–3 MPa) and 200–300 °C (Dever *et al.*, 2004; Anon., 2005).

In 2002, ethylene oxide was produced in more than 30 countries in Asia, Australia, Europe, the Middle East, North America and South America with a production capacity per year of 16.3 million tonnes (Lacson, 2003). Worldwide consumption of ethylene oxide was 14.7 million tonnes in 2002 (Dever *et al.*, 2004) and 18 million tonnes in 2006 (Devanney, 2007). Table 1 shows the number of producers by region as well as the production levels of ethylene oxide in 2004; approximately 17 million tonnes of ethylene oxide were produced worldwide. Production in Canada increased from 625 000 tonnes in 1996 (WHO, 2003) to 1 084 000 tonnes in 2004.

1.2.2   *Use*

Ethylene oxide is an important raw material used in the manufacture of chemical derivatives that are the basis for major consumer goods in virtually all industrialized countries. Figure 1 gives an overview of global industry demand for ethylene oxide by application. More than half of the ethylene oxide produced worldwide is used in the manufacture of monoethylene glycol (Occupational Safety and Health Administration, 2005; Devanney, 2007). The percentage of total ethylene oxide that is used domestically to manufacture ethylene glycols varies widely between regions: North America (66%), western Europe (43%), Japan (68%) and the Middle East (99%) (Lacson, 2003).

Other derivatives of ethylene oxide include: diethylene glycol, which is used in the production of polyurethanes, polyesters, softeners (cork, glue, casein and paper), plasticizers and solvents and in gas drying; triethylene glycol, which is used in the manufacture of lacquers, solvents, plasticizers and humectants (moisture-retaining agents) and in gas drying; poly(ethylene) glycols, which are reacted with other materials and used in cosmetics, ointments, pharmaceutical preparations, lubricants (finishing of textiles, ceramics), solvents (paints and drugs) and plasticizers (adhesives and printing inks); ethylene glycol ethers, which are frequently a component of brake fluids, detergents and solvents (paints and lacquers) and are used to treat natural and refinery gas; ethanolamines, which are used in textile finishing, cosmetics, soaps, detergents and natural gas purification; and ethoxylation products of fatty alcohols, fatty amines, alkyl phenols, cellulose and poly(propylene) glycol, which are used in the production of detergents and surfactants (non-ionic), biodegradable detergents, emulsifiers and dispersants (Occupational Safety and Health Administration, 2005; Devanney, 2007).

A very small proportion (0.05%) of the annual production of ethylene oxide is used directly in the gaseous form as a sterilizing agent, fumigant and insecticide, either alone or in non-explosive mixtures with nitrogen, carbon dioxide or dichlorofluoromethane (Dever *et al.*, 2004).

Table 1.   Production of ethylene oxide by region in 2004

Region	No. of producers	Production (thousand tonnes)
North America		
USA	10	4009
Canada	3	1084
Mexico	3	350
South America		
Brazil	2	312
Venezuela	1	82
Europe		
Belgium	2	770
France	1	215
Germany	4	995
Netherlands	2	460
Spain	1	100
Turkey	1	115
United Kingdom	1	300
Eastern Europe	NR	950
Middle East		
Iran	2	201
Kuwait	1	350
Saudi Arabia	2	1781
Asia/Pacific	>15	
China, mainland	NR	1354
China (Province of Taiwan)	4	820
India	> 2	488
Indonesia	1	175
Japan	4	949
Malaysia	1	385
Republic of Korea	3	740
Singapore	1	80

From Anon. (2004)
NR, not reported

Figure 1. Industrial products made from ethylene oxide
(globally, 17 million tonnes per annum)

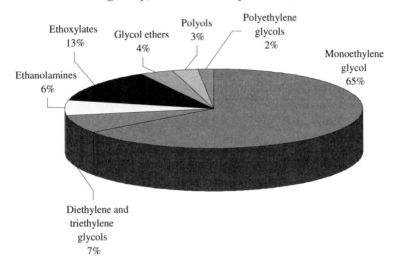

From Devanney (2007)

Ethylene oxide is also used as a fumigant and sterilant for microbial organisms in a variety of applications. An estimated 9–10 million pounds [4–5 million tonnes] of ethylene oxide were used in 2002 to sterilize drugs, hospital equipment, disposable and re-usable medical items, packaging materials, foods, books, museum artefacts, scientific equipment, clothing, furs, railcars, aircraft, beehives and other items (Lacson, 2003).

1.3   Occurrence

1.3.1   *Natural occurrence*

Ethylene oxide occurs endogenously as a metabolite of ethylene in certain plants and micro-organisms (see Section 4.1). Ethylene oxide can be generated from water-logged soil, manure and sewage sludge, but emissions are expected to be negligible (WHO, 2003).

1.3.2   *Occupational exposure*

Most of the data on occupational exposure are related to the production of ethylene oxide and its use in industrial and hospital sterilization.

Data were not available on exposures that are incurred outside North America and Europe, where almost half of the global amount of ethylene oxide is produced (Table 1).

The National Occupational Exposure Survey conducted by the National Institute for Occupational Safety and Health in the USA between 1981 and 1983 indicated that 270 000 employees in the USA were potentially exposed to ethylene oxide at work (NOES, 1993). This implies that, with an estimated labour force (aged 16 years and over) of 106 million (US Census, 1980), fewer than 0.3% of employees was exposed. Of this number, 22% was estimated to be exposed to ethylene oxide and 78% to materials that contain ethylene oxide. Workers in hospitals and in the chemical and allied products industry (manufacture of plastics, synthetic materials and drugs) accounted for half of that number.

More recent data on employment in the industrial sectors that use ethylene oxide have been reported by the Occupational Safety and Health Administration (2005). Approximated employment figures were: ethylene oxide production workers, 1100; ethoxylators (use of ethylene oxide to make derivatives), 4000; and sterilant or fumigant use in hospitals, 40 000. In addition, approximately 2700 workers were employed in commercial sterilization by medical and pharmaceutical product manufacturers, in commercial sterilization by spice manufacturers, as contract sterilizers and in other sterilization and fumigation facilities.

The CAREX exposure information system (see General Remarks) includes estimates of the numbers of exposed workers in the 15 member states of the European Union in 1990–93. The estimates were based on expert judgments and did not involve exposure measurements. According to CAREX, 47 000 workers were exposed to ethylene oxide, which is under 0.1% of the 139 million employed who are covered by CAREX (Kauppinen *et al.*, 2000). The major industries in which exposure occurred were medical, dental and other health and veterinary services (22 000 exposed) and the manufacture of industrial chemicals and other chemical products (7000 exposed).

The Finnish Register of occupational exposure to carcinogens reported that 126 workers were notified as having been exposed to ethylene oxide in 2004. This is below 0.01% of the 2.4 million people employed in Finland. Most of the workers exposed were employed in medical occupations. The Register does not include any information on exposure levels, and is based on annual notifications of employers; its completeness is unknown (Saalo *et al.*, 2006).

(a)   *Production of ethylene oxide and its derivatives*

Area samples taken in the 1960s throughout a plant in the USA where ethylene oxide was produced by direct oxidation of ethylene showed concentrations of 0–55 ppm [0–

100 mg/m³]. On the basis of these results, the general long-term exposure of operators to ethylene oxide was estimated to be 5–10 ppm [9–18 mg/m³] (Joyner, 1964).

Area and personal samples were taken by the National Institute for Occupational Safety and Health during 1977 and 1978 in five plants in the USA where ethylene oxide and its derivatives were produced. In most of the 95 personal samples taken, which were representative of whole shifts, the concentration of ethylene oxide was below the detection limit (which varied from 0.1 to 8 mg/m³); a few samples contained between 1 and 148 mg/m³. Similarly, in most area samples, the concentration was below the detection limit or was in the range < 1–1.5 ppm [2–3 mg/m³], apart from exceptional situations such as leaks (Lovegren & Koketsu, 1977a,b,c; Oser et al., 1978a,b, 1979). The fact that full-shift concentrations in these plants were usually well below the standards at that time (50 ppm [90 mg/m³]) has been attributed to three main factors: the use of completely closed systems for the storage, transfer and production of ethylene oxide; the implementation of measures to prevent fire; and operation outdoors which resulted in dilution by natural air (Morgan et al., 1981).

Estimates of exposure to ethylene oxide were made for a Swedish company where ethylene oxide and its derivatives were produced by the chlorohydrin process. Average exposure was estimated to be less than 25 mg/m³ during the period 1941–47 and 10–50 mg/m³ during the 1950s and early 1960s, with occasional peaks above the odour threshold of 1300 mg/m³. After manufacture of ethylene oxide was stopped in this company in 1963, exposure to 1–10 mg/m³ (with occasional higher values) continued to occur because of its use in the manufacture of other compounds (Högstedt et al., 1979a).

At a plant in Germany where ethylene oxide was manufactured, 2-h area samples taken in 1978–79 contained less than 5 ppm [9 mg/m³] under normal working conditions. Concentrations rose to 1900 ppm [3400 mg/m³] for several minutes in exceptional cases during plant breakdown (Thiess et al., 1981).

The typical average daily exposures of workers in a 1979 survey of plants in the USA where ethylene oxide was manufactured and used were 0.3–4 ppm [0.5–7.3 mg/m³]; worst-case peak exposures of maintenance workers were up to 9600 ppm [17 300 mg/m³] for less than 1 min (Flores, 1983).

In one chemical manufacturing complex in the USA, yearly time-weighted average (TWA) exposures to ethylene oxide in 1977–80 were reported to have been below 1 ppm [1.8 mg/m³] in all jobs except loading, during which technicians were exposed to up to 1.7 ppm [3 mg/m³] yearly and 5.7 ppm [10 mg/m³] individually. Peak exposures were usually < 20 ppm [< 36 mg/m³], except in loading, during which concentrations of up to 235 ppm [420 mg/m³] were reported (Currier et al., 1984).

In an ethylene oxide manufacturing plant in the Netherlands, geometric mean concentrations in 8-h personal samples were calculated to be < 0.01 ppm [< 0.02 mg/m³] in 1974, 1978 and 1980 and 0.12 ppm [0.2 mg/m³] in 1981; individual values ranged from not detected (< 0.05 ppm [< 0.1 mg/m³]) to 8 ppm [14 mg/m³] (van Sittert et al., 1985).

At another plant in Sweden where ethylene oxide was produced by oxygenation of ethylene, the 8-h TWA exposure to ethylene oxide was 9–15 mg/m³ [5–8 ppm] in 1963–

76 and 2–4 mg/m^3 [1–2 ppm] in 1977–82 during the production of ethylene oxide and ethylene glycol, 6 mg/m^3 [3 ppm] in 1963–76 and 2 mg/m^3 [1 ppm] in 1977–82 during the processing of ethylene oxide and 2–6 mg/m^3 [1–3 ppm] in 1963–76 and 1–3 mg/m^3 [0.6–1.7 ppm] in 1977–82 during maintenance and technical service work. Certain workers in each category were reported to have had higher exposures (up to 600–1800 mg/m^3 [333–1000 ppm]) during periods of minutes (Högstedt *et al.*, 1986).

In former Czechoslovakia, the 8-h TWA concentrations of ethylene oxide measured in 1982–84 in the working environment of an ethylene oxide production plant were 0–8.25 mg/m^3 [4.6 ppm] (Karelová *et al.*, 1987).

Under the sponsorship of the Chemical Manufacturers' Association, company data were collected on current exposures to ethylene oxide of workers in 11 ethylene oxide production units and 24 ethoxylation units in the USA in 1987 (Table 2). Respirators were reported to be used in specific operations, such as rail car loading and unloading, maintenance and product sampling, during which engineering controls are not feasible (Heiden Associates, 1988a).

Table 2. Exposure of workers to ethylene oxide by type of unit and job category in the chemical manufacturing industry in the USA, 1987

Unit and job category	No. of samples	8-h TWA (mg/m^3)		No. of samples	Short-term (10–150 min) exposure (mg/m^3)	
		Mean[a]	Range		Mean[a]	Range
Ethylene oxide production						
Production workers	402	0.7	0.11–3.2	171	7.7	1.62–19.8
Maintenance workers	439	1.3	0.14–5.6	59	19.6	0.20–35.3
Supervisors	123	0.2	0.04–0.18	3	1.3	1.3–1.4
Distribution workers	218	2.9	0.36–6.8	111	11.7	3.6–17.6
Laboratory workers	189	0.7	0.12–4.3	39	1.4	0.4–2.2
Other workers	97	0.2	0.05–0.72			
Ethoxylation						
Production workers	640	0.4	0.12–1.26	172	2.0	0.02–9.9
Maintenance workers	191	1.1	0.02–4.7	56	13.3	0.11–54.9
Supervisors	54	0.4	0.05–0.72	5	8.6	0.9–23.8
Distribution workers	105	0.7	0.20–2.7	100	3.4	0.9–21.6
Laboratory workers	52	0.4	0.02–0.9	19	5.0	0.4–11.0
Other workers	24	0.4	0.18–0.54			

Adapted from Heiden Associates (1988a)
TWA, time-weighted average
[a] Weighted by number of workers exposed

Gardner *et al.* (1989) reported that monitoring since 1977 in four British plants where ethylene oxide and derivatives were produced indicated average exposures to less than

5 ppm [9 mg/m³] in almost all jobs and to < 1 ppm [1.8 mg/m³] in many jobs; occasional peaks up to several hundred parts per million occurred as a result of operating difficulties. In earlier years, peak exposures above the odour threshold of 700 ppm [1260 mg/m³] were reported.

In industries in which ethylene oxide and its derivatives are manufactured, exposure to a large variety of chemicals other than ethylene oxide may occur, depending on the types of process and job. These include unsaturated aliphatic hydrocarbons (e.g. ethylene, propylene; see IARC, 1994), other epoxides (e.g. propylene oxide; see IARC, 1994), chlorohydrins (e.g. epichlorohydrin; see IARC, 1999a; and ethylene chlorohydrin), chlorinated aliphatic hydrocarbons (e.g. dichloromethane, dichloroethane; see IARC, 1999a), glycols and ethers (e.g. ethylene glycol, glycol ethers, bis(2-chloroethyl)ether; see IARC, 1999a, 2006), aldehydes (e.g. formaldehyde; see IARC, 2006), amines (e.g. aniline; see IARC, 1987), aromatic hydrocarbons (e.g. benzene, styrene; see IARC, 1987), alkyl sulfates and other compounds (Shore *et al.*, 1993).

(b)   Use of ethylene oxide for industrial sterilization

Industrial workers may be exposed to ethylene oxide during sterilization of a variety of products such as medical equipment and products (e.g. surgical products, single-use medical devices), disposable health care products, pharmaceutical and veterinary products, spices and animal feed.

In an extensive survey of the industry in the USA conducted by the National Institute for Occupational Safety and Health, exposure to ethylene oxide was estimated on the basis of data collected in 1976–85 by 21 of 36 companies, most of which were involved in the sterilization of medical supplies and spices. Individual 8-h TWA concentrations of samples collected by active sampling on charcoal tubes in the personal breathing zones of workers were included in a model in which regression analysis was used to link exposure concentrations to seven significant variables: year of operation, volume of sterilizer or treatment vessel, period since the product was sterilized, product type, aeration procedure, presence of a rear exhaust valve in the sterilizer and exposure category (sterilizer, chamber area, maintenance, production, warehouse, clean room, quarantine and laboratory) (Greife *et al.*, 1988; Stayner *et al.*, 1993; Hornung *et al.*, 1994). When the model was applied in a cohort study to the job histories of exposed workers in 13 of the companies surveyed, the estimated historical average concentrations ranged from 0.05 to 77.2 ppm [0.1–139 mg/m³], with a mean of 5.5 ppm [9.9 mg/m³] and a median of 3.2 ppm [5.8 mg/m³] (Stayner *et al.*, 1993). Wong and Trent (1993) used the industrial hygiene data from the same companies and estimated that sterilizer operators were exposed to an 8-h TWA concentration of 16 ppm [29 mg/m³] before 1978 and of 4–5 ppm [7–9 mg/m³] after 1978, while production workers were exposed to about 5 ppm [9 mg/m³] before 1978 and 2 ppm [3.6 mg/m³] after that year.

In a Swedish factory where hospital equipment was sterilized, area samples taken in 1977 in the storage area showed concentrations of ethylene oxide that ranged from 2 to 70 ppm [3.6–126 mg/m³]; the 8-h TWA concentration in the breathing zone of workers in the same area was 20 ppm [36 mg/m^3] (Högstedt *et al.*, 1979b). In 1978, full-shift personal sampling indicated that sterilizing room operators had an exposure concentration of 2.4 ppm [4.3 mg/m^3]; area sampling indicated an exposure of 1.3 ppm [2.3 mg/m^3]. Personal sampling showed a concentration of 0.1 ppm [0.2 mg/m^3] in the packing room, and area sampling showed a concentration of 0.8 ppm [1.4 mg/m^3] in the stockroom (Högstedt *et al.*, 1983). In another Swedish study, sterilization workers and a laboratory technician in the production of disposable medical equipment were reported to have been exposed to bursts of ethylene oxide at concentrations of 5–10 ppm [9–18 mg/m^3] for a total of 1 h per working day, while packers were exposed at an average of 0.5–1 ppm [1–2 mg/m^3] for the entire week (Pero *et al.*, 1981). Sterilization workers, packers and truck drivers at another Swedish factory, where single-use medical equipment was produced, were reported to be exposed to an 8-h TWA concentration of 0.5–1 ppm [1–2 mg/m^3] (Pero *et al.*, 1982). In two Swedish disposable medical equipment plants, sterilizers and packers were the most heavily exposed, but levels decreased steadily from 35–40 ppm [about 70 mg/m^3] in 1970 to < 0.2–0.75 ppm [< 1.5 mg/m^3] in 1985; the average levels of exposure of store workers and development engineers decreased from 5–20 ppm [9–36 mg/m^3] to < 0.2 ppm [< 0.4 mg/m^3] in the same period, while those of people in other job categories (repairmen, laboratory technicians, controllers and foremen) decreased from 1–4 ppm [2–7 mg/m^3] to < 0.2 ppm [< 0.4 mg/m^3] (Hagmar *et al.*, 1991).

Engineering controls and new work practices designed to lower the exposure of workers to ethylene oxide were generally adopted in the USA in 1978 and 1979 (Steenland *et al.*, 1991). Stolley *et al.* (1984) estimated that the 8-h TWA concentrations of sterilizer operators in three facilities in the USA before 1980 had been 0.5, 5–10 and 5–20 ppm [1, 9–18 and 9–36 mg/m^3], while data collected in the two plants that were still operating in 1980–82 indicated concentrations of less than 1 ppm [2 mg/m^3].

In Belgium, 12 workers involved in industrial sterilization in three plants were exposed to 8-h TWA concentrations of 0.1–9.3 ppm [0.2–16.7 mg/m^3], with averages in each plant of 1.7, 3.7 and 4.5 ppm [3.1, 6.7 and 8.1 mg/m^3] (Wolfs *et al.*, 1983).

In a plant in eastern Germany where disposable medical equipment was sterilized, workers were found to have been exposed to an average concentration of about 60 mg/m^3 [27.1 ppm] in 1985 and about 30 mg/m^3 [13.6 ppm] from 1989 onwards (Tates *et al.*, 1991).

Under the sponsorship of the Health Industry Manufacturers' Association, company data were collected in 1987 on current exposures to ethylene oxide of workers in 71 facilities in the USA where medical devices and diagnostic products were sterilized. The workers included sterilizer operators, maintenance workers, supervisors, warehouse workers, laboratory workers and quality control personnel. Respirators were reported to be used in specific operations, such as unloading the sterilizer, maintenance, quality control sampling, emergencies, loading aeration, and changing ethylene oxide bottles, cylinders and tanks. Concentrations were measured outside the respirators. The routine 8-h TWA concentration that occurred 2 or more days per week was > 1 ppm [> 1.8 mg/m^3] for 12.6% of workers, 0.5–1 ppm [0.9–1.8 mg/m^3] for 13.9%, 0.3–0.5 ppm

$[0.5–0.9 \text{ mg/m}^3]$ for 26.7% and < 0.3 ppm $[< 0.5 \text{ mg/m}^3]$ for 46.8%. Short-term sampling (for 5–120 min; average, 28 min; except in one factory where sampling was for 210 min for workers in other jobs) showed routine short-term exposures of > 10 ppm $[> 18 \text{ mg/m}^3]$ for 10.7% of workers, 5–10 ppm $[9–18 \text{ mg/m}^3]$ for 17.1% and < 5 ppm $[< 9 \text{ mg/m}^3]$ for 72.2%. Non-routine short-term exposure that occurred 1 day per week or near areas where there was exposure was > 10 ppm $[> 18 \text{ mg/m}^3]$ for 5.1% of workers, 5–10 ppm $[9–18 \text{ mg/m}^3]$ for 2.6% and < 5 ppm $[< 9 \text{ mg/m}^3]$ for 92.3% (Heiden Associates, 1988b).

At a commercial sterilization operation in the USA, workers were exposed to 8-h TWA concentrations of 1–10 ppm $[1.8–18 \text{ mg/m}^3]$ in 1993–2001 and to 1.3–2.4 ppm $[2.3–4.3 \text{ mg/m}^3]$ in 2002, according to measurements carried out by the employer. The Occupational Safety and Health Administration monitored personal exposures in the same workplace and found 8-h TWA concentrations of 0.6–9.3 ppm $[1.1–17 \text{ mg/m}^3]$. After improvement of working conditions, 8-h TWA concentrations of 0.2–1.2 ppm $[0.4–2.2 \text{ mg/m}^3]$ were found during follow-ups (Daniel et al., 2004).

Exposures in 10 factories in Taiwan (China) that used ethylene oxide as a sterilant in the manufacture of medical supplies were measured in 2005 (Chien et al., 2007). Sterilizer operators had an average short-term exposure level of 27.6 ppm $[50 \text{ mg/m}^3]$ during unloading of the sterilizer, and the mean 8-h TWA exposure was 7.4 ppm $[13 \text{ mg/m}^3]$. High concentrations were measured particularly in the aeration area, near the sterilizer and in the warehouse. Increasing the number of post-sterilization purge cycles and improvements to ventilation in the aeration area and warehouse decreased the average short-term exposures to 55% of the earlier values.

Other substances to which workers involved in the sterilization of medical products may be exposed include gases that are present with ethylene oxide in the sterilizing mixture, such as chlorofluorocarbons and carbon dioxide (Heiden Associates, 1988b), and methyl formate in Sweden (Hagmar et al., 1991).

(c)   Use of ethylene oxide in hospitals

Ethylene oxide is used widely in hospitals as a gaseous sterilant for heat-sensitive medical items, surgical instruments and other objects and fluids that come into contact with biological tissues. The National Institute for Occupational Safety and Health estimated that there were more than 10 000 sterilizers in use in health care facilities in the USA in 1977. Large sterilizers are found in central supply areas of most hospitals, and smaller sterilizers are found in clinics, operating rooms, tissue banks and research facilities (Glaser, 1979).

Exposure to ethylene oxide may result during any of the following operations and conditions: changing pressurized ethylene oxide gas cylinders; leaking valves, fittings and piping; leaking sterilizer door gaskets; opening the sterilizer door at the end of a cycle; improper ventilation at the sterilizer door; improperly ventilated or unventilated air gap between the discharge line and the sewer drain; removal of items from the sterilizer and transfer of the sterilized load to an aerator; improper ventilation of aerators and aeration areas; incomplete aeration of items; inadequate general room ventilation; and passing near or working in the same room as sterilizers and aerators during operation (Mortimer & Kercher, 1989).

Levels of exposure to ethylene oxide in hospitals are summarized in Table 3.

The National Institute for Occupational Safety and Health conducted a series of studies between 1977 and 1990 to document the exposure to ethylene oxide of hospital sterilization staff in the USA. The main results are summarized in Table 4. The more recent studies from Japan and France (see Table 3) suggest that 8-h TWA concentrations are often < 1 mg/m^3 [0.6 ppm] in hospitals.

From 1984 to 2001, a total of 256 666 ethylene oxide samples were analysed by a major vendor of passive ethylene oxide monitoring devices in the USA. Most of the measurements (86%) were taken in hospitals. Workshift measurements were taken from 28 373 hospital workers in 2265 hospitals and short-term measurements from 18 894 workers in 1735 hospitals. The percentage of hospitals in which the 8-h TWA exposure limit of 1 ppm [1.8 mg/m^3] was exceeded once or more times in a year decreased from 21% in 1988 to 0.9% in 2001 (La Montagne et al., 2004).

In most studies, exposure to ethylene oxide appears to result mainly from peak emissions during operations such as opening the door of the sterilizer and unloading and transferring sterilized material. Proper engineering controls and work practices have been reported to result in full-shift exposure levels of less than 0.1 ppm [0.18 mg/m^3] and short-term exposure levels of less than 2 ppm [3.6 mg/m^3] (Mortimer & Kercher, 1989). In a survey of 125 hospitals in the USA, however, use of personal protective equipment was found to be limited to the wearing of various types of gloves while transferring sterilized items. No respirators were used (Elliott et al., 1988).

In a unit in Argentina that was equipped with old gas sterilizers with no mechanical ventilation, the 8-h TWA concentration of ethylene oxide was 60–69 ppm [108–124 mg/m^3] (Lerda & Rizzi, 1992).

Other substances to which sterilizer operators in hospitals may be exposed include other gases present in the sterilizing mixture such as chlorofluorocarbons (see IARC, 1999a; banned by the Montreal Protocol in 1989) and carbon dioxide (Wolfs et al., 1983; Deschamps et al., 1989). Some operating room personnel exposed to ethylene oxide may also be exposed to anaesthetic gases and X-rays (Sarto et al., 1984a; see IARC, 2000; Chessor et al., 2005), and some may have occasional exposure to low concentrations of formaldehyde (Gardner et al., 1989; see IARC, 2006).

(d)   Other uses

In a wastewater treatment plant in the USA, ethylene oxide was used as a reaction chemical to modify starch in the starch processing area; in this area, full-shift personal breathing zone concentrations ranged from undetectable to 0.43 mg/m^3 [0.24 ppm] for operators and from undetectable to 2.5 mg/m^3 [1.4 ppm] for mechanics (McCammon et al., 1990).

Table 3. Concentrations of ethylene oxide observed in hospitals in various countries

Reference	Country	Year of sampling	No. of sites	Job or operation	Duration of sampling	No. of samples	Concentration (mg/m³) Range	Concentration (mg/m³) Mean
Hemminki et al. (1982)	Finland	1981	24	Sterilizer operators	8-h TWA	NR	0.2–0.0	
					Peaks	NR	≤ 450	
				Sterilizing chamber open	20 min	NR	9–18	
Mouilleseaux et al. (1983)	France	NR	4[a]	Loading, sterilizing, unloading, aerating; area sampling	Few minutes 6–8-h TWA	270 14	0.9–414 0.1–9	
Wolfs et al. (1983)	Belgium	NR	3	Sterilizer operators	8-h TWA	28	0.4–4.5	0.5–2.9
			1	Sterilizer operators; leaking equipment	8-h TWA	16	0.5–32.9	14.0
			1	Sterilizer operators; box sterilizer with capsules	8-h TWA	5	16.2–95.2	27.0
Hansen et al. (1984)	USA	NR	1			14 17 13	< 0.13–7.7 < 4.3–81 4–1430	
Sarto et al. (1984a,b)	Italy	NR	6	Old sterilizers				
				Opening sterilizer; area sampling	5 min	NR	23–288	113
				One sterilization cycle; personal sampling	Variable	NR	6.7–63.9	28.4
				Standard working day; personal sampling	8-h TWA	19 subjects	6.7–36	19.3
				Second-generation sterilizers				
				Opening sterilizer; area sampling	5 min	NR	9–47	15.5
				One sterilization cycle; personal sampling	Variable	NR	0.5–4.7	2.0
				Standard working day; personal sampling	8-h TWA	NR	0.4–0.9	0.63

Table 3 (contd)

Reference	Country	Year of sampling	No. of sites	Job or operation	Duration of sampling	No. of samples	Concentration (mg/m³)	
							Range	Mean
Brugnone et al. (1985)	Italy	NR	1	Sterilization workers	8-h TWA	10 subjects	1.90–4.71	
Karelová et al. (1987)	Former Czechoslovakia	1984	1	Sterilization workers; area sampling	8-h TWA	NR	0–4.8	
Sarto et al. (1987)	Italy	NR	1	Sterilizer workers Helpers	7–8-h TWA 7–8-h TWA	4 subjects 4 subjects	11.5–16.7 6.8–9.0	14.3 7.7
Deschamps et al. (1989)	France	1983–86	5	Opening sterilizer and handling sterilized material; personal samples	2.5–102 min	10	0.4–70	
Mayer et al. (1991)	USA	1985–86 1987 1988	1	Sterilizer operators; personal samples	8-h TWA	34 subjects NR 31	≤ 4.3 < 1.8 < 0.18	
Sarto et al. (1991)	Italy	NR	1	Sterilization workers Preparation workers	6.5-h TWA 6.5-h TWA	5 subjects 5 subjects	0.68[b] 0.045	
Schulte et al. (1992)	Mexico	NR	1	Sterilizer operators	8-h TWA	22 subjects	0–2.4	
Koda et al. (1999)	Japan	NR	2	Central supply division Working area (hospital A) Near sterilizer (hospital A) Working area (hospital B) Near sterilizer (hospital B)		322 322 298 35	0.2–1.1 0.2–1.1 0.5–1.4 2.0–2.3	0.7 0.5 0.9 2.2

Table 3 (contd)

Reference	Country	Year of sampling	No. of sites	Job or operation	Duration of sampling	No. of samples	Concentration (mg/m³)	
							Range	Mean
Sobaszek et al. (1999)	France	1988–95	2	Sterilization sites				
				Unloading; area samples	8-h TWA	5	0.05–0.72	
				Unloading; personal samples	14–34 min	5	0.09–11.1	
				Bottle changing; personal samples	7–9 min	5	0.18–162	
Hori et al. (2002)	Japan	NR	6	Sterilization, one laundry				
				Area samples	8-h TWA	37	< 0.05–10.3	
				Personal samples	NR	37	< 0.05–0.49	
	USA	NR	9	Sterilizer operators	8-h TWA	51 subjects	0–0.54	

NR, not reported; TWA, time-weighted average
[a] One was a municipal sterilization and disinfection facility.
[b] All samples had the same concentration.

Table 4. Exposure of hospital sterilizer operators to ethylene oxide (personal samples) in studies conducted by the National Institute for Occupational Safety and Health, in the USA, 1977–90

Reference	Period of measurements	No. of hospitals	Operation or conditions	Duration of sampling	No. of samples	Concentration (mg/m^3)
Kercher & Mortimer (1987)	NR	1	Before installation of controls (1984)	Full-shift TWA	NR	[0.43] (average)
				Short-term (15–20 min)	NR	[3.4] (average)
				Short-term (1–2 min)	NR	[4.3] (average)
			After installation of controls (1985)	Full-shift TWA	NR	[< 0.1] (average)
				Short-term (15–20 min)	NR	[< 0.4] (average)
				Short-term (1–2 min)	NR	[1]
Boeniger (1988a)	1987	1	Decontamination room	8-h TWA	2	[0.58–0.77]
			Sterile room	8-h TWA	6	[0.02–1.37]
Boeniger (1988b)	1987	1	Full shift	4–7 h TWA	8	[0.04–0.40]
			Cracking sterilizer door open	30 sec	6	[< 0.05–7.7]
			Transferring load to aerator	30 sec	15	[0.23–18.9]
Elliott et al. (1988)	[1984–85]	12	Good engineering controls and good work practice	8-h TWA	4	ND
				Short-term (2–30 min)	3	ND
			Good engineering controls and poor work practice	8-h TWA	15	[ND–0.29]
				Short-term (2–30 min)	19	[ND–5.4]
			No engineering controls and good work practices	8-h TWA	14	[ND–0.83]
				Short-term (2–30 min)	4	[0.43–7.2]
			No engineering controls and poor work practices	8-h TWA	24	[ND–8.3]
				Short-term (2–30 min)	8	[0.43–186]
Mortimer & Kercher (1989)	1984–86	8		Full-shift TWA (6–8 h)	50	[ND–0.5]
				Short-term (1–30 min)	59	[ND–10.4]
Newman & Freund (1989)	1988	1		8-h TWA	8	[< 0.02]
Shults & Seitz (1992)	1991	1		6–8-h TWA	3	[< 0.02]

ND, not detected; NR, not reported; TWA, time-weighted average

1.3.3 *Environmental occurrence*

Most ethylene oxide is released into the atmosphere (WHO, 2003). Ethylene oxide degrades in the atmosphere by reaction with photochemically produced hydroxyl radicals. The half-life of ethylene oxide in the atmosphere, assuming ambient concentrations of 5×10^5 hydroxy radicals/cm^3, is 211 days. Data suggest that neither rain nor absorption into aqueous aerosols remove ethylene oxide from the atmosphere (National Library of Medicine, 2005).

Releases of ethylene oxide (excluding sterilization) into the environment in Canada totalled 23 tonnes in 1996. The industry sectors that reported data were plastics and synthetics (0.24 tonnes), inorganic chemicals (6.1 tonnes), industrial organic chemicals (8.7 tonnes) and soap and cleaning compounds (8.0 tonnes) (WHO, 2003). An additional 3.0 tonnes per year are estimated to be released from the servicing of medical facilities that use ethylene oxide in sterilization processes and commercial sterilization operations (WHO, 2003). By 1997, the emissions had been reduced by 82% from the 1993 levels.

Emissions of ethylene oxide reported to the Environmental Protection Agency by industrial facilities in the USA declined from approximately 2900 tonnes in 1987 to 835 tonnes in 1991 and 135.3 tonnes in 2005 (National Library of Medicine, 2006). Ethylene oxide is one of the 33 hazardous urban air pollutants identified as those that pose the greatest threat to human health in the largest number of urban areas (Environmental Protection Agency, 2000).

In California, USA, concentrations of ethylene oxide in outdoor air were < 0.001– 0.96 mg/m^3 (128 samples) in Los Angeles, 0.032–0.40 µg/m^3 [0.018–0.22 ppb] (36 samples) in northern California and 0.03–0.36 µg/m^3 [0.017–0.20 ppb] in a remote coastal location (Havlicek *et al.*, 1992).

Three of 50 24-h air samples collected outside randomly selected residences in Alberta, Ontario and Nova Scotia in Canada contained 3.7–4.9 µg/m^3 ethylene oxide. Ethylene oxide was detected in only one sample (4 µg/m^3) taken inside these 50 residences. The limit of detection was 0.19 µg/m^3 (WHO, 2003).

1.3.4   *Other occurrence*

Food products, including herbs, spices, nuts, cocoa beans, cocoa, cocoa cake, raisins, dried vegetables and gums, were often treated with ethylene oxide in the 1980s. Of 204 food products from retail shops in Denmark that were examined for ethylene oxide residues in 1985, 96 samples were found to have concentrations of ethylene oxide that ranged from 0.05 to 1800 mg/kg. The food products surveyed included herbs and spices (14–580 mg/kg), dairy products (0.06–4.2 mg/kg), pickled fish (0.08–2.0 mg/kg), meat (0.05–20 mg/kg), cocoa products (0.06–0.98 mg/kg) and black and herb teas (3–5 mg/kg; one sample contained 1800 mg/kg). In a follow-up survey of 59 honey samples, no ethylene oxide residue was detected (Jensen, 1988).

A total of 200 samples of spices that are known to be consumed commonly without cooking (e.g. pepper, cinnamon/cassia, chilli, curry powder and paprika) were taken from wholesalers and retailers in New Zealand in 1999. Only two samples of cinnamon contained detectable amounts (limit of detection, 2 mg/kg) of ethylene oxide (6 and 15 mg/kg). Ethylene oxide intake, based on average spice consumption in New Zealand, was estimated to be 0.21 µg per person per day (conservative estimate) (Fowles *et al.*, 2001).

Ethylene oxide occurs as a contaminant of skin care products because current commercial preparations of polyglycol ethers may contain ethylene oxide monomer residues of up to 1 ppm (Filser *et al.*, 1994). This is in line with a study in which skin care products were reported to contain 0.08–1.5 mg/L ethylene oxide (Kreuzer, 1992).

Ethylene oxide is formed during the combustion of fossil fuel, but the amount is expected to be negligible (WHO, 2003).

Mainstream tobacco smoke contains 7 µg/cigarette ethylene oxide (IARC, 2004).

Patients may be exposed during dialysis when the equipment has been sterilized with ethylene oxide (IPCS-CEC, 2001).

1.4   Regulations and guidelines

Occupational exposure limits and guidelines for ethylene oxide in a number of countries, regions or organizations are presented in Table 5.

A tolerance of 50 ppm (mg/kg) has been established in the USA for residues of ethylene oxide when used as a post-harvest fumigant in or on raw black walnut meats, copra and whole spices (Environmental Protection Agency, 1992a). Ethylene oxide, either alone or with carbon dioxide or dichlorodifluoromethane, is permitted in the USA as a fumigant for the control of micro-organisms and insect infestation in ground spices and other processed natural seasoning materials, except mixtures to which salt has been added. Residues of ethylene oxide in ground spices must not exceed the established tolerance of 50 ppm (mg/kg) in whole spices (Environmental Protection Agency, 1992b).

Table 5.   Occupational exposure limits and guidelines for ethylene oxide

Country/region or organization	TWA (ppm)[a]	STEL (ppm)[a]	Carcinogenicity[b]	Notes
Australia	1		2	
Belgium	1		Ca	
Brazil	39			
Canada,				
British Columbia	0.1	1	1	ALARA; skin
Quebec	1		A2	Recirculation prohibited
China (mg/m³)	2	5		STEL based on ultra limit coefficient
China, Hong Kong SAR	1		A2	

Table 5 (contd)

Country/region or organization	TWA (ppm)[a]	STEL (ppm)[a]	Carcinogenicity[b]	Notes
China (Province of Taiwan)	1	2		
Czech Republic (mg/m³)	1	3		Skin
Finland	1			
France	1.8			
Germany	1 (TRK)		2 (MAK)	Skin
Ireland	5		Ca2	
Japan-JSOH	1		1	Skin sensitizer-2
Malaysia	1			
Mexico	1		A2	
Netherlands (mg/m³)	0.84		Ca	
New Zealand	1		A2	
Norway	1		Ca	
Poland (mg/m³)	1	3	Ca	
Romania	1			
South Africa-DOL CL	5			
Spain	1		Ca2	
Sweden	1	5	Ca	Skin
United Kingdom	5		R45	
USA				
ACGIH	1		A2	
NIOSH REL	0.1	5	Ca	Per day
OSHA PEL	1	5 (ceiling)	Ca	

From ACGIH® Worldwide (2005); SZW (2006); Chien *et al.* (2007)
ACGIH, American Conference of Governmental Industrial Hygienists; ALARA, as low as reasonably achievable; DOL CL, Department of Labour ceiling limits; JSOH, Japanese Society of Occupational Health; MAK, maximum allowed concentration; NIOSH, National Institute of Occupational Safety and Health; OSHA, Occupational Safety and Health Administration; PEL, permissible exposure limit; REL, recommended exposure limit; STEL, short-term exposure limit; TRK, technical guidance concentration; TWA, time-weighted average
[a] Unless otherwise specified
[b] 2 (Australia), probable human carcinogen; 2 (Germany), considered to be carcinogenic to humans; Ca (except Norway), carcinogen/substance is carcinogenic; Ca (Norway), potential cancer-causing agent; 1, substance which causes cancer in humans/carcinogenic to humans; A2, suspected human carcinogen/carcinogenicity suspected in humans; Ca2, suspected human carcinogen; R45, may cause cancer

2.   Studies of Cancer in Humans

The main findings of epidemiological studies of ethylene oxide and cancer risk are summarized in Table 6.

2.1   Case reports

Högstedt *et al.* (1979b) reported three cases of haematopoietic neoplasms that had occurred between 1972 and 1977 in workers at a Swedish factory where ethylene oxide and methyl formate had been used since 1968 to sterilize hospital equipment. Attention had been drawn to the case cluster by the factory safety committee. One woman with chronic myeloid leukaemia and another with acute myelogenous leukaemia had worked in a storage hall where they were exposed for 8 h per day to an estimated 20 ± 10 (standard deviation [SD]) ppm [36 ± 18 mg/m³] ethylene oxide. The third case was that of a man with primary Waldenström macroglobulinaemia who had been manager of the plant since 1965 and had been exposed to ethylene oxide for an estimated 3 h per week. [The Working Group noted that Waldenström macroglobulinaemia is classified in the WHO Classification of Diseases as lymphoplasmocytic lymphoma.]

Tompa *et al.* (1999) described a cluster of 16 cases of cancer (including eight women with breast cancer) over a 12-year period among 98 nurses who were exposed to ethylene oxide at a sterilizer unit in a hospital in Hungary. Airborne concentrations of ethylene oxide in the working area were reported to vary from 5 to 150 mg/m³.

2.2   Cohort studies

2.2.1   *Europe*

Högstedt *et al.* (1979a, 1986) and Högstedt (1988) examined workers at a Swedish chemical plant where ethylene oxide had been produced by the chlorhydrin process. The cohort comprised men who had taken part in a medical survey in 1959–61 and included 89 operators with regular exposure to ethylene oxide, 78 maintenance staff with inter-mittent exposure and 66 unexposed men. All of the men had been exposed or employed for at least 1 year. Average exposures to ethylene oxide during 1941–47 were estimated to have been below 25 mg/m³, but occasional peaks exceeded the odour threshold of 1300 mg/m³. During the 1950s and through to 1963, an average concentration of 10–50 mg/m³ was estimated. In 1963, production of ethylene oxide ceased, but the compound continued to be used in manufacturing processes, and random samples showed workplace concentrations of ethylene oxide in the range of 1–10 mg/m³, with occasional higher values. Other exposures in the plant included chloroform (IARC, 1999b), chlorinated acetals, chloral (IARC, 1995), DDT (IARC, 1991), ethylene glycol, surfactants, cellulose ethers, ethylene (IARC, 1994), ethylene chlorohydrin, ethylene dichloride, bis(2-chlorethyl)ether (IARC, 1987, 1999a) and propylene oxide (IARC, 1994, 1995, 1997).

Table 6. Epidemiological studies of exposure to ethylene oxide and cancer at various sites

Reference, location	Cohort description	Exposure assessment	Organ site (ICD code)	Exposure categories	No. of cases/ deaths	Relative risk (95% CI)	Adjustments and comments
COHORT STUDIES							
Europe							
Lymphohaematopoietic (LH)							
Högstedt et al. (1979a, 1986), Sweden	89 operators with regular exposure to ethylene oxide and 78 maintenance staff with intermittent exposure, employed for ≥ 1 year at a chemical plant, followed 1962–85		Leukaemia	Operators Maintenance staff	2 1	[10] [5]	Estimated average exposure before 1963, 5–25 ppm [9–45 mg/m³]; one CML, one acute leukaemia, one CLL
Thiess et al. (1981), Germany	602 male employees in a company in western Germany who worked for at least 6 months in ethylene oxide production, followed to June 1980		Myeloid leukaemia Lymphatic sarcoma		1 1	6.67 NR	
Högstedt et al. (1986), Sweden	203 workers employed ≥ 1 year in production of sterilized supplies, followed 1978–82		LH (200–209)	All cohort members	2	[15]	Estimated average past exposure in storeroom, 20 ppm [36 mg/m³]; one AML was part of a cluster which had originally prompted the study; one acute blastic leukaemia

Table 6 (contd)

Reference, location	Cohort description	Exposure assessment	Organ site (ICD code)	Exposure categories	No. of cases/ deaths	Relative risk (95% CI)	Adjustments and comments
Högstedt et al. (1986), Sweden	355 chemical workers and maintenance and technical personnel employed at a chemical plant, followed 1964–81	Air sampling and interview with experienced staff	CML	All cohort members	1	11.6 deaths expected from all causes	TWA exposures, 1–8 ppm [1.8–14.4 mg/m³] in 1963–76; 0.4–2.0 ppm [0.7–3.6 mg/m³] in 1977–82
Högstedt (1988), Sweden	Follow-up of Högstedt et al. (1979a,b, 1986)		Leukaemia Blood and lymphatic malignancies	All cohort Men All cohort Men	7 6 9 4	**SMR** 9.21 (NR) 3.54 (1.3–7.7) 4.59 (NR) 6.11 (1.7–15.7)	
Gardner et al. (1989), United Kingdom (updated by Coggon et al., 2004)	1471 workers employed in production or use of ethylene oxide at 4 chemical companies in 1956–85, followed to 31 December 2000	Environmental and personal monitoring since 1977	Leukaemia (204–208) Hodgkin lymphoma (201) NHL (200) Multiple myeloma (203)	All cohort members	4 1 4 3	1.41 (0.39–3.62) 1.40 (0.04–7.82) 1.38 (0.38–3.53) 2.03 (0.42–5.94)	Measured TWA concentrations < 5 ppm [9 mg/m³] in almost all jobs but with occasional peaks up to several hundred ppm; exposures probably higher in past
	1405 workers potentially exposed to ethylene oxide in sterilization units at 8 hospitals during 1964–86, followed to 31 December 2000		Leukaemia Hodgkin lymphoma NHL	All cohort members	1 1 3	0.55 (0.01–3.06) 2.98 (0.08–16.6) 1.59 (0.33–4.66)	

Table 6 (contd)

Reference, location	Cohort description	Exposure assessment	Organ site (ICD code)	Exposure categories	No. of cases/ deaths	Relative risk (95% CI)	Adjustments and comments
Kiesselbach et al. (1990), Germany	2658 employees from 6 chemical companies exposed to ethylene oxide for ≥ 12 months during 1928–82, followed to 31 December 1982		LH Leukaemia	All cohort members	5 2	1.00 (0.32–2.3) 0.85 (0.10–3.1)	No data on exposure levels; risk estimates may have been seriously biased since most deaths in cohort were not ascertained from death certificates.
Hagmar et al. (1991, 1995), Sweden	2170 workers employed for ≥ 12 months during 1964–85 at 2 plants where medical equipment was sterilized with ethylene oxide, followed for cancer incidence to 1990		LH Leukaemia	All cohort members All cohort members ≥ 0.14 ppm–years with induction period of 10 years	6 2 2	1.8 (0.65–3.88) 2.4 (0.30–8.81) 7.1 (0.87–25.8)	
Bisanti et al. (1993), Italy	1971 male chemical workers licensed to handle ethylene oxide for ≥ 1 year during 1938–84, followed 1940–84		LH Lymphosarcoma and reticulosarcoma Leukaemia	All cohort members	6 4 2	2.5 (0.91–5.5) 6.8 (1.9–17) 1.9 (0.23–7.0);	The 2 leukaemia deaths occurred in men with < 5 years of exposure and < 10 years after first exposure.
Kardos et al. (2003), Hungary	299 women employed on a hospital ward using ethylene oxide sterilizer in 1976–93, followed 1987–99		Leukaemia	All cohort members	1	4.38 deaths expected from all causes	Deaths in the cohort ascertained from a different source from the reference rates

Table 6 (contd)

Reference, location	Cohort description	Exposure assessment	Organ site (ICD code)	Exposure categories	No. of cases/ deaths	Relative risk (95% CI)	Adjustments and comments
Breast							
Gardner *et al.* (1989), United Kingdom (updated by Coggon *et al.*, 2004)	1011 women potentially exposed to ethylene oxide in sterilization units at 8 hospitals during 1964–86, followed to 31 December 2000		Breast	All cohort members Continual Unknown	11 5 6	0.84 (0.42–1.51) 0.70 (NR) 1.16 (NR)	
Hagmar *et al.* (1991, 1995), Sweden	2170 workers employed for ≥ 12 months in 1964–85 at 2 plants where medical equipment sterilized with ethylene oxide, followed for cancer incidence to 1990		Breast	All cohort members	5	0.46 (0.15–1.08)	
Kardos *et al.* (2003), Hungary	299 women employed on a hospital ward using ethylene oxide sterilizer in 1976–93, followed 1987–99		Breast	All cohort members	3	4.38 deaths expected from all causes	Deaths in the cohort ascertained from a different source from the reference rates; one or more breast cancer cases may have been part of a cluster that prompted the study.

Table 6 (contd)

Reference, location	Cohort description	Exposure assessment	Organ site (ICD code)	Exposure categories	No. of cases/ deaths	Relative risk (95% CI)	Adjustments and comments
Stomach							
Thiess et al. (1981), Germany	602 employees exposed to alkylene oxides and other substances, employed in 1928–80	Environmental monitoring	Stomach	All cohort members	4	[1.49] (NR)	
Högstedt et al. (1979a, 1986); Högstedt (1988), Sweden	89 operators with regular exposure to ethylene oxide and 78 maintenance staff with intermittent exposure, employed for ≥ 1 year at a chemical plant, followed 1962–85		Stomach	All cohort members	5	**SMR** 9.03 (2.9–21.1)	
Högstedt (1988), Sweden	539 men employed for ≥ 1 year at a chemical plant followed 1960–85		Stomach	*Length of employment* 1–9 years ≥ 10 years All	4 6 10	**SMR** 5.97 (NR) 6.08 (NR) 6.02 (2.9–11.1)	
Gardner et al. (1989), United Kingdom (updated by Coggon et al., 2004)	1471 workers in the production or use of ethylene oxide at 4 chemical companies during 1956–85, followed to 31 December 2000	Environmental and personal monitoring since 1977	Stomach	All cohort members Definite Probable Unknown	5 4 1 0	**SMR** [0.62 (0.20–1.46)] 0.78 (NR) 0.57 (NR) 0 (NR)	Measured TWA concentrations < 5 ppm [9 mg/m³] in almost all jobs but with occasional peaks up to several hundred ppm; exposures probably higher in the past

Table 6 (contd)

Reference, location	Cohort description	Exposure assessment	Organ site (ICD code)	Exposure categories	No. of cases/ deaths	Relative risk (95% CI)	Adjustments and comments
Kiesselbach et al. (1990), Germany	2658 employees from 6 chemical companies exposed to ethylene oxide for ≥ 12 months in 1928–82, followed to 31 December 1982		Stomach	All cohort members	14	**SMR** 1.38 (0.75–2.31)	No data on exposure levels; risk estimates may have been seriously biased since most deaths in cohort were not ascertained from death certificates.
Hagmar et al. (1991, 1995), Sweden	2170 workers employed for ≥ 12 months during 1964–85 at 2 plants using medical equipment sterilized with ethylene oxide, followed for cancer incidence to 1990		Stomach	All cohort members Induction period of 10 years	0 0	**SIR** 0 (0–4.55) 0 (0–8.38)	
Ambroise et al. (2005), France	181 male workers employed as pest-control workers 1979–94, followed for mortality through to 2000		Stomach	All cohort members	1	**SMR** 3.18 (0.08–17.70)	No information available on individual level of exposures to pesticides, rodenticides or formaldehyde

Table 6 (contd)

Reference, location	Cohort description	Exposure assessment	Organ site (ICD code)	Exposure categories	No. of cases/ deaths	Relative risk (95% CI)	Adjustments and comments
Brain							
Thiess *et al.* (1981), Germany	602 employees exposed to alkylene oxides and other substances, employed in 1928–80	Environmental monitoring	Malignant tumour of the brain	*Duration of exposure* 0.5–4 years 5–9 years 10–19 years ≥ 20 years	0 0 0 1	NR NR NR [41.7] (NR)	
Hagmar *et al.* (1991, 1995), Sweden	2170 workers employed for ≥ 12 months in 1964–85 at 2 plants using medical equipment sterilized with ethylene oxide, followed for cancer incidence to 1990		Brain	All cohort members All cohort members ≥ 0.14 ppm–years Induct on period of 10 years	4 3 3	**SIR** 1.69 (0.46–4.34) 3.80 (0.78–11.1) 2.80 (0.58–8.19)	

Table 6 (contd)

Reference, location	Cohort description	Exposure assessment	Organ site (ICD code)	Exposure categories	No. of cases/ deaths	Relative risk (95% CI)	Adjustments and comments
Pancreas							
Hagmar et al. (1991, 1995), Sweden	2170 workers employed for ≥ 12 months during 1964–85 at 2 plants where medical equipment was sterilized with ethylene oxide, followed for cancer incidence to 1990		Pancreas	All cohort members All cohort members ≥ 0.14 ppm–years Induction period of 10 years	2 1 1	**SIR** 2.47 (0.30–8.92) 2.86 (0.07–15.9) 2.22 (0.06–12.4)	
Ambroise et al. (2005), France	181 male workers employed as pest-control workers 1979–94, followed for mortality through to 2000		Pancreas	All cohort members	0	**SMR** 0 (0–10.77)	No information available on individual level of exposures to pesticides, rodenticides or formaldehyde
USA							
Lymphohaematopoeitic (LH)							
Morgan et al. (1981), eastern Texas (reported in Shore et al., 1993)	767 men employed in 1955–77 at a chemical plant for ≥ 5 years with potential exposure to ethylene oxide, followed 1955–85	Industrial hygiene survey in 1977	LH Leukaemia	All cohort members	3 0	10 (0.21–2.9) 0.0 (0.0–3.4)	Exposures in 1977 < 10 ppm [18 mg/m³]; included 2 cases of Hodgkin disease

Table 6 (contd)

Reference, location	Cohort description	Exposure assessment	Organ site (ICD code)	Exposure categories	No. of cases/deaths	Relative risk (95% CI)	Adjustments and comments
Steenland *et al.* (1991); Stayner *et al.* (1993); Steenland *et al.* (2004)	18 235 workers employed at 14 industrial plants that used ethylene oxide for sterilization since 1943 with ≥ 3 months exposure to ethylene oxide, followed to 1998		LH	All cohort members	79	**SMR** 1.00 (0.79–1.24)	Adjusted for age, race (white/non-white), date of birth (within 5 years); in an internal case–control analysis (excluding 1 small plant), log cumulative exposure to ethylene oxide lagged by 15 years significantly related to mortality from LH cancers in men (*p* = 0.02), but not in women; duration of exposure, peak exposure and average exposure less predictive of mortality from LH cancer; similar pattern observed for lymphoid-cell tumours
				Cumulative exposure in ppm–days			
				0–1199	18	0.77 (NR)	
				1200–3579	20	1.31 (NR)	
				3680–13 499	18	1.10 (NR)	
				≥ 13 500	18	0.94 (NR)	
			Lymphoid-cell	Men with 15- year lag (results from Cox regression)			
				Cumulative exposure in ppm–days			
				0		1.00	
				>0–1199		0.90 (0.16–5.24)	
				1200–3579		2.89 (0.65–12.86)	
				3680–13 499		2.74 (0.65–11.55)	
				≥ 13 500		3.76 (1.03–13.64) *p*-trend = 0.13	
			Hodgkin lymphoma	All cohort members	6	1.24 (0.53–2.43)	
				Cumulative exposure in ppm–days			
				0–1199	0	0 (NR)	
				1200–3579	1	0.99 (NR)	
				3680–13 499	3	2.97 (NR)	
				≥ 13 500	2	2.20 (NR)	

Table 6 (contd)

Reference, location	Cohort description	Exposure assessment	Organ site (ICD code)	Exposure categories	No. of cases/ deaths	Relative risk (95% CI)	Adjustments and comments
Steenland et al. (1991); Stayner et al. (1993); Steenland et al. (2004) (contd)			NHL	All cohort members	31	1.00 (0.72–1.35)	
				Cumulative exposure in ppm–days			
				0–1199	7	0.76 (NR)	
				1200–3679	8	1.34 (NR)	
				3680–13 499	6	0.85 (NR)	
				≥ 13 500	9	1.21 (NR)	
			Multiple myeloma	All cohort members	13	0.92 (0.54–0.87)	
				Cumulative exposure in ppm–days			
				0–1199	1	0.26 (NR)	
				1200–3679	5	1.89 (NR)	
				3680–13 499	3	0.92 (NR)	
				≥ 13 500	4	1.03 (NR)	
			Leukaemia	All cohort members	29	0.99 (0.71–1.36)	
				Cumulative exposure in ppm–days			
				0–1199	10	1.15 (NR)	
				1200–3679	6	1.06 (NR)	
				3680–13 499	6	0.93 (NR)	
				≥ 13 500	3	0.43 (NR)	
Benson & Teta (1993), West Virginia	278 men intermittently exposed to ethylene oxide in a chlorohydrin unit since 1949, followed to 1988		LH	All cohort members	8	2.94 (1.27–5.80)	Primarily exposed to ethylene chloro-hydrin, ethylene dichloride and bischloroethyl ether

Table 6 (contd)

Reference, location	Cohort description	Exposure assessment	Organ site (ICD code)	Exposure categories	No. of cases/ deaths	Relative risk (95% CI)	Adjustments and comments
Teta *et al.* (1993), West Virginia	1896 men potentially exposed to ethylene oxide since 1940 at 2 chemical plants but who never worked in chlorohydrin unit, followed to 1988		LH Lymphosarcoma and reticulosarcoma Leukaemia	All cohort members	7 2 5	0.6 (0.2–1.2) 1.0 (0.1–3.56) 1.1 (0.4–2.5)	
Norman *et al.* (1995), New York State	1132 workers employed in 1974–80 at a sterilizing plant that used ethylene oxide, followed for cancer incidence to 1957		Leukaemia	All cohort members	1	1.85 ($p = 0.42$)	
Olsen *et al.* (1997), Texas	1361 men employed for ≥ 1 year and potentially engaged for ≥ 1 month in ethylene or propylene chlorohydrin production since 1941 at 4 chemical plants, followed to 1992		LH	Ever in ethylene chlorohydrin product on Ever in ethylene chlorohydrin product on with allowance for 25-year induction period from first exposure	10 6	1.29 (0.62–2.38) 1.4 (0.52–3.12)	
Breast							
Norman *et al.* (1995), New York State	1132 workers employed during 1974–80 at a sterilizing plant that used ethylene oxide, followed for cancer incidence to 1957		Breast	All cohort members All cohort members	12 12	1.72* (0.99–3.00) 1.57** (0.90–2.75)	*Expected numbers from SEER rates for 1978–81 **Expected numbers from SEER rates for 1981–85

Table 6 (contd)

Reference, location	Cohort description	Exposure assessment	Organ site (ICD code)	Exposure categories	No. of cases/ deaths	Relative risk (95% CI)	Adjustments and comments
Steenland et al. (2003)	7576 women worked for ≥ 1 year at 13 plants, followed for breast cancer incidence to 1998		Breast	All cohort members	319	0.87* (0.77–0.97)	*Recognized to be an underestimate because of incomplete ascertainment of cases
			Breast excluding carcinoma in situ	All cohort members	299	0.94 ([0.84–1.05])	
			Breast	Exposures in ppm–days with 15-year lag			**Odds ratios calculated by Cox regression in a nested case–control analysis
				0	81	1.00** (lagged out)	
				< 647	45	1.07 (0.72–1.59)	
				647–2026	46	1.00 (0.67–1.50)	
				2027–4919	46	1.24 (0.85–1.90)	
				4920–14 620	45	1.17 (0.78–1.78)	
				> 14 620	48	1.74 (1.16–2.65)	***Analysis restricted to subset of 5139 women with data on potential confounders from interviews; adjusted for parity, breast cancer in first-degree relative
				Exposures in ppm–days with 15-year lag			
				0	81	1.00*** (lagged out)	
				< 647	45	1.06 (0.66–1.71)	
				647–2026	46	0.99 (0.61–1.60)	
				2027–4919	46	1.24 (0.76–2.00)	
				4920–14 620	45	1.42 (0.88–2.29)	
				> 14 620	48	1.87 (1.12–3.10)	
Steenland et al. (2004)	18 235 workers at 14 industrial plants that used ethylene oxide for sterilization since 1943 with ≥ 3 months' exposure to ethylene oxide, followed to 1998		Breast	All cohort members	103	0.99 (0.84–1.17)	At least one cancer occurred in a man.
				All female cohort members	NR	0.99 (0.81–1.20)	

Table 6 (contd)

Reference, location	Cohort description	Exposure assessment	Organ site (ICD code)	Exposure categories	No. of cases/ deaths	Relative risk (95% CI)	Adjustments and comments
Stomach							
Steenland *et al.* (1991); Stayner *et al.* (1993); Steenland *et al.* (2004)	18 254 workers at 14 industrial plants that used ethylene oxide for sterilization since 1943 with ≥ 3 months exposure to ethylene oxide, followed to 1998		Stomach	All cohort members (Steenland *et al.*, 2004) *Cumulative exposure in ppm–days* < 1200 1200–8500 > 8500 Total (Stayner *et al.*, 1993)	25 5 4 1 10	**SMR** 1.07 (0.74–1.49) 1.74 (0.57–4.07) 1.24 (0.29–2.60) 0.23 (0.11–1.32) 0.90 (0.43–1.66) *p* trend = 0.04	.
Benson & Teta (1993), West Virginia	278 men intermittently exposed to ethylene oxide in a chlorohydrin unit since 1949, followed to 1988		Stomach	All cohort members	1	[0.70] (0.2–3.92)	Primarily exposed to ethylene chloro-hydrin, ethylene dichloride and bischloroethyl ether
Teta *et al.* (1993), West Virginia	1896 men potentially exposed to ethylene oxide since 1940 at 2 chemical plants but who never worked in chlorohydrin unit, followed to 1988		Stomach	All cohort members	8	**SMR** 1.60 (0.69–3.15)	

Table 6 (contd)

Reference, location	Cohort description	Exposure assessment	Organ site (ICD code)	Exposure categories	No. of cases/ deaths	Relative risk (95% CI)	Adjustments and comments
Norman et al. (1995), New York State	1132 workers employed during 1974–80 at a sterilizing plant using ethylene oxide, followed for cancer incidence to 1957		Stomach	All cohort members	0	–	
Olsen et al. (1997), Texas	1361 men employed for ≥ 1 year and potentially engaged for ≥ 1 month in ethylene or propylene chlorohydrin production since 1941 at 4 chemical plants, followed to 1992		Stomach	Ever in ethylene chlorohydrin production	2	**SMR** 65 (8–234)	
				Ever in ethylene chlorohydrin production with allowance for 25-year induction period from first exposure	2	[1.17 (0.14–4.23)]	

Table 6 (contd)

Reference, location	Cohort description	Exposure assessment	Organ site (ICD code)	Exposure categories	No. of cases/ deaths	Relative risk (95% CI)	Adjustments and comments
Brain							
Steenland et al. (1991); Stayner et al. (1993); Steenland et al. (2004)	18 254 workers employed at 14 industrial plants using ethylene oxide for sterilization since 1943 with ≥ 3 months exposure to ethylene oxide, followed to 1998		Brain	All cohort members (Steenland et al., 2004) *Cumulative exposure in ppm–days* < 1200 1200–< 500 > 8500 Total (Stayner et al., 1993)	14 0 4 2 6	**SMR** 0.59 (0.36–0.91) 0.0 0.99 (0.27–2.53) 0.59 (0.07–2.12) 0.54 (0.20–1.18) *p*-trend = 0.43	
Benson & Teta (1993), West Virginia	278 men intermittently exposed to ethylene oxide in a chlorohydrin unit since 1949, followed to 1988		Brain and other nervous system	All cohort members	1	[1.17] (0.3–6.56)	Primarily exposed to ethylene chlorohydrin, ethylene dichloride and bischloroethyl ether
Teta et al. (1993), West Virginia	1896 men potentially exposed to ethylene oxide since 1940 at 2 chemical plants who never worked in chlorohydrin unit, followed to 1988		Brain and other nervous system	All cohort members		**SMR** 1.50 (0.55–3.27)	

Table 6 (contd)

Reference, location	Cohort description	Exposure assessment	Organ site (ICD code)	Exposure categories	No. of cases/ deaths	Relative risk (95% CI)	Adjustments and comments
Norman *et al.* (1995), New York State	1132 workers employed during 1974–80 at a sterilizing plant using ethylene oxide, followed for cancer incidence to 1957		Brain	All cohort members	0	–	
Olsen *et al.* (1997), Texas	1361 men employed for ≥ 1 year and potentially engaged for ≥ 1 month in ethylene or propylene chlorohydrin production since 1941 at 4 chemical plants, followed to 1992		Brain and other nervous system (191–192)	Ever in ethylene chlorohydrin production	3	**SMR** 1.23 (0.25–3.58)	
				Ever in ethylene chlorohydrin production with allowance for 25-year induction period from first exposure	3	[2.73 (0.56–7.97)]	

Table 6 (contd)

Pancreas

Reference, location	Cohort description	Exposure assessment	Organ site (ICD code)	Exposure categories	No. of cases/ deaths	Relative risk (95% CI)	Adjustments and comments
Steenland et al. (1991); Stayner et al. (1993); Steenland et al. (2004)	13 254 workers employed at 14 industrial plants using ethylene oxide for sterilization since 1943 with ≥ 3 months exposure to ethylene oxide, followed to 1998		Pancreas	All cohort members (Steenland et al., 2004)	38	**SMR** 0.92 (0.69–1.21)	.
				Cumulative exposure in ppm–days			
				< 1200	3	0.69 (0.14–2.03)	
				1200–≤500	10	1.70 (0.81–3.12)	
				> 850C	3	0.50 (0.10–1.47)	
				Total	16	0.98 (0.57–1.61)	
				(Stayner et al., 1993)		p-trend = 0.38	
Benson & Teta (1993), West Virginia	278 men intermittently exposed to ethylene oxide in a chlorohydrin unit since 1949, followed to 1988		Pancreas	All cohort members	8	4.92 (1.58–11.40)	Primarily exposed to ethylene chlorohydrin, ethylene dichloride and bischloroethyl ether
Teta et al. (1993), West Virginia	1896 men potentially exposed to ethylene oxide since 1940 at 2 chemical plants, who never worked in chlorohydrin unit, followed to 1988		Pancreas	All cohort members	4	**SMR** 0.61 (0.17–1.56)	

Table 6 (contd)

Reference, location	Cohort description	Exposure assessment	Organ site (ICD code)	Exposure categories	No. of cases/ deaths	Relative risk (95% CI)	Adjustments and comments
Norman et al. (1995), New York State	1132 workers employed in 1974–80 at a sterilizing plant using ethylene oxide, followed for cancer incidence to 1957		Pancreas	All cohort members	2	3.92 (p = 0.09)	
Olsen et al. (1997), Texas	1361 men employed for ≥ 1 year and potentially engaged for ≥ 1 month in ethylene or propylene chlorohydrin production since 1941 at 4 chemical plants, followed to 1992		Pancreas	Ever in ethylene chlorohydrin production	1	**SMR** 0.25 (0.1–1.40)	
				Ever in ethylene chlorohydrin production with allowance for 25-year induction period from first exposure	1	0.40 (0.1–2.26)	

Table 6 (contd)

Reference, location	Cohort description	Exposure assessment	Organ site (ICD code)	Exposure categories	No. of cases/deaths	Relative risk (95% CI)	Adjustments and comments
CASE–CONTROL STUDY							
Swaen et al. (1996), Belgium	210 employees of a chemical manufacturer between 1966 and 1992		Hodgkin lymphoma	All cohort members	3 exposed cases	**Odds ratio** 8.5 (1.4–39.9)	
META-ANALYSIS							
Teta et al. (1999), Germany, Italy, Sweden, United Kingdom, USA	Nearly 33 000 workers		Leukaemia		35	**Meta-SMR** 1.08 (0.61–1.93)	
			NHL		33	1.34 (0.96–1.89)	
			Stomach		59	1.23 (0.71–2.13)	
			Brain		25	0.96 (0.49–1.91)	
			Pancreas		37	0.95 (0.69–1.31)	

AML, acute myelogenous leukaemia; CI, confidence interval; CLL, chronic lymphocytic leukaemia; CML, chronic myelogenous leukaemia; ICD, International Classification of Diseases; NHL, non-Hodgkin lymphoma; NR, not reported; SEER, Surveillance, Epidemiology and End Results; SIR, standardized incidence ratio; SMR, standardized mortality ratio; TWA, time-weighted average

The cohort was followed from 1962 to 1985 through national registries. Among the ethylene oxide operators, 34 deaths from all causes occurred (25.0 expected), including 14 cancer deaths (6.1 expected) of which five were due to stomach cancer (0.6 expected) and two to leukaemia (0.2 expected; one chronic myelogenous and one acute leukaemia not further specified). No overall excess mortality from cancer was observed among the maintenance staff who had intermittent exposure or among the unexposed workers; however, four of the maintenance men had died from stomach cancer (0.6 expected) and one from chronic lymphocytic leukaemia (0.2 expected).

Two hundred and three workers employed for at least 1 year at the Swedish factory described in Section 2.1 were subsequently followed up for mortality through national census, death and emigration registries (Högstedt et al., 1986). During 1978–82, five deaths occurred (4.9 expected), four of which were from cancer (1.6 expected). Two of the deaths were from lymphatic and haematopoietic malignancies (0.13 expected), but one of these decedents (who had acute myelogenous leukaemia) had been part of the original case cluster that had prompted the study. The other died from acute blastic leukaemia.

The above reports also described a third cohort of Swedish workers who were exposed to ethylene oxide in a plant where the compound was produced by direct oxidation of ethylene (Högstedt et al., 1986; Högstedt, 1988). The cohort comprised 128 workers who were employed in the production of ethylene oxide or ethylene glycol and had had almost pure exposure to ethylene oxide; 69 workers who were employed in the processing of ethylene oxide and propylene oxide to non-ionic surfactants and polyols and whose principal exposure was to ethylene oxide and propylene oxide but who had also been exposed to various amines, sodium nitrate (IARC, 2009), formaldehyde (IARC, 2006) and 1,2-butene oxide; and 158 maintenance and technical personnel who had had multiple exposures that included ethylene oxide. Analyses of air samples and interviews with experienced staff indicated 8-h TWA exposures to ethylene oxide of 1–8 ppm [1.8–14.4 mg/m^3] during 1963–76, which fell to 0.4–2.0 ppm [0.7–3.6 mg/m^3] during 1977–82. Expected numbers of cancers and deaths were calculated from 5-year age-, sex- and calendar year-specific rates for the national population. During follow-up from 1964 to 1981 using national registries, eight deaths were observed in the entire cohort compared with 11.6 expected; one man in the maintenance and repair group died from chronic myelogenous leukaemia. During extended follow-up to 1985, a fatal case of reticular-cell sarcoma was recorded among the production workers [expected number not given]. [The Working Group noted that the cohort was not defined precisely.]

Högstedt (1988) also presented findings on cancer incidence (ascertained through the national cancer registry) for the three cohort studies described above. After exclusion of the three cases in the initial cluster at the sterilizing plant, seven leukaemias were observed (0.8 expected from national rates [standardized incidence ratio (SIR), 9.2]). For blood and lymphatic malignancies, nine deaths were observed (two expected; standardized mortality ratio [SMR], 4.59). Confidence intervals (CIs) were reported only for the SMRs of men.

Thiess *et al.* (1981) examined the mortality of 602 active and former male employees at a company in western Germany who had worked for at least 6 months in an area of alkylene oxide production. Until 1965, ethylene oxide had been made from ethylene chlorohydrin, but thereafter it was produced by direct oxidation of ethylene. Propylene oxide had been made since 1959 by a propylene chlorohydrin process. Industrial hygiene measurements in 1978 showed that the average concentration of ethylene oxide was < 4 ppm [7.2 mg/m^3], but no earlier measurement was available. Discussions with long-standing employees indicated that exposures before that time would have been higher. Other potential exposures included propylene oxide, butylene oxide, dioxane, epichlorohydrin, dichloropropane, ethylene chlorohydrin, propylene chlorohydrin, aniline, piperazine, cyclohexylamine, cyclohexane, formaldehyde, isobutyraldehyde, ethyleneimine, hydrocyanic acid, hydrogen sulfide, aluminium chloride, benzene, phenol, cyanuric acid, acrylic acid and acetylene alcohols (IARC, 1987, 1994, 1999a, 2006). The first worker was employed in 1928, and follow-up was from that year until 30 June 1980. The expected numbers of deaths in the cohort were calculated for each 5-year age group, using mortality rates for the populations of Ludwigshafen and Rhinehessia-Palatinate during 1970–75 and of Germany during 1971–74 as a reference. In addition, an internal comparison group of 1662 persons who were employed in a styrene production facility on the same site was used. During follow-up, 56 deaths were recorded in the exposed cohort, whereas the expected numbers were 71.5 (Ludwigshafen), 73.4 (Rhinehessia-Palatinate), 76.6 (Germany) and 57.9 (styrene cohort). Fourteen of the deaths were due to cancer, whereas 16.6 were expected from national statistics [SMR, 0.84]. The deaths from cancer included one case of myeloid leukaemia (< 0.15 expected) and one case of lymphatic sarcoma. [The Working Group noted that no indication of the completeness with which the cohort was identified was given, and that the methods of follow-up were not stated. It is not clear how losses to follow-up were handled in the analysis.]

Gardner *et al.* (1989) studied 2876 workers at four British chemical companies where ethylene oxide or its derivatives had been manufactured and in eight hospitals where ethylene oxide had been used as a sterilant. In one company, ethylene oxide had been produced by the chlorohydrin process during 1950–60 and by direct oxidation of ethylene from 1959 onwards; in the second company, the chlorohydrin process had been used during 1955–70 and direct oxidation was used thereafter; in the third company, ethylene oxide had been produced during 1960–81 only by direct oxidation; and in the fourth company, ethylene oxide had been used in the manufacture of derivatives since 1959. The eight hospitals had started using ethylene oxide between 1962 and 1972. The cohort comprised all workers at each factory and hospital who had had probable exposure to ethylene oxide during specified periods for which employment records were complete. Sixteen subjects had to be excluded because such information was not available in full. Jobs held by cohort members at the factories were classified as having involved definite, probable or possible exposure to ethylene oxide. At the hospitals, jobs were classed as involving continual, intermittent or possible exposure. Environmental and personal monitoring since 1977 had shown a TWA concentration of < 5 ppm [9 mg/m^3] in almost all jobs, but with occasional peaks of exposure up to several hundred parts per million as a result of operating difficulties in the chemical plants and during loading and unloading of sterilizers in the hospitals. Exposures were thought to have been higher in earlier years, and peak exposures above the odour threshold of 700 ppm [1260 mg/m^3] were reported both by the chemical manufacturers and at the hospitals. Cohort members at the manufacturing plants were potentially exposed to many other chemicals, including chlorohydrin, propylene oxide, styrene and benzene; some of the hospital workers had occasionally been exposed to formaldehyde and carbon tetrachloride. The cohort was followed for mortality through the National Health Service Central Register, with supplementary information from social security records for some subjects. In the most recently published analysis of this study (Coggon *et al.*, 2004), the results of which subsumed earlier findings, the cohort was followed for mortality to 2000. Follow-up for 51 untraced subjects was cut off at the last known date of employment. A further 206 subjects had emigrated or were otherwise lost to follow-up, and were considered to be at risk up to the date when they were last known to be alive. Observed mortality was compared with that expected from national death rates by sex, age and calendar period. No significant elevations of mortality were observed for any category of cancer either in the cohort as a whole, or separately in the chemical manufacturers and hospital workers. Among the 1471 chemical workers (all but one of whom were men), 366 deaths (366.9 expected) occurred from all causes, including 120 (108.6 expected; SMR, 1.11; 95% CI, 0.92–1.32) from all cancers combined. Increased non-significant risks were found for leukaemia, lymphoma and multiple myeloma. Lymphatic and haematopoietic cancer was more common in chemical workers who were classed as having had definite exposure to ethylene oxide (nine deaths versus 4.9 expected; SMR, 1.84), but there was no excess in the hospital workers who were classed as continually exposed (one death versus 2.6 expected).

Most of the above cohort was included in a larger study of employees from six chemical companies in western Germany (Kiesselbach *et al.*, 1990). The 2658 cohort members had been exposed to ethylene oxide for at least 12 months before 31 December 1982. The year of first exposure ranged from 1928 to 1981, but most had first been exposed after 1950. Other possible exposures included benzene (IARC, 1987), 4-aminobiphenyl and 2-naphthylamine (IARC, 1987), but no information was given on the extent of exposure to these substances. Subjects who had left employment were traced through local registries and, in the case of foreigners who had returned home, by letter or by asking fellow countrymen who were still working in the plant. Of the cohort members, 97.6% were traced successfully to 31 December 1982. For those who had died, the cause of death was ascertained from death certificates (27.6% of all deaths), lay statements, the physician who last treated the patient or hospital reports. Mortality was compared with that expected from 5-year age-, sex- and calendar period-specific rates in the national population; no statistics were available for periods before 1951, and the rates for 1951 were used. In total, 268 deaths were observed, whereas 307.6 were expected. There were

68 deaths from cancer (69.9 expected; SMR, 0.97; 95% CI, 0.76–1.24), including three from oesophageal cancer (1.5 expected), 14 from stomach cancer (10.2 expected; SMR, 1.38; 95% CI, 0.75–2.31) and five from lymphatic and haematopoietic cancer (5.0 expected; SMR, 1.00; 95% CI, 0.32–2.34). Two deaths were ascribed to leukaemia (2.4 expected). When expected numbers were calculated on the basis of rates in the states in which each plant was situated, the findings were very similar. Based on calculations in which the first 10 years of exposure for each subject were ignored, mortality ratios were similar to those in the main analysis. It was possible to classify exposure to ethylene oxide for 67.2% of subjects as 'weak', 'medium' or 'high'. The excess mortality from stomach cancer was greatest in those with weak or medium exposure and with less than 15 years of total exposure. When foreign workers were excluded from the analysis, there was no change in the observed number of deaths and mortality ratios were only slightly increased. [The Working Group noted that the full eligibility criteria for inclusion in the cohort were not reported, no data were given on probable levels of exposure to ethylene oxide or on the nature of the processes in which subjects worked, and risk estimates may have been seriously biased since certificates were available for only about one-quarter of deaths in the cohort.]

Hagmar *et al.* (1991) studied employees at two Swedish plants that produced disposable medical equipment that was sterilized with ethylene oxide. In plant A, a 50:50 mixture of ethylene oxide and methyl formate had been used since 1970. In 1973, personal sampling for two packers indicated an exposure to ethylene oxide of 24 ppm [43 mg/m^3]. After 1981, monitoring was carried out annually over 1–3 days for sterilizers and packers and showed a continuous decrease in exposure such that, after 1985, only sterilizers were exposed to concentrations greater than 0.2 ppm [0.4 mg/m^3] (the limit of detection of the method used). In plant B, a 50:50 mixture of ethylene oxide and methyl formate was used from 1964 but was replaced by an ethylene oxide:carbon dioxide mixture in 1978. In 1975, personal monitoring indicated exposures of 4–5 ppm [7–9 mg/m^3] ethylene oxide for four packers. After 1985, the 8-h TWA concentration was < 0.2 ppm [0.4 mg/m^3] for all employees except sterilizers and store workers. The authors estimated that sterilizers were exposed to up to 75 ppm [135 mg/m^3] in the earliest years of operation at this plant. On the basis of estimates of exposure in different job categories and time periods, the authors calculated individual cumulative exposures for 97% of subjects at plant A and 89% at plant B. The cohort comprised 594 men and 557 women who had been employed at plant A for at least 12 months between 1970 and 1985 and who were still working after 1 June 1975, and 267 men and 752 women who had been employed at plant B for at least 12 months between 1964 and 1985 and were still working after 1 January 1972. These subjects were followed through to 1986 for mortality and from 1972 to 1985 for cancer registration. None was lost to follow-up. Expected mortality was calculated on the basis of calendar year-, sex- and 5-year age-specific rates (cut-off at age 80 years) for the county in which the plants were located, and expected cancer incidence was calculated from corresponding registration rates in the same area. Fifteen deaths were observed (25.7 expected), including eight from cancer (9.0 expected), two from gastrointestinal cancer (2.1 expected) and one from haematopoietic and lymphatic cancer (1.0 expected). The observed/expected numbers of incident cancers were 21/26.8 for cancers at any site, 0/0.5 for stomach cancer, 1/1.6 for brain cancer, 2/1.3 for lymphoma and myeloma and one case of polycythaemia vera with 0.7 cases of leukaemia, polycythaemia vera and myelofibrosis expected. Among subjects with more than 1 ppm–year of cumulative exposure to ethylene oxide, two cases of cancer (3.3 expected) and no lymphatic or haematopoietic cancer (0.2 expected) were observed. Follow-up for cancer incidence was subsequently extended to 1990, again with no losses to follow-up (Hagmar et al., 1995). In total, 40 cases of cancer were recorded with 46.28 expected. No significant excesses in mortality were observed for any individual site of cancer, either with or without allowance for a 10-year induction period from first exposure. With no allowance for an induction period, the numbers of observed/expected cases were 5/10.8 (SIR, 0.5; 95% CI, 0.15–1.08) for cancer of the breast, 6/3.37 (SIR, 1.78; 95% CI, 0.65–3.88) for lymphatic and haematopoietic cancer and 2/0.82 (SIR, 2.44; 95% CI, 0.30–8.81) for leukaemia. Among 930 subjects with cumulative exposures of at least 0.14 ppm–years, after allowance for a minimum induction period of 10 years, two cases of leukaemia were observed compared with 0.28 expected (SIR, 7.1; 95% CI, 0.87–25.8).

Bisanti et al. (1993) studied a cohort that comprised all 1971 male chemical workers in the Lombardy and Piedmont regions of Italy who had held a licence to handle ethylene oxide for at least 1 year during 1938–84; 637 had held licences for ethylene oxide only and 1334 for ethylene oxide and other toxic gases. Some workers may have been exposed to ethylene oxide before they obtained a licence. The cohort was followed from 1 January 1940 to 31 May 1984, and vital status was ascertained at the census office at the place of residence of each subject. Sixteen subjects (0.8%) who were lost to follow-up were considered to be still alive. Expected numbers of deaths were calculated from 5-year age-, sex- and calendar period-specific rates for the regional (Lombardy) population. Seventy-six deaths were recorded (98.8 expected), including 43 from cancer (33.0 expected). The SMRs were 1.22 (95% CI, 0.40–2.87) for stomach cancer, 2.54 (95% CI, 0.52–7.44) for cancer of the pancreas, 1.61 (95% CI, 0.04–8.95) for cancer of the kidney, 6.82 (95% CI, 1.86–17.45) for lymphosarcoma and reticulosarcoma and 1.93 (95% CI, 0.23–6.99) for leukaemia. The two deaths from leukaemia occurred among men who had had less than 5 years of exposure and after a latency of less than 10 years since first exposure to ethylene oxide. Among the men who had held licences only for ethylene oxide, 27 deaths (30.1 expected) occurred (SMR, 0.87; 95% CI, 0.57–1.27), 15 of which were from cancer (10.5 expected; SMR, 1.42; 95% CI, 0.79–2.34), including one from stomach cancer (1.3 expected; SMR, 0.76; 95% CI, 0.02–4.26), three from lymphosarcoma and reticulo-sarcoma (0.2 expected; SMR, 16.93; 95% CI, 3.49–49.53) and two from leukaemia (0.3 expected; SMR, 6.50; 95% CI, 0.79–23.49). Results obtained from national mortality rates as the basis for expected numbers were similar. [The Working Group noted that no data were available on levels of exposure to ethylene oxide or on exposure to other chemicals.]

Following the observation of a cluster of breast cancer cases at a hospital in Hungary (Tompa *et al.*, 1999; see Section 2.1), Kardos *et al.* (2003) systematically followed 299 women who were employed on a ward where an ethylene oxide sterilizer was used during 1976–93. The cohort was followed from 1987 to 1999, and deaths among cohort members were ascertained from various databases, with personal contact to confirm the vital status of those who did not appear in any of these records. A total of 11 deaths from cancer were identified (three breast, two ovary, two lung and one each of large bowel, uterus, leukaemia and peritoneum) compared with 4.38 expected from national age- and calendar period-specific rates (SMR, 2.51; 95% CI, 1.25–4.49). Expected numbers based on local mortality rates were similar. [The Working Group noted that deaths in the cohort were ascertained from a different source from the reference rates. Also, it was unclear whether any of the cases from the original cluster were included in the study.]

Prompted by a perceived excess of cancer among pest-control officers of a large French city, Ambroise *et al.* (2005) conducted a historical cohort study of 181 men who had worked in the pest control department during 1979–84. The cohort was followed for mortality up to 2000 through registry offices of birthplaces and records held by the Institut National de la Statistique et des Etudes Economiques; causes of death were obtained by matching with a national file of death certificates or from records held by the personnel department (three cases). For three subjects who died abroad, vital status was established by interview with colleagues. Ethylene oxide had been used to sterilize hospital equipment, but no exposure measurements were reported. Individual exposures to ethylene oxide were assigned by application of a job–exposure matrix to occupational histories abstracted from administrative records. At least 140 subjects were classed as having worked with ethylene oxide. In the cohort as a whole, 39 deaths from all causes occurred, including 21 from cancer (9.36 expected from regional sex- and age-specific rates by calendar year). However, no statistically significant excess of mortality was observed for any specific site of cancer and no consistent trend of cancer mortality was observed in relation to estimated cumulative exposures to ethylene oxide. [The Working Group noted that less weight can be given to the overall excess of cancer in this study, since the investigation was prompted by a perceived excess of tumours.]

2.2.2   *USA*

Morgan *et al.* (1981) reported a retrospective cohort study of 767 men who had been employed between 1955 and 1977 at a chemical plant in eastern Texas where ethylene oxide was produced. All of the men had worked at the factory for at least 5 years and were 'potentially exposed' to the compound. Potential exposure to ethylene oxide was determined by personnel at the company on the basis of work histories. In an industrial hygiene survey in 1977, all samples taken in the production area contained less than 10 ppm [18 mg/m^3] ethylene oxide. Vital status was ascertained for more than 95% of the cohort members from a combination of plant records, 'personal knowledge' and telephone follow-up. Altogether, 46 deaths were recorded, whereas 80 were expected on the basis of US vital statistics. Death certificates were obtained for 42 of the 46 deceased subjects. Eleven deaths were from cancer (15.2 expected), and non-significant excesses were found for mortality from cancers of the pancreas (three versus 0.8 expected) and brain and central nervous system (two versus 0.7 expected) and from Hodgkin disease (two versus 0.4 expected); no deaths from leukaemia occurred. [The Working Group noted that details on the nature of the manufacturing process, the extent to which exposure readings were representative of earlier conditions in the plant and potential confounding exposures were lacking.] The results of an extended follow-up of this cohort to 1985 (follow-up rate, 99.7%) were reported by Shore *et al.* (1993) as part of a meta-analysis of cohort studies on ethylene oxide. Three deaths from brain cancer (1.1 expected), three from lymphatic and haematopoietic cancer (3.0 expected), none from leukaemia (1.1 expected) and none from stomach cancer [expected number not given] were observed.

A series of studies was carried out on a cohort of 2174 male employees at two chemical plants in West Virginia where ethylene oxide had been produced and used (Greenberg *et al.*, 1990; Benson & Teta, 1993; Teta *et al.*, 1993). It was produced by the chlorohydrin process during 1925–57 and by direct oxidation from 1937 to 1971. After 1971, the plants continued to use ethylene oxide that had been produced elsewhere. The cohort comprised men who had been employed at the plants during 1940–78 and assigned at any time before 1979 to a chemical production department in which ethylene oxide was judged to have been manufactured or used at the time of the assignment. The first large-scale environmental monitoring project at the plant began in 1976. The 8-h TWA concentration of ethylene oxide in departments where it was used was generally less than 1 ppm [1.8 mg/m^3] but ranged up to 66 ppm [120 mg/m^3]. The authors estimated that the 8-h TWA concentration in ethylene oxide production by direct oxidation in the 1960s ranged from 3 to 20 ppm [5.4–36 mg/m^3] and that exposures during production by the chlorohydrin process were probably higher. Departments were classified as having high, medium or low exposure concentrations according to the operations carried out, and the classification was validated by reference to reported incidents of acute exposure. The cohort was followed to the end of 1988, and vital status was ascertained for more than 98% of subjects. Death certificates were obtained for 99% of decedents, and expected numbers of deaths were calculated on the basis of national 5-year age- and calendar period-specific rates in white men.

A total of 278 men had worked in a chlorohydrin unit that primarily produced ethylene chlorohydrin, with ethylene dichloride and bischloroethyl ether as by-products (Benson & Teta, 1993). For part of the time, propylene chlorohydrin had also been produced. Ethylene oxide was handled only sporadically and in small volumes. Of these men, 147 had died while 140.8 deaths were expected. The deaths included 40 from cancer (30.8 expected; SMR, 1.30; 95% CI, 0.9–1.8), eight from lymphatic and haematopoietic cancer (2.7 expected; SMR, 2.9; 95% CI, 1.3–5.8) and eight from pancreatic cancer (1.6 expected; SMR, 4.9; 95% CI, 1.6–11.4). In a comparison with workers from other plants in the same locality, the risks for cancer of all types, for lymphatic and haematopoietic cancer, leukaemia and pancreatic cancer increased with duration of assignment to the chlorohydrin unit.

Among the 1896 men who had never been assigned to the chlorohydrin unit, 431 deaths occurred whereas 547.7 were expected (Teta *et al.*, 1993). The numbers of observed/expected deaths were 110/128.1 (SMR, 0.86; 95% CI, 0.7–1.0) for cancer at any site, 8/5.0 (SMR, 1.6; 95% CI, 0.7–3.2) for stomach cancer, 4/6.6 (SMR, 0.6; 95% CI, 0.2–1.6) for pancreatic cancer, 6/4.0 (SMR, 1.5; 95% CI, 0.6–3.3) for cancers of the brain and nervous system, 7/11.8 (SMR, 0.6; 95% CI, 0.2–1.2) for lymphatic and haemato-poietic cancer, 2/2.0 for lymphosarcoma and reticulosarcoma (International Classification of Diseases [ICD]-9 200), 5/4.7 (SMR, 1.1; 95% CI, 0.4–2.5) for leukaemia and aleu-kaemia and 0/1.2 for Hodgkin disease. No significant excess of mortality was observed for any cause of death. No excesses of mortality from leukaemia or stomach cancer were observed among men who had spent 2 or more years in high-exposure departments. Comparison with death rates of workers from plants in the same location who had never been assigned to ethylene oxide production or use showed no significant trend with duration of assignment for all cancers, leukaemia or pancreatic, brain or stomach cancers; however, a two- to threefold increase in the risk for leukaemia (based on three cases) was observed among workers with more than 10 years of assignment to ethylene oxide departments. This study confirmed and amplified the findings of an earlier case–control study at the same plants (Ott *et al.*, 1989).

Steenland *et al.* (1991) followed 18 254 employees at 14 industrial plants where ethylene oxide had been used to sterilize medical supplies or spices or in the testing of sterilizing equipment. The plants were selected because they held adequate records on personnel and exposure and their workers had accumulated at least 400 person–years at risk before 1978. Only workers with at least 3 months of exposure to ethylene oxide were included in the cohort. Forty-five per cent of the cohort were men, 79% were white, 1222 were sterilizer operators and 15 750 were employed before 1978. Analysis of 627 per-sonal 8-h TWA samples indicated that average exposure during 1976–85 was 4.3 ppm [7.7 mg/m^3] for sterilizer operators; on the basis of 1888 personal samples, the average level for other exposed workers was 2.0 ppm [3.6 mg/m^3]. Many companies began to install engineering controls in 1978, and exposures before that year were thought to have been higher. There was no evidence of potentially confounding exposure to other occupational carcinogens. The cohort was followed up to 1987 through the national death index and records of the Social Security Administration, the Internal Revenue Service and the US Postal Service; 95.5% were traced successfully. The expected numbers of deaths were calculated from rates in the US population, stratified according to age, race, sex and calendar year. In total, 1177 cohort members had died (1454.3 expected), including 40 for whom no death certificate was available. There were 343 deaths from cancer (380.3 expected; SMR, 0.9; 95% CI, 0.8–1.0). The observed/expected numbers of deaths were 36/33.8 (SMR, 1.07; 95% CI, 0.7–1.5) for all lymphatic and haematopoietic cancer, including 8/5.3 (SMR, 1.5; 95% CI, 0.7–3.0) for lymphosarcoma-reticulosarcoma [ICD-9 200], 4/3.5 (SMR, 1.1; 95% CI, 0.3–2.9) for Hodgkin lymphoma, 13/13.5 (SMR,

0.97; 95% CI, 0.5–1.7) for leukaemia, 8/6.7 (SMR, 1.2; 95% CI, 0.6–2.4) for non-Hodgkin lymphoma [ICD-9 202] and 3/5.1 (SMR, 0.6; 95% CI, 0.1–1.7) for myeloma; 6/11.6 (SMR, 0.5; 95% CI, 0.2–1.1) for cancer of the brain and nervous system; 11/11.6 (SMR, 0.95; 95% CI, 0.5–1.7) for cancer of the stomach; 16/16.9 (SMR, 0.95; 95% CI, 0.5–1.5) for cancer of the pancreas; 8/7.7 (SMR, 1.0; 95% CI, 0.4–2.1) for cancer of the oesophagus; and 13/7.2 (SMR, 1.8; 95% CI, 0.96–3.1) for cancer of the kidney. Mortality ratios for subjects who were first exposed before 1978 were virtually identical to those for the full cohort. No significant trend in mortality was observed in relation to duration of exposure, but the mortality ratios for leukaemia (1.79 based on five deaths) and non-Hodgkin lymphoma (1.92 based on five deaths) were higher after allowance for a latency of more than 20 years. Among the sterilizer operators, mortality ratios (and observed numbers of deaths) were 2.78 (two) for leukaemia and 6.68 (two) for lympho-sarcoma/reticulosarcoma; no death from stomach cancer was observed.

In a further analysis of the same study (Stayner *et al.*, 1993), an exposure–response analysis was conducted using previously derived quantitative estimates of individual exposure to ethylene oxide (Greife *et al.*, 1988). Analysis was limited to 13 of the facilities studied, since information on exposures at the other facility was inadequate. Mortality from lymphatic and haematopoietic cancer was greatest in the highest category of cumulative exposure to ethylene oxide (> 8500 ppm–days) (13 deaths; SMR, 1.24; 95% CI, 0.66–2.13), but the trend across three categories of cumulative exposure was weak (χ^2, 0.97; $p = 0.32$). A similar pattern was observed for non-Hodgkin lymphoma, but not for leukaemia. In addition, a Cox proportional hazard model was used to examine risk in relation to cumulative exposure (ppm–days), average exposure (ppm), maximal exposure (ppm) and duration of exposure (days) to ethylene oxide. A significant positive trend in risk with increasing cumulative exposure to ethylene oxide was observed for all neoplasms of the lymphatic and haematopoietic tissues [$p = 0.03$, two-tailed]. Moreover, this trend was strengthened [$p = 0.004$] when the analysis was restricted to neoplasms of lymphoid cell origin (lymphocytic leukaemia, ICD-9 204; non-Hodgkin lymphoma, ICD-9 200, 202). The exposure–response relationship between cumulative exposure to ethylene oxide and leukaemia was positive but non-significant [$p = 0.15$]. The regression coefficients for neoplasms of the lymphatic and haematopoietic tissues for duration of, average and maximal exposure were either weakly positive or negative. In this analysis, no significant increase was found for cancers of the stomach, pancreas, brain or kidney. [The Working Group gave greater weight to the internal exposure–response analyses using Cox regression than to those based on SMRs, since the latter are more vulnerable to bias.]

Wong and Trent (1993) reported a separate analysis of mortality in approximately the same population (Steenland & Stayner, 1993), with similar results. The cohort comprised 18 728 employees, and follow-up was to the end of 1988. [The Working Group noted that this report adds little useful information to that provided by Steenland *et al.* (1991).]

Norman *et al.* (1995) studied cancer incidence among 1132 workers (82% women) who were employed during 1974–80 at a plant in New York State that used ethylene oxide to sterilize medical equipment and supplies. The cohort included both regular employees (45%) and others who had worked only on a temporary basis and who were considered to have lower potential exposures. The investigation was prompted by the demonstration of elevated levels of sister chromatid exchange in the workforce. Leaks of ethylene oxide had been documented on several occasions. From three 2-h samples collected in 1980, the 8-h TWA exposures of sterilizer operators were estimated to be 50–200 ppm [90–360 mg/m³]. Hygiene at the plant was subsequently improved, and later 8-h TWA exposures were thought to be 5–20 ppm [9–36 mg/m³]. The cohort was followed for cancer incidence up to 1987, using data from various sources: health examinations (mostly conducted during 1982–85), telephone interviews (up to 1987), mailed surveys in 1987 and 1990, annual searches of the New York State Cancer Registry during 1985–89 and a search of the National Death Index in 1998. Expected numbers of cancers were derived from age- and sex-specific rates in the Surveillance, Epidemiology and End Result (SEER) programme for 1978–81. A small proportion of subjects (about 2%) had to be excluded from the analysis of cancer incidence because information was insufficient. A total of 28 cancers were identified (24 from the cancer registry and four from other sources), including 12 breast cancers (6.96 expected; SIR, 1.72; 95% CI, 0.99–3.00). When the expected number of breast cancers was calculated from SEER rates for 1981–85, it was slightly higher (7.64), and the excess fell just short of statistical significance (SIR, 1.57; 95% CI, 0.90–2.75). Among regular employees, nine cases of breast cancer occurred compared with 5.28 expected from SEER rates for 1981–85 (SIR, 1.70; 95% CI, 0.89–3.23). When analysis was restricted to workers who had completed at least one health examination or follow-up survey (approximately 79% of the total), the number of cases of breast cancer observed was again 12, but the expected number (from SEER rates for 1978–81) was reduced to 4.98. The time between first exposure and diagnosis of breast cancer was ≤ 11 years for each of the 12 observed breast cancer cases, and for one case was only 12 months. No statistically significant excess of mortality was observed for cancers at any other sites.

Lucas and Teta (1996) subsequently drew attention to the potential for early detection bias, among others, in this cohort, because the participants were under active health surveillance and the earlier investigation of cytogenetic abnormalities may have raised awareness of cancer risks. The authors acknowledged this concern, but noted that none of the cases of breast cancer was discovered by screening carried out at the health examinations that formed part of the study (Norman et al., 1996).

Olsen et al. (1997) analysed mortality from pancreatic and lymphatic and haematopoietic cancer at four chemical plants where ethylene oxide had been produced by the chlorohydrin process. Production of ethylene oxide had occurred during 1941–67 at one plant, 1951–71 and 1971–80 at the second, 1959–70 at the third and 1936–50 at the fourth. At other times, and sometimes in parallel with ethylene oxide, the plants had also produced propylene oxide by the chlorohydrin process. Workers engaged in the production of ethylene chlorohydrin and its conversion to ethylene oxide had potential exposure to ethylene oxide, but no data were reported on levels of exposure. The cohort comprised men who had been employed at the relevant facilities for at least 1 year and who had worked for at least 1 month in a job that had probably been in ethylene or propylene chlorohydrin production at some time since these processes began. Vital status was followed through to 1992 from date of entry into the cohort or (for those who entered the cohort before 1940) from 1940. This was achieved by record linkage with the Social Security Administration and the National Death Index, and causes of death were obtained for those cohort members who had died. In the main analysis, cause-specific mortality was compared with that expected from death rates in the US national population stratified by age, sex, race (white) and calendar year. Among the 1361 men eligible for study, 300 deaths occcurred in total, including 281 in the subset who had worked at some time in the ethylene chlorohydrin process. Within this subcohort, 70 deaths from cancer overall (73.8 expected) were observed, including one from pancreatic cancer (3.7 expected) and 10 from lymphatic and haematopoietic cancer (7.1 expected; SMR, 1.29; 95% CI, 0.62–2.38). With allowance for a 25-year induction period from first exposure, six lymphatic and haematopoietic cancers (4.2 expected; SMR, 1.44; 95% CI, 0.52–3.12) were observed. In internal analyses that used a control group of other male employees from the same company at two of the three sites where the study plants were located, there was a weak trend of increasing mortality from lymphatic and haematopoietic cancer in relation to duration of employment in any chlorohydrin production (ethylene or propylene), but this was not statistically significant. No data were presented on specific malignancies other than pancreatic and lymphatic and haematopoietic cancers.

In a report related to the study of Steenland et al. (1991), Steenland et al. (2003) examined the incidence of breast cancer in a subset of 7576 women who had worked for 1 year or longer at 13 of the 14 plants. The other plant was excluded because of its small size (only 19 women who were employed for 1 year). A postal questionnaire (supplemented by a telephone interview for non-responders) was used to collect information from cohort members (or, if they had died, from their next of kin) on history of breast cancer and various known and suspected risk factors for the disease. For plants that were still using ethylene oxide in the mid-1980s when the cohort had originally been assembled, individual work histories were updated with the assumption that women continued to work in the same job with the same level of exposure to ethylene oxide through to the date when they were last employed at the plant (in practice, this had little impact on estimates of cumulative exposures since, by the mid-1980s, exposure intensities were very low). Mortality follow-up for the cohort was extended to 1998 by the same methods that had been used previously. The incidence of breast cancer (also through to 1998) was established from a combination of questionnaire reports, death records and cancer registrations; the latter were available in nine of the 11 states in which the plants were located. Life-table analysis was used to compare overall incidence of breast cancer in the cohort with that in the general population of women covered by the (SEER) programme, with adjustment for age, calendar period and race (white/non-white). A total of 319 incident cases of breast cancer were identified including 20 with carcinoma in situ and 124 who had died by the end of 1998. This gave an SIR of 0.87 (95% CI, 0.77–0.97) for the cohort as a whole, which was recognized to be an underestimate because ascertainment of cases was incomplete for women who were not interviewed and for those who did not live in states that had cancer registries. When cases of carcinoma *in situ* were excluded, the SIR increased slightly to 0.94. With a 15-year lag, there was a significant trend of higher SIRs with higher cumulative exposures ($p = 0.002$), but this was less marked ($p = 0.16$) in an unlagged analysis. In addition to the external comparison, a nested case–control design with Cox regression was used to assess internal exposure–response relationships. In these analyses, risk sets matched on race were constructed for each case by randomly selecting 100 controls from the pool of all women who had survived without breast cancer to at least the same age as the index case. In an analysis that included all 319 cases and in which exposures were lagged by 15 years, the odds ratio for the highest fifth of cumulative exposure relative to no exposure was 1.74 (95% CI, 1.16–2.65). In a similar analysis that was restricted to the subset of 5139 women who were interviewed (233 cases) and adjusted for parity and history of breast cancer in a first degree relative (the two potential risk factors that were found to be important predictors of breast cancer), the corresponding odds ratio was 1.87 (95% CI, 1.12–3.10).

[The Working Group noted that, for cancers that have a high survival rate in the general population, such as breast cancer, studies based on incidence rather than mortality may be more sensitive in the detection of an elevated risk associated with an occupational exposure. In contrast, several methodological difficulties complicate the interpretation of studies on the incidence of breast cancer in occupational cohorts, including potential differences in reproductive histories associated with employment and the possibility of differential rates by occupational exposure. The Steenland *et al.* (2003) study was able to address some but not all of these potential limitations and was judged by the Working Group to provide the most pertinent evidence on the potential association of breast cancer with exposure to ethylene oxide.]

An updated analysis of mortality from cancer in the cohort of employees at 14 industrial plants was reported by Steenland *et al.* (2004) and included 18 235 subjects who were followed up to 1998. Work histories for individuals employed at plants that were still using ethylene oxide at the time the cohort had originally been assembled were extended to their last date of employment at the relevant plant, with an assumption that they did not change their job or exposure to ethylene oxide during the additional period of employment. Life-table analyses were conducted with the national population of the USA as a reference. In total, 2852 deaths from all causes (SMR, 0.90; 95% CI, 0.88–0.93) were observed, including 860 from cancer (SMR, 0.98; 95% CI, 0.92–1.03). The only category of malignancy for which mortality was significantly elevated was cancer of the bone (SMR, 2.82; 95% CI, 1.23–2.56). However, this finding was based on only six observed deaths, and there was no indication of an increase in risk with increasing cumulative exposure. Overall, mortality from cancer of the stomach (25 deaths; SMR, 0.98; 95% CI, 0.74–1.49), cancer of the breast (103 deaths; SMR, 0.99; 95% CI, 0.84–1.17), lymphatic and haematopoietic cancer (79 deaths; SMR, 1.00; 95% CI, 0.79–1.24), non-Hodgkin lymphoma (31 deaths; SMR, 1.00; 95% CI, 0.72–1.35), Hodgkin disease (six deaths;

SMR, 1.24; 95% CI, 0.53–2.43), myeloma (13 deaths; SMR, 0.92; 95% CI, 0.54–0.87) and leukaemia (28 deaths; SMR, 0.99; 95% CI, 0.71–1.36) was unremarkable. In an internal analysis (excluding one small plant for which exposure data were not available), cases of lymphatic and haematopoietic and breast cancer were matched for race, sex and date of birth with controls (100 per case) who had survived without these cancers to at least the age of the index case. When log cumulative exposures to ethylene oxide were lagged by 15 years, a statistically significant positive trend ($p = 0.02$) was observed for mortality from lymphatic and haematopoietic cancer in men but not in women. However, duration of, peak, average or cumulative exposure did not predict mortality from lymphatic and haematopoietic cancer. A similar pattern was observed for lymphoid-cell tumours specifically (including non-Hodgkin lymphoma, myeloma and lymphocytic leukaemia). With a lag of 20 years, mortality from breast cancer was highest in women who had the highest quarter of exposures (odds ratio, 3.13; 95% CI, 1.42–6.92 relative to no exposure).

2.3   Case–control study

Swaen *et al.* (1996) carried out a case–control study within the workforce of a chemical manufacturing plant in Belgium to investigate an increased incidence of Hodgkin lymphoma that had been noted by the medical director at the facility. Ten cases, diagnosed during 1968–91, were compared with a total of 200 individually matched controls. The controls had been employed at the plant for at least 3 consecutive months and were actively employed at the time that their matched case was diagnosed (a person could serve as a control for more than one case). The job histories of cases and controls were abstracted from personnel records and reviewed by a company industrial hygienist (blinded to health status), who assessed their potential exposure to a range of chemicals. For 24.3% of subjects who had inadequate occupational histories, additional data were then sought (unblinded to health status) from medical records. Three cases were classed as exposed to ethylene oxide (odds ratio, 8.5; 95% CI, 1.4–39.9), but one of these cases had been reclassified as a large-cell anaplastic carcinoma when pathology samples were reviewed.

2.4   Meta-analysis

Teta *et al.* (1999) updated the earlier meta-analysis of Shore *et al.* (1993) with inclusion of data from the study reported by Olsen *et al.* (1997) and the updated follow-up of Swedish sterilant workers reported by Hagmar *et al.* (1995). Thus, a total of 10 individual cohorts were studied. Altogether, 876 cases of cancer were recorded compared with 928 expected, giving a meta-SMR standardized for age, sex and calendar year of 0.94 (95% CI, 0.85–1.05). Observed/expected numbers for specific cancers were: pancreas, 37/39 (meta-SMR, 0.95; 95% CI, 0.69–1.31); brain, 25/26 (meta-SMR, 0.96; 95% CI, 0.49–1.91); stomach, 59/48 (meta-SMR, 1.23; 95% CI, 0.71–2.13); leukaemia,

35/32 (meta-SMR, 1.08; 95% CI, 0.61–1.93); and non-Hodgkin lymphoma, 33/25 (meta-SMR, 1.34; 95% CI, 0.96–1.89). None of the cancers analysed showed significant trends in risk with increasing duration or intensity of exposure; however, the risk for brain cancer increased with time since first exposure ($p < 0.05$ based on four studies).

3. Studies of Cancer in Experimental Animals

3.1   Inhalation exposure

Carcinogenicity bioassays of inhalation exposure to ethylene oxide in mice and rats are summarized in Tables 7 and 8, respectively.

3.1.1   *Mouse*

In a screening assay based on increased multiplicity and incidence of lung tumours in a strain of mice that is highly susceptible to the development of this neoplasm, groups of 30 female strain A/J mice, 8–10 weeks of age, were exposed by inhalation to 0, 70 or 200 ppm [0, 128 or 366 mg/m³] ethylene oxide (at least 99.7% pure) for 6 h per day on 5 days per week for up to 6 months in two independent experiments; in the second experiment, the 70-ppm group was omitted. Two groups of 30 female mice were exposed to room air and served as negative controls, and two groups of 20 female mice received a single intraperitoneal injection of 1000 mg/kg bw urethane and served as positive controls for both experiments. At the end of the 6th month, the survivors were killed and examined for pulmonary adenomas. In the first experiment, survival was 30/30 (0 ppm), 28/30 (70 ppm), 29/30 (200 ppm) and 19/20 (urethane); that in the second experiment was 29/30 (0 ppm), 28/30 (200 ppm) and 19/20 (urethane). The numbers of animals with pulmonary adenomas among survivors (and tumour multiplicity) in the first experiment were: untreated controls, 8/30 (0.46 ± 0.38 [± SD] adenomas/mouse); low-dose, 16/28 (0.86 ± 0.45); high-dose, 25/29 (2.14 ± 0.49); and urethane-treated, 19/19 (20.1 ± 1.77); those in the second experiment were: untreated controls, 8/29 (0.22 ± 0.38); ethylene oxide-treated, 12/28 (0.73 ± 0.98); and urethane-treated, 19/19 (23.5 ± 6.49). The tumour multiplicity increased significantly in each experiment ($p < 0.05$, Duncan's new multiple-range test); in the first experiment, it also increased significantly in a dose-dependent manner [$p < 0.001$, Cochran-Armitage trend test] (Adkins *et al.*, 1986).

Groups of 50 male and 50 female B6C3F₁ mice, 8 weeks of age, were exposed by inhalation to 0, 50 or 100 ppm [0, 92 or 183 mg/m³] ethylene oxide (> 99% pure) for 6 h per day on 5 days per week for up to 102 weeks, at which time the experiment was terminated. Mean body weights of treated males and females were similar to those of controls. At the end of the study, 28/50 control, 31/50 low-dose and 34/50 high-dose males, and 25/50 control, 24/50 low-dose and 31/50 high-dose females were still alive.

Table 7. Carcinogenicity studies of inhalation exposure to ethylene oxide in experimental mice

Strain	Sex	No./group at start	Purity	Dose and duration of exposure	Duration of study	Incidence of tumours	Result	Comments	Reference
Strain A/J	F	30	≥ 99.7%	0, 70, 200 ppm, 6 h/day, 5 days/week 0, 200 ppm, 6 h/day, 5 days/week	Up to 6 months Up to 6 months	Lung[a]: 8/30, 16/28, 25/29 Lung[a]: 8/29, 12/28	p < 0.001 (trend) NS	Two independent experiments; tumour multiplicities increased with dose in both experiments (p < 0.05)	Adkins et al. (1986)
B6C3F₁	M	50	> 99%	0, 50, 100 ppm, 6 h/day, 5 days/week	102 weeks	Lung[b]: 11/50, 19/50, 26/50 Harderian gland[c]: 1/43, 9/44, 8/42[d]	p = 0.002 (trend) p < 0.03 (trend)		National Toxicology Program (1987)
B6C3F₁	F	50	> 99%	0, 50, 100 ppm, 6 h/day, 5 days/week	102 weeks	Lung[b]: 2/49, 5/48, 22/49 Harderian gland[c]: 1/46, 6/46[d], 8/47 Lymphoma: 9/49, 6/48, 22/49 Uterus[e]: 0/49, 2/47, 5/49 Mammary gland[f]: 1/49, 8/48, 6/49	p < 0.001 (trend) p < 0.04 (trend) p = 0.023 (trend) p < 0.03 (trend) p = 0.012 (low dose only)		National Toxicology Program (1987); Picut et al. (2003)

F, female; M, male; NS, not significant

[a] Mice with one or more pulmonary adenomas/total mice at risk

[b] Mice with one or more tumours/total mice at risk, alveolar/bronchiolar adenomas and carcinomas combined

[c] Papillary cystadenomas

[d] A cystadenocarcinoma was also present in an animal with a cystadenoma.

[e] Adenocarcinomas, including one tumour in a low-dose mouse originally reported as an adenoma

[f] Carcinomas

Table 8. Carcinogenicity studies of inhalation exposure to ethylene oxide in experimental rats

Strain	Sex	No./group at start	Purity	Dose and duration of exposure	Duration of study	Incidence of tumours	Result	Comments	Reference
Fischer 344	M	80	99.7%	0, 50, 100 ppm, 7 h/day, 5 days/week	2 years	Brain[a]: 0/76, 2/77, 5/79 Mononuclear-cell leukaemia: 24/77, 38/79, 30/76 Peritesticular mesothelioma: 3/78, 9/79, 21/79	$p < 0.05$ (high dose) $p = 0.03$ (low dose) $p = 0.002$ (high dose)		Lynch et al. (1984a)
Fischer 344	M	120	> 99.9%	0, 10, 33, 100 ppm, 6 h/day, 5 days/week	2 years	Brain[b]: 1/181, 0/92, 3/85, 6/87 Mononuclear-cell leukaemia: 13/97, 9/51, 12/39, 9/30 Peritesticular mesothelioma: 2/97, 2/51, 4/39, 4/30 Subcutaneous fibroma: 3/97, 9/51, 1/39, 11/30	$p < 0.05$ (trend) $p < 0.05$ (trend) $p < 0.005$ (trend) $p < 0.01$ (high dose)	Early deaths due to viral sialo-dacryoadenitis; no increases in tumour incidence up to 18 months; sites other than brain include only necropsies after 24 months.	Snellings et al. (1984); Garman et al. (1985, 1986)
Fischer 344	F	120	> 99.9%	0, 10, 33, 100 ppm, 6 h/day, 5 days/week	2 years	Brain[b]: 0/187, 1/94, 2/90, 2/78 Mononuclear-cell leukaemia: 11/116, 11/54, 14/48, 15/26	$p < 0.05$ (trend) $p < 0.005$ (trend)		

F, female; M, male

[a] Brain tumours were gliomas. Focal proliferations of glial cells (termed 'gliosis') were also observed in two low-dose rats and four high-dose rats.

[b] Brain tumours included gliomas. Numbers include rats killed both at 18 months and at the conclusion of the 2-year study.

The incidence of alveolar/bronchiolar carcinomas in male mice was 6/50 control, 10/50 low-dose and 16/50 high-dose (p = 0.019, incidental tumour test for trend). A slight increase in the incidence of alveolar/bronchiolar adenomas also occurred. The combined incidence of lung tumours was 11/50 control, 19/50 low-dose and 26/50 high-dose (p = 0.002, incidental tumour test for trend). In females, the incidence of alveolar/bronchiolar adenomas (2/49 control, 4/48 low-dose and 17/49 high-dose) and alveolar/bronchiolar carcinomas (0/49 control, 1/48 low-dose and 7/49 high-dose) and the combined incidence of lung tumours (2/49 control, 5/48 low-dose and 22/49 high-dose) were all significantly increased (p < 0.001, incidental tumour test for trend). The incidence of papillary cystadenoma of the Harderian gland increased significantly in animals of each sex (males: 1/43 control, 9/44 low-dose and 8/42 high-dose; females: 1/46 control, 6/46 low-dose and 8/47 high-dose; p < 0.04, incidental tumour test for trend in both sexes). In addition, one papillary cystadenocarcinoma of the Harderian gland was observed in one high-dose male and one in a low-dose female. In females, the incidence of malignant lymphomas was 9/49 control, 6/48 low-dose and 22/49 high-dose mice (p = 0.023, life-table test for trend). An increase in the incidence of uterine adenocarcinomas was observed in 0/49 control, 2/47 low-dose and 5/49 high-dose females (p < 0.03, incidental tumour test for trend). The incidence of mammary gland carcinomas in females was 1/49 control, 8/48 low-dose (p = 0.012, incidental pair-wise tumour test) and 6/49 high-dose mice (National Toxicology Program, 1987). Because of the rarity of primary epithelial tumours of the uterus in long-term inhalation studies in mice, data on the pathology and incidence of uterine tumours in B6C3F$_1$ mice from 2-year National Toxicology Program inhalation bioassays of bromoethane, chloroethane and ethylene oxide were reviewed. Diagnoses of uterine adenocarcinoma in the 1987 bioassay of ethylene oxide were confirmed (Picut *et al.*, 2003). [The Working Group noted that the diagnosis of uterine adenoma in one low-dose female was revised to adenocarcinoma.]

3.1.2   *Rat*

Groups of 80 male weanling Fischer 344 rats were exposed by inhalation to 0 (control; filtered air), 50 or 100 ppm [92 or 180 mg/m^3] ethylene oxide (purity, 99.7%) vapour for approximately 7 h per day on 5 days per week for 2 years. The mortality rate was increased in the two treated groups over that in controls, and the increase was significant for the high-dose group (p < 0.01). Mononuclear-cell leukaemia was observed in 24/77 control rats, in 38/79 rats exposed to 50 ppm ethylene oxide and in 30/76 exposed to 100 ppm. The overall increase in the incidence of mononuclear-cell leukaemia was significant (p = 0.03) in the low-dose group, but the increase could not be ascertained in the high-dose group because of excessive mortality. Peritoneal mesotheliomas in the region of the testis developed in 3/78 control, 9/79 low-dose and 21/79 high-dose rats; the increase was significant for the high-dose group (p = 0.002). Gliomas (mixed cell type) were found in 0/76 control, 2/77 low-dose and 5/79 high-dose animals (p < 0.05, pair-wise comparison for the high dose). Focal proliferation of glial cells (termed 'gliosis') was observed in two rats exposed to 50 ppm and four rats exposed to 100 ppm ethylene oxide. [The Working Group noted that lesions such as those described as 'gliosis' are probably glial tumours, and that true gliosis is a reactive lesion and not a neoplasm.] The incidence of other neoplasms was comparable in the control and treated groups and was not associated with exposure to ethylene oxide. A high incidence of proliferative lesions described as 'multifocal cortical hyperplasia' and 'cortical nodular hyperplasia' was observed in the adrenal cortex of animals exposed to ethylene oxide (Lynch *et al.*, 1984a).

Three groups of 120 male and three groups of 120 female Fischer 344 rats, 8 weeks of age, were exposed by inhalation to 10, 33 or 100 ppm [18, 59 or 180 mg/m^3] ethylene oxide (purity, > 99.9%) vapour for 6 h per day on 5 days per week for up to 2 years. Two control groups (I and II), each of 120 male and 120 female rats, were exposed in inhalation chambers to room air. All animals that died or were killed when moribund and those killed at scheduled intervals of 6, 12, 18 and 24 (females)–25 (males) months were examined. During month 15 of exposure, mortality increased in both treated and control groups due to a viral sialodacryoadenitis. Mortality was higher in the groups exposed to 33 and 100 ppm ethylene oxide than in the other groups and was also higher in females than in males. Up to 18 months of exposure, no significant increase in tumour incidence was observed. In treated rats killed after 18 months, the incidence of brain tumours classified as 'gliomas, malignant reticulosis and granular-cell tumours' was increased in animals of each sex. The incidence of brain tumours (gliomas only) among rats killed at 18 and 24–25 months was: males: 1/181 (controls), 0/92 (10 ppm), 3/85 (33 ppm) and 6/87 (100 ppm) ($p < 0.05$, Cox's test for adjusted trend and Fisher's exact test for high-dose versus control); and females: 0/187 (controls), 1/94 (10 ppm), 2/90 (33 ppm) and 2/78 (100 ppm) ($p < 0.05$, Cox's test for adjusted trend). In females killed after 24 months of exposure, mononuclear-cell leukaemia was found in 5/60 (control I), 6/56 (control II), 11/54 (10 ppm), 14/48 (33 ppm) and 15/26 (100 ppm) animals; the incidence of leukaemia was reported by the authors to be significantly increased in the 100-ppm group ($p < 0.001$) and in a mortality-adjusted trend test ($p < 0.005$). In males, mononuclear-cell leukaemia was found in 5/48 (control I), 8/49 (control II), 9/51 (10 ppm), 12/39 (33 ppm) and 9/30 (100 ppm) animals ($p < 0.05$, mortality-adjusted trend test). Peritoneal mesotheliomas originating in the testicular serosa were found in 1/48 (control I), 1/49 (control II), 2/51 (10 ppm), 4/39 (33 ppm) and 4/30 (100 ppm) males ($p < 0.005$, trend test). The incidence of subcutaneous fibromas in male rats of the high-dose group was also significantly increased: 1/48 (control I), 2/49 (control II), 9/51 (10 ppm), 1/39 (33 ppm) and 11/30 (100 ppm) ($p < 0.01$) (Snellings *et al.*, 1984; Garman *et al.*, 1985, 1986).

3.2 Oral administration

Rat

Groups of 50 female Sprague-Dawley rats, approximately 100 days of age, were administered 7.5 or 30.5 mg/kg bw ethylene oxide (purity, 99.7%) in a commercial vegetable oil [composition unspecified] by gastric intubation twice weekly for 107 weeks (average total dose, 1186 or 5112 mg/kg bw, respectively). Controls comprised one group of 50 untreated female rats and a second group of 50 female rats treated with vegetable oil alone. The survival rate of rats in the high-dose group was lower than that of the control groups. Treatment with ethylene oxide resulted in a dose-dependent increase in the incidence of forestomach tumours, which were mainly squamous-cell carcinomas. Such tumours were not found in the untreated or vehicle controls. In the low-dose group, 8/50 animals developed squamous-cell carcinomas, 4/50 had carcinomas *in situ* and 9/50 had papillomas, hyperplasia or hyperkeratosis of the forestomach. In the high-dose group, 31/50 animals developed malignant tumours of the stomach; 29 were squamous-cell carcinomas of the forestomach and two were fibrosarcomas, one of which was located in the glandular stomach. In addition, 4/50 had carcinomas *in situ* and 11/50 had papillomas, hyperplasia or hyperkeratosis of the forestomach. Many of the stomach tumours found in the high-dose group metastasized or grew invasively into neighbouring organs. There was no increase in the incidence of tumours at other sites in the treated animals over that in controls (Dunkelberg, 1982).

3.3 Dermal application

Mouse

Thirty female ICR/Ha Swiss mice, 8 weeks of age at the start of treatment, received topical applications of approximately 100 mg of a 10% solution of ethylene oxide (purity, 99.7%) in acetone on the clipped dorsal skin three times a week for life. The median survival time was 493 days. No skin tumour was observed (Van Duuren *et al.*, 1965). [The Working Group noted the high volatility of ethylene oxide which would tend to reduce the dose that the animals received.]

3.4 Subcutaneous administration

Mouse

Groups of 100 female NMRI mice, 6–8 weeks of age, received subcutaneous injections of 0.1, 0.3 or 1.0 mg/mouse ethylene oxide (purity, 99.7%) in tricaprylin once a week for 95 weeks (mean total dose, 7.3, 22.7 or 64.4 mg/mouse). Groups of 200 untreated and 200 tricaprylin-treated mice served as controls. The survival rate of the group given the highest dose was reduced. Ethylene oxide induced a dose-dependent increase in the incidence of sarcomas at the injection site. Sarcomas occurred in 0/200 untreated controls, 4/200 animals treated with tricaprylin alone, and 5/100, 8/100 and 11/100 animals that received 0.1, 0.3 and 1 mg ethylene oxide, respectively [$p < 0.001$, Cochran-Armitage test for trend]. No significant increase in the incidence of tumours at other sites was observed (Dunkelberg, 1981).

3.5   Induction of enzyme-altered foci in a two-stage liver system

Rat

Litters of Sprague-Dawley rats, 3–5 days of age, were exposed with their dams by inhalation to 0 ppm (five male and nine female rats), 33 ppm (60 mg/m^3, 10 females), 55 ppm (100 mg/m^3, four males and seven females) or 100 ppm (183 mg/m^3, four males and eight females) ethylene oxide [purity unspecified] for 8 h per day on 5 consecutive days per week for 3 weeks. One week later, the offspring were administered, as a promoting agent, 10 mg/kg bw Clophen A 50 (a mixture of polychlorinated biphenyls [not otherwise specified]) orally by gavage twice a week for up to 8 additional weeks, at which time the experiment was terminated. The livers were examined for adenosine triphosphatase-deficient and γ-glutamyltranspeptidase-positive foci. In females that received the two highest doses, but not in males, the number and total area of adenosine triphosphatase-deficient foci increased significantly ($p < 0.05$, Student's t test) in comparison with the controls that received Clophen A 50 only. There was no significant difference in the number or total area of γ-glutamyltranspeptidase-positive foci between controls and animals given the high dose of ethylene oxide (Denk *et al.*, 1988).

4.   Mechanistic and Other Relevant Data

4.1   Absorption, distribution, metabolism and excretion

4.1.1   *Humans*

(a)   *Absorption, distribution and excretion*

Ethylene oxide is readily taken up by the lungs and is absorbed relatively efficiently into the blood. A study of workers exposed to ethylene oxide revealed an alveolar retention of 75–80%, calculated from hourly determinations of ethylene oxide concentrations in the environmental air that ranged from 0.2 to 24.1 mg/m^3 [0.11–13.2 ppm] and in alveolar air that ranged from 0.05 to 6 mg/m^3 [0.03–3.3 ppm] (Brugnone *et al.*, 1985, 1986). At steady state, therefore, 20–25% of inhaled ethylene oxide that reached the alveolar space was exhaled as the unchanged compound and 75–80% was taken up by the body and metabolized. Blood samples taken from workers 4 h after the workshift gave venous blood:alveolar air coefficients of 12–17 and venous blood:environmental air coefficients of 2.5–3.3. The difference from the value of 90 samples determined for the blood:air partition coefficient *in vitro* was explained by incomplete saturation of tissues and limitation of the metabolic rate by the rate of lung uptake (Brugnone *et al.*, 1986).

(b)   Metabolism

The following overall schema describes the mammalian metabolism of ethylene oxide (Figure 2). Ethylene oxide is converted (*a*) by enzymatic and non-enzymatic hydrolysis to ethylene glycol, which is partly excreted as such and partly metabolized further via glycolaldehyde, glycolic acid and glyoxalic acid to oxalic acid, formic acid and carbon dioxide; and (*b*) by conjugation with glutathione (GSH) followed by further metabolism to *S*-(2-hydroxyethyl)cysteine, *S*-(2-carboxymethyl)cysteine and *N*-acetylated derivatives (*N*-acetyl-*S*-(2-hydroxyethyl)cysteine (also termed *S*-(2-hydroxyethyl)mercapturic acid or HEMA) and *N*-acetyl-*S*-(2-carboxymethyl)cysteine) (Wolfs *et al.*, 1983; Popp *et al.*, 1994), which are partly converted to thiodiacetic acid (Scheick *et al.*, 1997).

Figure 2. Metabolism of ethylene oxide

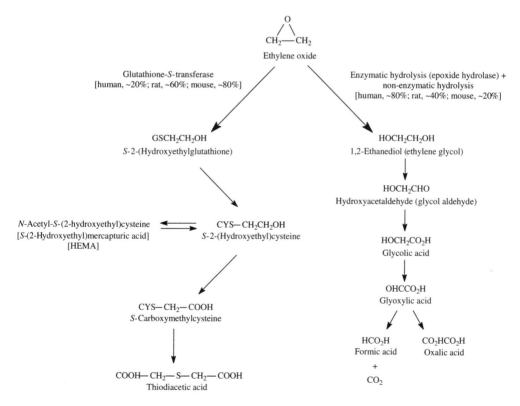

Adapted from Wolfs *et al.* (1983); Scheick *et al.* (1997)

Blood concentrations of ethylene glycol were determined at the end of day 3 of a normal working week in sterilization personnel who were exposed to ethylene oxide. TWA concentrations of ethylene oxide determined over 8 h ranged from 0.3 to 52 ppm [0.55–95.2 mg/m^3] (overall mean, 4.2 ppm [7.7 mg/m^3]). The mean concentrations of ethylene glycol in the blood of exposed subjects were twice as high (90 mg/L) as those in controls (45 mg/L) (Wolfs et al., 1983).

The concentration of thioethers excreted in urine collected at the end of sterilization processes was found to be twice as high in nonsmoking personnel (10.2 mmol/mol creatinine) exposed to peak concentrations of 1–200 ppm [1.83–366 mg/m^3] ethylene oxide as that in unexposed workers (5.46 mmol/mol creatinine). The concentration of ethylene oxide in air was not monitored routinely (Burgaz et al., 1992).

The glutathione-S-transferase (GST) activity for ethylene oxide in human liver cytosolic fractions was low (too low to determine the Michaelis-Menten constant [K_m] value). The maximum velocity (V_{max}) varied from 7.6 to 10.6 nmol/min/mg protein. Epoxide hydrolase (EH) activity in the microsomal fraction of the human liver averaged 1.8 nmol/min/mg protein. The K_m for hydrolysis has been estimated to be approximately 0.2 mM, but non-enzymatic hydrolysis was significant and precluded accurate determination (Fennell & Brown, 2001).

Metabolism of ethylene oxide to the GSH conjugate and ethylene glycol is generally considered to be the major pathway for the elimination of DNA-reactive ethylene oxide. However, strongly suggestive evidence in vitro was presented by Hengstler et al. (1994) that glycolaldehyde is formed by further metabolism of ethylene glycol and that this derivative leads to DNA–protein cross-links and to DNA strand breaks (as measured with the alkaline elution assay) after in-vitro incubation with human peripheral mononuclear blood cells.

(c)   GST polymorphisms

Ethylene oxide is a substrate of the GST isoenzyme T1 (Hayes et al., 2005). This isoenzyme is polymorphic and a relatively large population (in Caucasians about 20%, in Asians almost 50%) has a homozygous deletion (null genotype) (Bolt & Thier, 2006). As expected, these individuals show a significantly higher amount of hydroxyethyl valine in their haemoglobin due to the metabolism of endogenous ethylene to endogenous ethylene oxide (Thier et al., 2001). Nevertheless, the influence of this genetic trait on the formation of these haemoglobin adducts by workplace exposure to exogenous ethylene oxide is much less clear, as discussed below.

In the cytoplasm of erythrocytes obtained from 36 individuals, ethylene oxide was eliminated three to six times faster in samples from so-called conjugators (defined by a standardized conjugation reaction of methyl bromide and GSH; 75% of the population) than in those from the remaining 25% (who lack this GST-specific activity). In the latter samples, disappearance did not differ from that of controls. In this experiment, the disappearance of ethylene oxide was investigated in the gas phase of closed vials that contained GSH and cytoplasm of erythrocytes (Hallier et al., 1993).

In contrast, several publications reported no or an unclear association between GSTT1 status and hydroxyethyl adducts after workplace exposure to ethylene oxide (HEMA formation) (Haufroid *et al.*, 2007) or exposure to ethylene oxide from cigarette smoking (hydroxyethyl valine in haemoglobin) (Müller *et al.*, 1998). Other studies reported a relatively weak but significant association (0.17 ± 0.03 *N*-(2-hydroxy-ethyl)valine formed in haemoglobin versus 0.08 ± ≤ 0.01; $p \leq 0.02$) after exposure to ethylene oxide of individuals who had homozygous deletion of the *GSTT1* gene compared with those who had at least one copy of the gene (Yong *et al.*, 2001).

The different impact of the *GSTT1* polymorphism is due to the fact that, in the study of Hallier *et al.* (1993), cytoplasm of erythrocytes was exposed to ethylene oxide, while in the subsequent studies, the whole human organism was exposed to ethylene oxide. Similarly, Föst *et al.* (1995) also observed that, when ethylene oxide is added to whole blood of various individuals, the impact of the *GSTT1* polymorphism is significant.

In-vitro incubation of mononuclear blood cells from various individuals with polymorphisms in GSTs (*GSTM1, GSTT1* and *GSTP1*) did not demonstrate a significant influence on ethylene oxide-induced DNA strand breaks (measured by the Comet assay) and on micronucleus formation in binucleated cells (Godderis *et al.*, 2006). This lack of an effect is presumably due to the null or negligible contribution of GSTM1 and GSTP1 enzymes to ethylene oxide metabolism and to a too small (20%) contribution of GSTT1 activity in the human whole organism (Figure 2).

(d) Haemoglobin adducts

Ethylene oxide is an electrophilic agent that alkylates nucleophilic groups in biological macromolecules. Haemoglobin adducts have been used to monitor tissue doses of ethylene oxide (Calleman *et al.*, 1978; Farmer *et al.*, 1987; Osterman-Golkar & Bergmark, 1988; Ehrenberg, 1991; Ehrenberg & Törnqvist, 1992). The results have shown measurable increases in hydroxyethyl haemoglobin adducts that are dependent on the workplace exposure concentration (reported and discussed in IARC, 1994).

Cigarette smoke contains ethylene oxide, and hydroxyethyl valine in the haemoglobin of smokers correlates with the number of cigarettes smoked (Fennell *et al.*, 2000; Bono *et al.*, 2002; Wu *et al.*, 2004). The umbilical cord blood of smoking pregnant women contained increased levels of hydroxyethyl valine, which were quantitatively related to the increased levels in maternal blood (Farmer *et al.*, 1996a). Levels of this adduct were significantly higher in the haemoglobin of newborns from smoking compared with those from nonsmoking mothers (147 ± 68 compared with 42 ± 18 pmol/g haemoglobin; $p \leq 0.01$) (Tavares *et al.*, 1994). In *GSTT1*-null individuals, levels of hydroxyethyl valine were significantly elevated when normalized to smoking status or levels of cotinine. The lack of functional *GSTT1* was estimated to increase the internal dose of ethylene oxide derived from cigarette smoke by 50–70% (Fennell *et al.*, 2000). Ethylene oxide is also formed endogenously in humans (Bolt, 1996). This may limit the sensitivity of this adduct as a biomarker for cigarette smoking; indeed, the formation of hydroxyethyl valine was not associated with exposure to secondhand smoke or with tea or alcoholic beverage consumption, age or gender (Wu *et al.*, 2004).

(e)   Toxicokinetic modelling

A recent model by Fennell and Brown (2001) determined a half-life of ethylene oxide in the human body of 47.6 min, taking into account the enzymatic disposition of ethylene oxide by human liver microsomal EH (mEH) and cytosolic GST by their K_m and V_{max} characteristics, as well as a possible depletion of GSH. This half-life value was quite close to the 42-min value obtained by Filser *et al.* (1992). In this human model, the majority of ethylene oxide is metabolized by hydrolysis, and only approximately 20% is converted to GSH conjugates. There is little change in metabolism with increasing exposure concentration. At given exposure concentrations of ethylene oxide (1, 100 and 300 ppm [1.83, 183 and 549 mg/m^3]), blood concentration was sensitive to alveolar ventilation and to K_m and V_{max} for liver mEH but relatively insensitive to the liver GSH concentration and the rate of GSH synthesis in the liver.

4.1.2   Experimental systems

(a)   Absorption, distribution and excretion

Pulmonary uptake of ethylene oxide is expected to be rapid and dependent only upon the alveolar ventilation rate and concentration in the inspired air, since this compound is very soluble in blood (IPCS, 1985). Ethylene oxide is absorbed rapidly through the respiratory tract in rats (Filser & Bolt, 1984; Koga *et al.*, 1987; Tardif *et al.*, 1987), mice (Ehrenberg *et al.*, 1974; Tardif *et al.*, 1987) and rabbits (Tardif *et al.*, 1987). Close to 100% of inhaled ethylene oxide was absorbed by mice that were exposed for 1–2 h to 2–55 mg/m^3 (1.1–30 ppm) (Ehrenberg *et al.*, 1974).

The permeation rate of a solution of 1% ethylene oxide in water (w/v) through excised human skin at 30 °C was determined to be 0.125 mg/(cm^2 × h) (Baumbach *et al.*, 1987).

The pharmacokinetics of inhaled ethylene oxide have been investigated in male Sprague-Dawley (Filser & Bolt, 1984) and Fischer 344 rats (Krishnan *et al.*, 1992). The studies were carried out in closed exposure chambers of 6.4 and 9.5 L occupied by two and three rats, respectively. The initial concentrations of ethylene oxide vapour in the chamber atmospheres were up to about 1100 ppm [2000 mg/m^3]. Filser and Bolt (1984) showed that ethylene oxide is rapidly taken up by the lungs because the clearance due to uptake, which reflects the rate of transfer of ethylene oxide from the atmosphere into the organism, was 11 100 mL/h (185 mL/min) for two Sprague-Dawley rats that weighed 500 g. Johanson and Filser (1992) calculated a value of 58 mL/min for one Sprague-Dawley rat that weighed 250 g by allometric scaling, according to the method of Filser (1992). This value represents 50% of the alveolar ventilation (117 mL/min; Arms & Travis, 1988), which indicates that about 50% of the amount inhaled into the lung is exhaled again without becoming systemically available via the bloodstream. A possible explanation for this finding is that there is a 'wash in-wash out' effect in the upper airways (Johanson & Filser, 1992), which may be more effective in rats than in humans (Filser *et al.*, 1993). The maximal accumulation of ethylene oxide in the body of Sprague-Dawley rats, determined as the thermodynamic partition coefficient for whole body:air, was 30. Because of fast metabolic elimination, the concentration ratio at steady state for whole body:air, calculated for two animals that weighed 500 g, was only 1.52 over the entire dose range. A re-calculation of this parameter according to Filser (1992) for one Sprague-Dawley rat that weighed 250 g yielded a value of 1.88, which is similar to the coefficient for venous blood:environmental air found in workers exposed to ethylene oxide under steady-state conditions (see above).

An almost uniform distribution of ethylene oxide within the body was concluded from the similar tissue:air partition coefficients for organs of male Fischer 344 rats determined *in vitro*: fat, 44.1; muscle, 48.3; brain, 58.7; lung, 60.9; liver, 61.6; blood, 64.1; and testes, 83 (Krishnan *et al.*, 1992).

Elimination of ethylene oxide was described by first-order kinetics over the whole concentration range examined in both Sprague-Dawley (Filser & Bolt, 1984) and Fischer 344 rats (Krishnan *et al.*, 1992). At steady state, the clearance due to metabolism in relation to the concentration in the atmosphere was 10 600 mL/h (177 mL/min) for two Sprague-Dawley rats that weighed 500 g (Filser & Bolt, 1984). Re-calculation for one Sprague-Dawley rat that weighed 250 g according to the method of Filser (1992) gave a value of almost 55 mL/min. On the basis of the finding that clearance due to metabolism in relation to the concentration in the atmosphere is nearly identical to that due to uptake, uptake of ethylene oxide by inhalation was concluded to be the rate-limiting step for metabolism of this compound. Alveolar retention in one Sprague-Dawley rat that weighed 250 g was calculated as 47% on the basis of a ventilation rate of 117 mL/min and clearance of metabolism in relation to the concentration in the atmosphere of 55 mL/min. The half-life was reported to be 6 min in two animals that weighed 500 g (Bolt & Filser, 1987).

Clearance rates of ethylene oxide from the blood, brain, muscle and testes were nearly identical. Following a 4-h inhalation exposure of B6C3F$_1$ mice and Fischer 344 rats to 100 ppm [183 mg/m^3], the average blood elimination half-lives were 2.4–3.2 min in mice and 11–14 min in rats (Brown *et al.*, 1996, 1998).

In male Fischer 344/N rats exposed by nose-only inhalation for 60 min to 5 ppm [9.2 mg/m^3] ethylene oxide, a steady-state blood level of about 60 ng/g was reached after 15 min (Maples & Dahl, 1993).

After 4-h inhalation exposures of B6C3F$_1$ mice to 0, 50, 100, 200, 300 or 400 ppm [0, 91.5, 183, 366, 549 or 732 mg/m^3] ethylene oxide, concentrations of ethylene oxide in the blood increased linearly with inhaled concentrations of less than 200 ppm, but the blood concentration increased more rapidly than linearly above that level. GSH levels in the liver, lung, kidney and testes decreased as exposures increased above 200 ppm, which indicated that, at low concentrations, GSH conjugation is responsible for the disappearance of ethylene oxide but, at higher concentrations when tissue GSH begins to be depleted, the elimination occurs via a slower hydrolysis process, which leads to a greater than linear increase in blood concentrations of ethylene oxide (Brown *et al.*, 1998).

(b)   Metabolism

For an overview of mammalian metabolism of ethylene oxide, see Figure 2.

For early identification and quantification of mammalian metabolites of ethylene oxide, see IARC (1994).

After intravenous injection of 1 and 10 mg/kg bw ethylene oxide to male Sprague-Dawley rats, HEMA was excreted as a constant percentage of the dose: about 30% from 0 to 12 h and 5% from 12 to 24 h. Following administration of 100 mg/kg bw ethylene oxide, the corresponding percentages were 16% and 5%, respectively. These results indicate that the capacity for GSH conjugation at the high dose could have been exceeded within the first 12 h (Gérin & Tardif, 1986).

Ethylene glycol, 2-hydroxyethylmercapturic acid, 2-methylthioethanol and 2-mercaptoethanol were identified as metabolites in the urine of male Wistar rats exposed for 6 h to 500 ppm [915 mg/m^3] ethylene oxide (Koga *et al.*, 1987). The amounts of ethylene glycol in the urine of male Wistar rats collected during 6-h exposures to 50, 100, 200, 300 and 500 ppm [91.5, 183, 366, 549 and 915 mg/m^3] ethylene oxide and up to 20 h thereafter were 0.2, 0.35, 1.0, 2.5 and 4.2 mg, and thus increased disproportionately to the exposure concentrations (Koga *et al.*, 1985). These findings may indicate a relative decrease in GSH conjugation.

The pattern of excretion of ethylene oxide metabolites in mice, rats and rabbits was investigated in urine collected 24 h after treatment with ethylene oxide, either intravenously (20 and 60 mg/kg bw) or by inhalation for 6 h (about 200 ppm [366 mg/m^3]). Marked species differences were seen (Table 9), since metabolites that resulted from conjugation of ethylene oxide with GSH were found in the urine of male Swiss CD-1 mice and male Sprague-Dawley rats but not in that of rabbits [strain not given]. HEMA was excreted in the urine of mice and rats, but *S*-(2-hydroxyethyl)cysteine and *S*-(carboxymethyl)cysteine were present only in the urine of mice. Ethylene glycol, the reaction product of the enzymatic and non-enzymatic hydrolysis of ethylene oxide, was found in the urine of all three species (Tardif *et al.*, 1987).

(c)   GSH depletion

Treatment of animals with ethylene oxide lowered the concentration of GSH in various tissues. Immediately after a 4-h exposure of male Swiss-Webster mice and Fischer 344 rats to atmospheric concentrations of 100, 400 and 900 ppm [183, 732 and 1647 mg/m^3] (mice) and 100, 600 and 1200 ppm [183, 1098 and 2196 mg/m^3] (rats) ethylene oxide, concentration-related decreases in GSH levels were observed in the kidney, heart, lung, brain, stomach, spleen, testis and liver of both species, in the blood of mice but not of rats and in bone marrow, which was examined in rats only. In both species, the GSH levels were reduced to a greater extent in the liver, lung and stomach

Table 9. Urinary excretion of ethylene oxide metabolites within 24 h after treatment of mice, rats and rabbits with ethylene oxide intravenously or by inhalation

Treatment	Urinary metabolites (μmol/100 g bw) (mean values)			
	N-Acetyl-S-(2-hydroxy-ethyl)cysteine	S-(2-Hydroxy-ethyl)cysteine	S-(Carboxy-methyl)cysteine	Ethylene glycol
20 mg/kg intravenously				
Mouse	3.75	2.62	0.85	1.48
Rat	14.00	ND	ND	2.68
Rabbit	ND	ND	ND	0.95
60 mg/kg intravenously				
Mouse	9.53	6.80	4.30	3.55
Rat	32.28	ND	ND	8.59
Rabbit	ND	ND	ND	3.76
200 ppm [366 mg/m^3], 6 h inhalation				
Mouse	4.63	2.62	2.83	0.77
Rat	19.61	ND	ND	1.84
Rabbit	ND	ND	ND	2.56

Adapted from Tardif et al. (1987)
ND, not detected

than in other organs. After exposure to the highest concentrations, GSH levels in the tissues were depressed to 20–30% of the control values (McKelvey & Zemaitis, 1986).

Concentrations of GSH in the hepatic cytosol of male Wistar rats decreased to 37% of that of controls after a single exposure (4 h) to 500 ppm [915 mg/m^3] ethylene oxide, to 13% after exposure to 1500 ppm [2745 mg/m^3] (Katoh et al., 1990) and to 5% after exposure to 2500 ppm [4575 mg/m^3] (Nakashima et al., 1987). Immediately after the last of a series of repeated exposures of male Wistar rats to 500 ppm [915 mg/m^3] ethylene oxide for 6 h per day on 3 days per week for 6 weeks, the hepatic GSH concentration was decreased by 50%. Control values were reached again 12 h thereafter (Katoh et al., 1989).

The consequences of GSH depletion on the occurrence of non-linear increases in the concentration of ethylene oxide in the blood with increasing external doses of ethylene oxide is discussed in Section 4.1.2(a). Haemoglobin adduct formation in mice and rats exposed to 0, 3, 10, 33, 100 and 300 (rats only) ppm [0, 5.49, 18.3, 60.39, 183 and 549 mg/m^3] ethylene oxide for 6 h per day on 5 days per week for 4 weeks was linear in both species up to 33 ppm, after which the slope increased more than proportionately (Walker et al., 1992a). The dose-related decrease in hepatic GSH concentration (Brown *et al.*, 1998) provides a plausible explanation for the more than proportional increase in hydroxyethylated haemoglobin (see below). In both rats and mice, depletion of GSH was already considerable following a single exposure to high levels (i.e. 550 mg/m^3) of ethylene oxide (McKelvey & Zemaitis, 1986; Brown *et al.*, 1998).

(d)   Haemoglobin adducts

Binding of ethylene oxide to haemoglobin has been reviewed in some detail (IARC, 1994). In-vitro treatment of mouse, rat and human cells with ethylene oxide demonstrated the formation of adducts with *S*-cysteine, histidine and *N*-terminal valine in haemoglobin. The second-order rate constants were approximately the same for histidine and valine across the three species; however, large species differences were seen with respect to *S*-cysteine (Segerbäck, 1990). In studies of the fate of ethylene oxide in mice, single exposures to this epoxide produced in a dose-dependent manner haemoglobin adducts that disappeared at a rate predicted by the normal life-span of the red blood cells. These data suggested that stable haemoglobin adducts would accumulate over the lifetime of the erythrocyte during chronic exposures to ethylene oxide and provided the basis for the concept of using haemoglobin adducts to monitor integral doses of alkylating agents. Single intraperitoneal injections of and multiple inhalation exposures to ethylene oxide generally yielded linear dose–response relationships between dose and histidine and valine haemoglobin adduct levels. However, chronic inhalation exposures of male Fischer 344 rats to 10, 33 or 100 ppm [18.3, 60.4 or 183 mg/m^3] ethylene oxide under cancer bioassay conditions (6 h per day on 5 days per week for 2 years) resulted in a non-linear dose–response curve for N^τ-(2-hydroxyethyl)histidine (Osterman-Golkar *et al.*, 1983). Comparisons of the data from single-dose or 4-week inhalation exposure studies of rats versus a study of rats exposed for 2 years suggested that the dose–response relationship between the concentration of ethylene oxide and the formation of haemoglobin adducts can change over time during repeated exposure to this epoxide (Walker *et al.*, 1992a).

More recent studies on haemoglobin adducts in ethylene oxide-exposed mice and rats have focused on (*a*) potential species differences in the relationships between exposure, accumulation of haemoglobin adducts over time during repeated exposures and the dynamics in loss of adducts after discontinuation of exposures (Fennell *et al.*, 1992; Walker *et al.*, 1992a); and (*b*) comparisons of the formation and persistence of adducts in haemoglobin and DNA (Walker *et al.*, 1993), and the relationships between exposure, levels of haemoglobin adducts as a marker of dose and induction of somatic mutations (Tates *et al.*, 1999). Results of species comparisons of the formation and persistence of *N*-(2-hydroxyethyl)valine have been summarized previously (IARC, 1994). In brief, dose-related levels of *N*-(2-hydroxyethyl)valine were reported to be similar in mice and rats exposed to ethylene oxide (3–100 ppm [5.49–183 mg/m^3] for 4 weeks), while the adducts were lost in a species-specific pattern related to a differing life-span of red blood cells in each species. However, the relationships between *N*-(2-hydroxyethyl)valine in haemoglobin and *N*7-(2-hydroxyethyl)guanine in DNA varied with length of exposure, interval since exposure, species and tissue, which led the authors to conclude that the haemoglobin adducts were unlikely to provide accurate predictions of DNA adducts in tissues under conditions in which the actual scenario of exposure to ethylene oxide is unknown (Walker *et al.*, 1993). Tates *et al.* (1999) measured *N*-(2-hydroxyethyl)valine to determine blood levels of ethylene oxide in rats and then used the estimated blood doses to compare the mutagenic effects of ethylene oxide via three routes of exposure, including single intraperitoneal injections, ingestion via the drinking-water or inhalation; comparisons of the mutagenic responses from alternative treatments with ethylene oxide are considered below. Other studies that measured the formation of *N*-(2-hydroxy-ethyl)valine in mice and rats after inhalation of ethylene oxide have typically used this haemoglobin adduct as a marker of exposure for comparison with DNA adducts in the same animals (Walker *et al.*, 2000; Rusyn *et al.*, 2005). In general, the same relationships were found as those reported in the earlier rodent studies of ethylene oxide that are summarized above.

(e)   Toxicokinetic modelling

A physiologically based pharmacokinetic model has been developed for dosimetry of inhaled and intravenously injected ethylene oxide in rats (Krishnan *et al.*, 1992). The model enables the determination of tissue distribution, metabolic pathways, i.e. hydrolysis by EH and conjugation with GSH by GST, depletion of hepatic and extrahepatic GSH and binding of ethylene oxide to haemoglobin and DNA. The biochemical parameters used in the model were obtained by fitting data obtained after inhalation of ethylene oxide in closed chambers to data on tissue GSH concentrations (McKelvey & Zemaitis, 1986) and on levels of hydroxyethyl adducts in haemoglobin and tissue DNA (Potter *et al.*, 1989). The model was validated by comparing simulated and published data on urinary excretion of HEMA after inhalation and intravenous administration of ethylene oxide (Gérin & Tardif, 1986; Tardif *et al.*, 1987) and on levels of hydroxyethyl adducts in haemoglobin and tissue DNA after exposure for 6 h to 300 ppm [549 mg/m^3] ethylene oxide (Walker *et al.*, 1990, 1992a). The second-order rate constants obtained for the binding of ethylene oxide to amino acid residues in haemoglobin are similar to those published by Segerbäck (1990). According to the model, total adduct formation in haemoglobin and DNA accounted for 0.25% and 0.001% of the inhaled dose, respectively. After exposure to atmospheric concentrations of up to 500 ppm [915 mg/m^3] ethylene oxide, the model predicted first-order kinetics for whole-body elimination, but non-linearity in individual metabolic pathways and exhalation. Comparison of the predictions for low and 500-ppm exposures indicated that the share of GSH conjugation decreased from 38 to 27%, whereas the share of hydrolysis increased from 31 to 36% and that of exhalation from 23 to 28% (Krishnan *et al.*, 1992).

More recent physiologically based pharmacokinetic models of uptake and metabolism of ethylene oxide in mice, rats and humans were published by Csanády *et al.* (2000) and Fennell and Brown (2001). These models predicted adequately blood and tissue concentrations of ethylene oxide in rats and mice (with the exception of the testes). Simulations by the model of Fennell and Brown (2001) indicate that, in mice, rats and humans, about

80%, 60% and 20% of ethylene oxide, respectively, would be metabolized via GSH con-jugation. Nevertheless, modelling 6-h inhalation exposures gave simulated ethylene oxide areas under the curve and blood peak concentrations that were similar for mice, rats and humans (Fennell & Brown, 2001). Thus, exposure to a given concentration of ethylene oxide in air results in similar predicted blood ethylene oxide areas under the curve for mice, rats and humans.

4.1.3   *Comparison of rodent and human data*

A striking difference between rodents and humans in the metabolism of ethylene oxide is the predominance of the GSH pathway in mice and rats, while in humans (and in other larger animals tested to date), the pathway initiated by enzymatic and non-enzym-atic hydrolysis is of greater importance (Jones & Wells, 1981; Martis *et al.*, 1982; Gérin & Tardif, 1986; Tardif *et al.*, 1987; Brown *et al.*, 1996) which is consistent with the observed levels of the ethylene oxide that conjugate GSTT1 in the order mice > rats > humans. This leads to an onset of significant GSH depletion in rodents at exposure concentrations that were used in toxicological investigations, namely between 33 and 100 ppm [60.4 and 183 mg/m^3] ethylene oxide in ambient air (see above). However, it is important to note that carcinogenicity in rats was already observed at the lower exposure concentration of 10 ppm [18.3 mg/m^3] ethylene oxide in one study (see Section 3).

Although the physiologically based pharmacokinetic models constructed by Fennell and Brown (2001) indicated profound differences in the relative contribution of the different metabolic pathways, when differences in uptake and metabolism are taken into account, simulated blood peak concentrations and areas under the curve were similar for mice, rats and humans (human levels within about 15% of rat and mouse levels). Thus, exposure to a given concentration of ethylene oxide in air gives similar predicted blood levels of ethylene oxide and areas under the curve for mice, rats and humans (in the range of exposures used in the rodent cancer bioassays, i.e. 100 ppm [183 mg/m^3] and below; above these concentrations, the differences in GSH depletion may be expected to lead to significant differences in the levels of ethylene oxide in blood with comparable concen-trations in the ambient air).

Human erythrocytes are rich (but polymorphic) in the ethylene oxide-metabolizing enzyme GSTT1, but, in the experimental animals investigated, this protective enzyme is not present in the erythrocytes (Hallier *et al.*, 1993). This adds a further complexity to species differences in the metabolism of ethylene oxide.

4.2   Genetic and related effects

The direct reaction of ethylene oxide with DNA is thought to initiate the cascade of genetic and related events that lead to cancer (Swenberg *et al.*, 1990). Ethylene oxide is a direct alkylating agent and reacts with nucleophiles without the need for metabolic trans-formation. It uses the general S_N2 mechanism and has a high Swain-Scott substrate constant (Golberg, 1986), both of which favour efficient N7-alkylation of guanine (and other ring nitrogens to a lesser extent) due to the electron density distribution of purines and the steric availability of the N7-position of guanine (Kolman *et al.*, 2002). The reactivity of this agent is due to the strain of the oxirane ring and the partial positive charge on the carbon atoms, which give the compound its electrophilic character and predispose the ring to open and form a hydroxyethylcarbonium ion (Golberg, 1986). Several published reviews contain details of earlier studies of the reactivity and genetic toxicity of ethylene oxide in humans and experimental systems (Kolman *et al.*, 1986; Dellarco *et al.*, 1990; Walker *et al.*, 1990; IARC, 1994; Natarajan *et al.*, 1995; Health Canada, 1999; Preston, 1999; Thier & Bolt, 2000; Health Canada, 2001; Kolman *et al.*, 2002; WHO, 2003). This update is focused primarily upon recently published in-vivo studies of ethylene oxide-exposed humans and rodent models that shed light on the mode of action and the extent to which species comparisons may be pertinent to an evaluation of the carcinogenicity of this chemical in humans.

4.2.1   *Humans*

(a)   *DNA adducts*

For nearly 20 years, it has been known that the endogenous formation of ethylene and its conversion to ethylene oxide leads to 2-hydroxyethylation of DNA to yield background levels of N7-(2-hydroxyethyl)guanine (7-HEG) in unexposed humans (reviewed in Bolt, 1996; Farmer & Shuker, 1999; Walker *et al.*, 2000; Marsden *et al.*, 2007). Ethylene is generated *in vivo* during normal physiological processes such as lipid peroxidation, oxidation of methionine, oxidation of haeme in haemoglobin and/or through the metabolizing activity of intestinal bacteria (reviewed in Thier & Bolt, 2000). Walker *et al.* (2000) described a series of studies of background levels of these adducts in different tissues of unexposed humans, and showed that lower endogenous levels of 7-HEG have typically been found with more sensitive detection methods than those employed in reports on the impact of endogenously versus exogenously derived ethylene oxide (Bolt, 1996). Farmer and Shuker (1999) suggested that, in order to estimate the increase in cancer risk attributable to a given external exposure, it is clearly important to establish and consider background levels of corresponding DNA damage so that the scale of the incremental increase can be calculated. It is mainly for this reason that more sensitive and specific analytical methods have been developed for the measurement of background and treatment-induced levels of 7-HEG than for any other single DNA adduct (reviewed in Zhao *et al.*, 1999; Liao *et al.*, 2001; Kao & Giese, 2005).

Since endogenous DNA damage through lipid peroxidation is thought to contribute significantly to cancer in humans (Marnett, 2002), Zhao and Hemminki (2002) investigated the association between age and endogenous formation of 7-HEG in 34 younger and older healthy human subjects (mean ages, 39.8 and 82.8 years, respectively). Steady-state levels of 7-HEG in the DNA of peripheral blood lymphocytes were similar in the younger and older subjects (means, 3.8 ± 3.4 and 3.0 ± 2.7 adducts/10^7 nucleotides, respectively), which suggests that endogenous DNA damage by ethylene oxide that arises from ethylene generated by lipid peroxidation and the repair of such damage is in-dependent of age as a contributing factor to cancer risk.

A single study has been performed to examine the formation of 7-HEG in humans exposed to ethylene oxide in the workplace (Yong *et al.*, 2007). 7-HEG was quantified, using the method of Kao and Giese (2005), in peripheral blood granulocytes from 58 hospital workers exposed to ethylene oxide during the unloading of sterilizers or when working adjacent to sterilizers. Cumulative exposure to ethylene oxide (ppm–h) was estimated during the 4-month period before the collection of blood samples. There was considerable interindividual variation in the levels of 7-HEG in both unexposed control and ethylene oxide-exposed workers, ranging from 1.6 to 241 adducts/10^7 nucleotides. The mean levels in the unexposed, low-ethylene oxide exposure (< 32 ppm–h) [58.6 mg/m^3–h] and high-ethylene oxide exposure (> 32 ppm–h) groups were 3.8, 16.3 and 20.3 adducts/10^7 nucleotides, respectively, but the differences were not statistically significant after adjustment for cigarette smoking and other potential confounders. Since the life-span of granulocytes is less than 1 day compared with a life-span of up to several years for lymphocytes, the large inter-individual variation in 7-HEG levels as well as elevated values in individual ethylene oxide-exposed workers may have reflected very recent transient peak exposures that were not captured in the overall 4-month cumulative exposure estimates.

(b)   *Mutations and other genetic related effects* (see also Table 10)

Studies of human exposures to ethylene oxide have focused upon individuals who were employed in the operation of hospital or factory sterilization units and workers who were involved in ethylene oxide manufacturing or processing. Selected studies showed that exposure to ethylene oxide results in chromosomal alterations that are related to both the level and duration of exposure, while a single study suggested that exposure to ethylene oxide causes gene mutations. Several other biomarkers of DNA damage (un-scheduled DNA synthesis, DNA single-strand breaks, premature centromere division and DNA–protein cross-links) have been studied by only a few investigators; results are summarized at the end of this section.

Preston (1999) provided a critical assessment of the cytogenetic effects of ethylene oxide *in vitro* and *in vivo*, discussed the basic guidelines for cytogenetic assays in population monitoring and hazard identification, and exhaustively reviewed reports of human cytogenetic studies of ethylene oxide through to 1996. Occupational exposures to ethylene oxide have resulted in increased levels of chromosomal events, which included sister chromatid exchange, chromosomal aberrations and micronucleus formation in blood cells. Cytogenetic end-points can serve as markers of exposure to ethylene oxide and DNA damage. Moreover, several large prospective studies have demonstrated that, on a population basis, increased levels of chromosomal aberration or micronucleus for-mation are indicative of an increased risk for cancer development (Hagmar *et al.*, 1998;

Table 10. Cytogenetic observations in humans exposed to ethylene oxide

No. of exposed	No. of controls	Exposure time (years)		Ethylene oxide in air (ppm)[a]		Cytogenetic effects[b]			Reference
		Range	Mean	Range	Mean (TWA)	CA	MN	SCE	
12	8			0–36[c]				+	Garry et al. (1979)
12	11	1–8	4	0.5–1		–			Pero et al. (1981)
5	11	0.8–3	1.6	5–10		+			
18 (factory I)	11	0.5–8	3.2	<1		+	+[d]	–	Högstedt et al. (1983, 1990)
10 (factory II)	9	0.5–8	1.7	<1		+	–	–	
9 (low-dose task)	13				13[e]			–	Yager et al. (1983)
5 (high-dose task)	13				501[e]			+	
14	14			<0.07–4.3[f]				–	Hansen et al. (1984)
10 (nonsmokers)	15	0.5–10	5.7	[15–123]				+	Laurent et al. (1984)
15 (smokers)	7	0.5–10	4.5					+	
22 (low exposure)	22	1–4	3	0.2–0.5[f]	0.35	(+)		+	Sarto et al. (1984a,b; 1987)
10 (moderate exposure)	10			0–9.3[f]	1.84			+	
19 (high exposure)	19			3.7–20[f]	10.7	+		+	
13 (work site I)	12		3.2	0.5[f]		–		–	Stolley et al. (1984); Galloway et al. (1986)
22 (21)[g] (work site II)	19 (20)[g]		3.1	5–10[f]		–		(+)	
26 (25)[g] (work site III)	22 (21)[g]		4	5–20[f]		(+)		+	
33 (production workers)	32	1–14		≤0.05–8	≤0.01[h]	+		+	Clare et al. (1985)
50	141	1–10		1–40[f]		+		+	Richmond et al. (1985)
36	35	1–14		0.05–8	0.12	–			van Sittert et al. (1985)

Table 10 (contd)

No. of exposed	No. of controls	Exposure time (years)		Ethylene oxide in air (ppm)[a]		Cytogenetic effects[b]			Reference
		Range	Mean	Range	Mean (TWA)	CA	MN	SCE	
22 (sterilization unit)	10	1–8		0–2.6		+			Karelová et al. (1987)
21 (factory workers)	20	2–17		0–4.5		+			
25 (laboratory workers)	20	1–15		0–4.8		+			
9	27	0.5–12	5	0.025–0.38[f]			–		Sarto et al. (1990)
3	27			> 0.38[i]			+		
34	23		8	0.008–2.4[f]	< 0.3	–	–	+	Mayer et al. (1991)
5	10	0.1–4	8.6		0.025		–	–	Sarto et al. (1991)
5	10	4–12		< 1–4.4	0.38		–	+	
9 (hospital workers)	8	2–6	4	22–72	0.025[j]	+	–	+	Tates et al. (1991)
15 (factory workers)	15	3–27	12	14–400	5[j]	+	+	+	
10	10		3	60–69		+		+	Lerda & Rizzi (1992)
32	8		5.1	0–0.3[f]	0.04		–	+	Schulte et al. (1992)
11	8		9.5	0.13–0.3[f]	0.16		–	+	
47	47			< 1		–		–	Tomkins et al. (1993)
14 (hospital workers, nonsmokers)	14			0.5–208[f]				–	Popp et al. (1994)
11 (hospital workers, smokers)	11			0.5–417[f]				–	
75	22	3–14	7	2–5		+	+	+	Ribeiro et al. (1994)

Table 10 (contd)

No. of exposed	No. of controls	Exposure time (years)		Ethylene oxide in air (ppm)[a]		Cytogenetic effects[b]			Reference
		Range	Mean	Range	Mean (TWA)	CA	MN	SCE	
28 (hospital workers)	8			0–0.30	0.08		–	+	Schulte et al. (1995)
10 (hospital workers)				0.13–0.30	0.17		–	+	
7 (production workers)	7	Accidental		28–429			–	–	Tates et al. (1995)
7 (production workers)		< 5		< 0.005–0.02			–	–	
7 (production workers)		> 15		< 0.005–0.01			–		
9 (low exposure, hospital workers)	48		4	2.7–10.9	2.7	+		–	Major et al. (1996)
27 (high exposure, hospital workers)	10		15	2.7–82	5.5	+		+	

CA, chromosomal aberrations; MN, micronuclei; SCE, sister chromatid exchange; TWA, time-weighted average

Blanks not studied

[a] 1 ppm = 1.83 mg/m^3 ethylene oxide

[b] +, positive; –, negative

[c] Maximum concentration measured during purge cycle

[d] Positive for erythroblasts and polychromatic aberrations; negative for peripheral blood lymphocytes

[e] Average 6-month cumulative dose in mg ethylene oxide

[f] TWA

[g] Numbers in parentheses are for chromosomal aberrations evaluated by Galloway et al. (1986)

[h] Calculated by linear extrapolation

[i] Exposed acutely from sterilizer leakage

[j] Estimated 40-h TWA based on haemoglobin adducts

Liou *et al.*, 1999; Smerhovsky *et al.*, 2001; Hagmar *et al.*, 2004; Boffetta *et al.*, 2007; Bonassi *et al.*, 2007).

The induction of increased frequencies of sister chromatid exchange has been found to be a sensitive indicator of genotoxic exposure to ethylene oxide in humans (Tates *et al.*, 1991). Evaluation of the impact of exposure to ethylene oxide on changes in the frequency of sister chromatid exchange should take into consideration the observation that the available studies assessed a wide range of exposure concentrations and conditions, including moderately high-dose acute exposures and chronic exposures at varying concentrations of ethylene oxide. Some interesting trends are apparent across studies. Those that failed to find significant increases in frequencies of sister chromatid exchange following exposure to ethylene oxide were primarily studies of workers who were exposed to approximately 5 ppm [9.15 mg/m^3] or less (TWA) (Högstedt *et al.*, 1983; Yager *et al.*, 1983; Hansen *et al.*, 1984; Stolley *et al.*, 1984; Sarto *et al.*, 1991; Tates *et al.*, 1995), although a number of studies report increased frequencies of sister chromatid exchange in workers exposed to less than 5 ppm (TWA) (Sarto *et al.*, 1984a, 1987; Mayer *et al.*, 1991; Tates *et al.*, 1991; Schulte *et al.*, 1992, 1995). Significant increases in frequencies of sister chromatid exchange were commonly found in studies that evaluated individuals who were exposed to concentrations of ethylene oxide > 5 ppm (TWA) (Garry *et al.*, 1979; Yager *et al.*, 1983; Laurent *et al.*, 1984; Sarto *et al.*, 1984a; Stolley *et al.*, 1984; Tates *et al.*, 1991; Lerda & Rizzi, 1992; Schulte *et al.*, 1992). It should be noted that comparisons among studies are complicated by differences in the methodology used to record and report exposure concentrations of ethylene oxide; this problem is further complicated by the fact that, although workers were generally exposed to low average levels in some studies, acute high exposures were noted to have occurred (Tates *et al.*, 1991). In spite of these complications, several studies found significant differences in sister chromatid exchange frequencies in individuals and/or groups exposed to levels of ethylene oxide higher than the designated low-exposure group from the same or similar environment (Yager *et al.*, 1983; Sarto *et al.*, 1984a; Stolley *et al.*, 1984; Tates *et al.*, 1991; Schulte *et al.*, 1992). These findings support the observation that sister chromatid exchange frequencies varied with level and frequency of exposure to ethylene oxide. Two studies investigated changes in frequencies of sister chromatid exchange over time and found that they remained elevated for at least 6 months even when exposures were decreased or ceased after the first assessment (Sarto *et al.*, 1984b; Stolley *et al.*, 1984). A relationship between changes in frequencies of sister chromatid exchange and cigarette smoking has also been found by several investigators (Sarto *et al.*, 1991); because data on exposure to cigarette smoke as a potential confounding factor was not consistently included in all studies, it is not always possible to determine the primary cause for the observed changes in sister chromatid exchange frequency (Sarto *et al.*, 1991).

Because increased frequencies of some classes of chromosomal aberration are associated with an increased risk for the development of cancer (Sorsa *et al.*, 1990), several studies have investigated the induction of increased frequencies of chromosomal aberrations in individuals exposed to ethylene oxide. Workers exposed to a range of concentrations from 0.01 ppm to 200 ppm [0.02–366 mg/m^3] have been evaluated; the majority of the studies found significant increases in chromosomal aberrations (Pero *et al.*, 1981; Högstedt *et al.*, 1983; Sarto *et al.*, 1984b; Richmond *et al.*, 1985; Galloway *et al.*, 1986; Karelová *et al.*, 1987; Högstedt *et al.*, 1990; Tates *et al.*, 1991; Lerda & Rizzi, 1992; Ribeiro *et al.*, 1994; Major *et al.*, 1996). One study found significant increases in chromosomal aberrations in individuals exposed to concentrations of ethylene oxide of approximately 1 ppm [1.83 mg/m^3] and below (Högstedt *et al.*, 1983), although the majority of positive studies evaluated exposure conditions in which higher concentrations of ethylene oxide were present. Other studies of workers exposed to concentrations of ethylene oxide of approximately 1 ppm [1.83 mg/m^3] TWA and below did not find evidence of increased chromosomal aberrations (van Sittert *et al.*, 1985; Mayer *et al.*, 1991). Chromosomal aberration frequencies have been found to correlate with exposure concentrations of ethylene oxide and/or duration of exposure (Clare *et al.*, 1985; Galloway *et al.*, 1986; Tates *et al.*, 1991; Lerda & Rizzi, 1992). As noted for studies of sister chromatid exchange, chromosomal aberrations can be influenced by concurrent exposure to cigarette smoke and by ageing; these factors, combined with differences in the methods used to determine the magnitude of the exposures to ethylene oxide, limit the conclusions that can be drawn from comparisons between studies (Preston, 1999). As reported for sister chromatid exchange, the validity of these comparisons is supported by the observation that some investigators found significant increases in chromosomal aberrations in high-dose groups but not in low-dose groups exposed in the same or similar environments (Sarto *et al.*, 1984b; Galloway *et al.*, 1986).

Fewer investigators have evaluated the impact of exposure to ethylene oxide on the frequencies of micronucleated cells, and comparisons are therefore limited for this cyto-genetic marker. The available studies showed a combination of positive and negative effects. Högstedt *et al.* (1990) and Ribeiro *et al.* (1994) found increased frequencies of micronucleated lymphocytes in workers while Tates *et al.* (1991) found significant increases in micronucleus frequencies in workers exposed to high but not to low doses. Exposure concentrations in all of these studies varied, but ranged from < 1 ppm to 400 ppm [1.83–732 mg/m^3] ethylene oxide. Studies that evaluated individuals exposed to levels of ethylene oxide ≤ 1 ppm gave negative results (Högstedt *et al.*, 1983; Sarto *et al.*, 1990, 1991; Tates *et al.*, 1995).

Two studies determined micronucleus frequencies in tissues other than lymphocytes. Ribeiro *et al.* (1994) evaluated both peripheral blood lymphocytes and exfoliated buccal cells in individuals exposed to 2–5 ppm [3.66–9.15 mg/m^3] ethylene oxide (TWA); micronucleus frequencies in buccal cells had a negative association while lymphocytes had a significantly positive association with the effects of ethylene oxide. Sarto *et al.* (1990) found significant increases in micronucleus frequencies in nasal mucosal cells but not in exfoliated buccal cells of workers exposed to ethylene oxide at concentrations below 0.38 ppm [0.7 mg/m^3] (TWA) (some workers experienced acute exposure to ethylene). Exposure to cigarette smoke and age were not discussed as potential con-founders in these studies. These mixed results led to the conclusion by Tates *et al.* (1991)

that the relative sensitivity of end-points for the detection of exposure to ethylene oxide in humans was in the following order: haemoglobin adducts > sister chromatid exchange > chromosomal aberrations > micronucleus formation > hypoxanthine–guanine phosphoribosyl transferase gene (*HPRT*) mutants. However, *HPRT* mutation is a marker of heritable DNA change and thus should not be expected to be sensitive as an indicator of exposure.

Several studies reported individual differences in the magnitude of response for one or more biomarkers that were not accounted for by adjusting for known confounders such as smoking or age (Laurent *et al.*, 1984; Sarto *et al.*, 1984a). Yong *et al.* (2001) evaluated the relationship between levels of haemoglobin adducts, sister chromatid exchange frequencies and *GSTT1* genotype and found that individuals who had the null *GSTT1* genotype had significantly higher levels of haemoglobin adducts and lower frequencies of sister chromatid exchange than individuals who had at least one positive allele. Because these findings were made after most of the above reports, the impact of individual genotype upon the markers listed above is not known. The results of Yong *et al.* (2001) suggest that studies that found significant variations between individuals may have detected the impact of *GSTT1* genotype upon the study end-points, and support the need to consider genotype in future studies of ethylene oxide-induced effects.

Only three reports have addressed the issue of whether occupational exposure to ethylene oxide is associated with the induction of gene mutations. In the first study, the T-cell cloning assay was used to measure *HPRT* mutant frequencies in peripheral blood lymphocytes from nine ethylene oxide-exposed hospital workers and 15 ethylene oxide-exposed factory workers (Tates *et al.*, 1991). Hospital workers included nurses and technicians who were involved in the sterilization of medical equipment and were exposed to ethylene oxide once or twice a week for about 10 min. The concentrations of ethylene oxide ranged from 20 to 25 ppm [36.6–45.8 mg/m^3] in the sterilization room and from 22 to 72 ppm [40.3.–131.8 mg/m^3] in front of the sterilizer immediately after opening (as measured by GC). The hospital workers were matched for age, sex and smoking habits with a control group of eight unexposed administrative workers. The factory workers were employed at a plant that was involved in the production of ethylene oxide-sterilized disposable medical equipment, and were similarly matched with a group of 15 unexposed controls in the same factory. During a 4-month monitoring period (equivalent to the lifespan of erythrocytes in humans), five workers were engaged in 'daily' sterilization activities, two workers were involved in 'daily' sterilization except for leave periods of 7 or 11 days and eight remaining workers were 'occasionally' exposed to ethylene oxide during exposure control, packing and quality control of sterilized products. Before the collection of samples in early 1990, the mean duration of exposure of factory workers was 12 years (range, 3–27 years), with average ambient exposure levels from 1989 onwards that were estimated to be about 17 ppm [~31 mg/m^3] ethylene oxide. Based on measurements of *N*-(2-hydroxyethy)valine haemoglobin adducts that integrate exposure over time, average exposures to ethylene oxide in the 4 months before blood sampling were estimated to be a 40-h TWA of 0.025 ppm [0.046 mg/m^3] for hospital workers and 5 ppm [9.15 mg/m^3] for factory workers (Tates *et al.* 1991).

The average *HPRT* mutant frequencies in hospital workers (12.4 ± 9.9 × 10^{-6}) and factory workers (13.8 ± 4.4 × 10^{-6}) were remarkably similar and showed increases of 55% and 60%, respectively, above background in their respective control groups (8.0 ± 3.6 × 10^{-6} and 8.6 ± 4.4 × 10^{-6}); however, the mutagenic response was significantly elevated only in the factory workers. Tates *et al.* (1991) suggested that the statistically significant increase in the mutant frequency in the factory workers, and not the hospital workers, may have been due to some extent to the larger study populations of factory workers and their controls, but the investigators concluded that the difference was more probably due to the higher exposure concentrations and tissue doses of ethylene oxide in factory workers. The mean cloning efficiency was uniformly lower in the exposed factory workers than in their control group (as well as the hospital workers exposed and their control groups), which might exaggerate the effect of exposure to ethylene oxide on *HPRT* mutant frequency in factory workers; however, adjustments (using multiplicative and additive models) for the observed effect of cloning efficiency, age and smoking status in factory workers appeared to justify the conclusion that the increased *HPRT* mutant frequency in this group was due to exposure to ethylene oxide. [While the Working Group recognized the importance of this study, it also noted inconsistencies in the results with regard to the response in relation to the exposure concentrations and duration of exposure, as well as the apparent similarity of the mutational spectrum of the exposed group and that of control populations.]

In a follow-up study of workers in an ethylene oxide production plant, Tates *et al.* (1995) again used the T-cell cloning assay to measure *HPRT* mutant frequencies in three exposed and one unexposed groups (seven subjects per group). Group I workers were incidentally exposed to acute high concentrations of ethylene oxide, while group II and III workers were chronically exposed to low concentrations of ethylene oxide for < 5 years and > 15 years, respectively. No significant differences in mutant frequencies were observed between any combination of worker or control groups, which implies that incidental exposure to high levels of ethylene oxide (28–429 ppm [52–785 mg/m^3]) or chronic exposure to low concentrations of ethylene oxide (< 0.005–0.02 ppm [< 0.01–0.04 mg/m^3]) did not cause any measurable permanent gene mutations in lymphocytes.

A few investigations extended the number of biomarkers evaluated to characterize ethylene oxide-induced effects to include unscheduled DNA synthesis and induction of DNA single-strand breaks, premature centromere division and DNA–protein cross-links. Induction of unscheduled DNA synthesis was decreased compared with controls in workers exposed to a range of concentrations of ethylene oxide that included levels below 1 ppm [mg/m^3] (TWA) (Pero *et al.*, 1981; Sarto *et al.*, 1987; Mayer *et al.*, 1991); the significance of this finding was not clear, but one investigator considered the decrease to reflect diminished DNA repair capacity (Pero *et al.*, 1981). DNA single-strand breaks were not found to be increased in ethylene oxide-exposed workers in one study (Mayer *et al.*, 1991), but were shown to be increased by alkaline elution in peripheral blood mononuclear cells from hospital and factory workers occupied in sterilizing medical devices (Fuchs *et al.*, 1994). In nonsmokers, significantly higher elution was observed in ethylene oxide-exposed workers than controls, with remarkable individual differences in susceptibility according to *GSTT1* polymorphism. In smokers, a similar trend was observed in ethylene oxide-exposed subjects but the response was smaller and non-significant. Only one study evaluated premature centromere division as a potential indicator of genomic instability (Major *et al.*, 1999); an increase in this phenomenon was observed in ethylene oxide-exposed subjects that correlated with increased chromosomal aberrations. Another study measured DNA–protein cross-links by alkaline filter elution in hospital workers and found a significant correlation between reduced elution rates and exposure to ethylene oxide (Popp *et al.*, 1994).

4.2.2   *Experimental systems*

(a)   *DNA adducts*

The relative amounts of adducts found in two independent studies of the reactivity of ethylene oxide with double-stranded DNA *in vitro* (Segerbäck, 1990; Li *et al.*, 1992) are compared in tables in Segerbäck (1994) and Kolman *et al.* (2002). *In vitro*, the reaction of ethylene oxide with nucleic acids occurs mainly at ring nitrogens, and leads to the formation of 7-HEG, O^6-(2-hydroxyethyl)guanine (O^6-HEG) and reaction products with $N1$, $N3$, $N7$ and N^6 of adenine and $N3$ of cytosine, uracil and thymine. Depending upon the in-vitro study, 7-HEG accounted for up to 90% of alkylation products and smaller amounts of other DNA adducts were formed. Segerbäck (1990) reported that treatment of calf thymus DNA with ^{14}C-labelled ethylene oxide resulted in the formation of 7-HEG, $N3$-(2-hydroxyethyl)adenine (3-HEA) and O^6-HEG at a ratio of 100:4.4:0.5. In contrast, Walker *et al.* (1992b) found that the ratio of the steady-state concentrations of 7-HEG, 3-HEA and O^6-HEG was 100:0.3:0.4 following repeated exposures of rats to ethylene oxide, which indicates that 3-HEA and O^6-HEG do not accumulate *in vivo* at levels predicted by the in-vitro ratios of these adducts and 7-HEG.

Many studies have evaluated DNA adducts as a molecular dosimeter following single or repeated exposures of mice and rats to ethylene oxide by intraperitoneal injection or inhalation. 7-HEG has consistently been found to be the predominant adduct; relatively small amounts of O^6-HEG and 3-HEA were identified in a single investigation of in-vivo adduct formation in tissues of ethylene oxide-exposed rats (Walker *et al.*, 1992b). Time-course studies have demonstrated that 7-HEG accumulated at steady-state levels after 4 weeks of inhalation exposure of mice and rats to high concentrations of ethylene oxide (100 ppm [183 mg/m^3] in mice and 100 or 300 ppm [183 or 549 mg/m^3] in rats) for 6 h per day on 5 days per week (Walker *et al.*, 1990, 1992b; Rusyn *et al.*, 2005); in contrast, adducts reached a plateau after 1 week of exposure during in-vivo conversion of exogenous ethylene to low levels of ethylene oxide (~6 ppm [~11 mg/m^3]) in most tissues of mice and rats exposed to 3000 ppm ethylene by inhalation 6 h per day on 5 days per week for 4 weeks (Walker *et al.*, 2000; Rusyn *et al.*, 2005). These data support the hypothesis that, after repeated exposures of rodents to high concentrations of ethylene oxide, the discrepancies between the time to steady state (i.e. $\geq$ 28 days) and the DNA adduct half-life values [cited in the previous review of ethylene oxide (IARC, 1994); i.e. half-life of 1.0–2.3 days in most mouse tissues and 2.9–4.8 days in most rat tissues (Walker *et al.*, 1992b)] were most probably related to a greater dependence on spontaneous depurination for loss of 7-HEG than at lower levels of exposures to ethylene oxide at which DNA repair is not saturated (Walker *et al.*, 2000). In contrast, the patterns of elimination of 7-HEG adducts after a single 6-h exposure of rats to 40 or 3000 ppm ethylene exhibited slow linear loss of adducts from the brain, liver and spleen in animals exposed to endogeneously formed low-level ethylene oxide equivalents of ~1–6 ppm [1.83–11 mg/m^3] (Rusyn *et al.*, 2005).

Dose–response studies in mice and rats exposed to 3, 10, 33 or 100 ppm [5.49, 18.3, 60.4 or 183 mg/m^3] ethylene oxide for 6 h per day on 5 days per week for 4 weeks showed that the formation of 7-HEG at any given exposure level was similar for all tissues (brain, liver, lung, spleen) except the testis (within a factor of three) (Walker *et al.*, 1992b; Wu *et al.*, 1999a; Rusyn *et al.*, 2005), which suggests that, since not all of these tissues are targets for cancer, other critical factors may be involved in the species and tissue specificity for tumour induction by this chemical (Walker *et al.*, 1992b). Nevertheless, in rats exposed by inhalation for 6 h per day on 5 days per week for 4 weeks to 0, 50, 100 or 200 ppm [0, 91.5, 183 or 366 mg/m^3] ethylene oxide, statistically significant linear relationships were found between mean levels of 7-HEG and increases in *Hprt* mutant frequencies and between 7-HEG and elevations in sister chromatid exchange or so-called high-frequency cells (van Sittert *et al.*, 2000). Similar relationships between levels of 7-HEG and *Hprt* mutant frequencies were observed in mice exposed for 4 weeks to the same concentrations of ethylene oxide, except that the dose–response curves were sublinear and showed a greater effect per unit dose for both biomarkers with increasing exposure (see Fig. 4 in Walker *et al.*, 1997a). Thus, while levels of ethylene oxide-induced 7-HEG do not correlate directly with species/tissue susceptibility, they appear to predict the occurrence of increased frequencies of gene mutations and sister chromatid exchange in the lymphocytes of ethylene oxide-exposed rodents.

Background levels of 7-HEG in mice and rats have been investigated in numerous reports on the validation of sensitive methods to measure this adduct and/or establish the relative contribution of DNA damage that arises from endogenously and exogenously derived ethylene oxide (Föst *et al.*, 1989; Walker *et al.*, 1992b; Eide *et al.*, 1999; Wu *et al.*, 1999a,b; Zhao *et al.*, 1999; van Sittert *et al.*, 2000; Walker *et al.*, 2000; Rusyn *et al.*, 2005; Marsden *et al.*, 2007). Most recently, Marsden *et al.* (2007) developed a highly sensitive LC–MS/MS assay with selected reaction monitoring and established the lowest background levels of 7-HEG (1.1–3.5 adducts/10^8 nucleotides) reported to date for multiple tissues (colon, heart, kidney, liver, lung, spleen and stomach) in male Fischer 344 rats, which corroborated and extended an earlier report of ~2.6 7-HEG adducts/10^8 nucleotides in liver DNA from unexposed male Lewis rats (van Sittert *et al.*, 2000). Marsden *et al.* (2007) also measured exogenously derived 7-HEG following intraperitoneal administration of a single dose or three daily doses of 0.01–1.0 mg/kg ethylene oxide. These relatively low doses resulted in modest but generally dose-related increases in the observed concentrations of 7-HEG (i.e. background levels from endogenous ethylene oxide plus levels from exogenous ethylene oxide) in various tissues, except at the lowest concentration for which the measured amounts of 7-HEG in various tissues did not differ from those detected in control animals. The latter finding indicates that any increase in 7-HEG was negligible compared with the endogenous DNA damage already present.

> (b)   *Mutations and other genetic effects* (see Table 11 for details and references)

As a direct-acting alkylating agent, ethylene oxide has displayed genotoxic activity in nearly all studies in experimental systems, with a few notable dose-related exceptions in ethylene oxide-exposed rodents. *In vitro*, ethylene oxide caused DNA damage and gene mutations in bacteriophage, bacteria, fungi, insects and mammalian cells, and gene conversion in yeast (IARC, 1994). Given the general consistency of the in-vitro data in Table 11, only studies conducted in in-vivo systems are detailed here.

In-vivo exposure to ethylene oxide induced DNA damage and heritable mutations in germ cells of rodents, which caused alkali-labile sites and single-strand breaks in mouse sperm and spermatids, and chromosomal aberrations in mouse spermatocytes. It also induced dominant lethal effects in mice and rats, and heritable translocations in mice. Reviews of these studies have been published (Health Canada, 1999, 2001; WHO, 2003). It should be noted that these (mostly dose-related) effects were observed at relatively high concentrations of ethylene oxide (165–300 ppm [302–549 mg/m^3]; lower doses not tested) that exceeded the high dose used in the rodent carcinogenicity studies of this chemical.

Results of in-vivo gene mutation studies in rodents have given consistently positive results following ingestion, injection or inhalation of ethylene oxide. The in-vivo mutagenicity of ethylene oxide at the *Hprt* locus of somatic cells was demonstrated following intraperitoneal injection and after repeated inhalation exposures of mice. The impact of age-dependent trafficking on the 'manifestation' of mutant T-cells in rodents was taken into consideration in designing the *Hprt* mutation studies (Walker *et al.*, 1999). In young adult male *lacI* transgenic mice of B6C3F$_1$ origin, inhalation exposures for 4 weeks to ethylene oxide resulted in significant non-linear increases in the frequencies of *Hprt* mutations in splenic T cells. The average induced mutant frequencies (i.e. the average observed mutant frequency after treatment minus the average background mutant frequency) following exposures to 50, 100 or 200 ppm [91.5, 183 or 366 mg/m^3] ethylene oxide were 1.6, 4.6 and 11.9 × 10^{-6}; greater relative mutagenic efficiencies (mutations per unit dose) were observed at higher than at lower concentrations. The small but significant mutagenic response induced at 50 ppm ethylene oxide (the low-dose concentration in the carcinogenicity bioassay in mice) was only 73% above the average control animal value of 2.2 ± 0.3 × 10^{-6} ($p = 0.009$). In a follow-up study of rodents exposed for 4 weeks to

Table 11. Genetic and related effects of ethylene oxide

Test system	Result[a] Without exogenous metabolic system	Result[a] With exogenous metabolic system	Dose[b] (LED or HID)	Reference
DNA single-strand breaks, Chinese hamster V79 cells *in vitro*	+	NT	0.5 mM 1 h[c]	Herrero *et al.* (1997)
Gene mutation, Chinese hamster ovary cells, *Hprt* locus *in vitro*	+	+	0.5 mM 5 h[c]	Tan *et al.* (1981)
Gene mutation, Chinese hamster ovary cells, *Hprt* locus *in vitro*	+	NT	≤ 2000 ppm 1h	Zamora *et al.* (1983)
Micronucleus formation, Chinese hamster V79 cells *in vitro*	+	NT	12 344 ppm 30 min	Zhong *et al.* (1992)
Chromosomal aberrations, Chinese hamster V79 cells *in vitro*	+	NT	3500 ppm 30 min	Zhong *et al.* (1992)
Cell transformation, mouse C3H/10T1/2 cells	+	NT	2.5 mM 1 h[c]	Kolman *et al.* (1989)
DNA single-strand breaks, human diploid fibroblasts *in vitro*	+	NT	2.5 mM 1 h[c]	Nygren *et al.* (1994)
DNA double-strand breaks, human diploid fibroblasts *in vitro*	+	NT	10 mM 1 h[c]	Nygren *et al.* (1994)
DNA single-strand breaks, human lymphocytes *in vitro*	+	NT	0.5 mM 1 h[c]	Hengstler *et al.* (1997)
Unscheduled DNA synthesis, human lymphocytes *in vitro*	+	NT	0.1mM 24 h[c]	Pero *et al.* (1981)
Gene mutation, human fibroblasts *in vitro*	+	NT	2.5 mM 1 h[c]	Kolman *et al.* (1992)
Gene mutation, human fibroblasts *in vitro*	+	NT	5 mM 1 h[c]	Bastlová *et al.* (1993)
Sister chromatid exchange, human fibroblasts *in vitro*	+	NT	36 ppm 24 h[c]	Star (1980)
Sister chromatid exchange, human lymphocytes *in vitro*	+	NT	0.22 mM 20 min	Garry *et al.* (1982)
Sister chromatid exchange, human lymphocytes *in vitro*	+	NT	~1 mM 3 s[c]	Tucker *et al.* (1986)
Sister chromatid exchange, human lymphocytes *in vitro*	+[d]	NT	~2.5 mM 1 h[c]	Agurell *et al.* (1991)
Sister chromatid exchange, human lymphocytes *in vitro*	+	NT	1000 ppm 90 min	Hallier *et al.* (1993)
Chromosomal aberrations, human amniotic cell line *in vitro*	+	NT	≥ 5 mM 1 h	Poirier & Papadopoulo (1982)
DNA single-strand breaks, mouse spermatids *in vivo*	+		1800 ppm inh 1 h	Sega *et al.* (1988)

Table 11 (contd)

Test system	Result[a] Without exogenous metabolic system	Result[a] With exogenous metabolic system	Dose[b] (LED or HID)	Reference
DNA single-strand breaks, mouse spermatids *in vivo*	+		100 mg/kg × 1 ip	Sega & Generoso (1988)
Gene mutation, mouse spleen T lymphocytes, *Hprt* locus *in vivo*	+		600 mg/kg ip	Walker & Skopek (1993)
Gene mutation, mouse spleen T lymphocytes, *Hprt* locus *in vivo*	+		50 ppm inh[e] × 4 wk	Walker et al. (1997a)
Gene mutation, mouse and rat spleen T lymphocytes, *Hprt* locus *in vivo*	+		200 ppm inh[e] × 4 wk	Walker et al. (1997b, 2000)
Gene mutation, mouse lung, *LacI* transgene *in vivo*	+		200 ppm inh[e] × 4 wk	Sisk et al. (1997)
Gene mutation, mouse bone marrow, spleen, *LacI* transgene *in vivo*	−		200 ppm inh[e] × 4 wk	Sisk et al. (1997)
Gene mutation, male Lewis rat spleen T lymphocytes, *Hprt* locus *in vivo*	+		20 mg/kg × 1 ip	Tates et al. (1999)
Gene mutation, male Lewis rat spleen T lymphocytes, *Hprt* locus *in vivo*	+		2 mM dw, 30 d	Tates et al. (1999)
Gene mutation, male Lewis rat spleen T lymphocytes, *Hprt* locus *in vivo*	+		50 ppm inh[e] × 4 wk	Tates et al. (1999)
Gene mutation, male Lewis rat spleen T lymphocytes, *Hprt* locus *in vivo*	+		200 ppm inh[e] × 4 wk	van Sittert et al. (2000)
Gene mutation, mouse bone marrow, *LacI* transgene *in vivo*	+		100 ppm inh[e] × 48 wk	Recio et al. (2004)
Gene mutation, mouse testis, *LacI* transgene *in vivo*	+		25 ppm inh[e] × 48 wk	Recio et al. (2004)
Mouse specific locus, spermatogonial stem cells *in vivo*	−		255 ppm inh 6 h/d[f]	Russell et al. (1984)

Table 11 (contd)

Test system	Result[a] Without exogenous metabolic system	Result[a] With exogenous metabolic system	Dose[b] (LED or HID)	Reference
Mouse specific locus, spermatogonial stem cells *in vivo*	(+)		200 ppm inh 6 h/d[g]	Lewis *et al.* (1986)
Sister chromatid exchange, rabbit lymphocytes *in vivo*	+		50 ppm inh[e] × 12 wk	Yager & Benz (1982)
Sister chromatid exchange, male Fischer 344 rat lymphocytes *in vivo*	+		451 ppm inh 6 h	Kligerman *et al.* (1983)
Sister chromatid exchange, monkey lymphocytes *in vivo*	+		50 ppm inh 7 h/d[h], 5 d/wk, 2 years	Lynch *et al.* (1984b); Kelsey *et al.* (1988)
Sister chromatid exchange, rabbit lymphocytes *in vivo*	+		200 ppm inh 6 h/d, 40 days	Yager (1987)
Sister chromatid exchange, Swiss mouse bone-marrow cells *in vivo*	+		30 mg/kg ip × 1	Farooqi *et al.* (1993)
Sister chromatid exchange, male Fischer 344 rat bone-marrow cells and spleen *in vivo*	+		100 ppm inh[e], 3 mo	Ong *et al.* (1993)
Sister chromatid exchange, male Fischer 344 rat lymphocytes *in vivo*	+		150 ppm inh[e] × 1–4 wk	Preston & Abernethy (1993)
Sister chromatid exchange, male Lewis rat splenic lymphocytes *in vivo*	(+)		50–200 ppm inh[e] × 4 wk	van Sittert *et al.* (2000); Lorenti Garcia *et al.* (2001)
Micronucleus formation, mouse and rat bone-marrow cells *in vivo*	+		100 mg/kg × 1 iv	Appelgren *et al.* (1978)
Micronucleus formation, mouse bone-marrow cells *in vivo*	+		125 mg/kg × 1 ip	Jenssen & Ramel (1980)
Micronucleus formation, rat bone-marrow cells *in vivo*	+		100 ppm inh[e], 3 mo	Hochberg *et al.* (1990)
Micronucleus formation, Swiss mouse bone-marrow cells *in vivo*	+		30 mg/kg ip × 1	Farooqi *et al.* (1993)

Table 11 (contd)

Test system	Result[a] Without exogenous metabolic system	With exogenous metabolic system	Dose[b] (LED or HID)	Reference
Micronucleus formation, male Fischer 344 rat and B6C3F$_1$ mouse bone marrow *in vivo*	+		200 ppm inh[e] × 4 wk	Vergnes & Pritts (1994)
Micronucleus formation, male Lewis rat splenic lymphocytes *in vivo*	–		50–200 ppm inh[e] × 4 wk	van Sittert et al. (2000); Lorenti Garcia et al. (2001)
Chromosomal aberrations, male Swiss mouse bone-marrow cells *in vivo*	+		200 ppm inh 6 h/d	Ribeiro et al. (1987a)
Chromosomal aberrations, Swiss mouse bone-marrow cells *in vivo*	+		30 mg/kg × 1 ip	Farooqi et al. (1993)
Chromosomal aberrations, male Fischer 344 rat lymphocytes *in vivo*	–		450 ppm inh 6 h/d, 3 d	Kligerman et al. (1983)
Chromosomal aberrations, monkey lymphocytes *in vivo*	+		100 ppm inh 7 h/d, 5 d/wk, 2 years	Lynch et al. (1984b)
Chromosomal aberrations, male Fischer 344 rat lymphocytes *in vivo*	–		150 ppm inh[e] × 1–4 wk	Preston & Abernethy (1993)
Chromosomal aberrations, male Lewis rat lymphocytes *in vivo*	–		50–200 ppm inh[e] × 4 wk	van Sittert et al. (2000); Lorenti Garcia et al. (2001)
Chromosomal aberrations, mouse spermatocytes treated *in vivo*	+		400 ppm inh 6 h/d	Ribeiro et al. (1987a)
Dominant lethal mutation, mouse *in vivo*	–		25 mg/kg × 1 iv	Appelgren et al. (1977)
Dominant lethal mutation, mouse *in vivo*	+		150 mg/kg × 1 ip	Generoso et al. (1980)
Dominant lethal mutation, mouse *in vivo*	+		250 ppm inh[e] × 2 wk	Generoso et al. (1983)

Table 11 (contd)

Test system	Result[a]		Dose[b] (LED or HID)	Reference
	Without exogenous metabolic system	With exogenous metabolic system		
Dominant lethal mutation, mouse *in vivo*	+		300 ppm inh 6 h/d × 4 d	Generoso *et al.* (1986)
Dominant lethal mutation, mouse *in vivo*	+		204 ppm inh 6 h/d [j]	Generoso *et al.* (1990)
Dominant lethal mutation, rat *in vivo*	+		1000 ppm inh 4 h	Embree *et al.* (1977)
Mouse heritable translocation	+		30 mg/kg ip × 5 d/wk, 5 wk	Generoso *et al.* (1980)
Mouse heritable translocation	+		165 ppm 6 h/d [j]	Generoso *et al.* (1990)
Binding (covalent) to calf thymus DNA *in vitro*	+	NT	2M 10 h	Li *et al.* (1992)
Binding (covalent) to human DNA *in vitro*	+	NT	1 mM 3 h	Pauwels & Veulemans (1998)
Binding (covalent) to mouse DNA *in vivo*	+		1.15 ppm inh 75 min	Ehrenberg *et al.* (1974)
Binding (covalent) to rat DNA *in vivo*	+		20.4 µmol/kg × 1 ip	Osterman-Golkar *et al.* (1983)
Binding (covalent) to rat DNA *in vivo*	+		100 ppm inh 4 h	Föst *et al.* (1989)
Binding (covalent) to rat DNA *in vivo*	+		1 ppm inh 6 h	Potter *et al.* (1989)
Binding (covalent) to rat DNA *in vivo*	+		300 ppm inh[e] × 4 wk	Walker *et al.* (1990)
Binding (covalent) to mouse DNA *in vivo*	+		300 ppm inh 1 h	Sega *et al.* (1991)
Binding (covalent) to mouse DNA *in vivo*	+		33 ppm inh[e] × 4 wk	Walker *et al.* (1992b)
Binding (covalent) to rat DNA *in vivo*	+		10 ppm inh[e] × 4 wk	Walker *et al.* (1992b)
Binding (covalent) to rat DNA *in vivo*	+		~ 4.6 ppm inh 6 h × 1	Bolt & Leutbecher (1993)
Binding (covalent) to rat DNA *in vivo*	+		300 ppm inh 12 h/d × 3	Eide *et al.* (1995)
Binding (covalent) to mouse DNA *in vivo*	+		10 ppm inh[e] × 4 wk	Wu *et al.* (1999a)
Binding (covalent) to rat DNA *in vivo*	+		3 ppm inh[e] × 4 wk	Wu *et al.* (1999a)
Binding (covalent) to rat DNA *in vivo*	+		50 ppm inh[e] × 4 wk	van Sittert *et al.* (2000)

Table 11 (contd)

Test system	Result[a] Without exogenous metabolic system	Result[a] With exogenous metabolic system	Dose[b] (LED or HID)	Reference
Binding (covalent) to mouse and rat DNA *in vivo*	+		~ 1 ppm inh[e] × 4 wk	Walker *et al.* (2000); Rusyn *et al.* (2005)
Binding (covalent) to rat DNA *in vivo*	+		0.1 mg/kg × 1 ip	Marsden *et al.* (2007)
Binding (covalent) to rat haemoglobin *in vivo*	+		1 ppm inh 6 h	Potter *et al.* (1989)
Binding (covalent) to mouse haemoglobin *in vivo*	+		300 ppm inh 1 h	Sega *et al.* (1991)
Binding (covalent) to mouse haemoglobin *in vivo*	+		≥ 33 ppm inh[e] × 4 wk	Walker *et al.* (1993)
Binding (covalent) to rat haemoglobin in vivo	+		≥ 10 ppm inh[e] × 4 wk	Walker et al. (1993)
Sperm morphology, mouse *in vivo*	+		200 ppm inh 6 h/d × 5	Ribeiro *et al.* (1987b)

[a] +, positive; –, negative; (+), weak positive; NT, not tested
[b] LED, lowest effective dose; HID, highest ineffective dose; d, day; dw, drinking-water; inh, inhalation; inj, injection; ip, intraperitoneal; iv, intravenous; mo, month; wk, week
[c] Concentration in the culture medium
[d] Single concentration, positive only for non-conjugators of glutathione
[e] 6 h/day, 5 days/week
[f] Sixty days total over a 5-month period
[g] Five days/week; 6–7 months; mating started 7th week of exposure and continued throughout exposure period
[h] Five days/week; 2 years (study group from Lynch *et al.*, 1984b)
[i] Five days/week; 16 days
[j] Five days/week; 6 weeks then daily 2.5 weeks

0 or 200 ppm [366 mg/m^3] ethylene oxide, *Hprt* mutant frequency measurements in splenic T cells of young adult male Fischer 344 rats and B6C3F$_1$ mice were significantly increased by five- to sixfold over background (1.7 and 1.3×10^{-6} in control mice and rats, respectively).

Ethylene oxide-induced mutagenesis at the *Hprt* locus in splenic T cells of rats was confirmed in two additional investigations in young adult male Lewis rats exposed to ethylene oxide by single intraperitoneal injection, in the drinking-water or by inhalation. Significant mutagenic effects were observed by all three routes of exposure; plots of the mutagenicity data against blood dose (estimated from haemoglobin adducts) were a common denominator, which showed that, at equal blood doses, injection of ethylene oxide led to higher mutant frequencies than treatment in the drinking-water, which was more mutagenic than exposure via inhalation. In a follow-up study of inhalation exposure of male Lewis rats to the same concentrations of ethylene oxide, modest dose-related increases in *Hprt* mutant frequencies were found but the only significant elevation was in the group exposed to the highest dose of ethylene oxide. The results of these studies of *Hprt* gene mutation led to the conclusion that ethylene oxide is only weakly mutagenic in adult rats.

Ethylene oxide-induced gene mutations have been demonstrated in multiple tissues of *LacI* transgenic mice. Following 4 weeks of inhalation exposure of male Big Blue™ mice to ethylene oxide, the frequencies of *LacI* gene mutations in exposed animals were significantly increased over control values in lung but not bone marrow or spleen. When Big Blue mice were exposed to ethylene oxide for 12, 24 and 48 weeks, clear dose-related mutagenic responses in bone marrow were observed only after 48 weeks of exposure, with *LacI* mutant frequencies significantly increased only in the 100- and 200-ppm [183- and 366-mg/m^3] exposure groups. In testes of the same mice, dose-related increases in mutant frequencies were found in the groups exposed to 25, 50 or 100 ppm [45.8, 91.5 or 183 mg/m^3] but not the group exposed to 200 ppm [366 mg/m^3] ethylene oxide.

Recent assessments of the carcinogenicity of ethylene oxide have included discussions and summary tables of the results from many studies on chromosomal effects in ethylene oxide-exposed humans (Health Canada, 1999, 2001; WHO, 2003), but no critical review of cytogenetic studies in ethylene oxide-exposed rodents has been made since 1990 (Dellarco *et al.*, 1990). Several studies have shown that repeated exposures of rats to levels equal to or greater than those used in rodent carcinogenicity studies of ethylene oxide (> 50 ppm [> 91.5 mg/m^3]) induced dose-related increases in sister chromatid exchange. Treatment of rats and mice with high acute doses of ethylene oxide by intraperitoneal or intravenous injection or orally (i.e. routes of exposure that are less relevant to humans) also caused increases in the frequencies of micronucleus formation and chromosomal aberrations.

In contrast, following inhalation exposure (i.e. a route of exposure relevant to humans), only concentrations of ethylene oxide that exceeded those used in rodent cancer bioassays induced micronucleus formation or chromosomal aberrations in mice and rats. Modest but significant increases in bone marrow micronuclei were observed in male

Fischer 344 rats and B6C3F$_1$ mice following 4 weeks of exposure for 6 h per day on 5 days per week to 200 ppm [366 mg/m^3] ethylene oxide, but not to 40, 1000 or 3000 ppm exogenous ethylene which is converted *in vivo* to about 1–6 ppm [1.83–11 mg/m^3] ethylene oxide (Vergnes & Pritts, 1994). In contrast, no increases in the frequencies of chromosomal aberrations or micronucleus formation were found in peripheral blood/splenic lymphocytes from rats exposed to ethylene oxide. Furthermore, another study showed that 4 weeks of exposure of rats to ethylene oxide failed to cause an increase in translocations (e.g. the percentage of translocations in controls and rats treated with 200 ppm [366 mg/m^3] was 0.1% and 0.09%, respectively). [The Working Group noted, however, that strong conclusions cannot be drawn about the clastogenic potential of the ethylene oxide treatment regimen used in the 4-week inhalation study (van Sittert *et al.*, 2000; Lorenti Garcia *et al.*, 2001) because cytogenetic studies were initiated 5 days after the final day of exposure, a suboptimal time, and the power of the fluorescent in-situ hybridization studies were limited by analysis of only a single chromosome and the small numbers of rats per group examined.] In studies of the potential clastogenicity of styrene, a group of rats exposed to 150 ppm [274.5 mg/m^3] ethylene oxide by inhalation for 6 h per day on 5 days per week for 1, 2, 3 or 4 weeks was included based upon the expectation that, with appropriate sampling times shortly after exposure, a positive response for chromosomal aberrations would be produced in lymphocytes of ethylene oxide-exposed animals. However, the frequency of chromosomal aberrations in ethylene oxide-exposed rats was not increased over that in air controls at any sampling time.

(c)   *Mutational spectra*

Walker and Skopek (1993) reported limited data on mutational spectra for *Hprt* mutant T-cell clones from B6C3F$_1$ mice given repeated intraperioneal injections of ethylene oxide. Molecular analyses using polymerase chain reaction-based denaturing gradient gel electrophoresis and sequencing for mutations in the exon 3 region of *Hprt* suggested the involvement of both modified guanine and adenine bases in ethylene oxide-induced mutagenesis. Additional data on *Hprt* gene mutational spectra were presented in a preliminary report following 4-week inhalation exposures of mice to 0, 50, 100 or 200 ppm [0, 91.5, 183 or 366 mg/m^3] ethylene oxide or rats to 0 or 200 ppm [366 mg/m^3] ethylene oxide for 6 h per day on 5 days per week (Walker *et al.*, 1997b). The types of mutation in ethylene oxide-exposed mice or rats were independent of the route of exposure; these mutations included a combination of base substitutions, frameshifts and small deletions; the most common lesions were a +1G in a run of six guanines (base pairs 207–212) and several different small deletions in the region of base pairs 275–280. These data suggest that ethylene oxide mutagenesis may involve similar mechanisms in mice and rats.

In ethylene oxide-exposed Big Blue™ mice, molecular analyses of mutations in the *lacI* transgene of bone marrow showed a decrease in mutations at G:C base pairs and an increase at A:T base pairs, which were exclusively A:T→T:A transversions and accounted for 25.4% (14/55) of the mutations isolated (Recio *et al.*, 2004). In contrast,

A:T→T:A transversions occurred at a frequency of 1.4% (1/70) in concurrent control mice. The mutational spectrum in the testes of ethylene oxide-exposed mice indicated that small increases across most mutational types were sufficient to produce an overall increase in the *LacI* mutation frequency, although this was not significant for a specific type compared with controls.

4.2.3   *Mechanism of mutation induction*

Although abundant data *in vitro* and *in vivo* indicate that genotoxicity plays a major role in the carcinogenicity of ethylene oxide, and its mutagenicity is deemed to be a consequence of high reactivity with DNA, the lesions responsible for ethylene oxide-induced mutations *in vivo* have not yet been identified. Possible precursor lesions for the induction of mutations by ethylene oxide are thought to include the formation of (*a*) 7-HEG and other *N*-alkylated bases that may 'predispose' to mutational events, (*b*) O^6-HEG as a promutagenic adduct, (*c*) hydroxyethyl adducts of the DNA backbone and (*d*) secondary reactive oxygen species. Systematic studies of oxidative damage from exposure to ethylene oxide *in vivo* have not been performed and this potential source of mutation is not considered in depth here. Since the publication of the first data on mutational spectra following exposure of human cells *in vitro* (Bastlová *et al.*, 1993) and exposure of mice to ethylene oxide *in vivo* (Walker & Skopek, 1993), several lines of research have been pursued in a limited fashion (*a*) to assess the hypothesis that adducts that lead to abasic (apurinic/apyrimidinic) sites may contribute to the mutagenesis of ethylene oxide; (*b*) to identify and characterize promutagenic adducts that may account for certain types of mutations induced by ethylene oxide; and (*c*) to evaluate the means by which adducts could cause large deletions and chromosomal alterations produced by ethylene oxide.

As the major DNA adduct of ethylene oxide, 7-HEG is unlikely to be directly promutagenic because *N*7-alkylguanine adducts formed from small epoxides such as ethylene oxide and propylene oxide do not cause distortion of the double helix and do not interfere with hydrogen bonding (Albertini & Sweeney, 2007); rather, *N*7-alkylguanine adducts are hypothesized to result in mutation by loss of the adduct via depurination or the action of DNA glycosylases. The resulting abasic sites are non-coding and may result in base substitutions and strand breaks. The action of apurinic endonuclease creates a single-strand break which, if unresolved, can lead to DNA double-strand breaks and, possibly, chromosomal alterations (Vogel & Natarajan, 1982). Current data suggest that depurination of *N*7-alkylguanine adducts results largely in G→T transversions and, to a lesser extent, G→A transitions and G→C transversions (Loeb & Preston, 1986; Takeshita *et al.*, 1987). Approximately half of the base substitutions at the *Hprt* locus of splenic T cells of mice and rats exposed to ethylene oxide were at A:T base pairs (Walker & Skopek, 1993; Walker *et al.*, 1997b), and it is feasible that these mutations could originate from spontaneous or glycosylase-mediated depurination of 3-HEA and other *N*-hydroxyethyl adducts of adenine/thymine, with subsequent by-pass replication of abasic sites. While chemically induced abasic sites have been found to be important in the mutagenic

mechanisms for only a few exogenous chemicals (Loeb & Preston, 1986), the fact that
> 98% of the DNA adducts produced by ethylene oxide lead to abasic sites denoted the
need to investigate their role in the mutagenesis of this agent (Walker & Skopek, 1993).
In order for these mutagenic events to occur at a rate sufficient to result in ethylene oxide-
induced changes in mutational spectra (including increases in base substitutions and
deletions), accumulation of abasic sites that arise from high levels of 7-HEG would be
expected to occur over time (Rusyn et al., 2005).

A study was recently completed to test the hypothesis that exposure to ethylene oxide
results in the accumulation of abasic sites and induces changes in the expression of genes
for base-excision DNA repair, which predisposes to point mutations and chromosomal
aberrations in Fischer 344 rats exposed by inhalation for 6 h per day on 5 days per week
for 4 weeks to 0 or 100 ppm [183 mg/m^3] ethylene oxide or 0 to 3000 ppm ethylene
(~ 6 ppm ethylene oxide) (Rusyn et al., 2005). The resulting data demonstrated that, while
7-HEG accumulates with repeated exposures, N-hydroxyethylation of DNA by ethylene
oxide is repaired without accumulation of abasic sites, and that the mechanisms proposed
above probably play a minor role in the mutagenicity of this agent. The same conclusions
would apply to the minor accumulation of 3-HEA and other N-hydroxyethyl adducts of
adenine/thymine, and the induction of strand-breaks or point mutations at A:T base pairs
by ethylene oxide.

Several investigators have proposed that the mutagenicity of ethylene oxide may involve the action of minor promutagenic adducts, such as O^6-HEG, $N3$-(2-hydroxyethyl)-
2′-deoxyuridine (3-HEdU) and possibly ring-opened 7-HEG (Solomon, 1999; van Sittert
et al., 2000; Rusyn et al., 2005; Marsden et al., 2007). O^6-HEG is considered to be a
miscoding lesion due to mispairing with thymine during DNA replication (Ellison et al.,
1989); however, this adduct is formed at extremely low levels in vivo in ethylene oxide-
exposed rats (and presumably other species) and is efficiently removed from DNA by the
repair protein O^6-alkylguanine–DNA alkyltransferase and excision repair (Ludeke &
Kleihues, 1988). In addition, only a few G→A mutations were found in p53 exons 6 and
7 of ethylene oxide-induced mammary gland carcinomas (Houle et al., 2006) and these
transitions were not significantly increased in reporter genes of ethylene oxide-exposed
mice and rats. While O^6-HEG may contribute minimally to the mutagenicity of ethylene
oxide in vivo, O^6-alkylguanine adducts are probably important promutagenic lesions for
epoxides with an S_N1 character, such as styrene oxide (Latif et al., 1988; Solomon, 1999).
$N3$-(2-Hydroxyethyl)-2′-cytidine in DNA rapidly deaminates to stable, potentially mutagenic 3-HEdU lesions (Solomon, 1999). This lesion has been shown to block DNA
replication by bacterial polymerases in vitro and to cause G:C→A:T and G:C→T:A base
substitutions (Bhanot et al., 1994; Zhang et al., 1995). In contrast, the formation of
cytosine or uracil adducts has not been shown in rodents exposed to ethylene oxide, and,
if formed, 3-HEdU would be expected to be at very low levels and to contribute to a
minor extent to the mutagenicity of ethylene oxide in vivo. 7-HEG can undergo imidazole
ring-opening to chemically stable, potentially mutagenic lesions (Solomon, 1999).
Formation of ethylene oxide-induced ring-opened 7-HEG has not been demonstrated in

vivo but is worthy of investigation in the future. Exploration of other potential pro-mutagenic adducts of ethylene oxide should not only include site-directed mutagenesis studies to characterize the mutagenic specificity and efficiency of these adducts, but also experiments *in vivo* to demonstrate whether or not these adducts occur at biologically relevant concentrations in ethylene oxide-exposed rodents.

Because exposure to ethylene oxide is associated with cytogenetic effects in humans and induces deletions in human cells *in vitro* and in rodents *in vivo*, it is also essential to determine which DNA adducts and mechanism(s) are responsible for large-scale mutational events. The suspected metabolite of ethylene oxide, glycolaldehyde, has been shown to form DNA–protein crosslinks and single-strand breaks *in vitro* (Hengstler *et al.*, 1994), but no information is available on the formation of this intermediate *in vivo* or its potential effects following exposures to ethylene oxide. The lack of accumulation of abasic sites during repeated high-dose exposures of rats to ethylene oxide (Rusyn *et al.*, 2005) does not favour a mechanism that involves the induction of strand breaks via abasic sites that result from labile DNA adducts (Lindahl, 1979). Another postulated mechanism for ethylene oxide-induced strand scissions is via the formation of a β-hydroxyethyl phosphotriester adduct that requires the interaction of the β-hydroxyethyl group with the phosphate backbone (Agurell *et al.*, 1991). 2-Hydroxyethylation of phosphate groups introduces extreme instability into the sugar–phosphate backbone, since the resultant phosphotriester breaks down through a dioxaphospholane ring intermediate (Eisenbrand *et al.*, 1986). This alternative mechanism for ethylene oxide-induced strand breaks and chromosomal damage deserves further investigation both *in vitro* and *in vivo*.

4.2.4   *Alterations in oncogenes and suppressor genes in tumours*

The ability of ethylene oxide to induce alterations in *ras* proto-oncogenes and the *p53* tumour-suppressor gene has been investigated in immunohistochemical and molecular studies of mutations in control and chemically induced neoplasms of B6C3F$_1$ mice. In the first investigation of spontaneous and ethylene oxide-induced mammary gland carci-nomas, the *p53* and H-*ras* genes were selected for study because they are among the most commonly altered genes in human cancers, mutations in both often occur in the same cancer cell and several lines of evidence support an interaction between these genes during the multistep process of oncogenesis (Houle *et al.*, 2006). Immunohistochemistry results showed that p53 protein expression was detected in 42% (8/19) of spontaneous and 67% (8/12) of ethylene oxide-induced carcinomas. Further semiquantitative evaluations revealed that the protein levels were sixfold higher in cancers from exposed mice than in those from control mice (i.e. the average scores by the 'quickscore method' were 3.83 and 0.63, respectively). Mutations in *p53* exons 5–8 were detected in eight of 12 (67%) ethylene oxide-induced carcinomas; five of the eight mutations had two or more base changes. Fourteen base substitutions were identified, including eight silent muta-tions, five missense mutations and one nonsense mutation; no, four, seven and three mutations occurred in exons 5, 6, 7 and 8, respectively. Nine of 14 alterations (64%)

involved guanine bases, including mutations in codons 241 and 264 that occurred in more than one neoplasm from mice treated with 50 and 100 ppm [91.5 and 183 mg³] ethylene oxide. Ethylene oxide-induced mammary carcinomas exhibited a clear dose-related response in relation to the level of p53 protein expression and the number of *p53* gene mutations. Base substitutions were found in the *p53* gene in 58% (7/12) of spontaneous mammary carcinomas, including five silent mutations, seven missense mutations and one nonsense mutation. However, in contrast to the results seen in the tumours of ethylene oxide-exposed animals, nine of the 13 mutations occurred in exon 5, none was found in exon 6 and seven were C→T transitions. H-*ras* Mutations in codon 61 (bases CAA) were detected in 33% (4/12) and 26% (5/19) of ethylene oxide-induced and spontaneous mammary carcinomas, respectively. All ethylene oxide-induced alterations were missense mutations localized to the second base (or mutations at adenine), whereas 80% (4/5) of spontaneous mutations occurred in the first base of codon 61 (or mutations at cytosine) with the remaining mutation found in the third base of codon 61 (Houle *et al.*, 2006).

Analyses for cancer gene mutations were extended to other target tissues by evaluating the occurrence K-*ras* gene mutations in lung, Harderian gland and uterine neoplasms from ethylene oxide-exposed and control B6C3F₁ mice (Hong *et al.*, 2007). Specifically, the base triplets for codons 12 (GGT), 13 (GGC) and 61 (CAA) were examined for mutations. K-*ras* Gene mutations were identified in 100% (23/23) of the ethylene oxide-induced lung neoplasms and 25% (27/108) of the spontaneous lung neoplasms. Codon 12 mutations were most common in the lung neoplasms from both exposed and control mice; however, 97% (21/23) of the ethylene oxide-induced tumours had a G→T transversion at the second base compared with only one in 108 spontaneous tumours that exhibited this mutation, while 11 spontaneous tumours had a G→A transition in the second base compared with only two ethylene oxide-induced tumours. In Harderian gland neoplasms, 86% (18/21) of ethylene oxide-induced tumours compared with 7% (2/27) of spontaneous tumours contained K-*ras* gene mutations. Codon 13 G→C and codon 12 G→T transversions were the predominant mutations in ethylene oxide-induced Harderian gland neoplasms, but these did not occur in the spontaneous counterparts. Spontaneous uterine carcinomas were not examined, but 83% (5/6) of such neoplasms from ethylene oxide-exposed mice had K-*ras* gene mutations, all of which were codon 13 C→T transitions. Dose-related trends for K-*ras* gene mutations were found for all three cancer types in mice treated with 50 and 100 ppm [91.5 and 183 mg/m³] in the cancer bioassay of ethylene oxide.

These data on *p53* and *ras* gene mutational spectra show distinct differences in the locations and types of base substitutions in spontaneous versus ethylene oxide-induced neoplasms in mice. Futhermore, the profile of K-*ras* gene mutations in ethylene oxide-induced lung and Harderian gland neoplasms was different from that described for other chemically induced tumours of the same tissues, which suggests that ethylene oxide induces a chemical-specific signature for base substitutions (Hong *et al.*, 2007). Based upon the spectra of *p53* and H-*ras* gene mutations in mammary gland neoplasms, Houle *et al.* (2006) suggested that purine bases (guanine and adenine) serve as the primary targets for mutation by ethylene oxide while mutation that involves mostly cytosine appears to be a more common spontaneous event. The larger data set for cancer gene mutations in spontaneous and ethylene oxide-induced neoplasms of the lung, Harderian gland, uterus and mammary gland indicates that ethylene oxide probably increases the mutant fraction for most types of base substitution across proto-oncogenes and tumour-suppressor genes, as was found in the *Hprt* gene of T cells and the *LacI* gene of testes from ethylene oxide-exposed mice. The overall data suggest that a common mechanism for ethylene oxide is as a point mutagen in oncogenes and tumour-suppressor genes of multiple tissues in mice.

4.3   Mechanisms of carcinogenesis

Ethylene oxide is a direct-acting alkylating agent that has been shown to have genotoxic and mutagenic activity in numerous assays in both somatic and germ cells, and in both prokaryotic and eukaryotic organisms (IARC, 1994). It is active in a wide range of in-vitro and in-vivo systems. Increases in both gene mutations and chromosomal alterations, two general classes of cancer-related genetic changes, have been observed. In-vitro and in-vivo studies have shown that ethylene oxide can bind to cellular macromolecules, which results in a variety of DNA, RNA and protein adducts. The major DNA adduct recovered *in vivo* is 7-HEG and additional adducts such as 3-HEA and O^6-HEG are detected at much lower levels (Walker *et al.*, 1992b). In-vitro studies indicate that other minor adducts can also be formed from the reaction of ethylene oxide with the $N1$ and N^6 of adenine and the $N3$ of cytosine, uracil and thymine (IARC, 1994; Tates *et al.*, 1999; Kolman *et al.*, 2002). While the exact mechanism by which these adducts lead to mutation is unknown, a number of mechanisms could be involved, including the mis-pairing of altered bases or the formation of apurinic/apyrimidinic sites via DNA repair or chemical depurination/depyrimidination combined with the insertion of another base, which would typically be an adenine opposite an apurinic site (Tates *et al.*, 1999; Houle *et al.*, 2006). These lesions can also lead to the formation of single-strand breaks and, subsequently, to chromosomal breakage. In addition, the putative ethylene oxide metabolite, glycolaldehyde, has been shown to form DNA–protein cross-links and DNA single-strand breaks (Hengstler *et al.*, 1994).

In-vivo studies using reporter genes such as *Hprt* or the *LacI* transgene have shown that ethylene oxide can significantly increase the frequency of mutations following exposure in both mice and rats (Walker *et al.*, 1993; Sisk *et al.*, 1997; Walker *et al.*, 1997a,b; Tates *et al.*, 1999; Recio *et al.*, 2004). The type of mutation that is recovered appears to be influenced by the assay system involved. In mouse splenic and/or thymic T lymphocytes, mutations in *Hprt* could be detected after shorter exposures (4-week inhalation exposure or multiple intraperitoneal injections over 1 week) and appeared to consist of larger deletion mutations as well as base-pair substitutions and frameshift mutations (Walker *et al.*, 1993, 1997a,b). The latter point mutations appeared to originate primarily from either altered G or altered A bases (Walker *et al.*, 1993; IARC, 1994). In the inhalation study, significant increases in *LacI* mutations were not seen in the spleen, bone marrow or germ cells of mice after 4 weeks of exposure to ethylene oxide (Sisk *et al.*, 1997). A modest but significant increase in *LacI* mutants was seen in the lungs of mice exposed to 200 ppm [366 mg/m^3] ethylene oxide. In a follow-up study with prolonged exposure (up to 48 weeks), significant increases in *LacI* mutants were seen in the bone marrow and testes of ethylene oxide-exposed transgenic mice (Recio *et al.*, 2004). DNA sequence analysis of mutants obtained from the bone marrow showed that only AT→TA transversions were recovered at a significantly increased frequency in the exposed mice. A unique mutational spectrum was not seen in the testes.

Only limited information is available on the mutagenicity of ethylene oxide in humans. A significant increase in *HPRT* mutation frequency was reported in one group of workers with prolonged higher exposures to ethylene oxide (~5 ppm [~ 9.15 mg/m^3] TWA) but not in another group with lower exposure levels (0.025 ppm [0.046 mg/m^3] TWA) (Tates *et al.*, 1991; Kolman *et al.*, 2002).

In two recent studies, an elevated frequency of mutations or a change in mutational spectra has been seen in the tumours of ethylene oxide-treated mice (Houle *et al.*, 2006; Hong *et al.*, 2007). In the Hong *et al.* (2007) study, K-*ras* mutations were detected in 100% (23/23) of ethylene oxide-induced lung tumours compared with 25% (27/108) of spontaneous tumours. Codon 12 G→T transversions occurred frequently in the ethylene oxide-induced lung neoplasms (21/23) but infrequently in spontaneous lung neoplasms (1/108). Similarly, K-*ras* mutations were present in 86% (18/21) of Harderian gland tumours from ethylene oxide-treated animals but were only seen in 7% (2/27) of the spontaneous tumours in this organ. Codon 13 G→C and codon 12 G→T transversions were common in the ethylene oxide-induced but absent in the spontaneous Harderian gland tumours (0/27). K-*ras* Mutations were also seen in 83% (5/6) of ethylene oxide-induced uterine tumours, all of which exhibited a G→C transition in codon 13. The incidence in spontaneous uterine tumours was not reported. A similar study by Houle *et al.* (2006) provided evidence of the involvement of H-*ras* and *p53* mutations in mammary gland tumours induced by ethylene oxide in mice. The mutation frequency was only slightly elevated for H-*ras* (33% in treated versus 26% in spontaneous) or *p53* (67% in the ethylene oxide-treated versus 58% in the control animals), but the mutational spectra of tumours obtained from control and treated animals differed significantly. The mutational spectra were generally consistent with a targeting of G and A bases by ethylene oxide (Houle *et al.*, 2006; Hong *et al.*, 2007). The high frequencies of mutation present in these genes, particularly mutations in the critical codons of K-*ras* and inactivation of *p53*, indicate that mutations are induced in the tumours of ethylene oxide-treated mice and that the changes probably play an important role in ethylene oxide-induced tumorigenesis in these tissues.

Little is known about the mechanisms that might lead to ethylene oxide-induced tumours in humans. However, activating mutations in the *ras* family of oncogenes and inactivation of *p53* have been shown to play critical roles in the development of both spontaneous and chemically induced cancers (Pedersen-Bjergaard *et al.*, 2006; Zarbl,

2006). For example, activating mutations in *ras* genes have been shown to occur in up to 30% of cases of acute myelogenous leukaemia (Byrne & Marshall, 1998). In most cases, N-ras is activated, although activation of K-ras is occasionally seen (Byrne & Marshall, 1998; Bowen *et al.*, 2005; Christiansen *et al.*, 2005). The mutations typically occur in codons 12, 13 and 61, sites that are critical for the normal regulation of ras activity. The activating mutations lead to the generation of constitutively activated ras proteins that cannot be switched off and inappropriately generate proliferative signals within the cell (Byrne & Marshall, 1998). Some patients who lack *ras* mutations still exhibit an overexpression of *ras* genes and this has been considered as further evidence for the involvement of dysregulated ras signalling in leukaemogenesis (Byrne & Marshall, 1998).

Acute myelogenous leukaemia in patients who have previously been treated with alkylating agents frequently exhibits distinctive characteristics that allow it to be distinguished from acute myelogenous leukaemia induced by other agents (such as topoisomerase II inhibitors) or that occurs spontaneously (Pedersen-Bjergaard & Rowley, 1994; Pedersen-Bjergaard *et al.*, 2006). One of the hallmarks of leukaemias induced by alkylating agents is that they frequently exhibit loss of chromosomes 5 or 7 (-5, -7) or loss of part of the long arms of these chromosomes (5q-, 7q-). In addition, mutations in *p53* are frequently seen in leukaemias with the -5/5q- karyotype, and mutations in *p53* and *ras* are seen in a subset of those that exhibit the -7/7q- karyotype (Christiansen *et al.*, 2001; Pedersen-Bjergaard *et al.*, 2006). Although ethylene oxide has not been investigated specifically for its ability to induce losses in chromosomes 7 and 5 or deletions of the long arms of chromosomes 7 and 5 (7q- or 5q-), it has been reported to induce similar types of chromosomal alterations and deletions in a variety of experimental models and/or in the lymphocytes of exposed workers (IARC, 1994; Major *et al.*, 1996, 1999). The detection of elevated levels of chromosomal aberrations and micronuclei in the peripheral blood lymphocytes of ethylene oxide-exposed workers is of particular note, as multiple prospective studies have reported that individuals with increased levels of chromosomal aberrations or micronuclei in these cells are at increased risk for developing cancer (Hagmar *et al.*, 1998; Liou *et al.*, 1999; Smerhovsky *et al.*, 2001; Hagmar *et al.*, 2004; Boffetta *et al.*, 2007; Bonassi *et al.*, 2007).

A comparison of the evidence for ethylene oxide-induced genetic and related changes in experimental animals and humans is summarized in Table 12.

Table 12. Comparison of the evidence for key ethylene oxide-induced genetic and related changes in humans, human cells and experimental animals

End-point	In-vivo exposure		In-vitro exposure
	Animals	Humans	Human cells
Haemoglobin adduct formation	Strong	Strong	Strong
DNA adduct formation	Strong	Weak*	Strong
Mutations in reporter genes in somatic cells	Strong	Weak*	Strong
Mutations in cancer-related genes in tumours	Strong	NI	NA
Increased levels of cancer-related proteins in tumours	Strong	NI	NA
Chromosomal alterations in somatic cells			
Sister chromatid exchange	Strong	Strong	Strong
Structural chromosomal aberrations	Strong+	Strong	Moderate
Micronucleus formation	Strong+	Strong	NI

NA, not applicable; NI, no information
* Possibly due to a lack of adequate studies
+ Positive responses were seen only at exposure concentrations above those used in rodent cancer bioassays.

5. Summary of Data Reported

5.1 Exposure data

Ethylene oxide is a flammable gas. It was first produced in the 1910s by the chlorohydrin process, which has gradually been replaced by the direct oxidation of ethylene since the 1930s. Ethylene oxide is used predominantly for the production of other chemicals, such as ethylene glycols, ethoxylates, ethanol amines and glycol ethers, and its use is increasing. It is also used as a sterilant to treat hospital equipment, disposable medical items, spices and other products. The highest human exposures occur in occupational settings. Historically, 8-h time-weighted average exposures above 20 mg/m³ were common when the chlorohydrin process was used, while average exposures of 2–20 mg/m³ were reported during direct oxidation of ethylene and in plants that produce sterilized medical items. The largest group of exposed workers is hospital personnel who perform sterilization operations. The average levels of exposure in hospitals and production facilities have decreased significantly (on average to below 1 ppm [2 mg/m³]) in western Europe and North America following the introduction of new occupational exposure limits in the mid-1980s. High peak exposures may still occur in some short-term work tasks. Ethylene oxide may occur in indoor air at levels generally < 0.2 mg/m³, probably due to small amounts in tobacco smoke. Ethylene oxide residues have also been detected in some spices and other food products.

5.2   Cancer in humans

Epidemiological evidence of the risk for human cancer from ethylene oxide derives principally from the follow-up of 14 cohorts of exposed workers either in chemical plants where ethylene oxide was produced or converted into derivatives or in facilities where it was used as a sterilant. Data from 10 of the cohorts were collated in a meta-analysis that was published in 1999, but this did not include updates of two cohorts that were published after that time. Many of the cohort members employed at chemical factories were also exposed to other chemicals.

By far the most informative epidemiological investigation was a study by the National Institute of Occupational Safety and Health of more than 18 000 employees at 14 industrial facilities in the USA where ethylene oxide was used to sterilize medical supplies or food spices, or to test the sterilizing equipment. This investigation benefited not only from greater statistical power than other studies (as a consequence of its large size), but also from a lower potential for confounding by concomitant exposure to other chemicals and from incorporation of detailed quantitative assessments of individual exposures to ethylene oxide. For these reasons, the Working Group gave greatest weight to the National Institute for Occupational Safety and Health study when assessing the balance of epidemiological evidence on ethylene oxide, although findings from other studies were also taken into account.

In examining the epidemiological evidence, the Working Group focused in particular on lymphatic and haematopoietic cancers and on cancers of the breast, stomach, pancreas and brain. These sites were selected because excess risks had been suggested by one or more epidemiological study or because tumours at the same site had been reported in rodent bioassays.

Evaluation of the possible risks for lymphatic and haematopoietic cancer was hampered by temporal changes and inconsistencies in the histopathological classification of diagnoses. The interpretation of results for these malignancies was constrained by the diagnostic groupings that had been used by researchers when the studies were conducted and possible errors in the exact specification of tumours on death certificates.

The Working Group found some epidemiological evidence for associations between ethylene oxide and lymphatic and haematopoietic cancers, and specifically lymphoid tumours (i.e. non-Hodgkin lymphoma, multiple myeloma and chronic lymphocytic leukaemia). In the most recent follow-up of the National Institute for Occupational Safety and Health cohort, no overall excess of deaths from non-Hodgkin lymphoma or multiple myeloma was observed in comparison with national death rates. However, in an internal analysis, mortality from lymphoid tumours (as defined above) was associated with measures of cumulative exposure to ethylene oxide among men. No corresponding association was found among women. Other studies did not point consistently to an increase in the risk for non-Hodgkin lymphoma or multiple myeloma in comparisons with external reference populations, although moderate elevations of risk were reported in some investigations.

Early reports of an excess risk for all types of leukaemia combined have not been confirmed by later studies. In the latest analysis of the National Institute for Occupational Safety and Health cohort, mortality from all types of leukaemia combined was close to that expected from national rates. Weak evidence for an exposure–response relationship between cumulative exposure to ethylene oxide and leukaemia was observed in a previous analysis of this cohort. Results from other cohort studies did not point clearly or consistently to an increased risk for leukaemia.

The numbers of cases of Hodgkin lymphoma in published studies were too few to draw meaningful conclusions.

Four of the cohort studies provided useful information on the association between exposure to ethylene oxide and breast cancer. The National Institute for Occupational Safety and Health study and a cohort study of hospital sterilization workers in the United Kingdom examined mortality from breast cancer and found no overall excess risk. Three studies examined the incidence of breast cancer: the National Institute for Occupational Safety and Health study and a cohort study from Sweden found no overall excess risk for breast cancer, while another cohort study from New York State, USA, found a borderline significant excess risk of about 60%. Cancer incidence was recognized to be underestimated in the National Institute for Occupational Safety and Health study, which was thus negatively biased for the investigation of overall cancer incidence.

A study conducted within the National Institute for Occupational Safety and Health cohort was designed to investigate the association between exposure to ethylene oxide and the risk for breast cancer in greater detail. Internal analyses in this study found increased relative risks for breast cancer in the higher categories of cumulative exposure to ethylene oxide and a significant exposure–response relationship, both of which persisted in analyses that controlled for parity and history of breast cancer in a first-degree relative. The risk for the highest category of cumulative exposure was almost doubled.

While early epidemiological studies had suggested increased risks for stomach and pancreatic cancer in workers exposed to ethylene oxide, these findings were not supported by more recent, larger studies (including the National Institute for Occupational Safety and Health investigation); nor did the balance of epidemiological evidence point to an increased risk for brain cancer in humans exposed to ethylene oxide.

5.3   Cancer in experimental animals

Ethylene oxide was tested for carcinogenicity in one experiment by intragastric intubation in female rats, by inhalation in female mice in one experiment and in both sexes of mice in another experiment, by inhalation in both sexes of rats in one experiment and in male rats of the same strain in another experiment. It was also tested in single studies in female mice by skin application and by subcutaneous injection.

In the experiment of intragastric intubation in female rats, ethylene oxide produced tumours of the forestomach, which were mainly squamous-cell carcinomas. In one study in both sexes of mice, inhalation of ethylene oxide resulted in increases in the incidence of alveolar/bronchiolar lung tumours and tumours of the Harderian gland in animals of each sex and of uterine adenocarcinomas, mammary carcinomas and malignant lymphomas in females. In a pulmonary tumour bioassay in female strain A/J mice, inhalation of ethylene oxide increased the number of pulmonary adenomas per mouse. In both experiments in which male and female rats of one strain were exposed by inhalation, ethylene oxide increased the incidence of mononuclear-cell leukaemia and brain tumours in animals of each sex and of peritoneal mesotheliomas in the region of the testis and subcutaneous fibromas in males. Ethylene oxide produced local sarcomas in female mice following subcutaneous injection. In a limited study in female mice treated by skin application, no skin tumours were observed.

5.4   Mechanistic and other relevant data

Inhaled ethylene oxide is readily taken up by the lungs, is absorbed efficiently into the blood and is systemically distributed in rodents and in humans. Ethylene oxide is converted by both enzymatic and non-enzymatic hydrolysis to ethylene glycol, which is excreted or further metabolized, and by conjugation with glutathione mediated by the polymorphic glutathione-S-transferase T1. Glycolaldehyde, which is potentially formed by further metabolism of ethylene glycol, can cause DNA–protein crosslinks and DNA strand breaks. A striking difference in the metabolism of ethylene oxide between rodents and humans is the predominance of the glutathione conjugation pathway in mice and rats, while the pathway initiated by enzymatic and non-enzymatic hydrolysis is of greater importance in humans. Simulations indicated that, in mice, rats and humans, about 80%, 60% and 20%, respectively, would be metabolized via glutathione conjugation. Despite these differences, physiologically based pharmacokinetic models of uptake and metabolism of ethylene oxide in the range of exposures used in rodent bioassays (100 ppm [180 mg/m^3] and below) yielded simulated blood peak concentrations and areas under the curve that were similar for mice, rats and humans.

Ethylene oxide is a direct-acting alkylating agent that forms adducts with proteins and DNA. Haemoglobin adducts have been used for biomonitoring purposes, in view of the significant correlation between cumulative exposure over 4 months (the lifespan of human erythrocytes) and levels of adducts in the haemoglobin of ethylene oxide-exposed workers. Endogenous hydroxyethyl adducts of haemoglobin and DNA are also found in both humans and experimental animals in the absence of known exogenous exposure to ethylene oxide. N7-Hydroxyethylguanine is quantitatively the major DNA adduct formed, but does not appear to be directly promutagenic. Minor promutagenic adducts proposed for ethylene oxide are either induced at very low levels or have not been shown to occur in humans or experimental animals.

Studies of workers exposed to ethylene oxide in hospital and factory sterilization units and in ethylene oxide manufacturing and processing plants have been fairly consistent in showing chromosomal damage in peripheral blood lymphocytes, which included sister chromatid exchange in 21 of 33 study groups, chromosomal aberrations in 18 of 24 study groups and micronucleus formation in four of 18 study groups. In ethylene oxide-exposed workers, the frequency of micronucleus formation was also elevated in the bone marrow in one study and in nasal mucosal cells in another study, but not in exfoliated buccal cells in two studies. In general, the degree of chromosomal damage was correlated with level and duration of exposure, and the majority of positive results were found in studies that evaluated individuals who were exposed to time-weighted average concentrations greater than 5 ppm [9 mg/m^3] ethylene oxide. Elevated levels of chromosomal aberrations and micronucleus formation in peripheral blood lymphocytes have been associated with increased risks for cancer in humans. One study suggested an elevation in gene mutations in one of two groups of ethylene oxide-exposed workers. Several other biomarkers of DNA damage, which include unscheduled DNA synthesis, DNA single-strand breaks, premature centromere divisions and DNA–protein crosslinks, have been studied by only a few investigators.

Collectively, the genotoxicity data in experimental systems consistently demonstrate that ethylene oxide is a mutagen and clastogen across all phylogenetic levels tested. Ethylene oxide induced unscheduled DNA synthesis, DNA strand breaks, gene mutation, sister chromatid exchange and chromosomal aberrations in cultured human cells, as well as mutations, chromosomal aberrations, micronucleus formation and cell transformation in rodent cells *in vitro*. It also induced gene mutation, specific locus mutation, sister chromatid exchange, chromosomal aberrations, micronucleus formation, dominant lethal mutation and heritable translocation in somatic and/or germ cells in rodents treated *in vivo*. Analogous genetic and related effects of ethylene oxide were observed in non-mammalian systems. Unequivocal data show that ethylene oxide caused dose-related increases in point mutations in both reporter genes and cancer genes of multiple tissues from mice and rats exposed to 25–200 ppm [45–360 mg/m^3] ethylene oxide, doses that encompassed all but the lowest concentration used in rodent cancer bioassays. In these in-vivo studies, ethylene oxide was consistently a relatively weak point mutagen. Ethylene oxide induced sister chromatid exchange but not chromosomal aberrations or micronucleus formation in rodents exposed by inhalation to concentrations that were used in carcinogenicity studies. In contrast, assays for the potential clastogenic effects of inhalation of this concentration range of ethylene oxide by rodents have not been performed uniformly in an optimal fashion. Rodent studies that were positive for clastogenicity following exposure to higher doses of ethylene oxide or via a less relevant route of exposure may also be informative for a risk for chromosomal events under some exposure scenarios in ethylene oxide-exposed humans. With regard to the mode of action of ethylene oxide as a genotoxic carcinogen in rodents, there is clear evidence that point mutations in *ras* proto-oncogenes and the *p53* tumour-suppressor gene (which are involved in a range of human cancers) are key events in the development of cancers, but the role of chromosomal alterations as primary mutational events in the carcinogenicity of ethylene oxide in mice and rats is still uncertain.

6. Evaluation and Rationale

6.1 Carcinogenicity in humans

There is *limited evidence* in humans for the carcinogenicity of ethylene oxide.

6.2 Carcinogenicity in experimental animals

There is *sufficient evidence* in experimental animals for the carcinogenicity of ethylene oxide.

6.3 Overall evaluation

Ethylene oxide is *carcinogenic to humans (Group 1)*.

6.4 Rationale

In making the overall evaluation, the Working Group also took into consideration the following supporting evidence:

(*a*) Ethylene oxide is a direct-acting alkylating agent that reacts with DNA.

(*b*) Ethylene oxide induces a dose-related increase in the frequency of ethylene oxide-derived haemoglobin adducts in exposed humans and rodents.

(*c*) Ethylene oxide induces a dose-related increase in the frequency of ethylene oxide-derived DNA adducts in exposed rodents.

(*d*) Ethylene oxide consistently acts as a mutagen and clastogen at all phylogenetic levels.

(*e*) Ethylene oxide induces heritable translocations in the germ cells of exposed rodents.

(*f*) Ethylene oxide induces a dose-related increase in the frequency of sister chromatid exchange, chromosomal aberrations and micronucleus formation in the lymphocytes of exposed workers.

(*g*) Prospective studies have shown that elevated levels of chromosomal aberrations and micronucleus formation in peripheral blood lymphocytes are associated with increased risks for cancer in humans.

7.   References

ACGIH® Worldwide (2005) *Documentation of the TLVs® and BEIs® with Other Worldwide Occupational Exposure Values — 2005 CD ROM,* Cincinnati, OH, American Conference of Governmental Industrial Hygienists

Adkins, B., Jr, Van Stee, E.W., Simmons, J.E. & Eustis, S.L. (1986) Oncogenic response of strain A/J mice to inhaled chemicals. *J. Toxicol. environ. Health*, **17**, 311–322

Agurell, E., Cederberg, H., Ehrenberg, L., Lindahl-Kiessling, K., Rannug, U. & Törnqvist, M. (1991) Genotoxic effects of ethylene oxide and propylene oxide: A comparative study. *Mutat. Res.*, **250**, 229–237

Albertini, R.A. & Sweeney, L.M. (2007) Propylene oxide: Genotoxicity profile of a rodent nasal carcinogen. *Crit. Rev. Toxicol.*, **37**, 489–520

Allied Signal Chemicals (1993) *Ethylene Oxide*, Morristown, NJ

Ambroise, D., Moulin, J.-J., Squinazi, F., Protois, J.-C., Fontana, J.-M. & Wild, P. (2005) Cancer mortality among municipal pest-control workers. *Int. Arch. occup. environ. Health,* **78**, 387–393

Anon. (2004) Product focus — EO-EG, *Chem. Week*, **April 28**, 38

Anon. (2005) Chemical profile: Ethylene oxide. *Eur. chem. News,* **25 July** (electronic archive)

Appelgren, L.-E., Eneroth, G. & Grant, C. (1977) Studies on ethylene oxide: Whole-body auto-radiography and dominant lethal test in mice. *Proc. Eur. Soc. Toxicol.*, **18**, 315–317

Appelgren, L.-E., Eneroth, G., Grant, C., Landström, L.-E. & Tenghagen, K. (1978) Testing of ethylene oxide for mutagenicity using the micronucleus test in mice and rats. *Acta pharmacol. toxicol.*, **43**, 69–71

Arms, A.D. & Travis, C.C. (1988) *Reference Physiological Parameters in Pharmacokinetic Modeling* (Report No EPA 600 6-88/004), Washington DC, US Environmental Protection Agency.

Bailey, E., Farmer, P.B. & Shuker, D.E.G. (1987) Estimation of exposure to alkylating carcinogens by the GC–MS determination of adducts to hemoglobin and nucleic acid bases in urine. *Arch. Toxicol.*, **60**, 187–191

Bastlová, T., Andersson, B., Lambert, B. & Kolman, A. (1993) Molecular analysis of ethylene oxide-induced mutations at the HPRT locus in human diploid fibroblasts. *Mutat. Res.*, **287**, 283–292

Baumbach, N., Herzog, V. & Schiller, F. (1987) [In vitro studies on the permeation of ethylene oxide through human skin]. *Dermatol. Monatsschr.*, **173**, 328–332 (in German)

Benson, L.O. & Teta, M.J. (1993) Mortality due to pancreatic and lymphopoietic cancers in chlorohydrin production workers. *Br. J. ind. Med.*, **50**, 710–716

Bhanot, O.S., Singh, U.S. & Solomon, J.J. (1994) The role of 3-hydroxethyluridine in mutagenesis by ethylene oxide. *J. biol. Chem.*, **269**, 30056–30064

Bisanti, L., Maggini, M., Raschetti, R., Alegiani, S.S., Ippolito, F.M., Caffari, B., Segnan, N. & Ponti, A. (1993) Cancer mortality in ethylene oxide workers. *Br. J. ind. Med.*, **50**, 317–324

Boeniger, M. (1988a) *Health Hazard Evaluation Report, University of Cincinnati Hospital, Cincinnati, OH* (Report No. HETA 86-508), Cincinnati, OH, National Institute for Occupational Safety and Health

Boeniger, M. (1988b) *Health Hazard Evaluation Report, Humana Audubon Hospital, Louisville, KY* (Report No. HETA 87-378), Cincinnati, OH, National Institute for Occupational Safety and Health

Boffetta, P., van der Hel, O., Norppa, H., Fabianova, E., Fucic, A., Gundy, S., Lazutka, J., Cebulska-Wasilewska, A., Puskailerova, D., Znaor, A., Kelecsenyi, Z., Kurtinaitis, J., Rachtan, J., Forni, A., Vermeulen, R. & Bonassi, S. (2007) Chromosomal aberrations and cancer risk: Results of a cohort study from Central Europe. *Am. J. Epidemiol.*, **165**, 36–43

Bolt, H.M. (1996) Quantification of endogenous carcinogens: The ethylene oxide paradox. *Biochem. Pharmacol.*, **52**,1–5

Bolt, H.M. & Filser, J.G. (1987) Kinetics and disposition in toxicology. Example: Carcinogenic risk estimate for ethylene. *Arch. Toxicol.*, **60**, 73–76

Bolt, H.M. & Leutbecher, M. (1993) Dose–DNA adduct relationship for ethylene oxide. *Arch. Toxicol.*, **67**, 712–713

Bolt, H.M. & Thier, R. (2006) Relevance of the deletion polymorphisms of the glutathione S-transferases GSTT1 and GSTM1 in pharmacology and toxicology. *Curr. Drug Metab.*, **7**, 613–628

Bolt, H.M., Peter, H. & Föst, U. (1988) Analysis of macromolecular ethylene oxide adducts. *Int. Arch. occup. environ. Health*, **60**, 141–144

Bonassi, S., Znaor, A., Ceppi, M., Lando, C., Chang, W.P., Holland, N., Kirsch-Volders, M., Zeiger, E., Ban, S., Barale, R., Bigatti, M.P., Bolognesi, C., Cebulska-Wasilewska, A., Fabianova, E., Fucic, A., Hagmar, L., Joksic, G., Martelli, A., Migliore, L., Mirkova, E., Scarfi, M.R., Zijno, A., Norppa, H. & Fenech, M. (2007) An increased micronucleus frequency in peripheral blood lymphocytes predicts the risk of cancer in humans. *Carcinogenesis*, **28**, 625–631

Bono, R., Vincenti, M., Saglia, U., Pignata, C., Russo, R., & Gilli, G. (2002) Tobacco smoke and formation of N-(2-hydroxyethyl)valine in human hemoglobin. *Arch. environ. Health*, **57**, 416–421

Bowen, D.T., Frew, M.E., Hills, R., Gale, R.E., Wheatley, K., Groves, M.J., Langabeer, S.E., Kottaridis, P.D., Moorman, A.V., Burnett, A.K. & Linch, D.C. (2005) RAS mutation in acute myeloid leukemia is associated with distinct cytogenetic subgroups but does not influence outcome in patients younger than 60 years. *Blood*, **106**, 2113–2119

Brown, C.D., Wong, B.A. & Fennell, T.R. (1996) In vivo and in vitro kinetics of ethylene oxide metabolism in rats and mice. *Toxicol. appl. Pharmacol.*, **136**, 8–19

Brown, C.D., Asgharian, B., Turner, M.J. & Fennell, T.R. (1998) Ethylene oxide dosimetry in the mouse. *Toxicol. appl. Pharmacol.*, **148**, 215–221

Brugnone, F., Perbellini, L., Faccini, G. & Pasini, F. (1985) Concentration of ethylene oxide in the alveolar air of occupationally exposed workers. *Am. J. ind. Med.*, **8**, 67–72

Brugnone, F., Perbellini, L., Faccini, G.B., Pasini, F., Bartolucci, G.B. & DeRosa, E. (1986) Ethylene oxide exposure. Biological monitoring by analysis of alveolar air and blood. *Int. Arch. occup. environ. Health*, **58**, 105–112

Burgaz, S., Rezanko, R., Kara, S. & Karakaya, A.E. (1992) Thioethers in urine of sterilization personnel exposed to ethylene oxide. *J. clin. pharm. Ther.*, **17**, 169–172

Byrne, J.L. & Marshall, C.J. (1998) The molecular pathophysiology of myeloid leukaemias: Ras revisited. *Br. J. Haematol.*, **100**, 256–264

Calleman, C.J., Ehrenberg, L., Jansson, B., Osterman-Golkar, S., Segerbäck, D., Svensson, K. & Wachtmeister, C.A. (1978) Monitoring and risk assessment by means of alkyl groups in hemoglobin in persons occupationally exposed to ethylene oxide. *J. environ. Pathol. Toxicol.*, **2**, 427–442

Chessor, E., Verhoeven, M., Hon, C.-Y. & Teschke, K. (2005) Evaluation of a modified scavenging system to reduce occupational exposure to nitrous oxide in labor and delivery rooms. *J. occup. environ. Hyg.*, **2**, 314–322

Chien, Y.C., Liu, H.H., Lin Y.C., Su, P.C., Li, L.H., Chang, C.P. Dang, D.T. & Chen C.Y. (2007) Ethylene oxide sterilization in the medical-supply manufacturing industry: Assessment and control of worker exposure. *J. biomed. Mat. Res. B, appl. Biomat.*, **83**, 527–537

Christiansen, D.H., Andersen, M.K. & Pedersen-Bjergaard, J. (2001) Mutations with loss of heterozygosity of p53 are common in therapy-related myelodysplasia and acute myeloid leukemia after exposure to alkylating agents and significantly associated with deletion or loss of 5q, a complex karyotype, and a poor prognosis. *J. clin. Oncol.*, **19**, 1405–1413

Christiansen, D.H., Andersen, M.K., Desta, F. & Pedersen-Bjergaard, J. (2005) Mutations of genes in the receptor tyrosine kinase (RTK)/RAS-BRAF signal transduction pathway in therapy-related myelodysplasia and acute myeloid leukemia. *Leukemia*, **19**, 2232–2240

Clare, M.G., Dean, B.J., de Jong, G. & van Sittert, N.J. (1985) Chromosome analysis of lymphocytes from workers at an ethylene oxide plant. *Mutat. Res.*, **156**, 109–116

Coggon, D., Harris, E.C., Poole, J. & Palmer, K.T. (2004) Mortality of workers exposed to ethylene oxide: Extended follow up of a British cohort. *Occup. environ. Med.*, **61**, 358–362

Csanády, G.A., Denk, B., Pütz, C., Kreuzer, P.E., Kessler, W., Baur, C., Gargas, M.L. & Filser, J.G. (2000) A physiological toxicokinetic model for exogenous and endogenous ethylene and ethylene oxide in rat, mouse, and human: Formation of 2-hydroxyethyl adducts with hemoglobin and DNA. *Toxicol. appl. Pharmacol.*, **165**, 1–26

Cummins, K.J., Schultz, G.R., Lee, J.S., Nelson, J.H. & Reading, J.C. (1987) The development and evaluation of a hydrobromic acid-coated sampling tube for measuring occupational exposures to ethylene oxide. *Am. ind. Hyg. Assoc. J.*, **48**, 563–573

Currier, M.F., Carlo, G.L., Poston, P.L. & Ledford, W.E. (1984) A cross sectional study of employees with potential occupational exposure to ethylene oxide. *Br. J. ind. Med.*, **41**, 492–498

Dahlgran, J.R. & Shingleton, C.R. (1987) Determination of ethylene oxide in ethoxylated surfactants and demulsifiers by headspace gas chromatography. *J. Assoc. off. anal. Chem.*, **70**, 796–798

Daniel, G., Hoffman, W. & McDonald, B. (2004) OSHA compliance issues: Ethylene oxide in a commercial sterilization operation. *J. occup. environ. Hyg.*, **1**, D121–D125

Danielson, J.W., Snell, R.P. & Oxborrow, G.S. (1990) Detection and quantitation of ethylene oxide, 2-chloroethanol, and ethylene glycol with capillary gas chromatography. *J. chromatogr. Sci.*, **28**, 97–101

Dellarco, V.L., Generoso, W.M., Sega, G.A., Fowle, J.R., III & Jacobson-Kram, D. (1990) Review of the mutagenicity of ethylene oxide. *Environ. mol. Mutag.*, **16**, 85–103

Denk, B., Filser, J.G., Oesterle, D., Deml, E. & Greim, H. (1988) Inhaled ethylene oxide induces preneoplastic foci in rat liver. *J. Cancer Res. clin. Oncol.*, **114**, 35–38

Deschamps, D., Laurent, A.-M., Festy, B. & Conso, F. (1989) [Study of six ethylene oxide sterilization units in the Poor Law Administration of Paris.] *Arch. Mal. prof.*, **50**, 641–649 (in French)

Devanney, M.T. (2007) *CEH Marketing Research Report – Ethylene Oxide* (Abstract), Zürich, SRI Consulting [available at http://www.sriconsulting.com/CEH/Public/Reports/654.5000/ accessed 26.02.2008]

Dever, J.P., George, K.F., Hoffman, W.C. & Soo, H. (2004) Ethylene oxide. In: Kroschwitz, J.I. & Howe-Grant, M., eds, *Kirk Othmer Encyclopedia of Chemical Technology*, Vol. 10, New York, John Wiley & Sons, pp. 632–673 (on line)

Dunkelberg, H. (1981) [Carcinogenic activity of ethylene oxide and its reaction products 2-chloro-ethanol, 2-bromoethanol, ethylene glycol and diethylene glycol. I. Carcinogenicity of ethylene oxide in comparison with 1,2-propylene oxide after subcutaneous administration in mice.] *Zbl. Bakt. Hyg. I. Abt. Orig. B*, **174**, 383–404 (in German)

Dunkelberg, H. (1982) Carcinogenicity of ethylene oxide and 1,2-propylene oxide upon intragastric administration to rats. *Br. J. Cancer*, **46**, 924–933

Ehrenberg, L. (1991) Detection and measurement of protein adducts: Aspects of risk assessment. *Prog. clin. biol. Res.*, **372**, 79–87

Ehrenberg, L. & Törnqvist, M. (1992) Use of biomarkers in epidemiology: Quantitative aspects. *Toxicol. Lett.*, **64–65**, 485–492

Ehrenberg, L., Hiesche, K.D., Osterman-Golkar, S. & Wennberg, I. (1974) Evaluation of genetic risks of alkylating agents: Tissue doses in the mouse from air contaminated with ethylene oxide. *Mutat. Res.*, **24**, 83–103

Eide, I., Hagemann, R., Zahlsen, K., Tabreke, E., Törnqvist, M., Kumar, R., Vodicka, P. & Hemminki, K. (1995) Uptake, distribution, and formation of hemoglobin and DNA adducts after inhalation of C2–C8 1-alkenes (olefins) in the rat. *Carcinogenesis*, **16**, 1603–1609

Eide, I, Zhao, C., Kumar, R., Hemminki, K., Wu, K.-Y. & Swenberg, J.A. (1999) Comparison of ^{32}P-postlabeling and high-resolution GC/MS in quantifying N7-(2-hydroxyethyl)guanine adducts. *Chem. Res. Toxicol.*, **12**, 979–984

Eisenbrand, G., Muller, N., Denkel, E. & Sterzel, W. (1986) DNA adducts and DNA damage by antineoplastic and carcinogenic N-nitrosocompounds. *J. Cancer Res. clin. Oncol.*, **112**, 196–204

Elliott, L.J., Ringenburg, V.L., Morelli-Schroth, P., Halperin, W.E. & Herrick, R.F. (1988) Ethylene oxide exposures in hospitals. *Appl. ind. Hyg.*, **3**, 141–145

Ellison, K.S., Dogliotti, E., Connors, T.D., Basu, A.K. & Essigmann, J.M. (1989) Site-specific mutagenesis by O^6-alkylguanines located in the chromosomes of mammalian cells: Influence of the mammalian O^6-alkylguanine–DNA alkyltransferase. *Proc. natl Acad. Sci. USA*, **86**, 8620–8624

Embree, J.W., Lyon, J.P. & Hine, C.H. (1977) The mutagenic potential of ethylene oxide using the dominant-lethal assay in rats. *Toxicol. appl. Pharmacol.*, **40**, 261–267

Environmental Protection Agency (1992a) Ethylene oxide; tolerances for residues. *US Code fed. Regul.*, **Title 40**, Part 180.151, p. 311

Environmental Protection Agency (1992b) Ethylene oxide. *US Code fed. Regul.*, **Title 40**, Part 185.2850, p. 456

Environmental Protection Agency (2000) *Control of Emissions of Hazardous Air Pollutants from Motor Vehicles and Motor Vehicle Fuels. EPA Technical Support Document* (EPA 420-R-00-023), Washington DC

Farmer, P.B. & Shuker, D.E.G. (1999) What is the significance of increases in background levels of carcinogen-derived protein and DNA adducts? Some considerations for incremental risk assessment. *Mutat. Res.*, **424**, 275–286

Farmer, P.B., Bailey, E., Gorf, S.M., Törnqvist, M., Osterman-Golkar, S., Kautiainen, A. & Lewis-Enright, D.P. (1986) Monitoring human exposure to ethylene oxide by the determination of haemoglobin adducts using gas chromatography–mass spectrometry. *Carcinogenesis*, **7**, 637–640

Farmer, P.B., Neumann, H.G., & Henschler, D. (1987) Estimation of exposure of man to substances reacting covalently with macromolecules. *Arch Toxicol.*, **60**, 251–260

Farmer, P.B., Cordero, R., & Autrup, H. (1996a) Monitoring human exposure to 2-hydroxy-ethylating carcinogens. *Environ Health Perspect.*, **104**, 449–452

Farmer, P.B., Sepai, O., Lawrence, R., Autrup, H., Sabro Nielsen, P., Vestergard, A.B., Waters, R., Leuratti, C., Jones, N.J., Stone, J., Baan, R.A., van Delft, J.H., Steenwinkel, M.J., Kyrtopoulos, S.A., Souliotis, V.L., Theodorakopoulos, N., Bacalis, N.C., Natarajan, A.T., Tates, A.D., Haugen, A., Andreassen, A., Ovrebo, S., Shuker, D.E., Amaning, K.S., Schouft, A., Ellul, A., Garner, R.C., Dingley, K.H., Abbondandolo, A.A., Merlo, F., Cole, J., Aldrich, K., Beare, D., Capulas, E., Rowley, G., Waugh, A.P.W., Povey, A.C., Haque, K., Kirsch-Volders, M., van Hummelen, P. & Castelain, P. (1996b) Biomonitoring human exposure to environmental carcinogenic chemicals. *Mutagenesis*, **11**, 363–381

Farooqi, Z., Tornqvist, M., Ehrenberg, L. & Natarajan, A.T. (1993) Genotoxic effects of ethylene oxide and propylene oxide in mouse bone marrow cells. *Mutat. Res.*, **288**, 223–228

Fennell, T.R. & Brown, C.D. (2001) A physiologically based pharmacokinetic model for ethylene oxide in mouse, rat, and human. *Toxicol. appl. Pharmacol.*, **173**, 161–175

Fennell, T.R., Sumner, S.C. & Walker, V.E. (1992) A model for the formation and removal of hemoglobin adducts. *Cancer Epidemiol. Biomarkers Prev.*, **1**, 213–219

Fennell, T.R., MacNeela, J.P., Morris, R.W., Watson, M., Thompson, C.L. & Bell, D.A. (2000) Hemoglobin adducts from acrylonitrile and ethylene oxide in cigarette smokers: Effects of glutathione S-transferase T1-null and M1-null genotypes. *Cancer Epidemiol. Biomarkers Prev.*, **9**, 705–712

Filser, J.G. (1992) The closed chamber technique-uptake, endogenous production, excretion, steady-state kinetics and rates of metabolism of gases and vapors. *Arch. Toxicol.*, **66**, 1–10

Filser, J.G. & Bolt, H.M. (1984) Inhalation pharmacokinetics based on gas uptake studies. VI. Comparative evaluation of ethylene oxide and butadiene monoxide as exhaled reactive metabolites of ethylene and 1,3-butadiene in rats. *Arch. Toxicol.*, **55**, 219–223

Filser, J.G., Denk, B., Törnqvist, M., Kessler, W. & Ehrenberg, L. (1992) Pharmacokinetics of ethylene in man; body burden with ethylene oxide and hydroxyethylation of hemoglobin due to endogenous and environmental ethylene. *Arch. Toxicol.*, **66**, 157–163

Filser, J.G., Schwegler, U., Csanády, G.A., Greim, H., Kreuzer, P.E. & Kessler, W. (1993) Species-specific pharmacokinetics of styrene in rat and mouse. *Arch. Toxicol.*, **67**, 517–530

Filser, J.G., Kreuzer, P.E., Greim, H. & Bolt H.M. (1994) New scientific arguments for regulation of ethylene oxide residues in skin-care products. *Arch. Toxicol.*, **68**, 401–405

Flores, G.H. (1983) Controlling exposure to alkylene oxides. *Chem. Eng. News*, **79**, 39–43

Föst, U., Marczynsk, B., Kasemann, R. & Peter, H. (1989) Determination of 7-(2-hydroxy-ethyl)guanine with gas chromatography/mass spectrometry as a parameter for genotoxicity of ethylene oxide. *Arch. Toxicol.*, **Suppl. 13**, 250–253

Föst, U., Hallier, E., Ottenwälder, H., Bolt, H.M. & Peter, H. (1991) Distribution of ethylene oxide in human blood and its implications for biomonitoring. *Hum. exp. Toxicol.*, **10**, 25–31

Föst, U., Törnqvist, M., Leutbecher, M., Granath, F., Hallier, E., & Ehrenberg, L. (1995) Effects of variation in detoxification rate on dose monitoring through adducts. *Hum. exp. Toxicol.*, **14**, 201–203

Fowles, J., Mitchell, J. & McGrath, H. (2001) Assessment of cancer risk from ethylene oxide residues in spices imported into New Zealand. *Food. chem. Toxicol.*, **39**, 1055–1062

Fuchs, J., Wullenweber, U., Hengstler, J.G., Bienfait, H.G., Hiltl, G. & Oesch. F. (1994) Genotoxic risk for humans due to work place exposure to ethylene oxide: Remarkable individual differences in susceptibility. *Arch. Toxicol.*, **68**, 343–348

Galloway, S.M., Berry, P.K., Nichols, W.W., Wolman, S.R., Soper, K.A., Stolley, P.D. & Archer, P. (1986) Chromosome aberrations in individuals occupationally exposed to ethylene oxide and in a large control population. *Mutat. Res.*, **170**, 55–74

Gardner, M.J., Coggon, D., Pannett, B. & Harris, E.C. (1989) Workers exposed to ethylene oxide: A follow up study. *Br. J. ind. Med.*, **46**, 860–865

Garman, R.H., Snellings, W.M. & Maronpot, R.R. (1985) Brain tumors in F344 rats associated with chronic inhalation exposure to ethylene oxide. *Neurotoxicology*, **6**, 117–138

Garman, R.H., Snellings, W.M. & Maronpot, R.R. (1986) Frequency, size and location of brain tumours in F-344 rats chronically exposed to ethylene oxide. *Food chem. Toxicol.*, **24**, 145–153

Garry, V.F., Hozier, J., Jacobs, D., Wade, R.L. & Gray, D.G. (1979) Ethylene oxide: Evidence of human chromosomal effects. *Environ. Mutag.*, **1**, 375–382

Garry, V.F., Opp, C.W., Wiencke, J.K. & Lakatua, D. (1982) Ethylene oxide induced sister chromatid exchange in human lymphocytes using a membrane dosimetry system. *Pharmacology*, **25**, 214–221

Generoso, W.M., Cain, K.T., Krishna, M., Sheu, C.W. & Gryder, R.M. (1980) Heritable translocation and dominant-lethal mutation induction with ethylene oxide in mice. *Mutat. Res.*, **73**, 133–142

Generoso, W.M., Cumming, R.B., Bandy, J.A. & Cain, K.T. (1983) Increased dominant-lethal effects due to prolonged exposure of mice to inhaled ethylene oxide. *Mutat. Res.*, **119**, 377–379

Generoso, W.M., Cain, K.T., Hughes, L.A., Sega, G.A., Braden, P.W., Gosslee, D.G. & Shelby, M.D. (1986) Ethylene oxide dose and dose-rate effects in the mouse dominant-lethal test. *Environ. Mutag.*, **8**, 1–7

Generoso, W.M., Cain, K.T., Cornett, C.V., Cacheiro, N.L.A. & Hughes, L.A. (1990) Concentration–response curves for ethylene-oxide-induced heritable translocations and dominant lethal mutations. *Environ. mol. Mutag.*, **16**, 126–131

Gérin, M. & Tardif, R. (1986) Urinary N-acetyl-S-2-hydroxyethyl-L-cysteine in rats as biological indicator of ethylene oxide exposure. *Fundam. appl. Toxicol.*, **7**, 419–423

Glaser, Z.R. (1979) Ethylene oxide: Toxicology review and field study results of hospital use. *J. environ. Pathol. Toxicol.*, **12**, 173–208

Godderis, L., Aka, P., Mateuca, R., Kirsch-Volders, M., Lison, D. & Veulemans, H. (2006) Dose-dependent influence of genetic polymorphisms on DNA damage induced by styrene oxide, ethylene oxide and gamma-radiation. *Toxicology*, **219**, 220–229

Golberg, L. (1986) *Hazard Assessment of Ethylene Oxide*, Boca Raton, FL, CRC Press, pp. 3–7

Greenberg, H.L., Ott, M.G. & Shore, R.E. (1990) Men assigned to ethylene oxide production or other ethylene oxide related chemical manufacturing: A mortality study. *Br. J. ind. Med.*, **47**, 221–230

Greife, A.L., Hornung, R.W., Stayner, L.G. & Steenland, K.N. (1988) Development of a model for use in estimating exposure to ethylene oxide in a retrospective cohort mortality study. *Scand. J. Work Environ. Health*, **14** (Suppl. 1), 29–30

Hagmar, L., Welinder, H., Lindén, K., Attewell, R., Osterman-Golkar, S. & Törnqvist, M. (1991) An epidemiological study of cancer risk among workers exposed to ethylene oxide using hemoglobin adducts to validate environmental exposure assessments. *Int. Arch. occup. environ. Health*, **63**, 271–277

Hagmar, L., Mikoczy, Z. & Welinder, H. (1995) Cancer incidence in Swedish sterilant workers exposed to ethylene oxide. *Occup. environ. Med.*, **52**, 154–156

Hagmar, L., Bonassi, S., Strömberg, U., Brogger, A., Knudsen, L.E., Norppa, H. & Reuterwall, C. (1998) Chromosomal aberrations in lymphocytes predict human cancer: A report from the European Study Group on Cytogenetic Biomarkers and Health (ESCH). *Cancer Res.*, **58**, 4117–4121

Hagmar, L., Strömberg, U., Bonassi, S., Hansteen, I.L., Knudsen, L.E., Lindholm, C. & Norppa, H. (2004) Impact of types of lymphocyte chromosomal aberrations on human cancer risk: Results from Nordic and Italian cohorts. *Cancer Res.*, **64**, 2258–2263

Hallier, E., Langhof, T., Dannappel, D., Leutbecher, M., Schröder, K., Goergens, H.W., Müller, A. & Bolt, H.M. (1993) Polymorphism of glutathione conjugation of methyl bromide, ethylene oxide and dichloromethane in human blood: Influence on the induction of sister chromatid exchanges (SCE) in lymphocytes. *Arch. Toxicol.*, **67**, 173–178

Hansen, J.P., Allen, J., Brock, K., Falconer, J., Helms, M.J., Shaver, G.C. & Strohm, B. (1984) Normal sister chromatid exchange levels in hospital sterilization employees exposed to ethylene oxide. *J. occup. Med.*, **26**, 29–32

Haufroid, V., Merz, B., Hofmann, A., Tschopp, A., Lison, D., & Hotz, P. (2007) Exposure to ethylene oxide in hospitals: Biological monitoring and influence of glutathione S-transferase and epoxide hydrolase polymorphisms. *Cancer Epidemiol. Biomarkers Prev.*, **16**, 796–802

Havlicek, C.S., Hilpert, L.R., Dal, G. & Perotti, D. (1992) *Assessment of Ethylene Oxide Concentrations and Emissions from Sterilization and Fumigation Processes. Final Report*, Sacramento, CA, Prepared for Research Division, California Air Resources Board

Hayes, J.D., Flanagan, J.U. & Jowsey, I.R. (2005) Glutathione transferases. *Annu. Rev. Pharmacol. Toxicol.*, **45**, 51–88

Health Canada (1999) *Priority Substances List Assessment Report, Ethylene Oxide*, (Canadian Environmental Protection Act, 1999), Ottawa

Health Canada (2001) *Priority Substances List; Assessment Report Ethylene Oxide*, Ottawa [available at: http://www.ec.gc.ca/substances/ese/eng/psap/final/ethyleneoxide.cfm]

Heiden Associates (1988a) *An Estimate of Industry Costs for Compliance with Two Ethylene Oxide Workplace STEL Scenarios: Ethylene Oxide Production and Ethoxylation Plants*, Washington DC

Heiden Associates (1988b) *A Medical Products Industry Profile for Evaluating Compliance with Two Ethylene Oxide Workplace STEL Scenarios: 10 ppm STEL and 5 ppm STEL*, Washington DC

Hemminki, K., Mutanen, P., Saloniemi, I., Niemi, M.-L. & Vainio, H. (1982) Spontaneous abortions in hospital staff engaged in sterilising instruments with chemical agents. *Br. med. J.*, **285**, 1461–1463

Hengstler, J.G., Fuchs, J., Gebhard, S. & Oesch, F. (1994) Glycolaldehyde causes DNA–protein crosslinks: A new aspect of ethylene oxide genotoxicity. *Mutat. Res.*, **304**, 229–234

Hengstler, J.G., Fuchs, J., Tanner, B., Oesch-Bartomowicz, B., Hölz, C. & Oesch, F. (1997) Analysis of DNA single-strand breaks in human venous blood: A technique which does not require isolation of white blood cells. *Environ. mol. Mutag.*, **29**, 58–62

Herrero, M.E., Arand, M., Hengstler, J.G. & Oesch, F. (1997) Recombinant expression of human microsomal epoxide hydrolase protects V79 chinese hamster cells from styrene oxide- but not from ethylene oxide-induced DNA strand breaks. *Environ. mol. Mutag.*, **30**, 429–439

Hochberg, V., Shi, X.-C., Moorman, W. & Ong, T. (1990) Induction of micronuclei in rat bone marrow and spleen cells by varied dose-rate of ethylene oxide (Abstract No. 91). *Environ. mol. Mutag.*, **15**, 26

Hoechst Celanese Corp. (1992) *Material Safety Data Sheet: Ethylene Oxide*, Dallas, TX

Högstedt, L.C. (1988) Epidemiological studies on ethylene oxide and cancer: An updating. In: Bartsch, H., Hemminki, K. & O'Neill, I.K., eds, *Methods for Detecting DNA Damaging Agents in Humans: Applications in Cancer Epidemiology and Prevention* (IARC Scientific Publications No. 89), Lyon, IARC, pp. 265–270

Högstedt, C., Rohlén, O., Berndtsson, B.S., Axelson, O. & Ehrenberg, L. (1979a) A cohort study of mortality and cancer incidence in ethylene oxide production workers. *Br. J. ind. Med.*, **36**, 276–280

Högstedt, C., Malmqvist, N. & Wadman, B. (1979b) Leukemia in workers exposed to ethylene oxide. *J. Am. med. Assoc.*, **241**, 1132–1133

Högstedt, B., Gullberg, B., Hedner, K., Kolnig, A.-M., Mitelman, F., Skerfving, S. & Widegren, B. (1983) Chromosome aberrations and micronuclei in bone marrow cells and peripheral blood lymphocytes in humans exposed to ethylene oxide. *Hereditas*, **98**, 105–113

Högstedt, C., Aringer, L. & Gustavsson, A. (1986) Epidemiologic support for ethylene oxide as a cancer-causing agent. *J. Am. med. Assoc.*, **255**, 1575–1578

Högstedt, B., Bergmark, E., Törnqvist, M. & Osterman-Golkar, S. (1990) Chromosomal aberrations and micronuclei in lymphocytes in relation to alkylation of hemoglobin in workers exposed to ethylene oxide and propylene oxide. *Hereditas*, **113**, 133–138

Hong, H.-H.L., Houle, C.D., Ton, T.-V.T. & Sills, R.C. (2007) K-ras Mutations in lung tumors and tumors of other organs are consistent with a common mechanism of ethylene oxide tumorigenesis in the B6C3F1 mouse. *Toxicol. Pathol.*, **35**, 81–85

Hori, H., Yahata, K., Fujishiro, K., Yoshizumi, K., Li, D., Goto, Y. & Higashi, T. (2002) Personal exposure level and environmental ethylene oxide gas concentration in sterilization facilities of hospitals in Japan. *Appl. occup. environ. Hyg.*, **17**, 634–639

Hornung, R.W., Greife, A.L., Stayner, L.T., Steenland, N.K., Herrick, R.F., Elliott, L.J., Ringenburg, V.L. & Morawetz, J. (1994) Statistical model for prediction of retrospective exposure to ethylene oxide in an occupational mortality study. *Am. J. ind. Med.*, **25**, 825–836

Houle, C.D., Ton, T.-V.T., Clayton, N., Huff, J., Hong, H.-H.L. & Sills, R.C. (2006) Frequent *p53* and H-*ras* mutations in benzene- and ethylene oxide-induced mammary gland carcinomas from B6C3F1 mice. *Toxicol. Pathol.*, **34**, 752–762

IARC (1976) *IARC Monographs on the Evaluation of Carcinogenic Risk of Chemicals to Man*, Vol. 11, *Cadmium, Nickel, Some Epoxides, Miscellaneous Industrial Chemicals and General Considerations on Volatile Anaesthetics*, Lyon, pp. 157–167

IARC (1985) *IARC Monographs on the Evaluation of the Carcinogenic Risk of Chemicals to Humans*, Vol. 36, *Allyl Compounds, Aldehydes, Epoxides and Peroxides*, Lyon, pp. 189–226

IARC (1987) *IARC Monographs on the Evaluation of Carcinogenic Risks to Humans*, Suppl. 7, *Overall Evaluations of Carcinogenicity: An Updating of* IARC Monographs *Volumes 1 to 42*, Lyon

IARC (1991) *IARC Monographs on the Evalution of Carcinogenic Risks to Humans*, Vol. 53, *Occupational Exposures in Insecticide Application, and Some Pesticides*, Lyon, pp. 179–249

IARC (1994) *IARC Monographs on the Evaluation of Carcinogenic Risks to Humans*, Vol. 60, *Some Industrial Chemicals*, Lyon, pp. 73–159

IARC (1995) *IARC Monographs on the Evaluation of Carcinogenic Risks to Humans*, Vol. 63, *Dry Cleaning, Some Chlorinated Solvents and Other Industrial Chemicals*, Lyon

IARC (1997) *IARC Monographs on the Evaluation of Carcinogenic Risks to Humans*, Vol. 69, *Polychlorinated Dibenzo-para-Dioxins and Polychlorinated Dibenzofurans*, Lyon

IARC (1999a) *IARC Monographs on the Evaluation of Carcinogenic Risks to Humans*, Vol. 71, *Re-evaluation of Some Organic Chemicals, Hydrazine and Hydrogen Peroxide*, Lyon

IARC (1999b) *IARC Monographs on the Evaluation of Carcinogenic Risks to Humans*, Vol. 73, *Some Chemicals that Cause Tumours of the Kidney or Urinary Bladder in Rodents and Some Other Substances*, Lyon, pp. 131–182

IARC (2000) *IARC Monographs on the Evaluation of Carcinogenic Risks to Humans*, Vol. 75, *Ionizing Radiation, Part 1: X- and γ-Radiation, and Neutrons*, Lyon, pp. 121–359

IARC (2004) *IARC Monographs on the Evaluation of Carcinogenic Risks to Humans*, Vol. 83, *Tobacco Smoking*, Lyon, p. 51–1187

IARC (2006) *IARC Monographs on the Evaluation of Carcinogenic Risks to Humans*, Vol. 88, *Formaldehyde, 2-Butoxyethanol and 1*-tert-*Butoxypropan-2-ol*, Lyon

IARC (2009) *IARC Monographs on the Evaluation of Carcinogenic Risks to Humans*, Vol. 94, *Ingested Nitrates and Nitrites, and Cyanobacterial Peptide Toxins*, Lyon (in press)

IPCS (1985) *Ethylene Oxide* (Environmental Health Criteria 55), Geneva, World Health Organization, International Programme on Chemical Safety

IPCS-CEC (2001) *International Chemical Safety Card 0155*, Geneva, World Health Organization

IRSST (2005) [Guide to Sampling Contaminants in Workplace Air], 8th rev. Ed. [www.irsst.qc.ca/fr/_outil_100038.html] (in French)

Jensen, K.G. (1988) Determination of ethylene oxide residues in processed food products by gas–liquid chromatography after derivatization. *Z. Lebensmitt. Untersuch. Forsch.*, **187**, 535–540

Jenssen, D. & Ramel, C. (1980) The micronucleus test is part of a short-term mutagenicity test program for the prediction of carcinogenicity evaluated by 143 agents tested. *Mutat. Res.*, **75**, 191–202

Johanson, G. & Filser, J.G. (1992) Experimental data from closed chamber gas uptake studies in rodents suggest lower uptake rate of chemical than calculated from literature values on alveolar ventilation. *Arch. Toxicol.*, **66**, 291–295

Jones, A.R. & Wells, G. (1981) The comparative metabolism of 2-bromoethanol and ethylene oxide in the rat. *Xenobiotica*, **11**, 763–770

Joyner, R.E. (1964) Chronic toxicity of ethylene oxide. *Arch. environ. Health*, **8**, 700–710

Kao, C.-Y. & Giese, R.W. (2005) Measurement of N7-(2'-hydroxyethyl)guanine in human DNA by gas chromatography electron capture mass spectrometry. *Chem. Res. Toxicol.*, **18**, 70–75

Kardos, L., Széles, G., Gombkötö, G., Szeremi, M., Tompa, A. & Ádány, R. (2003) Cancer deaths among hospital staff potentially exposed to ethylene oxide: An epidemiological analysis. *Environ. mol. Mutag.*, **42**, 59–60

Karelová, J., Jablonická, A. & Vargová, M. (1987) Results of cytogenetic testing of workers exposed to ethylene oxide. *J. Hyg. Epidemiol. Microbiol. Immunol.*, **31**, 119–126

Katoh, T., Higashi, K., Inoue, N. & Tanaka, I. (1989) Lipid peroxidation and the metabolism of glutathione in rat liver and brain following ethylene oxide inhalation. *Toxicology*, **58**, 1–9

Katoh, T., Higashi, K., Inoue, N. & Tanaka, I. (1990) Different responses of cytosolic and mitochondrial glutathione in rat livers after ethylene oxide exposure. *Toxicol. Lett.*, **54**, 235–239

Kauppinen, T., Toikkanen, J., Pedersen, D., Young, R., Ahrens, W., Boffetta, P., Hansen, J., Kromhout, H., Maqueda Blasco, J., Mirabelli, D., de la Orden-Rivera, V., Pannett, B., Plato, N., Savela, A., Vincent, R. & Kogevinas, M. (2000) Occupational exposure to carcinogens in the European Union. *Occup. environ. Med.*, **57**, 10–18 [data partially available on the CAREX web site: http://www.ttl.fi/NR/rdonlyres/407B368B-26EF-475D-8F2B-DA0024B853E0/0/5_exposures_by_agent_and_industry.pdf]

Kautiainen, A. & Törnqvist, M. (1991) Monitoring exposure to simple epoxides and alkenes through gas chromatographic determination of hemoglobin adducts. *Int. Arch. occup. environ. Health*, **63**, 27–31

Kelsey, K.T., Wiencke, J.K., Eisen, E.A., Lynch, D.W., Lewis, T.R. & Little, J.B (1988) Persistently elevated sister chromatid exchanges in ethylene oxide-exposed primates: The role of a sub-population of high frequency cells. *Cancer Res.*, **48**, 5045–5050

Kercher, S.L. & Mortimer, V.D. (1987) Before and after: An evaluation of engineering controls for ethylene oxide sterilization in hospitals. *Appl. ind. Hyg.*, **2**, 7–12

Kiesselbach, N., Ulm, K., Lange, H.J. & Korallus, U. (1990) A multicentre mortality study of workers exposed to ethylene oxide. *Br. J. ind. Med.*, **47**, 182–188

Kligerman, A.D., Erexson, G.L., Phelps, M.E. & Wilmer, J.L. (1983) Sister-chromatid exchange induction in peripheral blood lymphocytes of rats exposed to ethylene oxide by inhalation. *Mutat. Res.*, **120**, 37–44

Koda, S., Kumagai, S. & Ohara, H. (1999) Environmental monitoring and assessment of short-term exposures to hazardous chemicals of a sterilization process in hospital working environments. *Acta med. Okayama*, **53**, 217–223

Koga, M., Hori, H., Tanaka, I., Akiyama, T. & Inoue, N. (1985) [Quantitative analysis of urinary ethylene glycol in rats exposed to ethylene oxide]. *J. UOEH.*, **7**, 45–49 (in Japanese)

Koga, M., Hori, H., Tanaka, I., Akiyama, T. & Inoue, N. (1987) [Analysis of urinary metabolites of rats exposed to ethylene oxide]. *J. UOEH.*, **9**, 167–170 (in Japanese)

Kolman, A., Näslund, M. & Calleman, C.J. (1986) Genotoxic effects of ethylene oxide and their relevance to human cancer. *Carcinogenesis*, **7**, 1245–1250

Kolman, A., Näslund, M., Osterman-Golkar, S., Scalia-Tomba, G.-P. & Meyer, A. (1989) Comparative studies of in vitro transformation by ethylene oxide and gamma-radiation of C3H/10T1/2 cells. *Mutagenesis*, **4**, 58–61

Kolman, A., Bohušová, T., Lambert, B. & Simons, J.W.I.M. (1992) Induction of 6-thioguanine-resistant mutants in human diploid fibroblasts *in vitro* with ethylene oxide. *Environ. mol. Mutag.*, **19**, 93–97

Kolman, A., Chovanec, M., & Osterman-Golkar, S. (2002) Genotoxic effects of ethylene oxide, propylene oxide and epichlorohydrin in humans: Update review (1990–2001). *Mutat. Res.*, **512**, 173–194

Kreuzer, P.E. (1992) [Permeation Kinetics of Ethylene Oxide in Gaseous Form and Dissolved Other Matrices Through the Skin of Rats, Hamsters and Humans] (GSF-Bericht 19/92), Neuherberg, GSF-Forschungszentrum für Umwelt und Gesundheit (in German)

Kring, E.V., Damrell, D.J., Basilio, A.N., Jr, McGibney, P.D., Douglas, J.J., Henry, T.J. & Ansul, G.R. (1984) Laboratory validation and field verification of a new passive air monitoring badge for sampling ethylene oxide in air. *Am. ind. Hyg. Assoc. J.*, **45**, 697–707

Krishnan, K., Gargas, M.L., Fennell, T.R. & Andersen, M.E. (1992) A physiologically based description of ethylene oxide dosimetry in the rat. *Toxicol. ind. Health*, **8**, 121–140

Lacson, J. (2003) *CEH Marketing Research Report — Ethylene Oxide*, Zurich, SRI Consulting

La Montagne, A.D., Oakes, J.M. & Lopez Turley, R.N. (2004) Long term ethylene oxide exposure trends in US hospitals: Relationship with OSHA regulatory and enforcement actions. *Am. J. public Health*, **94**, 1614–1619

Latif, F., Moschel, R.C., Hemminki, K. & Dipple, A. (1988) Styrene oxide as a stereochemical probe for the mechanism of aralkylation at different sites on guanosine. *Chem. Res. Toxicol.*, **1**, 364–369

Laurent, C., Frederic, J. & Leonard, A.Y. (1984) Sister chromatid exchange frequency in workers exposed to high levels of ethylene oxide in a hospital sterilization service. *Int. Arch. occup. environ. Health*, **54**, 33–43

Lerda, D. & Rizzi, R. (1992) Cytogenetic study of persons occupationally exposed to ethylene oxide. *Mutat. Res.*, **281**, 31–37

Lewis, S.E., Barnett, L.B., Felton, C., Johnson, F.M., Skow, L.C., Cacheiro, N. & Shelby, M.D. (1986) Dominant visible and electrophoretically expressed mutations induced in male mice exposed to ethylene oxide by inhalation. *Environ. Mutag.*, **8**, 867–872

Li, F., Segal, A. & Solomon, J.J. (1992) In vitro reaction of ethylene oxide with DNA and characterization of DNA adducts. *Chem.-biol. Interact.*, **83**, 35–54

Liao, P.-C., Li, C.-M., Hung, C.-W. & Chen S.-H. (2001) Quantitative detection of N^7-(2-hydroxyethyl)guanine adducts in DNA using high-performance liquid chromatography/electrospray ionization tandem mass spectrometry. *J. mass Spectrom.*, **36**, 336–343

Lide, D.R., ed. (2005) *CRC Handbook of Chemistry and Physics*, 86th Ed., Boca Raton, FL, CRC Press, pp. 3–408

Lindahl, T. (1979) DNA glycosylases, endonucleases for apurinic/apyrimidinic sites, and base excision-repair. *Prog. Nucleic Acid Res. mol. Biol.*, **22**, 135–192

Liou, S.H., Lung, J.C., Chen, Y.H., Yang, T., Hsieh, L.L., Chen, C.J. & Wu, T.N. (1999) Increased chromosome-type chromosome aberration frequencies as biomarkers of cancer risk in a blackfoot endemic area. *Cancer Res.*, **59**, 1481–1484

Loeb, L.A. & Preston, B.D. (1986) Mutagenesis by apurinic/apyrimidinic sites. *Ann. Rev. Genet.*, **20**, 201–230

Lorenti Garcia, C., Darroudi, F., Tates, A.D. & Natarajan, A.T. (2001) Induction and persistence of micronuclei, sister-chromatid exchanges and chromosomal aberrations in splenocytes and bone-marrow cells of rats exposed to ethylene oxide. *Mutat. Res.*, **492**, 59–67

Lovegren, B.C. & Koketsu, M. (1977a) *BASF-Wyandotte Corporation, Geismar, Louisiana, Task II, Ethylene Oxide Survey Report of the Plant Contact, June 27–28, 1977* (PB81-229775), Springfield, VA, National Technical Information Service

Lovegren, B.C. & Koketsu, M. (1977b) *Union Carbide Corporation, Institute, West Virginia, Task II, Ethylene Oxide Survey Report of the Plant Contact, July 15–16, 1977* (PB82-106709), Springfield, VA, National Technical Information Service

Lovegren, B.C. & Koketsu, M. (1977c) *Union Carbide Corporation, Texas City, Texas, Task II, Ethylene Oxide Survey Report of the Plant Contact, June 8–9, 1977* (PB82-108218), Springfield, VA, National Technical Information Service

Lucas, L.J. & Teta, M.J. (1996) Breast cancer and ethylene oxide exposure. *Int. J. Epidemiol.*, **25**, 685–686

Ludeke, B.I. & Kleihues, P. (1988) Formation and persistence of O^6-(2-hydroxyethyl)-2′-deoxy-guanosine in DNA for various rat tissues following a single dose of *N*-nitroso-*N*-(2-hydroxy-ethyl)urea. An immuno-slot-blot study. *Carcinogenesis*, **9**, 147–151

Lynch, D.W., Lewis, T.R., Moorman, W.J., Burg, J.R., Groth, D.H., Khan, A., Ackerman, L.J. & Cockrell, B.Y. (1984a) Carcinogenic and toxicologic effects of inhaled ethylene oxide and pro-pylene oxide in F344 rats. *Toxicol. appl. Pharmacol.*, **76**, 69–84

Lynch, D.W., Lewis, T.R., Moorman, W.J., Burg, J.R., Gulati, D.K., Kaur, P. & Sabharwal, P.S. (1984b) Sister-chromatid exchanges and chromosome aberrations in lymphocytes from mon-keys exposed to ethylene oxide and propylene oxide by inhalation. *Toxicol. appl. Pharmacol.*, **76**, 85–95

Major, J., Jakab, M.G. & Tompa, A. (1996) Genotoxicological investigation of hospital nurses occupationally exposed to ethylene-oxide: I. Chromosome aberrations, sister-chromatid ex-changes, cell cycle kinetics, and UV-induced DNA synthesis in peripheral blood lymphocytes. *Environ. mol. Mutag.*, **27**, 84–92

Major, J., Jakab, M.G. & Tompa, A. (1999) The frequency of induced premature centromere divi-sion in human populations occupationally exposed to genotoxic chemicals. *Mutat. Res.*, **445**, 241–249

Maples, K.R. & Dahl, A.R. (1993) Levels of epoxides in blood during inhalation of alkenes and alkenes oxides. *Inhal. Toxicol.*, **5**, 43–54

Margeson, J.H., Steger, J.L. & Homolya, J.B. (1990) Chromatographic methods for analysis of ethylene oxide in emissions from stationary sources. *J. chromatogr. Sci.*, **28**, 204–209

Marlowe, D.E., Lao, N.T., Eaton, A.R., Page, B.F.J. & Lao, C.S. (1987) Interlaboratory compari-son of analytical methods for residual ethylene oxide in medical device materials. *J. pharm. Sci.*, **76**, 333–337

Marnett, L.J. (2002) Oxy radicals, lipid peroxidation and DNA damage. *Toxicology*, **181–182**, 219–222

Marsden, D.A., Jones, D.J.L., Lamb, J.H., Tompkins, E.M., Farmer, P.B. & Brown, K. (2007) Determination of endogenous and exogenously derived N7-(2-hydroxyethyl)guanine adducts in ethylene oxide-treated rats. *Chem. Res. Toxicol.*, **20**, 290–299

Martis, L., Kroes, R., Darby, T.D., & Woods, E.F. (1982) Disposition kinetics of ethylene oxide, ethylene glycol, and 2-chlorethanol in the dog. *J. Toxicol. environ. Health*, **10**, 847–856

Mayer, J., Warburton, D., Jeffrey, A.M., Pero, R., Walles, S., Andrews, L., Toor, M., Latriano, L., Wazneh, L., Tang, D., Tsai, W.-Y., Kuroda, M. & Perera, F. (1991) Biologic markers in ethylene oxide-exposed workers and controls. *Mutat. Res.*, **248**, 163–176

McCammon, J., Orgel, D. & Hill, B. (1990) *Health Hazard Evaluation Report, A.E. Staley Manufacturing Co., Decatur, IL* (Report No. HETA-88-348-2081), Cincinnati, OH, National Institute for Occupational Safety and Health

McKelvey, J.A. & Zemaitis, M.A. (1986) The effects of ethylene oxide (EO) exposure on tissue glutathione levels in rats and mice. *Drug chem. Toxicol.*, **9**, 51–66

Morgan, R.W., Claxton, K.W., Divine, B.J., Kaplan, S.D. & Harris, V.B. (1981) Mortality among ethylene oxide workers. *J. occup. Med.*, **23**, 767–770

Mortimer, V.D., Jr & Kercher, S.L. (1989) *Control Technology for Ethylene Oxide Sterilization in Hospitals* (NIOSH Publ. No. 89–120), Cincinnati, OH, National Institute for Occupational Safety and Health

Mouilleseaux, A., Laurent, A.-M., Fabre, M., Jouan, M. & Festy, B. (1983) [Atmospheric levels of ethylene oxide in the occupational environment of sterilization and disinfection facilities.] *Arch. Mal. prof.*, **44**, 1–14 (in French)

Müller, M., Krämer, A., Angerer, J. & Hallier, E. (1998) Ethylene oxide–protein adduct formation in humans: Influence of glutathione-S-transferase polymorphisms. *Int. Arch. occup. environ. Health*, **71**, 499–502

Nakashima, K., Furutani, A., Higashi, K., Okuno, F. & Inoue, N. (1987) Glutathione contents in rat livers after acute and chronic exposure to ethylene oxide. *J. UOEH*, **9**, 355–359

Natarajan, A.T., Preston, R.J., Dellarco, V., Ehrenberg, L., Generoso, W., Lewis, S. & Tates, A.D. (1995) Ethylene oxide: Evaluation of genotoxicity data and an exploratory assessment of genetic risk. *Mutat. Res.*, **330**, 55–70

National Institute for Occupational Safety and Health (1987) *NIOSH Manual of Analytical Methods*, 3rd Ed., Suppl. 2 (DHHS (NIOSH) Publ. No. 84–100), Washington DC, US Government Printing Office, pp. 1614-1–1614-6

National Institute for Occupational Safety and Health (1998) *NIOSH Manual of Analytical Methods*, 4th Ed., Suppl. 2 (DHHS (NIOSH) Publ. No. 98–119), Washington DC, US Government Printing Office

National Library of Medicine (2005) *Hazardous Substances Data Bank Database*, Bethesda, MD [available at http://toxnet.nlm.nih.gov/cgi-bin/sis/search]

National Library of Medicine (2006) *Toxic Chemical Release Inventory (TRI) Data Banks* [TRI87, TRI88, TRI89, TRI90, TRI91, TRI05], Bethesda, MD

National Toxicology Program (1987) *Toxicology and Carcinogenesis Studies of Ethylene Oxide (CAS No. 75-21-8) in B6C3F₁ Mice (Inhalation Studies)* (NTP Technical Report No. 326; NIH Publication No. 88-2582), Research Triangle Park, NC

Newman, M.A. & Freund, E. (1989) *Health Hazard Evaluation Report, Washington Hospital, Washington, PA* (Report No. HETA 89-006-2002), Cincinnati, OH, National Institute for Occupational Safety and Health

NOES (1993) *National Occupational Exposure Survey (1981–1983)*, Cincinnati, OH, National Institute for Occupational Safety and Health

Norman, S.A., Berlin, J.A., Soper, K.A., Middendorf, B.F. & Stolley, P.D. (1995) Cancer incidence in a group of workers potentially exposed to ethylene oxide. *Int. J. Epidemiol.*, **24**, 276–284

Norman, S.A., Berlin, J.A., Soper, K.A., Middendorf, B.F. & Stolley, P.D. (1996) Authors' response: Cancer incidence in a group of workers potentially exposed to ethylene oxide. *Int. J. Epidemiol.*, **25**, 686

Nygren, J. Cedervall, B., Eriksson, S., Dušinská, M. & Kolman, A. (1994) Induction of DNA strand breaks by ethylene oxide in human diploid fibroblasts. *Environ. mol. Mutag.*, **24**, 161–167

O'Neil, M.J., ed. (2006) *Merck Index*, 14th Ed., Whitehouse Station, NJ, Merck, p. 651

Occupational Safety and Health Administration (2005) *Regulatory Review of the Occupational Safety and Health Administration's Ethylene Oxide Standard* (29 CFR 1910.1047), Washington DC

Olsen, G.W., Lacy, S.E., Bodner, K.M., Chau, M., Arceneaux, T.G., Cartmill, J.B., Ramlow, J.M. & Boswell, J.M. (1997) Mortality from pancreatic and lymphopoietic cancer among workers in ethylene and propylene chlorohydrin production. *Occup. environ. Med.*, **54**, 592–598

Ong, T., Bi, H.-K., Xing, S., Stewart, J. & Moorman, W. (1993) Induction of sister chromatid exchange in spleen and bone marrow cells of rats exposed by inhalation to different dose rates of ethylene oxide. *Environ. mol. Mutag.*, **22**, 147–151

Oser, J.L., Crandall, M., Phillips, R. & Marlow, D. (1978a) *Indepth Industrial Hygiene Report of Ethylene Oxide Exposure at Union Carbide Corporation, Institute, West Virginia* (PB82-114786), Springfield, VA, National Technical Information Service

Oser, J.L., Crandall, M. & Rinsky, R. (1978b) *Industrial Hygiene Survey of Dow Chemical Company, Plaquemine, Louisiana* (PB81-229924), Springfield, VA, National Technical Information Service

Oser, J.L., Young, M., Boyle, T. & Marlow, D. (1979) *Indepth Industrial Hygiene Report of Ethylene Oxide Exposure at Union Carbide Corporation, South Charleston, West Virginia* (PB82-110024), Springfield, VA, National Technical Information Service

Osterman-Golkar, S. & Bergmark, E. (1988) Occupational exposure to ethylene oxide. Relation between in vivo dose and exposure dose. *Scand. J. Work Environ. Health*, **14**, 372–377

Osterman-Golkar, S., Farmer, P.B., Segerbäck, D., Bailey, E., Calleman, C.J., Svensson, K. & Ehrenberg, L. (1983) Dosimetry of ethylene oxide in the rat by quantitation of alkylated histidine in hemoglobin. *Teratog. Carcinog. Mutag.*, **3**, 395–405

Ott, M.G., Teta, M.J. & Greenberg, H.L. (1989) Lymphatic and hematopoietic tissue cancer in a chemical manufacturing environment. *Am. J. ind. Med.*, **16**, 631–643

Pauwels, W. & Veulemans, H. (1998) Comparison of ethylene, propylene, and styrene 7,8-oxide in vitro adduct formation on N-terminal valine in human haemoglobin and on N-7-guanine in human DNA. *Mutat. Res.*, **418**, 21–33

Pedersen-Bjergaard, J. & Rowley, J.D. (1994) The balanced and the unbalanced chromosome aberrations of acute myeloid leukemia may develop in different ways and may contribute differently to malignant transformation. *Blood*, **83**, 2780–2786

Pedersen-Bjergaard, J., Christiansen, D.H., Desta, F. & Andersen, M.K. (2006) Alternative genetic pathways and cooperating genetic abnormalities in the pathogenesis of therapy-related myelodysplasia and acute myeloid leukemia. *Leukemia*, **20**, 1943–1949

Pero, R.W., Widegren, B., Högstedt, B. & Mitelman, F. (1981) In vivo and in vitro ethylene oxide exposure of human lymphocytes assessed by chemical stimulation of unscheduled DNA synthesis. *Mutat. Res.*, **83**, 271–289

Pero, R.W., Bryngelsson, T., Widegren, B., Högstedt, B. & Welinder, H. (1982) A reduced capacity for unscheduled DNA synthesis in lymphocytes from individuals exposed to propylene oxide and ethylene oxide. *Mutat. Res.*, **104**, 193–200

Picut, C.A., Aoyama, H., Holder, J.W., Gold, L.S., Maronpot, R.R. & Dixon, D. (2003) Bromoethane, chloroethane and ethylene oxide induced uterine neoplasms in B6C3F1 mice from 2-year NTP inhalation bioassays: Pathology and incidence data revisited. *Exp. Toxicol. Pathol.*, **55**, 1–9

Poirier, V. & Papadopoulo, D. (1982) Chromosomal aberrations induced by ethylene oxide in a human amniotic cell line *in vitro*. *Mutat. Res.*, **104**, 255–260

Popp, W., Wahrenholz, C., Przygoda, H., Brauksiepe, A., Goch, S., Müller, G., Schell, C. & Norporth, K. (1994) DNA–protein cross-links and sister chromatid exchange frequencies in lymphocytes and hydroxyethyl mercapturic acid in urine of ethylene oxide-exposed hospital workers. *Int. Arch. occup. environ. Health*, **66**, 325–332

Potter, D., Blair, D., Davies, R., Watson, W.P. & Wright, A.S. (1989) The relationships between alkylation of haemoglobin and DNA in Fischer 344 rats exposed to [^{14}C]ethylene oxide. *Arch. Toxicol.*, **Suppl. 13**, 254–257

Preston, R.J. (1999) Cytogenetic effects of ethylene oxide, with an emphasis on population monitoring. *Crit. Rev. Toxicol.*, **29**, 263–282

Preston, R.J. & Abernethy, D.J. (1993) Studies on the induction of chromosomal aberration and sister chromatid exchange in rats exposed to styrene by inhalation. In: Sorsa, M., Peltonen, K., Vainio, N. & Hemminki, K, eds, *Butadiene and Styrene: Assessment of Health Hazards* (IARC Scientific Publications No. 127), Lyon, IARC, pp. 225–233

Puskar, M.A. & Hecker, L.H. (1989) Field validation of passive dosimeters for the determination of employee exposures to ethylene oxide in hospital product sterilization facilities. *Am. ind. Hyg. Assoc. J.*, **50**, 30–36

Puskar, M.A., Nowak, J.L. & Hecker, L.H. (1990) Generation of ethylene oxide permissible exposure limit data with on-site sample analysis using the EO Self-Scan™ passive monitor. *Am. ind. Hyg. Assoc. J.*, **51**, 273–279

Puskar, M.A., Szopinski, F.G. & Hecker, L.H. (1991) Development and validation of a protocol for field validation of passive dosimeters for ethylene oxide excursion limit monitoring. *Am. ind. Hyg. Assoc. J.*, **52**, 145–150

Rebsdat, S. & Mayer, D. (2005) Ethylene oxide. In: *Ullmann's Encyclopedia of Industrial Chemistry*, 7th Ed., Weinheim, Wiley–VCH Publishers (on line)

Recio, L., Donner, M., Abernethy, D., Pluta, L., Steen, A.-M., Wong, B.A., James, A. & Preston, R.J. (2004) In vivo mutagenicity and mutation spectrum in the bone marrow and testes of B6C3F1 lacI transgenic mice following inhalation exposure to ethylene oxide. *Mutagenesis*, **19**, 215–222

Ribeiro, L.R., Rabello-Gay, M.N., Salvadori, D.M.F., Pereira, C.A.B. & Beçak, W. (1987a) Cytogenetic effects of inhaled ethylene oxide in somatic and germ cells of mice. *Arch. Toxicol.*, **59**, 332–335

Ribeiro, L.R., Salvadori, D.M.F., Pereira, C.A.B. & Beçak, W. (1987b) Activity of ethylene oxide in the mouse sperm morphology test. *Arch. Toxicol.*, **60**, 331–333

Ribeiro, L.R., Salvadori, D.M.F., Rios, A.C.C., Costa, S.L., Tates, A.D., Törnqvist, M. & Natarajan, A.T. (1994) Biological monitoring of workers occupationally exposed to ethylene oxide. *Mutat. Res.*, **313**, 81–87

Richmond, G.W., Abrahams, R.H., Nemenzo, J.H. & Hine, C.H. (1985) An evaluation of possible effects on health following exposure to ethylene oxide. *Arch. environ. Health*, **40**, 20–25

Russell, I.B., Cumming, R.B. & Hunsicker, P.R. (1984) Specific-locus mutation rates in the mouse following inhalation of ethylene oxide and application of the results to estimation of human genetic risk. *Mutat. Res.*, **129**, 381–388

Rusyn, I., Asakura, S., Li, Y., Kosyk, O., Koc, H., Nakamura, J., Upton, P.B. & Swenberg, J.A. (2005) Effects of ethylene oxide and ethylene inhalation on DNA adducts, apurinic/apyrimidinic sites and expression of base excision DNA repair gene in rat brain, spleen, and liver. *DNA Repair*, **4**, 1099–1110

Saalo, A., Soosaar, A., Vuorela, R. & Kauppinen, T. (2006) [ASA 2004], Helsinki, Finnish Institute of Occupational Health. [available at: http://www.ttl.fi/NR/rdonlyres/5A54A452-7350-4255-8DF3-AF632D9D2775/0/ASA_2004.pdf] (in Finnish)

Sadtler Research Laboratories (1991) *Sadtler Standard Spectra. 1981–1991 Supplementary Index*, Philadelphia, PA

Sangster, J. (1989) Octanol–water partition coefficients of simple organic compounds. *J. phys. chem. Ref. Data*, **18**, 1144

Sarto, F., Cominato, I., Pinton, A.M., Brovedani, P.G., Faccioli, C.M., Bianchi, V. & Levis, A.G. (1984a) Workers exposed to ethylene oxide have increased incidence of sister chromatid exchange. In: Berlin, A., Draper, M., Hemminki, K. & Vainio, H., eds, *Monitoring Human Exposure to Carcinogenic and Mutagenic Agents* (IARC Scientific Publications No. 59), Lyon, IARC, pp. 413–419

Sarto, F., Cominato, I., Pinton, A.M., Brovedani, P.G., Faccioli, C.M., Bianchi, V. & Levis, A.G. (1984b) Cytogenetic damage in workers exposed to ethylene oxide. *Mutat. Res.*, **138**, 185–195

Sarto, F., Clonfero, E., Bartolucci, G.B., Franceschi, C., Chiricolo, M. & Levis, A.G. (1987) Sister chromatid exchanges and DNA repair capability in sanitary workers exposed to ethylene oxide: evaluation of the dose–effect relationship. *Am. J. ind. Med.*, **12**, 625–637

Sarto, F., Tomanin, R., Giacomelli, L., Iannini, G. & Cupiraggi, A.R. (1990) The micronucleus assay in human exfoliated cells of the nose and mouth: Application to occupational exposures to chromic acid and ethylene oxide. *Mutat. Res.*, **244**, 345–351

Sarto, F., Törnqvist, M.A., Tomanin, R., Bartolucci, G.B., Osterman-Golkar, S.M. & Ehrenberg, L. (1991) Studies of biological and chemical monitoring of low-level exposure to ethylene oxide. *Scand. J. Work Environ. Health*, **17**, 60–64

Scheick, C., Spiteller, G., & Dasenbrock, C. (1997) Thiodiacetic acid—a metabolite of ethylene oxide. *Z. Naturforsch.*, **52C**, 70–76

Schettgen, T., Broding, H.C., Angerer, J. & Drexler, H. (2002) Hemoglobin adducts of ethylene oxide, propylene oxide, acrylonitrile and acrylamide-biomarkers in occupational and environmental medicine. *Toxicol. Lett.*, **134**, 65–70

Schulte, P.A., Boeniger, M., Walker, J.T., Schober, S.E., Pereira, M.A., Gulati, D.K., Wojciechowski, J.P., Garza, A., Froelich, R., Strauss, G., Halperin, W.E., Herrick, R. & Griffith, J. (1992) Biologic markers in hospital workers exposed to low levels of ethylene oxide. *Mutat. Res.*, **278**, 237–251

Schulte, P.A., Walker, J.T., Boeniger, M.F., Tsuchiya, Y. & Halperin, W.E. (1995) Molecular, cytogenetic, and hematologic effects of ethylene oxide on female hospital workers. *J. occup. med. Health*, **37**, 313–320

Sega, G.A. & Generoso, E.E. (1988) Measurement of DNA breakage in spermiogenic germ-cell stages of mice exposed to ethylene oxide, using an alkaline elution procedure. *Mutat. Res.*, **197**, 93–99

Sega, G.A., Generoso, E.E. & Brimer, P.A. (1988) Inhalation exposure-rate of ethylene oxide affects the level of DNA breakage and unscheduled DNA synthesis in spermiogenic stages of the mouse. *Mutat. Res.*, **209**, 177–180

Sega, G.A., Brimer, P.A. & Generoso, E.E. (1991) Ethylene oxide inhalation at different exposure-rates affects binding levels in mouse germ cells and hemoglobin. Possible explanation for the effect. *Mutat. Res.*, **249**, 339–349

Segerbäck, D. (1990) Reaction products in hemoglobin and DNA after in vitro treatment with ethylene oxide and *N*-(2-hydroxyethyl)-*N*-nitrosourea. *Carcinogenesis*, **11**, 307–312

Segerbäck, D. (1994) DNA alkylation by ethylene oxide and some mono-substituted epoxides. In: Hemminki, K., Dipple, A., Shuker, D.E.G., Kadlubar, F.F., Segerbäck, D. & Bartsch, H., eds, *DNA Adducts: Identification and Biological Significance* (IARC Scientific Publications No. 125), Lyon, IARC, pp. 37–47

Shell Chemicals (2005) *MSDS Ethylene Oxide 28.3.2005* [available at http://shellchemicals.com/msds/1,1098,1136,00.html accessed 30/10/07]

Shore, R.E., Gardner, M.J. & Pannett, B. (1993) Ethylene oxide: An assessment of the epide-miological evidence on carcinogenicity. *Br. J. ind. Med.*, **50**, 971–997

Shults, R.A. & Seitz, T.A. (1992) *Health Hazard Evaluation Report, Valley Hospital, Palmer, Alaska* (Report No. HETA 91-293-2203), Cincinnati, OH, National Institute for Occupational Safety and Health

Sisk, S.C., Pluta, L.J., Meyer, K.G., Wong, B.C. & Recio, L. (1997) Assessment of the in vivo mutagenicity of ethylene oxide in the tissues of B6C3F1 *lacI* transgenic mice following inha-lation exposure. *Mutat. Res.*, **391**, 153–164

van Sittert, N.J., de Jong, G., Clare, M.G., Davies, R., Dean, B.J., Wren, L.J. & Wright, A.S. (1985) Cytogenetic, immunological, and haematological effects in workers in an ethylene oxide manu-facturing plant. *Br. J. ind. Med.*, **42**, 19–26

van Sittert, N.J., Beulink, G.D.J., van Vliet, E.W.N. & van der Waal, H. (1993) Monitoring occupational exposure to ethylene oxide by the determination of hemoglobin adducts. *Environ. Health Perspect.*, **99**, 217–220

van Sittert, N.J., Boogaard, P.J., Natarajan, A.T., Tates, A.D., Ehrenberg, L.G. & Törnqvist, M.A. (2000) Formation of DNA adducts and induction of mutagenic effects in rats following 4 weeks inhalation exposure to ethylene oxide as a basis for cancer risk assessment. *Mutat. Res.*, 447, 27–48

Smerhovsky, Z., Landa, K., Rössner, P., Brabec, M., Zudova, Z., Hola, N., Pokorna, Z., Mareckova, J. & Hurychova, D. (2001) Risk of cancer in an occupationally exposed cohort with increased level of chromosomal aberrations. *Environ. Health Perspect.*, **109**, 41–45

Snellings, W.M., Weil, C.S. & Maronpot, R.R. (1984) A two-year inhalation study of the carcinogenic potential of ethylene oxide in Fischer 344 rats. *Toxicol. appl. Pharmacol.*, **75**, 105–117

Sobaszek, A., Hache, J.C., Frimat, P., Akakpo, V., Victoire, G. & Furon D. (1999) Working conditions and health effects of ethylene oxide exposure at hospital sterilization sites. *J. occup. environ. Med.*, **41**, 492–499

Solomon, J. (1999) Cyclic adducts and intermediates induced by simple epoxides. In: Singer, B. & Bartsch, H., eds, *Exocyclic Adducts in Mutagenesis and Carcinogenesis* (IARC Scientific Publications No. 150), Lyon, IARC, pp. 123–125

Sorsa, M., Ojajärvi, A. & Salomaa, S. (1990) Cytogenetic surveillance of workers exposed to genotoxic chemicals: Preliminary experiences from a prospective cancer study in a cytogenetic cohort. *Teratog. Carcinog. Mutag.*, **10**, 215–221

Star, E.G. (1980) [Mutagenic and cytotoxic effect of ethylene oxide on human cell cultures.] *Zbl. Bakt. Hyg. I. Abt. Orig. B*, **170**, 548–556 (in German)

Stayner, L., Steenland, K., Greife, A., Hornung, R., Hayes, R.B., Nowlin, S., Morawetz, J., Ringenburg, V., Elliot, L. & Halperin, W. (1993) Exposure–response analysis of cancer mortality in a cohort of workers exposed to ethylene oxide. *Am. J. Epidemiol.*, **138**, 787–798

Steenland, K. & Stayner, L. (1993) An epidemiological study of workers potentially exposed to ethylene oxide. *Br. J. ind. Med.*, **50**, 1125–1126

Steenland, K., Stayner, L., Greife, A., Halperin, W., Hayes, R., Hornung, R. & Nowlin, S. (1991) Mortality among workers exposed to ethylene oxide. *New Engl. J. Med.*, **324**, 1402–1407

Steenland, K., Whelan, E., Deddens, J., Stayner, L. & Ward, E. (2003) Ethylene oxide and breast cancer incidence in a cohort study of 7576 women (United States). *Cancer Causes Control*, **14**, 531–539

Steenland, K., Stayner, L. & Deddens, J. (2004) Mortality analyses in a cohort of 18 235 ethylene oxide exposed workers: Follow up extended from 1987 to 1998. *Occup. environ. Med.*, **61**, 2–7

Steger, J. (1989) *Analytical Method Evaluation for Measuring Ethylene Oxide Emissions from Commercial Dilute-acid Hydrolytic Control Units* (EPA Report No. EPA-600/3-89-016; US NTIS PB89-155253), Research Triangle Park, NC, US Environmental Protection Agency, Office of Research and Development

Stolley, P.D., Soper, K.A., Galloway, S.M., Nichols, W.W., Norman, S.A. & Wolman, S.R. (1984) Sister-chromatid exchanges in association with occupational exposure to ethylene oxide. *Mutat. Res.*, **129**, 89–102

Swaen, G.M.H., Slangen, J.M.M., Ott, M.G., Kusters, E., Van Den Langenbergh, G., Arends, J.W. & Zober, A. (1996) Investigation of a cluster of ten cases of Hodgkin's disease in an occupational setting. *Int. Arch. occup. environ. Health*, **68**, 224–228

Swenberg, J.A., Fedtke, N., Fennell, T.R. & Walker, V.E. (1990) Relationships between carcinogen exposure, DNA adducts and carcinogenesis. In: Clayson, D.B., Munro, I.C., Shubik, P. & Swenberg, J.A. eds, *Progress in Predictive Toxicology*, Amsterdam, Elsevier Scientific Publications, pp. 161–184

Szopinski, F.G., Puskar, M.A. & Hecker, L.H. (1991) Field validation of three passive dosimeters for excursion limit monitoring of ethylene oxide. *Am. ind. Hyg. Assoc. J.*, **52**, 151–157

Sociale Zaken & Werkgelegenheid (2006) [Modification of the rules concerning work conditions.] *Off. State J.*, **28 December, 252**, 23 (in Dutch)

Takeshita, M., Chang, C.-N., Johnson, F., Will, S. & Grollman, A.P. (1987) Oligodeoxynucleotides containing synthetic abasic sites. *J. biol. Chem.*, **262**, 10171–10179

Tan, E.-L., Cumming, R.B. & Hsie, A.W. (1981) Mutagenicity and cytotoxicity of ethylene oxide in the CHO/HGPRT system. *Environ. Mutag.*, **3**, 683–686

Tardif, R., Goyal, R., Brodeur, J., & Gérin, M. (1987) Species differences in the urinary disposition of some metabolites of ethylene oxide. *Fundam. appl. Toxicol.*, **9**, 448–453

Tates, A.D., Grummt, T., Törnqvist, M., Farmer, P.B., van Dam, F.J., van Mossel, H., Schoemaker, H.M., Osterman-Golkar, S., Uebel, C., Tang, Y.S., Zwinderman, A.H., Natarajan, A.T. & Ehrenberg, L. (1991) Biological and chemical monitoring of occupational exposure to ethylene oxide. *Mutat. Res.*, **250**, 483–497

Tates, A.D., Boogaard, P.J., Darroudi, F., Natarajan, A.T., Caubo, M.E. & van Sittert, N.J. (1995) Biological effect monitoring in industrial workers following incidental exposure to high concentrations of ethylene oxide. *Mutat. Res.*, **329**, 63–77

Tates, A.D., van Dam, F.J., Natarajan, A.T., van Teylingen, C.M.M., de Zwart, F.A., Zwinderman, A.H., van Sittert, N.J., Nilsen, A., Nilsern, O.G., Zahlsen, K., Magnusson, A.-L. & Törnqvist, M. (1999) Measurement of HPRT mutations in splenic lymphocytes and haemoglobin adducts in erythrocytes of Lewis rats exposed to ethylene oxide. *Mutat. Res.*, **431**, 397–415

Tavares, R., Ramos, P., Palminha, J., Bispo, M.A., Paz, I., Bras, A., Rueff, J., Farmer, P.B. & Bailey, E. (1994) Transplacental exposure to genotoxins. Evaluation in haemoglobin of hydroxyethylvaline adduct levels in smoking and non-smoking mothers and their newborns. *Carcinogenesis*, **15**, 1271–1274

Teta, M.J., Benson, L.O. & Vitale, J.N. (1993) Mortality study of ethylene oxide workers in chemical manufacturing: A 10 year update. *Br. J. ind. Med.*, **50**, 704–709

Teta, M.J., Sielken, R.L., Jr & Valdez-Flores, C. (1999) Ethylene oxide cancer risk assessment based on epidemiological data: Application of revised regulatory guidelines. *Risk Anal.*, **19**, 1135–1155

Thier, R. & Bolt, H.M. (2000) Carcinogenicity and genotoxicity of ethylene oxide: New aspects and recent advances. *Crit. Rev. Toxicol.*, **30**, 595–608

Thier, R., Balkenhol, H., Lewalter, J., Selinski, S., Dommermuth, A. & Bolt, H.M. (2001) Influence of polymorphisms of the human glutathione transferases and cytochrome P450 2E1 enzyme on the metabolism and toxicity of ethylene oxide and acrylonitrile. *Mutat. Res.*, **482**, 41–46

Thiess, A.M., Schwegler, H., Fleig, I. & Stocker, W.G. (1981) Mutagenicity study of workers exposed to alkylene oxides (ethylene oxide/propylene oxide) and derivatives. *J. occup. Med.*, **23**, 343–347

Tomkins, D.J., Haines, T., Lawrence, M. & Rosa, N. (1993) A study of sister chromatid exchange and somatic cell mutation in hospital workers exposed to ethylene oxide. *Environ. Health Perspect.*, **101** (Suppl. 3), 159–164

Tompa, A., Major, J. & Jakab, M.G. (1999) Is breast cancer cluster influenced by environmental and occupational factors among hospital nurses in Hungary? *Pathol. oncol. Res.*, **5**, 117–121

Tucker, S.P. & Arnold, J.E. (1984) *Evaluation of OSHA Method No. 30 for Ethylene Oxide in Air with 400-mg/200-mg Charcoal Tubes* (NIOSH Report No. 84/02/00; US NTIS PB84-242049), Cincinnati, OH, National Institute for Occupational Safety and Health

Tucker, J.D., Xu, J., Stewart, J., Baciu, P.C., & Ong, T.M. (1986) Detection of sister chromatid exchanges induced by volatile genotoxicants. *Teratog. Carcinog. Mutag.*, **6**, 15–21

US Census (1980) [http://www2.census.gov/prod2/decennial/documents/1980a_vsC-01.pdf]

Van Duuren, B.L., Orris, L. & Nelson, N. (1965) Carcinogenicity of epoxides, lactones, and peroxy compounds. Part II. *J. natl Cancer Inst.*, **35**, 707–717

Vergnes, J.S. & Pritts, I.M. (1994) Effects of ethylene on micronucleus formation in the bone marrow of rats and mice following four week of inhalation exposure. *Mutat. Res.*, **324**, 87–91

Vogel, E. & Natarajan, A.T. (1982) The relation between reaction kinetics and mutagenic action of mono-functional alkylating agents in higher eukaryotic systems: Interspecies comparisons. In: Hollaender, A. & De Serres, F.J. eds, *Chemical Mutagens VII*, New York, Plenum, pp. 295–336

Walker, V.E. & Skopek, T.R. (1993) A mouse model for the study of in vivo mutational spectra: Sequence specificity of ethylene oxide at the *hprt* locus. *Mutat. Res.*, **288**, 151–162

Walker, V.E., Fennell, T.R., Boucheron, J.A., Fedtke, N., Ciroussel, F. & Swenberg, J.A. (1990) Macromolecular adducts of ethylene oxide: A literature review and a time-course study on the formation of 7-(2-hydroxyethyl)guanine following exposures of rats by inhalation. *Mutat. Res.*, **233**, 151–164

Walker, V.E., MacNeela, J.P., Swenberg, J.A., Turner, M.J. & Fennell, T.R. (1992a) Molecular dosimetry of ethylene oxide: Formation and persistence of N-(2-hydroxyethyl)valine in hemoglobin following repeated exposures of rats and mice. *Cancer Res.*, **52**, 4320–4327

Walker, V.E., Fennell, T.R., Upton, P.B., Skopek, T.R., Prevost, V., Shuker, D.E.G. & Swenberg, J.A. (1992b) Molecular dosimetry of ethylene oxide: Formation and persistence of 7-(2-hydroxyethyl)guanine in DNA following repeated exposures of rats and mice. *Cancer Res.*, **52**, 4328–4334

Walker, V.E., Fennell, T.R., Upton, P.B., MacNeela, J.P. & Swenberg, J.A. (1993) Molecular dosimetry of DNA and hemoglobin adducts in mice and rats exposed to ethylene oxide. *Environ. Health Perspect.*, **99**, 11–17

Walker, V.E., Sisk, S.C., Upton, P.B., Wong, B.A. & Recio, L. (1997a) In vivo mutagenicity of ethylene oxide at the hprt locus in T-lymphocytes of B6C3F1 lacI transgenic mice following inhalation exposure. *Mutat. Res.*, **392**, 211–222

Walker, V.E., Meng, Q. & Clement, N.L. (1997b) Spectra of mutations in *hprt* exon 3 of T-cells from F344 rats and *lacI* transgenic and nontransgenic B6C3F1 mice exposed by inhalation to ethylene oxide. *Environ. mol. Mutag.*, **29** (Suppl. 28), 54

Walker, V.E., Jones, I.M., Crippen, T.L., Meng, Q., Walker, D.M., Bauer, M.J., Reilly, A.A., Tates, A.D., Nakamura, J., Upton, P.B. & Skopek, T.R. (1999) Relationships between exposure, cell loss and proliferation, and manifestation of *HPRT* mutant T-cells following treatment of preweanling, weanling, and adult male mice with N-ethyl-N-nitrosourea. *Mutat. Res.*, **431**, 371–388

Walker, V.E., Wu, K.-Y., Upton, P.B., Ranasinghe, A., Scheller, N., Cho, M.-H., Vergnes, J.S., Skopek, T.R. & Swenberg, J.A. (2000) Biomarkers of exposure and effect as indicators of potential carcinogenic risk arising from in vivo metabolism of ethylene to ethylene oxide. *Carcinogenesis*, **21**, 1661–1669

Weast, R.C. & Astle, M.J. (1985) *CRC Handbook of Data on Organic Compounds*, Vol. I, Boca Raton, FL, CRC Press, p. 627

WHO (2003) *Ethylene Oxide* (Concise International Chemical Assessment Document 54), Geneva, World Health Organization [available at http://www.inchem,org/documents/cicads/cidads/cicad54.htm]

Wojcik-O'Neill, K.M. & Ello, M. (1991) Equivalency of hydrochloric acid and distilled water extraction media for determining residual ethylene oxide in medical devices. *J. pharm. Sci.*, **80**, 783–784

Wolfs, P., Dutrieux, M., Scailteur, V., Haxhe, J.-J., Zumofen, M. & Lauwerys, R. (1983) [Monitoring of workers exposed to ethylene oxide in a plant distributing sterilizing gases and in units for sterilizing medical equipment.] *Arch. Mal. prof.*, **44**, 321–328 (in French)

Wong, O. & Trent, L.S. (1993) An epidemiological study of workers potentially exposed to ethylene oxide. *Br. J. ind. Med.*, **50**, 308–316

Wu, K.-Y., Ranasinghe, A., Upton, P.B., Walker, V.E. & Swenberg, J.A. (1999a) Molecular dosimetry of endogenous and ethylene oxide-induced N7-(2-hydroxyethyl)guanine formation in tissues of rodents. *Carcinogenesis*, **30**, 1787–1792

Wu, K.-Y., Scheller, N., Ranasinghe, A., Yen, T.-Y., Sangaiah, R., Giese, R. & Swenberg, J.A. (1999b) A gas chromatography/electron capture/negative chemical ionization high-resolution mass spectrometry method for analysis of endogenous and exogenous N7-(2-hydroxy-ethyl)guanine in rodents and its potential for human biological monitoring. *Chem. Res. Toxicol.*, **12**, 722–729

Wu, K.Y., Chiang, S.Y., Huang, T.H., Tseng, Y.S., Chen, Y.L., Kuo, H.W. & Hsieh, C.L. (2004) Formation of N-(2-hydroxyethyl)valine in human hemoglobin-effect of lifestyle factors. *Mutat. Res.*, **559**, 73–82

Yager, J.W. (1982) Sister chromatid exchanges induced in rabbit lymphocytes by ethylene oxide after inhalation exposure. *Environ. Mutag.*, **4**, 121–134

Yager, J.W. (1987) Effect of concentration-time parameters on sister-chromatid exchanges induced in rabbit lymphocytes by ethylene oxide inhalation. *Mutat. Res.*, **182**, 343–352

Yager, J.W. & Benz, R.D. (1982) Sister chromatid exchanges induced in rabbit lymphocytes by ethylene oxide after inhalation exposure. *Environ. Mutag.*, **4**, 121–134

Yager, J.W., Hines, C.J. & Spear, R.C. (1983) Exposure to ethylene oxide at work increases sister chromatid exchanges in human peripheral lymphocytes. *Science*, **219**, 1221–1223

Yong, L.C., Schulte, P.A., Wiencke, J.K., Boeniger, M.F., Connally, L.B., Walker, J.T., Whelan, E.A. & Ward, E.M. (2001) Hemoglobin adducts and sister chromatid exchanges in hospital workers exposed to ethylene oxide: Effects of glutathione S-transferase T1 and M1 genotypes. *Cancer Epidemiol. Biomarkers Prev.*, **10**, 539–550

Yong, L.C., Schulte, P.A., Kao, C.-Y., Giese, R.W., Boeniger, M.F., Strauss, G.H.S., Petersen, M.R. & Wiencke, J.K. (2007) DNA adducts in granulocytes of hospital workers exposed to ethylene oxide. *Am. J. ind. Med.*, **50**, 293–302

Zamora, P.O., Benson, J.M., Li, A.P. & Brooks, A.L. (1983) Evaluation of an exposure system using cells grown on collagen gels for detecting highly volatile mutagens in the CHO/HGPRT mutation assay. *Environ. Mutag.*, **5**, 795–801

Zarbl, H. (2006) Cellular oncogenes and carcinogenesis. *In:* Warshawsky, D. & Landolph, J.R., Jr, eds, *Molecular Carcinogenesis and the Molecular Biology of Cancer,* New York, Taylor and Francis, pp. 103–129

Zhang, W., Johnson, F., Grollman, A.P. & Shibutani, S. (1995) Miscoding by the exocyclic and related DNA adducts 3,N^4-etheno-2′-deoxycytidine, 3,N^4-ethano-2′-deoxycytidine, and 3-(2-hydroxyethyl)-2′-deoxyuridine. *Chem. Res. Toxicol.*, **8**, 157–163

Zhao, C. & Hemminki, K. (2002) The *in vivo* levels of DNA alkylation products in human lymphocytes are not age dependent: An assay of 7-methyl- and 7-(2-hydroxyethyl)-guanine DNA adducts. *Carcinogenesis*, **23**, 307–310

Zhao, C., Tyndyk, M., Eide, I. & Hemminki, K. (1999) Endogenous and background DNA adducts by methylating and 2-hydroxyethylating agents. *Mutat. Res.*, **424**, 117–125

Zhong, B.-Z., Gu, Z.-W., Whong, W.-Z., Wallace, W.E. & Ong, T.-M. (1992) Comparative study of micronucleus assay and chromosomal aberration analysis in V79 cells exposed to ethylene oxide. *Teratog. Carcinog. Mutag.*, **11**, 227–233

VINYL CHLORIDE

This substance was considered by previous IARC Working Groups in June 1974 (IARC, 1974), February 1978 (IARC, 1979) and March 1987 (IARC, 1987). Since that time new data have become available, and these have been incorporated into the monograph and taken into account in the present evaluation.

1.   Exposure Data

1.1   Chemical and physical data

From IARC (1999), WHO (1999), IPCS-CEC (2000), Lide (2005), ATSDR (2006), Cowfer and Gorensek (2006) and O'Neil (2006), unless otherwise specified

1.1.1   *Nomenclature*

Chem. Abstr. Services Reg. No.: 75-01-4
Chem. Abstr. Name: Chloroethene; chloroethylene; monochloroethylene; VC; VCM; vinyl C monomer
RTECS No.: KU9625000
UN TDG No.: 1086 (stabilized)
EC Index No.: 602-023-00-7
EINECS No.: 200-831-0

1.1.2   *Structural and molecular formulae and relative molecular mass*

C$_2$H$_3$Cl

Relative molecular mass: 62.5

1.1.3   *Chemical and physical properties of the pure substance*

(a)   *Description*: Colourless gas
(b)   *Boiling-point*: −13 °C
(c)   *Melting-point*: −154 °C
(d)   *Relative density*: d_4^{20} 0.9106 (as liquid)
(e)   *Relative vapour density*: 2.2 (air = 1)
(f)   *Refractive index*: n_D^{20} 1.3700
(g)   *Spectroscopy data*: Infrared, nuclear magnetic resonance and mass spectral data have been tabulated (Grasselli & Ritchey, 1975).
(h)   *Solubility*: Slightly soluble in water (1.1 g/L at 25 °C); soluble in ethanol; very soluble in ether, carbon tetrachloride and benzene
(i)   *Volatility*: Vapour pressure, 2530 mm Hg at 20 °C
(j)   *Flash-point*: −78 °C (closed cup)
(k)   *Stability*: The substance can, under specific circumstances, form peroxides and initiate explosive polymerization. The substance decomposes on burning to produce toxic and corrosive fumes (hydrogen chloride, phosgene).
(l)   *Octanol/water partition coefficient*: log P_{ow}, 0.6
(m)   *Auto ignition temperature*: 472 °C
(n)   *Explosion limit in air*: 3.6–33%
(o)   *Henry's law constant*: 18.8 at 20 °C
(p)   *Conversion factor*: mg/m^3 = 2.6 × ppm[1]

1.1.4   *Technical products and impurities*

Vinyl chloride is generally supplied as a compressed liquefied gas.

1.1.5   *Analysis*

Several reviews of methods of sampling and analysis of vinyl chloride in the workplace atmosphere, ambient air, water, water piping, food and cigarette smoke, and of polyvinyl chloride (PVC) are available (Environmental Protection Agency, 1975; Laramy, 1977; Egan *et al.*, 1978).

Several methods for the analysis of vinyl chloride in ambient air have been developed. The Environmental Protection Agency method TO-1 analyses volatile organic compounds in ambient air using Tenax® and detection by gas chromatography (GS)–mass spectrometry (MS); method TO-14 analyses volatile organic compounds in ambient air using canister sampling followed by high-resolution GC (Environmental Protection Agency, 1999).

---

[1] Calculated from: mg/m^3 = (relative molecular mass/24.45) × ppm, assuming normal temperature (25 °C) and pressure (101.3 kPa)

A GC analytical method has been used since 1978 to determine vinyl chloride concentrations in foodstuffs and in vinyl chloride polymers and copolymers that are intended to come into contact with food (Directive 78-142-EEC; European Commission, 1978).

The Department of Labor (1989) of the USA published the Occupational Safety and Health Administration method 75 that detects vinyl chloride in air with a reliable quantitation limit of 0.020 ppm [0.051 mg/m^3]. More recently, Charvet *et al.* (2000) proposed the use of a solid-phase microextraction/GS/MS to analyse vinyl chloride in materials and aqueous samples.

1.2   Production and use

1.2.1   *Production*

The most common method for the production of vinyl chloride monomer (VCM) is by thermal cracking of ethylene dichloride (1,2-dichloroethane). Over 95% of the VCM produced worldwide in 2006 was made by this method. A less common method is by hydrochlorination of acetylene (WHO, 1999; Cowfer & Gorensek, 2006).

In the ethylene-based process, ethylene dichloride is synthesized by the reaction of elemental chlorine with ethylene over a catalyst. The crude ethylene dichloride is washed, dried and purified. Pure, dry ethylene dichloride is thermally cracked to produce VCM and hydrogen chloride. Hydrogen chloride recovered from the cracking of ethylene dichloride is recycled in the process via reaction with oxygen and ethylene over a copper catalyst to make more ethylene dichloride. This process is known as oxychlorination. VCM is purified by distillation, and side-products can be recovered for the manufacture of chlorinated solvents, or combusted or catalytically oxidized usually with recovery of hydrogen chloride (WHO, 1999; Cowfer & Gorensek, 2006).

VCM was initially produced commercially by the acetylene-based process, in which acetylene (usually produced by the reaction of water with calcium carbide) is reacted with hydrogen chloride over a mercury-based catalyst. VCM is again purified by distillation (WHO, 1999; Cowfer & Gorensek, 2006). Acetylene-based plants continue to operate solely in China. In 2001, the chemical corporation Borden stopped production at its acetylene plant in Louisiana, USA (Borruso, 2006).

The ethylene dichloride/VCM/PVC production chain represents the largest single consumer of chlorine (European Commission, 2003).

Vinyl chloride has been produced commercially in the USA for over 70 years (Tariff Commission, 1928). In 1988, the production of vinyl chloride in the USA was 9.1 billion pounds [4.1 million tonnes] and increased to around 13.75 billion pounds [6.2 million tonnes] in 1993 (ACGIH® Worldwide, 2005). In Taiwan, China, production has increased from 12 000 tonnes in 1971 (Luo *et al.*, 1999) to 1.7 million tonnes in 2005 (Borruso, 2006).

In 1999, worldwide production capacity was around 30 million tonnes (SIDS, 2001). Worldwide production capacity of VCM in 2005 was 35 million tonnes (Dow Chemical

Company, 2007). Table 1 gives production levels in various countries and regions (Borruso, 2006).

Table 1. World production capacity for vinyl chloride monomer in 2005

Region/country	Capacity (thousands of tonnes)
North America	
USA/Canada	8 934
Mexico	270
South America	
Brazil	635
Other	410
Western Europe	6 650
Central and eastern Europe	2 195
Africa and the Middle East	1 557
Asia	
Japan	3 050
China	3 443
China, Province of Taiwan	1 710
Korea, Republic of	1 466
Other Asia[a]	2 304
Oceania	0
Total	32 624

From Borruso (2006)
[a] Includes India, Indonesia, Korea (People's Democratic Republic of), Malaysia and Thailand

1.2.2   *Use*

Vinyl chloride is used primarily (> 95%) in the manufacture of PVCs, which comprise about 12% of plastic usage (WHO, 1999). The largest use of PVC resins is in the production of plastic piping. Other important uses are in floor coverings, consumer goods, electrical applications and transport applications. About 1% of PVC capacity is used to produce vinyl chloride/vinyl acetate copolymer. Other minor uses of VCM include the manufacture of chlorinated solvents (primarily 10 000 tonnes per year of 1,1,1-trichloroethane) and ethylene diamine production for the manufacture of resins (WHO, 1999; European Commission, 2003).

Vinyl chloride has been used in the past as a refrigerant, as an extraction solvent for heat-sensitive materials, in the production of chloroacetaldehyde, as an aerosol propellant and in drug and cosmetic products; these uses were banned in the USA by the Environmental Protection Agency in 1974 (ATSDR, 2006).

1.3   Occurrence

1.3.1   *Natural occurrence*

Vinyl chloride is not known to occur naturally.

1.3.2   *Occupational exposure*

According to the 1990–93 CAREX database for 15 countries of the European Union (Kauppinen *et al.*, 2000) and the 1981–83 National Occupational Exposure Survey in the USA (NOES, 1997), approximately 40 000 workers in Europe and 80 000 workers in the USA were potentially exposed to vinyl chloride (see General Remarks).

The major categories of industries that entail exposure to VCM in Europe comprise the manufacture of industrial chemicals (10 400 persons), plastic products (9100 persons) and other chemical products (7600) (Kauppinen *et al.*, 2000). In the USA, the major categories of industries were the production of chemicals and allied products (15 400), business services (10 000) and the production of rubber and miscellaneous plastic products (9600) (NOES, 1997).

The Finnish Register of occupational exposure to carcinogens reported that 90 workers were notified as being exposed to vinyl chloride in 2004. This is below 0.01% of the 2.4 million people employed in Finland. Most of the exposed were employed in the chemical industry. The register is based on annual notifications of employers and its completeness is unknown (Saalo *et al.*, 2006).

In Taiwan, China, where production has increased dramatically in recent decades, thousands of workers could be exposed to VCM (Luo *et al.*, 1999).

The main route of occupational exposure is by inhalation, which occurs primarily in vinyl chloride/PVC plants and in PVC processing plants. Few measured exposure data have been reported but estimates from the chemical industry indicate that exposure to VCM amounted to several thousands of milligrams per cubic metre in the 1940s and 1950s, and were several hundreds of milligrams per cubic metre in the 1960s and early 1970s. After its recognition as a carcinogen, occupational exposure standards were set at approximately 13–26 mg/m^3 [5–10 ppm] in most countries in the 1970s (Fleig & Thiess, 1974; WHO, 1999).

A report from the Centers for Disease Control and Prevention (CDC) in the USA concluded that the development and acceptance by the PVC industry of a closed-loop polymerization process in the late 1970s "almost completely eliminated worker exposures" and that "new cases of hepatic angiosarcoma in vinyl chloride polymerization workers have been virtually eliminated" (CDC, 1997; see also Section 1.4). Even after the late 1970s, however, high concentrations were reported and may still be encountered in some countries (see Table 2).

Table 2. Levels of vinyl chloride reported in workplace air samples in vinyl chloride/polyvinyl chloride (PVC) production plants

Reference	Year of study	Country	Workplace	Concentration (mg/m^3)
Filatova & Gronsberg (1957)	NR	Former USSR	PVC producing plant	50–800 (occasionally 87 300)
Anghelescu et al. (1969)	1965–67	Romania	PVC production plant	112–554
Baretta et al. (1969)	NR	USA	PVC plant	≤ 650 (weekly TWA)
Fleig & Theiss (1974)	1974	Germany	PVC production department	< 65–81
Ott et al. (1975)	1950–59	USA	PVC plant	≤ 10 400; 13–2140 (8-h TWA)
	1960–63			≤ 1300; 13–620 (8-h TWA)
Rowe (1975)	1973	USA	Vinyl chloride/PVC plants	≤ 390 (TWA); peaks 2600–10 400
Barnes (1976)	'Early days'	United Kingdom	PVC production plant (full-time autoclave cleaner)	7800
Orusev et al. (1976)	1974	Former Yugoslavia	PVC production plant	> 195
German Environmental Office (1978)	1977	Germany	PVC production plant	1.3–91
Hansteen et al. (1978)	1974	Norway	PVC plant	65
Haguenoer et al. (1979)	1977–78	France	PVC production plant	2.3–7.3 (range of monthly means)
Heger et al. (1981)	1979	Germany	PVC production plant	12 (12-h TWA, stationary); 15.5 (12-h TWA, personal)
Bao et al. (1988)	1981	China	PVC production plant	9.9–229
Holm et al. (1982)	1974–81	Sweden	PVC production plant	0.26–114 (8-h TWA)
	1974–80			0.26–5.7 (6-h TWA)
Coenen (1986); BIA (1996)	1981–84	Germany	24 plants	3% of 33 samples > 5 (90th percentile, < 1) (shift means)
	1989–1992		46 plants	All of 117 samples < 5 (90th percentile < 0.1) (shift means)

Table 2 (contd)

Reference	Year of study	Country	Workplace	Concentration (mg/m^3)
De Jong et al. (1988)	1976–77	The Netherlands	PVC plant	2.6–26 (8-h TWA)
Smulevich et al. (1988)	Early 1950s	Former USSR	Vinyl chloride/PVC plants	100–800
Studniarek et al. (1989)	1974	Poland	Vinyl chloride/PVC plant (several departments)	(30–600)[a]
	1975			(30–270)[a]
	1976			(15–60)[a]
	1977			(6–150)[a]
	1978			(1–30)[a]
	1979			(1–15)[a]
	1981			(0.1–36)[a]
	1982			(0.1–12)[a]
	1974		(autoclave cleaners)	(990)[a]
	1982			(9–180)[a]
Fucic et al. (1990)	NR	Croatia	Plastics industry	Mean, 13; 5200 (occasional peak)
Hrivnak et al. (1990)	NR	Former Czechoslovakia	NR	2–41
Ho et al. (1991)	1976	Singapore	PVC production plant	2.6–54 (15.3)[a]
	After 1983			≤26 (short-term) (3.9)[a]
Pirastu et al. (1991)	1950–85	Italy	Vinyl chloride/PVC plants	<13–≥1300
Dobecki & Romaniwicz (1993)	1986	Poland	Vinyl chloride synthesis mechanic, breathing zone	21.3
	1987			66.9
	1988			43.7
	1989			0.7
	1990			0.2
Viinanen (1993)	1981-85	Finland	PVC production plant, breathing zone	1.6 (8-h TWA); range, <0.3–57
	1986–89			1.6 (8-h TWA); range, <0.3–46
	1993			0.3 (8-h TWA); range, <0.3–26

Table 2 (contd)

Reference	Year of study	Country	Workplace	Concentration (mg/m³)
Gáliková et al. (1994)	1990–93	Russian Federation	Vinyl chloride/PVC plant	
			Whole plant (16 probes)	1–9 (range of annual means)
			Under the reactor	≤ 200 (range of annual means)
			In compressor room	≤ 400 (range of annual means)
Rashad et al. (1994)	NR	Egypt	Vinyl chloride/PVC plant	0.05–18 (8-h TWA)
Du et al. (1996)	NR	Taiwan, China	5 PVC plants	
			15 different operation units	Range (114 samples), ND (0.13)–1009
			Outside reaction tank[b]	Range (4 samples), 6–1009 (mean, 296; median, 86)
			15 different job titles	Range of TWA (85 samples), ND–3680
			Tank supplier[b]	Range (9 samples), 5.7–3680 (mean, 660; median, 23.7)
Hozo et al. (1996, 1997)	1949–87	Croatia	Vinyl chloride/PVC plant	Mean, 543; up to 1300 (peak)
Zhu et al. (2005a)	NR	China	PVC plant	Geometric mean, 7.1; range, 0.8–48.4

Updated from WHO (1999)
ND, not detected; NR, not reported; TWA, time-weighted average
[a] Geometric means
[b] Highest mean concentrations of vinyl chloride

(a) Production of vinyl chloride and its derivatives

Measured levels of VCM concentrations in vinyl chloride/PVC production are summarized in Table 2 (WHO, 1999). Only one recent study was found in which levels of exposure to vinyl chloride were reported (Zhu *et al.*, 2005a).

Zhu *et al.* (2005a) reported the exposure to VCM of workers in a plant in China. Ambient air levels of VCM at different worksites in the plant ranged from 0.3 to 17.8 ppm [0.8–48.4 mg/m^3]; the geometric average concentration was 2.6 ppm [7.1 mg/m^3]. In another study in Taiwan, China (Du *et al.*, 1996), the highest median concentration was reported for short-term exposure (15–40 min) of a tank cleaner was 70 mg/m^3 [27 ppm].

In former socialist countries in eastern Europe, the stringent regulations for PVC production that were introduced in western Europe and the USA in the 1970s could not be met for socioeconomic reasons, and large plants with old-fashioned technologies continued to function with concentrations of VCM that remained at levels of former standards (Hozo *et al.*, 1996).

In vinyl chloride production, workers may be exposed to ethylene dichloride and to catalysts such as iron(III) chloride. In PVC production, concurrent exposure to PVC dust may occur (Casula *et al.*, 1977). The polymerization inhibitor bisphenol-A has been reported to leach from polycarbonate flasks during autoclaving (Krishnan *et al.*, 1993).

(b) PVC processing

Measured levels of VCM in plants where PVC was being processed are considerably lower than those in vinyl chloride and PVC producing plants (Table 3; WHO, 1999). Improvements in PVC production in the 1970s resulted in a much lower content of residual VCM in PVC resin. The lower monomer content led automatically to concentrations in the ambient air of PVC processing factories < 0.1 ppm [0.26 mg/m^3] (Holm *et al.*, 1982).

In PVC processing, the polymer may be mixed with antixodants (such as *p*-nonylphenol), stabilizers (such as organic tin compounds), plasticizers (phthalates) and colouring agents (pigments) (reviewed in Summers, 2006) and occupational exposure to these compounds, as well as to PVC dust, may occur (Boraiko & Batt, 2005).

1.3.3 Environmental occurrence

(a) Ambient air

Vinyl chloride has been reported in landfill gas and groundwater as a degradation product of chlorinated solvents that were deposited in landfills (WHO, 1999).

In recent years, the industrial release of vinyl chloride into the air in the USA slowly decreased from 734 259 pounds [333 tonnes] in 2001 to 670 992 pounds [305 tonnes] in 2002, 645 804 pounds [293 tonnes] in 2003, 653 837 pounds [297 tonnes] in 2004 and 545 252 pounds [248 tonnes] in 2005 (National Library of Medicine, 2007).

Table 3. Levels of vinyl chloride reported for workplace air samples in polyvinyl chloride (PVC) processing plants

Reference	Country	Workplace	Year	Concentration (mg/m^3)
Bol'shakov (1969)	Russia	PVC processing plant (synthetic leather plant)	Before 1966	< 114
Fleig & Thiess (1974)	Germany	PVC processing department	1974	< 2.6–68
Murdoch & Hammond (1977)	United Kingdom	PVC processing plants (cable factories)	NR	0.4–0.9
Holm et al. (1982)	Sweden	PVC processing plant	1974	< 0.26–0.8
Bao et al. (1988)	China	PVC processing plant	1981–85	≤ 30
Solionova et al. (1992)	Russia	PVC processing plant (rubber footwear plant)	Before 1990	0.007–1.26
Lundberg et al. (1993)	Sweden	PVC processing plant Mixing	Before 1975 After 1975	< 26 <<< 26
		Others	Before 1975 After 1975	< 13 < 2.6
Nelson et al. (1993)	USA	Automotive assembly plant(s)	1970s	0.13–7.8 (2 personal samples)
BIA (1996)	Germany	Polymer extrusion (17 plants)	1989–92	All of 33 samples < 8 (90 percentile, < 0.15) (shift means)

From WHO (1999)
NR, not reported; TWA, time-weighted average

Atmospheric concentrations of VCM in ambient air are low (usually < 3 μg/m³). A monitoring programme in the 1970s that measured VCM in the air around vinyl chloride and PVC production plants found some relatively high concentrations of vinyl chloride in ambient air. Maximum 24-h average concentrations ranged from 0.32 to 10.6 ppm [0.8–28 mg/m³]. Levels of VCM were much lower in the vicinity of PVC product manufacturing plants than near vinyl chloride and PVC production plants (Dimmick, 1981).

(b)   Accidental releases

In June 1996, 10 of 18 tank wagons filled with vinyl chloride were derailed on the Magdeburg–Halle railway line just outside the Schönebeck station in Germany. One wagon exploded and four others ignited; 28 people received in-patient treatment in a nearby hospital and 268 others were treated as outpatients. Vinyl chloride concentrations of 0.06–8 ppm [0.16–20.8 mg/m³] were measured in residential areas. Almost 300 urine samples that were taken from rescue workers, residents and a control group were analysed for the vinyl chloride metabolite thiodiacetic acid. The measured values appeared to be in the range of those of unexposed people (Thriene *et al.*, 2000).

(c)   Residues in PVC resin and products

PVC products contain VCM as a residue from production (WHO, 1999). In a survey from 1976 to 1977, the following articles contained VCM at levels > 0.05 ppm [0.13 mg/m³]: bathroom tiles, piping, plastic bottles for table oil and kitchen wrapping film. The highest concentrations were found in vinyl music records. The VCM content of toys, kitchen utensils, food wrappings, wallpaper and car interiors was < 0.05 ppm (German Environmental Office, 1978). The introduction of improved manufacturing practices has considerably reduced the residual content of VCM in PVC products (WHO, 1999).

(d)   Other occurrences

VCM was identified in mainstream smoke of cigarettes (1.3–16 ng/cigarette) and cigars (14–27 ng/cigar). The measured levels correlated with chloride content of the tobacco (Hoffmann *et al.*, 1976; IARC, 2004).

There has been no report of vinyl chloride levels found in food, pharmaceutical or cosmetic products in recent years (WHO, 1999).

1.4   Regulations and guidelines

Historically, the American Conference of Government Industrial Hygienists threshold limit values (ACGIH TLV®) were lowered from a maximum allowed concentration–time-weighted average (MAC–TWA) of 500 ppm in 1946–47 to a TLV–TWA of 200 ppm in 1972. In 1978–79, the carcinogenic classification A1c was added. In 1980, a

TLV–TWA value of 5 ppm was recommended together with the carcinogen classification of A1c, which changed to A1a and then to A1 in 1987. In 1999, a TLV–TWA value of 1 ppm was accepted with the A1 carcinogen classification (ACGIH, 2001).

Many countries, regions or organizations have established exposure guidelines for vinyl chloride in the workplace (Table 4).

The international, national and state regulations and guidelines regarding vinyl chloride in air, water and other media have been summarized by ATSDR (2006).

Since 1978, the European Union has controlled the presence of vinyl chloride in polymers and copolymers that are intended to come into contact with food (78/142/EEC; European Commission, 1978).

Table 4. Exposure guidelines for vinyl chloride in the workplace

Country/region or organization	TWA (ppm)[a]	STEL (ppm)[a]	Carcinogenicity[b]	Notes
Australia	5		1	
Belgium	3		Ca	
Brazil		156 (ceiling)		
Canada				
Alberta	1			
British Columbia	1		1	ALARA
Ontario	1			
Quebec	1	5	A1	Recirculation prohibited
China	10 mg/m^3	25 mg/m^3		STEL based on ultra limit coefficient
China, Hong Kong SAR	5		A1	
Czech Republic	7.5 mg/m^3	15 mg/m^3		
Finland	3			MAC
Germany-MAK			1	
Ireland	3		Ca1	
Japan JSOH		2.5 (ceiling)	1	
Malaysia	1			Medical surveillance is appropriate
Mexico	5		A1	
Netherlands	7.77 mg/m^3		Ca	
New Zealand	5		A1	
Norway	1		Ca[a]	
Poland	5 mg/m^3	30 mg/m^3	Ca	
South Africa-DOL-RL	7			
Spain	3		Ca1	
Sweden	1	5	Ca	Skin

Table 4 (contd)

Country/region or organization	TWA (ppm)[a]	STEL (ppm)[a]	Carcinogenicity[b]	Notes
United Kingdom	3		R45	
USA				
ACGIH	1		A1	
NIOSH REL			Ca	
OSHA PEL	1	5		STEL is an average not to exceed 15 minutes

From ACGIH® Worldwide (2005)
ACGIH, American Conference of Governmental Industrial Hygienists; ALARA, as low as reasonably achievable; DOL-RL, Department of Labour-recommended limit; JSOH, Japanese Society of Occupational Health; MAC, maximum acceptable concentration; MAK, maximum allowed concentration; NIOSH, National Institute of Occupational Safety and Health; OSHA, Occupational Safety and Health Administration; PEL, permissible exposure limit; REL, recommended exposure limit; STEL, short-term exposure limit; TWA, time-weighted average
[a] Unless otherwise specified
[b] 1, established human carcinogen/substance which causes cancer in humans/carcinogenic to humans; Ca, Carcinogen/substance is carcinogenic; Ca[a], potential cancer-causing agent; A1, confirmed human carcinogen; Ca1, substance known to be carcinogenic to humans; R45, may cause cancer

2. Studies of Cancer in Humans

2.1 Case reports

A case report of three cases of angiosarcoma of the liver in men who had been employed in the manufacture of PVC resins provided the first evidence of an association between vinyl chloride and cancer in humans (Creech & Johnson, 1974). The case report was particularly informative because of the rarity of the tumour. Case reports of hepato-cellular carcinoma in workers exposed to vinyl chloride have been published since the mid-1970s in France (Saurin *et al.*, 1997), Germany (Gokel *et al.*, 1976; Koischwitz *et al.*, 1981; Dietz *et al.*, 1985; Lelbach, 1996; Weihrauch *et al.*, 2000), China (Hong Kong SAR) (Evans *et al.*, 1983), Italy (Pirastu *et al.*, 1990), Japan (Makita *et al.*, 1997) and the USA (Bond *et al.*, 1990).

2.2   Methods and main results of epidemiological cohort studies of workers exposed to vinyl chloride

Two epidemiological multicentric investigations of workers who were employed in the vinyl chloride industry have been carried out: one in North America and one in Europe. In addition to reports that related to these cohorts in their entirety, a number of studies reported findings from individual subcohorts. In this section, results for subcohorts are described only when they provide important information that is not available in analyses of the full cohorts. Six cohort studies have also been reported in addition to and separately from the two multicentric investigations.

2.2.1   *North American multicentric study*

The North American multicentric cohort was originally assembled under the sponsorship of the Chemical Manufacturers' Association (now known as the American Chemistry Council). The first published report of this study (Cooper, 1981) included 10 173 workers from 37 plants, whose vital status was updated through to 31 December 1972. Among the 37 plants included in the study, 11 plants with 1214 workers produced only VCM, 18 plants with 6848 workers produced only PVC, three plants with 935 workers produced both VCM and PVC and five plants with 1176 workers produced homo-polymers and copolymers. To be eligible for inclusion into the cohort, male employees at the 37 participating plants were required to have been exposed to VCM for at least 1 year before 31 December 1972 and to have been employed in or after 1942. The time at which the employees were included in the study depended on the date at which the plant where they worked began making or using VCM and the earliest date at which personnel records were complete for all employees, whichever was later. A second major follow-up of this cohort was published by Wong *et al.* (1991), at which time vital status had been updated through to 31 December 1989; this update included 10 173 individuals who satisfied the original entry criteria for this study. A third major update included the same eligibility criteria; after minor corrections to study records, 10 109 subjects were included in the analysis and vital status was updated through to 31 December 1995 (Mundt *et al.*, 2000). On the basis of state reference rates, the standardized mortality ratio (SMR) was 0.83 (95% confidence interval [CI], 0.80–0.86) for all causes, 0.96 (95% CI, 0.90–1.03) for all malignant neoplasms and 3.59 (80 deaths; 95% CI, 2.84–4.46) for cancer of the liver and biliary tract. Results for cancer at other sites were given for brain and central nervous system (36 deaths; SMR, 1.42; 95% CI, 1.00–1.97), lung (303 deaths; SMR, 0.82; 95% CI, 0.73–0.92), lymphatic and haematopoeitic tissue (71 observed; SMR, 0.86; 95% CI, 0.67–1.08), lymphosarcoma and reticulosarcoma (International Classification of Diseases (ICD)-9 code 200; 12 deaths; SMR, 1.20; 95% CI, 0.62–2.09) and skin (ICD-9 code 172–173; 12 deaths; SMR, 0.64; 95% CI, 0.33–1.12).

A separate analysis for a plant located in Louisville, KY (USA), that was included in the multicentric cohort was published by Lewis *et al.* (2003). The plant was the site at which an excess of deaths from angiosarcoma had first been detected in workers exposed to vinyl chloride; it had opened in 1942 and has produced VCM, PVC resin and nitrile rubber copolymers. Among 2200 workers who had been employed for at least 1 year in jobs that entailed exposure to VCM in 1942–72 and who were followed-up during 1942–95, mortality from all causes was below that expected (903 deaths versus 1008.8 expected; SMR, 0.88), while that for all cancers combined was above expectation (264 deaths versus 248.2 expected; SMR, 1.06); mortality from cancer of the liver and biliary tract was also greater than that expected (24 deaths versus six expected; SMR, 4.00).

A subsequent study at this plant compared the exposure histories of cases of liver angiosarcoma and brain cancer with those of 1817 workers who had been exposed for at least 1 year and had been hired before 1967 (Lewis & Rempala, 2003). Exposure variables included history of employment in various PVC and nitrile rubber production buildings, ranked peak exposure to VCM and estimated cumulative exposure to VCM, acrylonitrile (IARC, 1999), 1,3-butadiene (see this volume) and styrene (IARC, 2002). In a nested case–control study, each case was individually matched to controls by year of birth, year of hire and duration of employment. The matched case–control analysis considered ranked exposure to VCM, vinylidene chloride (IARC, 1999), vinyl acetate (IARC, 1995), PVC, acrylonitrile (IARC, 1999), 1,3-butadiene (see this volume) and styrene (IARC, 2002). The occurrence of angiosarcoma was strongly associated with exposure to vinyl chloride but not with exposure to the other chemicals; the risk for brain cancer was highest among workers who had been hired before 1950 but was not associated with exposure to vinyl chloride.

2.2.2 *European multicentric study*

The European multicentric cohort was conducted in four countries (Italy, Norway, Sweden and the United Kingdom). The first report of the study results (Simonato *et al.*, 1991) included follow-up of vital status through to 31 December 1986; an update of the study (Ward *et al.*, 2001) analysed incidence and mortality through to the latest year for which data were available in each country, which ranged between 1993 and 1997. The study included a total of 19 factories; 11 of these produced VCM/PVC, two produced VCM only, five produced PVC only and one was a PVC processing plant. Male workers who had been employed for at least 1 year in 1942–72 in jobs that entailed exposure to VCM were included. The observation period for the cohort began in 1955, the year for which reference rates were first available. The most recent report provided updated information on vital status for 17 of the 19 factories and on cancer incidence for 13 factories in three countries. In addition, results for most of the national cohorts were published separately (Byren *et al.*, 1976; Fox & Collier, 1977; Molina *et al.*, 1981; Heldaas *et al.*, 1984, 1987; Jones *et al.*, 1988; Hagmar *et al.*, 1990; Pirastu *et al.*, 1990, 1998; Langård *et al.*, 2000).

Of the 12 700 men included in the updated analysis of the full cohort (Ward *et al.*, 2001), 9688 (76.3%) were alive (range by country, 66–89%), 2665 (21.0%; range by country, 10–33%) had died, 63 (0.5%) were lost to follow-up and 284 (2.2%) had emigrated. Overall, the follow-up was 97.3% complete.

Age- and calendar period-specific (men only) national mortality rates were used as the reference for the SMR analysis. These were computed using the WHO mortality database, in which only three-digit ICD codes have been stored consistently since 1955. A search for the best available data for a diagnosis of liver cancer was conducted by reviewing all available documentation. For Sweden and Norway, this included histology on the death certificate, if noted, and morphology coded by the cancer registry. For Italy, where cancer registry data were not available, information was obtained from the death certificate or from medical records. In the United Kingdom, sources of histological diagnosis included the death certificate, cancer registry, medical records and a registry of angiosarcomas developed by the Health and Safety Executive (Baxter, 1981). Records of cases of liver cancer from all of the countries were also matched by indirect identifiers to records of an angiosarcoma registry maintained by the Association of European Plastics Manufacturers (Forman et al., 1985).

Analysis by production process was based on the type of plant. The majority of workers (8032) were employed in mixed VCM/PVC production facilities, followed by PVC production (3047), PVC processing (1353) and VCM production (206). Calendar period-specific job–exposure matrices were provided by industrial hygienists for 13 of the 19 factories, and matrices that provided job- and calendar time-specific estimates of exposure to vinyl chloride in parts per million were created. Each job–exposure matrix was checked and validated as being generally accurate by two other industrial hygienists, one from Sweden and one from the United Kingdom, both of whom had had several years of experience in the vinyl chloride industry.

In general, exposure estimates for the study plants were highest in the earliest years of operation. For example, estimates of exposure to VCM in the highest exposure categories, including reactor operators, were as high as > 500 ppm [> 1300 mg/m^3] in 1950–65 in several of the Italian plants, 2000 ppm [5200 mg/m^3] in 1950–54 in a Norwegian plant, approximately 3000 ppm [7800 mg/m^3] in 1940–44 in one of the Swedish plants and 770 ppm [2000 mg/m^3] in 1944–50 in one of the British plants. Exposure estimates for high-exposure jobs in the 1960s were substantially lower in most plants, and the majority were below 200 ppm [520 mg/m^3]. By the mid-1970s, very few plants had estimated exposures > 5 ppm [> 13 mg/m^3]. Exposure variables in the analysis were autoclave worker (ever/never), duration of employment, and ranked level of exposure and cumulative exposure to VCM in air in ppm–years. Exposures to vinyl chloride in the study plants were estimated to be < 1 ppm [< 2.6 mg/m^3] for all jobs between 1976 and 1988. Most factories had a specific job category for autoclave workers, and the classification of individuals as 'ever autoclave worker' was based on ever having held a job in this category. For these workers, three categories were created: 1, known to have been an autoclave worker; 2, not known to have been an autoclave worker, and from a factory with a specific job code for autoclave worker; and 3, from a factory in which work as an autoclave worker could not be determined.

In addition to the job–exposure matrix with job- and calendar time-specific estimated exposures to vinyl chloride in parts per million, an index of ranked level of exposure was developed. Classification of subjects in this index was based on the maximum exposure level for any job held by an individual, based on the job- and the calendar time-specific exposure estimates given for that job in the job–exposure matrix. In order to examine the potential association of exposure to PVC dust with lung cancer and non-malignant respiratory disease, stratified analyses were conducted for those workers who had only, ever or never been employed in curing, filtering and packing jobs.

Using national mortality and incidence rates as the reference, mortality from all causes (SMR, 0.85; 95% CI, 0.82–0.88) and from all cancers (SMR, 0.99; 95% CI, 0.93–1.06) was below the reference, as was total cancer incidence (standardized incidence ratio [SIR], 0.85; 95% CI, 0.79–0.91). An increase in the occurrence of primary liver cancer was observed (53 deaths and 29 incident cases; SMR, 2.40; 95% CI, 1.80–3.14; SIR, 3.98; 95% CI, 2.67–5.72). From the best available data on diagnosis, 71 cases of liver cancer were identified and used in the internal analysis for latency, duration of employment, cumulative exposure and employment as autoclave cleaner. On the same basis, 37 cases of angiosarcoma and 10 cases of hepatocellular carcinoma were ascertained for which detailed analyses of latency, duration of exposure, cumulative exposure and ever versus never having worked as an autoclave cleaner were conducted. The results of these internal analyses are presented in Section 2.3. Results for other cancer sites (Ward et al., 2001) were: brain cancer — SMR, 0.93 (24 deaths; 95% CI, 0.60–1.39) and SIR, 0.91 (19 cases; 95% CI, 0.55–1.42); lung cancer — SMR, 0.95 (272 deaths; 95% CI, 0.84–1.07) and SIR, 0.80 (154 cases; 95% CI, 0.68–0.94); and lymphatic and haematopoeitic cancer — SMR, 0.94 (62 deaths; 95% CI, 0.72–1.21) [SIR not reported]; no significant excess was reported in any category of leukaemia or lymphoma. A non-significantly elevated SMR was found for malignant melanoma (15 deaths; SMR, 1.60; 95% CI, 0.90–2.65) but the analysis of incidence did not show an excess (18 observed cases; SIR, 1.06; 95% CI, 0.63–1.68) (Ward et al., 2001). Results of internal analyses for selected sites are presented in Sections 2.3–2.9.

The European study found evidence of a significant association between exposure to VCM and mortality from liver cirrhosis. The relative risks for cumulative exposures of < 524 (reference), 524–998, 999–3429, 3430–5148 and ≥ 5149 ppm–years were 1.00, 9.38 (eight cases; 95% CI, 3.52–25.0), 4.01 (nine cases; 95% CI, 1.55–10.4), 9.77 (eight cases; 95% CI, 3.66–26.1) and 8.28 (nine cases; 95% CI, 3.15–21.8), respectively.

In a Swedish study of 2031 workers employed for ≥ 3 months in a PVC processing plant during 1961–80 (Hagmar et al., 1990), mortality and cancer incidence in 1961–85 were studied; vital status was established for 95.5% of cohort members. Work activities were classified for estimated exposure to VCM as none, low, moderate or high. The cohort was later included in the European multicentric study. The incidence of all cancers was higher than expected (SIR, 1.16; 95% CI, 0.99–1.36). Two incident cases of cancer of the liver and biliary tract were observed among workers with 10 or more years latency, an incidence that was higher than expected (SIR, 2.44; 95% CI, 0.30–8.80).

A Swedish cohort of 717 workers who had been employed for ≥ 3 months in three PVC processing plants in 1964–74 was followed up for mortality in 1964–86 and for incidence of disease in 1964–84; work activities were classified as having high, intermediate or low potential exposure to VCM and national reference rates were used for comparison. Mortality from all causes was as expected (SMR, 1.0; 95% CI, 0.8–1.2), and no cases of liver cancer were observed (Lundberg *et al.*, 1993).

A prospective follow-up study of French VCM workers was initiated in 1980 (Laplanche *et al.*, 1992). The study population included exposed and unexposed workers from 12 plants; 1096 employees, aged 44–55 years, had been exposed to VCM in 1980–81 or earlier and were free of disease at the time of enrolment; the unexposed group included 1093 employees who were individually matched to the exposed group by age, plant and plant physician. Interviews and data collection were conducted by plant physicians. Occupational and medical histories, parental history of cancer, employment status, nationality, tobacco smoking status and alcoholic beverage consumption were recorded. The follow-up period ended in December 1988. During the study period, 20 deaths from cancer were observed among the exposed and 22 among the unexposed. Cancer morbidity was higher among the exposed (38 cases observed) than the unexposed (32 cases observed; relative risk, 1.3; 95% CI, 0.8–2.1).

In an Italian plant in Porto Marghera that was included in the European multicentric study, an internal analysis was completed with mortality follow-up for 1972–95 and employment histories for 1972–85 (Gennaro *et al.*, 2003). The relative risks for mortality from all causes and all cancers for autoclave workers versus all other workers were 1.32 (11 deaths; 95% CI, 0.55–3.15) and 1.09 (six deaths; 95% CI, 0.36–3.31), respectively; an increase was also observed for mortality from liver cancer (four deaths; relative risk, 9.57; 95% CI, 1.69–54.1).

In the same plant, mortality and occupational history were updated until 1999 (Pirastu *et al.*, 2003). On the basis of job- and time-specific exposure estimates, cumulative exposure was calculated and classified into six exposure categories (0–735, 735–2379, 2379–5188, 5188–7531 and 7531–9400 ppm–years); employment as an autoclave worker (ever/never) was also considered in the analyses. Data (clinical and pathological) that gave the best diagnosis were used to identify cases of liver angiosarcoma and hepatocellular carcinoma. Regional rates were used as a reference, mortality from primary liver cancer was determined and internal analyses for duration, latency and exposure were completed. A comparison of mortality in the cohort with local reference rates was made for all causes (SMR, 0.75; 90% CI, 0.68–0.83) and all cancers (SMR, 0.94; 90% CI, 0.81–1.09), both of which were lower than expected. For all causes, the analysis by time since leaving employment and adjusted for latency showed that the SMR in the first year after leaving employment was 2.76 (90% CI, 1.94–3.91). Mortality rates for liver angiosarcoma (six cases) increased with latency and cumulative exposure; no cases were associated with duration of employment of < 12 years, latency of < 10 years or cumulative exposure of < 2379 ppm–years. Mortality rates for hepatocellular carcinoma (12 cases) and liver cirrhosis (20 cases) showed a similar pattern.

A cross-sectional study in the same plant examined occupational and non-occupational risk factors for cirrhosis of the liver and hepatocellular carcinoma among 13 individuals who had liver cancer (eight confirmed histologically), 40 individuals who had liver cirrhosis (24 confirmed histologically) and 139 referents who had been examined in a medical surveillance programme in 1999–2002 and were found not to have had any evidence of liver disease or cancer at any site (Mastrangelo et al., 2004). Among the 13 cases of hepatocellular carcinoma, 11 also had liver cirrhosis and were included in both groups. [The Working Group noted that it was not clear how the 139 referent subjects with no evidence of liver disease were selected from among the 643 persons examined in the medical surveillance programme.] Exposure to VCM was evaluated using a job–exposure matrix developed by Pirastu et al. (1990); history of alcoholic beverage consumption was ascertained from clinical or health surveillance records and chronic infection with hepatitis B (HBV) or hepatitis C virus was examined by serological markers. An association between exposure to VCM and both liver cirrhosis and hepatocellular carcinoma was found with much higher odds ratios among those exposed to multiple risk factors.

2.2.3   Other studies

A proportionate mortality study of workers employed in 1964–73 at 55 PVC processing plants in the USA used national mortality rates for comparison; six deaths from primary liver cancer were observed versus an expected 4.19 (Chiazze & Ference, 1981).

Thériault and Allard (1981) compared the mortality of a small cohort of 451 male workers who had been employed for 5 or more years in 1948–72 in a Canadian VCM production and polymerization plant with that of a group of 870 workers who had been employed for ≥ 5 months at a nearby industrial complex that was not involved in the production of VCM or PVC and who were considered to be unexposed, and also with the mortality of the Québec general population in 1971. Occupational histories were obtained by interview either at home or at work with the worker himself or his next of kin. Vital status was ascertained as at the end of 1977. The relative risk for exposed versus unexposed workers for mortality from all causes was 1.48 (95% CI, 0.84–2.61). Eight cases of liver cancer were observed with only 0.14 expected in comparison with the general population; all of these were angiosarcomas. Two deaths from cancer of the 'bone, skin, connective tissue' (ICD codes 170–173) were observed compared with 0.38 expected.

Weber et al. (1981) reported findings in a historical cohort of 7021 VCM/PVC production workers in Germany. The cohort included German and Austrian men who had been employed from the beginning of VCM/PVC production in all German plants [no details given] to the end of 1974. Vital status and follow-up for cause of death [methods not described] were 93.2% and 92.7% complete, respectively. Mortality rates of the West German male population were used as the reference. To calculate expected numbers for person–years of observation before 1968, rates from 1968 were used. A method described by Tabershaw and Gaffey (1974) was used to take into account unknown causes of deaths. No information on exposure levels was available. The SMRs for mortality from all causes, all cancers and liver cancer (ICD-8 155) were 0.95 (414 deaths), 1.12 (94 deaths) and 15.23 (12 deaths), respectively. [The Working Group noted that an earlier cohort studied by Frentzel-Beyme *et al.* (1978) appeared to be included in this cohort.]

Smulevich *et al.* (1988) conducted a cohort study at the oldest PVC plants in the former Soviet Union. Overall, 3232 workers (2195 men) were identified as having held jobs that entailed exposure to VCM. Exposure levels were greater than 300 mg/m^3 [115 ppm] for part of the cohort [number unspecified]. Expected deaths were computed in strata of age (15–74 years) from death rates in the same city, based on follow-up for the years 1939–77. The total number of deaths was not in excess in the cohort. The SMR for all cancer was 1.07 (63 deaths). No cases of liver cancer were observed. The proportion of the cohort that was ever exposed to the highest estimated levels of VCM was not reported; however, 40 of 63 cancer deaths occurred in the high-exposure category. A statistically significant excess ($p < 0.05$) was detected for leukaemias and lymphomas (five deaths; SMR, 4.17), while excess mortality from for pancreatic cancer in both sexes (SMR, 1.43) and skin cancer (both melanoma and non-melanoma) in men (SMR, 1.67) were not statistically significant. Histological confirmation of causes of death was available for 60% of the cancer cases. A significant increase in the occurrence of lymphomas and leukaemias (seven deaths; SMR, 6.36) was noted at the highest level of exposure ($p < 0.05$). Although the number of cohort members per exposure level was not reported, 28 cancer deaths occurred in the highest-exposure group, 15 in the intermediate (30–300 mg/m^3 [11.5–115 ppm])-exposure group and one in the lowest (< 30 mg/m^3 [11.5 ppm])-exposure group. [The Working Group noted that few details were provided on the methods used for the computation of expected numbers of deaths.]

Du and Wang (1998) conducted a proportionate morbidity study in Taiwan, China, at five PVC plants that were operational in 1989–95. The 2224 workers who had been exposed to VCM (97% of the total) and who were traced were compared with two other cohorts who were unexposed to VCM—one of optical workers and one of motorcycle manufacturers (work histories were ascertained from records of the Labour Insurance Bureau). Hospital admissions for cancer at several sites were compared with admissions for cardiovascular and cerebrovascular disease as reference conditions and morbidity odds ratios were calculated. An excess of primary liver cancer was noted (morbidity odds ratio, 4.5; 95% CI, 1.5–13.3; or 6.5; 95% CI, 2.3–18.4, depending on the comparison cohort). An excess of deaths from haematopoietic cancer (morbidity odds ratio, 3.4; 95% CI, 1.0–11.8) was seen. Overall, 12 cases of primary liver cancer were observed in the PVC workers, including six hepatocellular carcinomas and six with unknown histology. [The Working Group noted that in a morbidity study, as in a proportionate mortality study, risk estimates may be influenced by differences in the occurrence of the reference diseases as well as those of the disease of interest.]

Wong, O. *et al.* (2002) conducted a retrospective mortality study of a cohort of workers from six vinyl chloride polymerization factories in Taiwan, China. A total of 3293 male workers met the eligibility criteria for the study: they must have been employed for at least 1 year between 1 January 1950 and 31 December 1992 and have been alive on 1 January 1985. The workers were followed for ascertainment of vital status from 1 January 1985 to 31 December 1997 through a national mortality registry. More than 99% of the study subjects was successfully traced using this method, and the remaining 1% was excluded from the analysis. SMRs were estimated using national rates for men as the reference. Exposure to VCM was estimated to be about 500 ppm [1300 mg/m^3] in the 1960s based on a previous report (Du *et al.*, 2001). The SMR for all causes was 0.78 (95% CI, 0.65–0.91) and the number of deaths from for all cancers combined was greater than that expected (SMR, 1.30; 95% CI, 0.99–1.69). A significant excess of mortality from liver cancer was observed in this study (25 cases; SMR, 1.78; 95% CI, 1.15–2.62). None of the deaths from liver cancer appeared to be due to angiosarcoma, although diagnosis of primary liver cancer was only histologically confirmed for five cases.

A study on risk factors for hepatocellular carcinoma was conducted at six PVC polymerization plants in Taiwan, China, an area that has a high prevalence of chronic HBV and hepatitis C virus infection and an associated high incidence of hepatocellular carcinoma (Wong *et al.*, 2003a). Among a cohort of 4096 workers, 25 cases of liver cancer were diagnosed in 1985–97. Of the 18 cases of liver cancer for whom medical records were available, all were considered to be hepatocellular carcinomas, although only five were confirmed histopathologically. Four control subjects were selected from among a pool of eligible workers who had known HBV status, no evidence of liver disease and provided information on questionnaires. Indices of exposure to VCM were developed based on job titles. HBV surface antigen (HBsAg)-negative subjects with history of tank cleaning had a 4.0-fold greater risk for liver cancer (95% CI, 0.2–69.1). HBsAg carriers with no history of tank cleaning had a 25.7-fold (95% CI, 2.9–229.4) increased risk, whereas the HBsAg carriers with a history of tank cleaning had the greatest risk (odds ratio, 396.0; 95% CI, 22.6–∞), which suggested an interaction between occupational exposure to VCM and HBV infections for the development of liver cancer.

A meta-analysis of cohort studies of vinyl choride-exposed workers that had been published up to 2002 was conducted (Boffetta *et al.*, 2003). The meta-analysis was based on eight independent studies, two multicentric investigations (Mundt *et al.*, 2000; Ward *et al.*, 2001) and six smaller additional studies (Thériault & Allard, 1981; Weber *et al.*, 1981; Smulevich *et al.*, 1988; Laplanche *et al.*, 1992; Huang, 1996; Wong, O. *et al.*, 2002). For a selection of cancer sites, a meta-SMR and 95% CIs were calculated using a random-effects model when the *p*-value for the test for heterogeneity was ≥ 0.01. Six of eight studies reported results for liver cancer, but these were considered to be too heterogeneous to be included in a meta-analysis because, for both liver cancer overall and for liver cancer other than angiosarcoma, the *p* value for heterogeneity was < 0.001. For the two multicentric studies (Mundt *et al.*, 2000; Ward *et al.*, 2001), the lack of heterogeneity allowed the calculation of meta-SMRs of 2.96 (95% CI, 2.00–4.39) for liver cancer overall (*p* value for heterogeneity = 0.03) and 1.35 (95% CI, 1.04–4.39) for liver cancer other than angiosarcoma (*p* value for heterogeneity = 0.7). [The Working Group noted that the meta-analysis did not evaluate the quality of the studies and that some heterogeneity between studies may have resulted from variable data quality. Excluding one study in China, other studies reported SMRs that ranged from 1.78 (95% CI, 1.15–2.62) to 57.1 (95% CI, 24.6–113) for liver cancer overall and from 1.27 (95% CI, 0.84–1.83) to 10.1 (95% CI, 4.37–20.0) for liver cancer other than angiosarcoma.]

2.3   Cancer of the liver

2.3.1   *Cohort studies* (Table 5)

(a)   *North American multicentric study*

The most recent update of the multicentric cohort study of men in the North American vinyl chloride industry (Mundt *et al.*, 2000) and reports relative to previous follow-up periods for the same cohort (Tabershaw & Gaffey, 1974; Cooper, 1981; Wong *et al.*, 1991) found, on the basis of state reference rates, an SMR for cancer of the liver and biliary tract of 3.59 (80 deaths; 95% CI, 2.84–4.46). SMRs increased with increasing duration of exposure: 0.83 (95% CI, 0.33–1.71), 2.15 (95% CI, 1.03–3.96), 6.79 (95% CI, 4.83–9.29) and 6.88 (95% CI, 4.40–10.23) for 1–4, 5–9, 10–19 and ≥ 20 years, respectively; and latency: 2.87 (95% CI, 1.31–5.44), 3.23 (95% CI, 2.00–4.93) and 4.34 (95% CI, 3.22–5.72) for 10–19, 20–29 and ≥ 30 years, respectively. In the Cox's proportional hazard model, duration of exposure had the strongest independent and significant effect in comparison with age and year of first exposure; adjusting for age and year of first exposure, and using 1–4 years as the reference, the relative risk values for 5–9, 10–19 and ≥ 20 years of duration were 2.8 (95% CI, 1.0–7.3), 9.0 (95% CI, 4.0–20.7) and 6.0 (95% CI, 2.5–14.4), respectively. For a total of 48 cases of angiosarcoma identified from both death certificates and the World Angiosarcoma Registry, Cox's proportional hazard analysis, adjusting for age and year of first exposure, showed an increase in risk for increasing duration of exposure: using 1–4 years duration as the reference, the relative risks for 5–9, 10–19 and ≥ 20 years of duration were 3.7 (95% CI, 0.9–14.7), 15.9 (95% CI, 4.6–54.8) and 9.7 (95% CI, 2.6–36.4), respectively. [It is not known whether the 32 deaths from liver cancer that were not identified as angiosarcoma were angiosarcoma or hepatocellular carcinoma; however, the number of expected deaths from liver and biliary tract cancer was 22.30.]

In a separate analysis of one plant located in Louisville, KY (USA), that was included in the multicentric cohort (Lewis *et al.*, 2003), mortality from cancer of the liver and biliary tract was higher than that expected on the basis of local rates (24 observed deaths versus six expected; SMR, 4.00). The analysis showed that SMRs for cancer of the liver and biliary tract increased with increasing duration of exposure (durations of 10–19 and ≥ 20 years had SMRs of 10.85 and 3.64, respectively; $p < 0.05$ for both categories) and latency (latencies of 10–19, 20–29 and ≥ 30 years had SMRs of 6.49, 6.94 and 2.55, respectively; $p < 0.05$ for all three categories). In this plant, a total of 28 liver angiosarcomas, 18 from deaths from liver cancer and 10 from other causes of death, were identified.

Table 5. Cohort studies of liver cancer in vinyl chloride monomer (VCM) and polyvinyl chloride (PVC) production workers

North American multicentric study

Name of study Reference, location	Cohort description	Exposure assessment	Type of cancer (ICD code)	Exposure categories	No. of cases/ deaths	Relative risk (95% CI)	Adjustment for potential confounders	Comments
Mundt et al. (2000), USA	10 109 white male workers (race unknown, 6%) employed ≥ 1 year in jobs that entailed exposure to VCM in 1942–72; mortality follow-up, 1942–95; vital status, 96.8%; cause of death, 99%; 37 plants	JEM	Liver and biliary tract (ICD-9 155–156)	Job exposed to VCM	80	**SMR** (state rates) 3.59 (2.84–4.46) (state rates)		Reference rates: state and USA population; in Cox model, duration of exposure strongest and significant versus age at and year of first exposure
				Duration of exposure (years)				
				1–4	7	0.83 (0.33–1.71)		
				5–9	10	2.15 (1.03–3.96)		
				10–19	39	6.79 (4.83–9.29)		
				≥ 20	24	6.88 (4.40–10.23)		
				Latency (years)				
				10–19	9	2.87 (1.31–5.44)		
				20–29	21	3.23 (2.00–4.93)		
				≥ 30	50	4.34 (3.22–5.72)		
				First exposure (year)				
				≤ 1950	48	4.99 (3.68–6.62)		
				1950–59	32	3.11 (1.97–4.67)		
			48 ASL (33 death certificate, 15 World Angiosarcoma Registry)	*Duration of exposure (years)*		**Hazard ratio**	Age at first exposure, duration of exposure and year of first exposure	
				1–4	3	Reference		
				5–9	6	3.7 (0.9–14.7)		
				10–19	26	15.9 (4.6–54.8)		
				≥ 20	13	9.7 (2.6–36.4)		

Table 5 (contd)

Name of study Reference, location	Cohort description	Exposure assessment	Type of cancer (ICD code)	Exposure categories	No. of cases/ deaths	Relative risk (95% CI)	Adjustment for potential confounders	Comments
Lewis et al. (2003), Lousville, KY, USA	2200 male workers employed ≥ 1 year in jobs that entailed exposure to VCM in 1942–72; mortality follow-up, 1942–95; vital status, 98.5%	JEM	Liver and biliary tract (ICD-9 155–156)	Job exposed to VCM	24	**SMR** 4.00 (p < 0.05; 6 exp.)		Reference rates: state of Kentucky
				Duration of exposure (years)				
				1–4	2	0.91 (2.19 exp.)		
				5–9	2	2.20 (0.91 exp.)		
				10–19	14	10.85 (p < 0.05; 1.29 exp.)		
				≥ 20	6	3.64 (p < 0.05; 1.65 exp.)		
				Latency (years)				
				1–9	0	0 (0.27 exp.)		
				10–19	5	6.49 (p < 0.05; 0.77 exp.)		
				20–29	10	6.94 (p < 0.05; 1.44 exp.)		
				≥ 30	9	2.55 (p < 0.05; 3.53 exp.)		
				First exposure (year)				
				< 1950	12	3.57 (p < 0.05; 3.36 exp.)		
				1950–59	10	4.76 (p < 0.05; 2.10 exp.)		
				1960–72	2	3.51 (0.57 exp.)		

Table 5 (contd)

European multicentric study

Name of study Reference, location	Cohort description	Exposure assessment	Type of cancer (ICD code)	Exposure categories	No. of cases/ deaths	Relative risk (95% CI)	Adjustment for potential confounders	Comments
Ward *et al.* (2001), Italy, Norway, Sweden, United Kingdom	12 700 male workers employed in 19 VCM/PVC plants for ≥ 1 year in 1950–85; mortality follow-up, 1955–97; incidence follow-up, 1955–96	Calendar period JEM for 13/19 factories grouped in 22 broad categories; factory-specific JEM with validated exposure estimates (ppm)	Liver cancer (ICD-9 155)			**SMR**		Reference rates: national
					53	2.40 (1.80–3.14)		Reference rates: national
					29	**SIR** 3.98 (2.67–5.72)		
				PVC production	10	**SMR** 2.28 (1.09–4.18)		
				VCM and PVC production	41	2.85 (2.05–3.87)		
				Duration (years)				
				1–9	15	1.00		
				10–16	17	2.58 (1.28–5.24)		
				17–20	9	3.48 (1.49–8.15)		
				21–25	18	8.21 (3.98–16.9)		
				≥ 26	12	9.39 (4.17–21.1)		
						Test for linear trend, *p* < 0.001		
				Latency (years)			Age, calendar period	Poisson regression analysis
				0–20	17	1.00		
				21–25	12	2.44 (1.09–5.45)		
				26–30	12	2.99 (1.26–7.09)		
				31–36	17	5.58 (2.34–13.3)		
				≥ 37	12	6.20 (2.30–16.7)		
						Test for linear trend, *p* < 0.001		

Table 5 (contd)

Name of study Reference, location	Cohort description	Exposure assessment	Type of cancer (ICD code)	Exposure categories	No. of cases/ deaths	Relative risk (95% CI)	Adjustment for potential confounders	Comments
Ward et al. (2001) (contd)				*Cumulative exposure (ppm–years)*				
				0–734	13	1.00		
				735–2379	12	3.97 (1.81–8.71)		
				2380–5188	15	7.55 (3.57–15.9)		
				5189–7531	13	14.0 (6.43–30.7)		
				≥ 7532	15	28.27 (12.84–62.25)		
						Test for linear trend, *p* < 0.001		
				Autoclave workers				
				Never	22	1.00		
				Ever	38	6.61 (3.90–11.2)		
				Unknown	11	5.43 (2.63–11.2)		
			ASL	*Duration (years)*				
				1–9	7	1.00		
				10–16	8	3.01 (1.06–8.54)		
				17–20	2	2.04 (0.41–10.3)		
				21–25	12	15.7 (5.60–44.0)		
				≥ 26	8	19.67 (6.28–61.59)		
						Trend test, *p* < 0.001		
				Latency (years)			Age, calendar period	Poisson regression analysis
				0–20	10	1.00		
				21–25	6	2.77 (0.89–8.69)		
				26–30	7	4.80 (1.47–15.7)		
				31–36	10	10.38 (3.09–34.9)		
				≥ 37	4	7.99 (1.71–37.3)		
						Trend test, *p* < 0.001		

Table 5 (contd)

Name of study Reference, location	Cohort description	Exposure assessment	Type of cancer (ICD code)	Exposure categories	No. of cases/ deaths	Relative risk (95% CI)	Adjustment for potential confounders	Comments
Ward et al. (2001) (contd)				*Cumulative exposure (ppm–years)*		1.00		
				0–734	4	1.00		
				735–2379	6	6.56 (1.85–23.3)		
				2380–5188	8	13.6 (4.05–45.5)		
				5189–7531	7	28.0 (8.00–98.2)		
				≥ 7532	12	88.2 (26.4–295)		
						Trend test, p < 0.001		
				Autoclave workers				
				Never	4	1.0		
				Ever	26	25.5 (8.86–73.2)		
				Unknown	7	19.3 (5.66–66.2)		
			HCC	*Duration (years)*				
				1–9	1	1.0		
				10–16	3	6.94 (0.71–67.5)		
				17–20	2	12.6 (1.11–143)		
				21–25	1	7.34 (0.44–122)		
				≥ 26	3	35.5 (3.34–377)		
						Trend test, p = 0.002	Age, calendar period	Poisson regression analysis
				Latency (years)				
				< 26	2	1.00		
				26–30	1	3.72 (0.29–48.3)		
				31–36	3	15.9 (1.86–135)		
				≥ 37	4	35.7 (3.56–359)		
						Trend test, p = 0.001		

Table 5 (contd)

Name of study Reference, location	Cohort description	Exposure assessment	Type of cancer (ICD code)	Exposure categories	No. of cases/ deaths	Relative risk (95% CI)	Adjustment for potential confounders	Comments
Ward et al. (2001) (contd)				*Cumulative exposure (ppm–years)*				
				0–734	3	1.0		
				735–2379	2	3.02 (0.50–18.1)		
				2380–5188	1	2.47 (0.26–23.9)		
				5189–7531	1	5.33 (0.54–52.5)		
				≥ 7532	2	20.27 (2.98–138)		
						Trend test, p = 0.004		
				Autoclave worker				
				Never	5	1.0		
				Ever	4	2.97 (0.80–11.1)		
				Unknown	1	2.04 (0.24–17.4)		
Gennaro et al.. (2003), Porto Marghera, Italy	1658 male workers employed in 1956–85; mortality follow-up, 1973–95	JEM	Liver cancer (ICD-9 155)	Autoclave workers	4	9.57 (1.69–54.1)	Age, calendar time, duration, latency	Internal comparison ; 'job title groups' versus other workers
				PVC baggers	4	3.44 (0.62–18.97)		
				Autoclave + PVC baggers + compound	9	4.08 (0.85–19.57)		
Pirastu et al. (2003), Porto Marghera, Italy	1658 male workers employed in 1956–99; mortality follow-up, 1973–99; vital status, 100%; cause of death, 99%	JEMs; job- and time-specific VCM estimates (ppm); ever/never autoclave worker	Primary liver cancer (ICD-9 155.0)		17	**SMR** 2.78 (1.86–4.14)[a]		Reference rates: regional
				Autoclave worker: ever/never		**Relative risk** 4.4 (1.9–10.0)[a]	Age, calendar time, latency	Internal comparison of rates

Table 5 (contd)

Name of study Reference, location	Cohort description	Exposure assessment	Type of cancer (ICD code)	Exposure categories	No. of cases/deaths	Relative risk (95% CI)	Adjustment for potential confounders	Comments
Pirastu et al. (2003) (contd)			ASL	Autoclave worker: ever/never	6	21.1 (3.5–128.7)[a]	Age, calendar time, latency	Best available clinical and pathological data; internal comparison of rates
			HCC	Autoclave worker: ever/never	12	3.5 (1.4–9.2)[a]		
			HCC and ASL	*Cumulative exposure (ppm–years)*		**Rate (× 100 000)**		
				0–735	3	10.0		
				735–2379	1	18.6		
				2379–5188	7	191.7		
				5188–7531	1	62.8		
				7531–9400	0	χ^2 14.52 Trend test, $p < 0.001$		
Other studies								
Thériault & Allard (1981), Québec, Canada	451 male workers exposed to VCM for ≥ 5 years in a polymerization plant, employed in 1948–72; mortality follow-up, 1948–77	JEM	Digestive tract cancer (ICD-7 150–159)		14 (6 deaths from liver cancer)	6.25 (2.69–14.52)		Reference rates: Canadian population in 1971; comparison population: 870 workers not exposed to VCM for ≥ 5 months

Table 5 (contd)

Name of study Reference, location	Cohort description	Exposure assessment	Type of cancer (ICD code)	Exposure categories	No. of cases/ deaths	Relative risk (95% CI)	Adjustment for potential confounders	Comments
Weber et al. (1981), Germany	7021 male VCM/PVC production workers from beginning of operation to 1974; mortality follow-up, from beginning of operation to 1974; vital status, > 90%; cause of death, 7–13%	JEM	Malignant tumour of the liver (ICD-8 155)		**12**	**SMR** 15.23		Reference rates: national
				Duration of exposure (months)				
				< 12	0	–		
				13–60	2	8.74		
				61–120	3	15.25		
				≥ 121	7	25.28		
Smulevich et al. (1988), former Soviet Union	3232 (2195 men, 1037 women) VCM/PVC production workers employed for ≥ 1 month in VCM-exposed jobs; mortality follow-up, 1939–77	Exposure data in 1953–66 from JEM	Malignant liver neoplasm (ICD-8 155)	Estimated area exposure: low, medium and high	0			City (Gorki) mean death rates in 1959, 1969 and 1975

Table 5 (contd)

Name of study Reference, location	Cohort description	Exposure assessment	Type of cancer (ICD code)	Exposure categories	No. of cases/ deaths	Relative risk (95% CI)	Adjustment for potential confounders	Comments
Laplanche et al. (1992), France	1100 VCM-exposed and 1100 unexposed subjects; matched on age, plant, physician, aged 40–55 years, identified in 1980; mortality and morbidity follow-up, 1980–88	JEM	Liver cancer (ICD-9 155)		3 exposed 0 unexposed	NR		Prospective study
Du & Wang (1998), Taiwan, China	2224 workers with occupational exposure to VCM; controls were optical or motor cycle equipment workers.		Liver cancer (ICD-9 155)	VCM versus optical workers		4.5 (1.5–13.3)		
				VCM versus motor cycle workers		6.5 (2.3–18.4)		

Table 5 (contd)

Name of study Reference, location	Cohort description	Exposure assessment	Type of cancer (ICD code)	Exposure categories	No. of cases/ deaths	Relative risk (95% CI)	Adjustment for potential confounders	Comments
Wong, O. et al. (2002); Wong et al. (2003a), Taiwan, China	3293 male workers in 6 PVC polymerization plants exposed to VCM ≥ 1 year in 1950–92; mortality follow-up, 1985–97; vital status, 99%		Malignant neoplasm of the liver (ICD-9 155)			**SMR**		Reference rates, national; cohort assembled from records of Labour Insurance Bureau
					25	1.78 (1.15–2.62)		
				Duration of exposure (years)				
				< 10	13	2.45 (1.30–4.19)		
				10–19	10	1.76 (0.84–3.24)		
				≥ 20	2	– (3.2 exp.)		
				Latency (years)				
				< 15	8	1.29 (0.56–2.54)		
				15–24	7	1.46 (0.58–3.61)		
				≥ 25	10	3.13 (1.50–5.75)		
				First exposure (year)				
				≤ 1970	11	4.82 (2.41–8.63)		
				1970–79	8	1.92 (0.83–3.79)		
				After 1980	6	0.78 (0.28–1.69)		
				Age at first exposure (years)				
				< 30	10	2.24 (1.07–4.12)		
				30–39	6	1.78 (0.65–3.88)		
				≥ 40	9	1.43 (0.65–2.71)		
						Odds ratio		
			HCC	Tank cleaners		2.9 (1.1–7.3)		

ASL, angiosarcoma of the liver; CI, confidence interval; exp., expected; HCC, hepatocellular carcinoma; ICD, International Classification of Diseases; JEM, job–exposure matrix; SIR, standardized incidence ratio; SMR, standardized mortality ratio
[a] 90% confidence interval

(b)   European studies

In the European multicentric cohort study of workers in the vinyl chloride industry, an increase in the incidence of primary liver cancer was observed (53 deaths and 29 incident cases; SMR, 2.40; 95% CI, 1.80–3.14; SIR, 3.98; 95% CI, 2.67–5.72) using national mortality and incidence rates as the reference. On the basis of the best available data for diagnosis, 71 cases of liver cancer were identified and used in the internal analysis for latency, duration of employment, cumulative exposure and employment as an autoclave cleaner. The risk increased with increasing duration and latency of employment with a significant trend (for both latency and duration, $p < 0.001$). For durations of exposure of 10–16, 17–20, 21–25 and $\geq$ 26 years (1–9 years as the reference), the relative risks for liver cancer were 2.58 (95% CI, 1.28–5.24), 3.48 (95% CI, 1.49–8.15), 8.21 (95% CI, 3.98–16.9) and 9.39 (95% CI, 4.17–21.1), respectively. For latencies of 21–25, 26–30, 31–36 and $\geq$ 37 years (0–20 years as reference), the relative risks were 2.44 (95% CI, 1.09–5.45), 2.99 (95% CI, 1.26–7.09), 5.58 (95% CI, 2.34–13.3) and 6.20 (95% CI, 2.30–16.7), respectively. The trend was also significant for cumulative exposure ($p < 0.001$); the risk was almost four times that for the reference category (0–734 ppm–years) starting with cumulative exposures of 735–1379 ppm–years (relative risk, 3.97; 95% CI, 1.81–8.71); for 2380–5188, 5189–7531 and $\geq$ 7532 ppm–years, the relative risks were 7.55 (95% CI, 3.57–15.9), 14.0 (95% CI, 6.43–30.7) and 28.27 (95% CI, 12.84–62.25), respectively. Analysis of the exposure–response trends at low doses (defined as < 1500 ppm–years and thus including 20 cases of liver cancer) yielded a relative risk of 2.0 (95% CI, 1.3–3.0) for one logarithmic unit of cumulative dose. From the best available data for diagnosis, 37 cases of angiosarcoma were ascertained for which a significant increasing trend ($p < 0.001$) was observed for latency, duration of exposure and cumulative exposure; for ever versus never autoclave cleaners, the relative risk was 25.5 (95% CI, 8.86–73.2). Ten cases of hepatocellular carcinoma were also used in the internal analysis. For latency and duration of exposure, the trend in risk was significant ($p = 0.001$ and $p = 0.002$, respectively); the risk was also significant for 7532 ppm–years of cumulative exposure (relative risk, 20.27; 95% CI, 2.98–137.71; $p = 0.004$); for ever versus never having been an autoclave cleaner, the relative risk was 2.97 (95% CI, 0.80–11.1).

In the study of the Porto Marghera plant in Italy (Pirastu *et al.*, 2003), mortality from primary liver cancer was higher than that expected from regional rates (SMR, 2.78; 90% CI, 1.86–4.14). In an internal comparison, death rates for primary liver cancer with latencies of 10–30 years (26.1/100 000) and $\geq$ 30 years (160.7/100 000) were higher than those for the reference (latency $\leq$ 10 years). In the internal analysis for employment as an autoclave worker (ever/never), the relative risk was 4.4 (90% CI, 1.9–10.0); a significant increasing trend was seen for increasing cumulative estimated exposure ($p <0.001$). The analyses of rates for both liver angiosarcoma (six cases) and hepatocellular carcinoma (12 cases) showed that longer latency implied higher rates; employment as an autoclave worker (ever/never) was associated with an increased risk for both angiosarcoma (relative risk, 21.1; 90% CI, 3.5–

128.7) and hepatocellular carcinoma (relative risk, 3.5; 90% CI, 1.4–9.2); for both histo-types, there was a significant increasing trend with increasing estimated exposure ($p < 0.001$).

In the same plant (Porto Marghera), an analysis that used internal reference groups (Gennaro *et al.*, 2003) showed that the relative risk for mortality from liver cancer of autoclave workers versus all other workers was 9.57 (four deaths; 95% CI, 1.69–54.1); for two job title groups, 'compound workers' and 'compound + autoclave + PVC bagger workers', the relative risks were 3.44 (four deaths; 95% CI, 0.62–18.97) and 4.08 (nine deaths; 95% CI, 0.85–19.57), respectively.

(c)   Other studies

In the Canadian cohort study (Thériault & Allard, 1981), histopathological confirmation was available from medical files at the hospitals for 19 of 20 causes of death from cancer: eight were angiosarcomas of the liver. Two more angiosarcomas of the liver were notified as cirrhosis on the death certificate and were considered as such throughout this study. In comparison with an unexposed cohort, the relative risk for digestive cancers (ICD codes 150–159) was 6.25 (14 observed deaths; 95% CI, 2.69–14.52). [No relative risks for more specific cancer sites were given.]

In the study by Weber *et al.* (1981), the SMRs for liver cancer by duration of exposure for < 12 months, 13–60 months, 61–120 months and > 121 months were 0, 8.74 (two deaths), 15.25 (three deaths) and 25.28 (seven deaths), respectively. [The Working Group noted that an increased mortality from liver cancer was briefly described in a cohort of PVC processing workers. This cohort probably included the data of Frentzel-Beyme *et al.* (1978).]

No deaths from liver cancer were reported in PVC plants in the former Soviet Union (Smulevich *et al.*, 1988).

In the French study (Laplanche *et al.*, 1992), three angiosarcomas of the liver and three liver cancers were observed among the exposed workers compared with none in the unexposed [no relative risk estimates given].

In a proportionate morbidity study in Taiwan, China (Du & Wang, 1998), an excess of primary liver cancer was noted (morbidity odds ratio, 4.5 or 6.5, depending on the comparison group).

In a retrospective cohort study of mortality in Taiwan, China (Wong, O. *et al.*, 2002), the risk for liver cancer decreased with duration of exposure; the authors suggested that this might be attributable to a higher turnover of workers in jobs that entailed high exposures or because workers with illnesses retired early. The excess mortality from liver cancer was most pronounced among workers who began employment before 1970 (SMR, 4.82; 95% CI, 2.41–8.63), when, according to the authors, exposures to VCM were higher, because permissible exposure limits for VCM were not established in Taiwan until 1981. The excess mortality from liver cancer was found to increase with time since first exposure and to reach a peak after more than 25 years (SMR, 3.13; 95% CI, 1.50–5.75). It was also found to be inversely related to age at first exposure; workers who were under 30 years of age at first exposure demonstrated the highest risk (SMR, 2.24; 95% CI, 1.07–4.12).

A study of risk factors for hepatocellular carcinoma that was conducted in Taiwan, China (Wong *et al.*, 2003a), reported an odds ratio of 15.7 (95% CI, 3.6–68.4) for HBsAg status. An odds ratio of 3.6 (95% CI, 1.4–9.2) was estimated for jobs that entailed high exposure to VCM; for tank cleaners specifically, the odds ratio was 2.9 (95% CI, 1.1–7.3). [The Working Group noted that, due to problems in the methodology of this study, the results were not considered to be useful for the evaluation of the potential relationship between exposure to vinyl chloride and hepatocellular carcinoma. These methodological problems included lack of histological confirmation for the majority of cases of hepatocellular carcinoma, the resulting potential that some of the cases were truly angiosarcomas, lack of detail in the methodology for selection of controls and exclusion of individuals with evidence of liver disease from the control group.]

[The Working Group considered that the evidence that exposure to VCM is associated with cirrhosis of the liver supports the likelihood that exposure to vinyl chloride increases the risk for hepatocellular carcinoma, although relative risks for hepatocellular carcinoma are smaller than those associated with angiosarcoma of the liver. Inflammatory and regenerative processes associated with HBV and hepatitis C viral infection and chronic alcoholism are considered to be an important pathway through which the risk for hepatocellular carcinoma is increased by these exposures in the general population.]

(d) Meta-analysis

In meta-analysis of cohort studies of vinyl chloride (Boffetta *et al.*, 2003), duration of employment was available in three studies (Weber *et al.*, 1981; Mundt *et al.*, 2000; Ward *et al.*, 2001): in the two multicentric investigations (Mundt *et al.*, 2000; Ward *et al.*, 2001), an increase in mortality from liver cancer was evident beginning at durations of ≥ 7 years and up to 25 years whereas, in the German study (Weber *et al.*, 1981), a sharp increase was found starting from 13–16 years of duration of exposure. Mortality from liver cancer by year of first employment was increased in the two multicentric studies (Mundt *et al.*, 2000; Ward *et al.*, 2001). [Adjustment for time since first employment would be advisable; the lack of adjustment could be misleading, as a very strong decrease in risk over calendar time was shown, while more recently exposed workers had not completed the latency time necessary for liver cancer to be expressed.]

2.3.2 Case–control studies (Table 6)

A case–control analysis of 23 liver angiosarcomas was conducted at the plant in Louisville, KY (USA), and confirmed a strong and significant association with exposure to vinyl chloride and PVC (exposure to vinyl chloride, $p < 0.001$; exposure to PVC, $p = 0.003$); in a case–cohort analysis that used exposure estimated on the basis of a six-point ranking scale of chemicals present in the plant, cases of angiosarcoma had significantly greater exposure to vinyl chloride than the reference cohort (Lewis & Rempala, 2003).

Table 6. Case–control studies of liver cancer in vinyl chloride monomer (VCM) and polyvinyl chloride (PVC) production workers

Reference, location	Organ site (ICD code)	Characteristics of cases	Characteristics of controls	Exposure assessment	Exposure categories	Relative risk (95% CI)	Adjustment for potential confounders	Comments
Lewis & Rempala (2003), Louisville, KY, USA	ASL	23 men; histologically confirmed	Matched by year of birth and duration of employment		CERM	Logistic regression analysis showed strong, highly significant association with exposure to VC ($p < 0.001$) and PVC ($p = 0.003$)		In Lewis et al. (2003), 28 ASL reported
			1817 white men hired before 1967 who had worked at least 1 year		CERM	ASL cases had significantly greater exposure to VC (69.9% > 1000 VC–CERM)		
Wong et al. (2003a), Taiwan, China	Liver cancer; HCC	18 men; 5 histologically confirmed; 5 AFP > 1000 µg/L + at least one positive image from angiography, sonography, liver scan and/or CT; 8 from clinical manifestation and imaging studies	68 randomly selected from a pool of eligible workers; matched on age and specific plant employment	Job titles; high VCM-exposure jobs: tank cleaning, unloading PVC, adding catalyst; HBsAg status from medical surveillance records	History of high-exposure job HBsAg-positive versus HBsAg-negative status History of tank cleaning versus r o history	2.9 (1.1–7.3) 15.7 (3.6–68.4) 3.6 (1.4–9.2)		Nested case–control; for deceased individuals, validation of exposure by next of kin versus co-workers and industrial hygienist

Table 6 (contd)

Reference, location	Organ site (ICD code)	Characteristics of cases	Characteristics of controls	Exposure assessment	Exposure categories	Relative risk (95% CI)	Adjustment for potential confounders	Comments
Wong et al. (2003a) (contd)					HBsAg-positive status and history of tank cleaning	4.0 (0.2–69.1)	Family history of chronic liver disease	Reference: HBsAg-negative status and no history of tank cleaning
					HBsAg-negative status and history of tank cleaning	396 (22.6–∞)		
					HBsAg-positive status and no history of tank cleaning	25.7 (2.9–229.4)		
					HBsAg-negative status and history of high exposure job	2.9 (0.2–50.0)		
					HBsAg-positive status and history of high exposure job	184.5 (15.0–∞)		
					HBsAg-positive status and no history of high exposure job	26.1 (2.9–235.1)		

Table 6 (contd)

Reference, location	Organ site (ICD code)	Characteristics of cases	Characteristics of controls	Exposure assessment	Exposure categories	Relative risk (95% CI)	Adjustment for potential confounders	Comments
Mastrangelo et al. (2004), Porto Marghera, Italy	HCC	13 men; 8 histologically confirmed; 5 focal hepatic lesions at sonography + AFP > 400 µg/L	139 workers with no clinical or biochemical evidence of chronic liver disease or cancer at any site from medical surveillance in 1999–2002	JEMs, job- and time-specific VCM estimates (ppm); information for cases from company files, from medical surveillance data for controls; alcoholic beverage consumption from hospital/clinical records and surveillance data; serological markers for HBsAg and anti-HCV antibodies	*Cumulative VCM exposure (ppm-years)*			Nested case–control
					< 500	Reference		
					500–2500	6.32 (0.48–336)		
					> 2500	29.3 (3.61–1298)		
					< 250/alcohol < 60 g/day	Reference	Adjusted for age, hepatitis infection	Odds ratio in univariate analysis
					> 250/alcohol < 60 g/day	18.8 (1.62–218.0)		
					< 250/alcohol > 60 g/day	42.9 (3.41–540.0)		
					> 250/alcohol > 60 g/day	409 (19.6–8553.0)		
					< 250/HBsAg/HCV-negative	Reference	Age, alcoholic beverage consumption	
					> 250/HBsAg/HCV-negative	25.0 (2.77–226.0)		
					< 250/HBsAg/HCV-positive	106.9 (4.43–2578.0)		
					> 250/HBsAg/HCV-positive	210.3 (7.13–6203.0)		

AFP, α-fetoprotein; ASL, angiosarcoma of the liver; CERM, cumulative exposure rank months; CI, confidence interval; CT, computed tomography; HBsAg, hepatitis B virus surface antigen; HCC, hepatocellular carcinoma; HCV, hepatitis C virus; ICD, International Classification of Diseases; JEM, job-exposure matrix; VC, vinyl chloride

In the case–control study of cases of liver cancer nested in the cohort in Taiwan, China (Wong *et al.*, 2003a), tobacco smoking, alcoholic beverage consumption and familial history of chronic liver disease were not found to be associated with liver cancer, which may be attributed to the low prevalence of these risk factors in the study population.

A history of employment in a high-exposure job was associated with an increased risk of 2.9 (95% CI, 1.1–7.3). A strong association was observed with HBsAg (odds ratio, 15.7; 95% CI, 3.6–68.4) or a history of tank cleaning (odds ratio, 3.6; 95% CI, 1.4–9.2). Models were also fitted that included both HBsAg and a history of tank cleaning, and a parameter for the potential interaction between the two. Strong evidence for an interaction between HBsAg and a history of tank cleaning was observed in this model; a history of tank cleaning and HBsAg negativity had an odds ratio of 4.0 (95% CI, 0.2–69.1), HBsAg positivity and no history of tank cleaning had an odds ratio of 25.7 (95% CI, 2.9–229.4) and combined HBsAg positivity and a history of tank cleaning had an odds ratio of 396 (95 % CI, 22.6–∞). Similar results were observed when the analysis was based on a history of high exposure to VCM rather than a history of tank cleaning. [The Working Group was concerned that the method used to select controls may have biased the study. The age at which controls were matched to cases was not clear. Of greater concern is that the controls were restricted to individuals who had no history of chronic liver disease. This may have biased the study towards the null since this restriction was not applied to the cases.]

A cross-sectional study of hepatocellular carcinoma in the Porto Marghera (Italy) cohort (Mastrangelo *et al.*, 2004) found an association between exposure to VCM and both liver cirrhosis and hepatocellular carcinoma. The odds ratio for cumulative exposure to VCM of > 2500 ppm × year was 29.3 (95% CI, 3.61–1298). Odds ratios tended to be higher for those subjects who were exposed to multiple risk factors. For example, the odds ratio for exposure to > 2500 ppm × year and consumption of > 60 g per day of alcohol was 409 (95% CI, 19.6–8553). These analyses controlled for age and hepatitis viral infection. Similar patterns were seen in analyses of the relationship between exposure to VCM and HBV/hepatitis C viral infection that controlled for alcoholic beverage consumption. [The Working Group noted that the methodology used to select controls for this analysis, which excluded individuals who had liver cirrhosis, may have resulted in a positive bias in the relative risk estimates.]

2.4   Cancer of the brain and central nervous system

2.4.1   *Cohort studies* (Table 7)

(a)   *North American multicentric study*

An update of the North American multicentric study found an overall SMR for cancer of the brain and central nervous system of 1.42 (36 exposed deaths; 95% CI, 1.00–1.97) (Mundt *et al.*, 2000). There was no apparent trend with increasing duration of exposure (9 observed deaths; hazard ratio, 1.9; 95% CI, 0.8–5.0). The risk for brain cancer was

Table 7. Cohort studies of brain cancer in vinyl chloride monomer (VCM) and polyvinyl chloride (PVC) production workers

Name of study Reference, location	Cohort description	Exposure assessment	Type of cancer (ICD code)	Exposure categories	No. of cases/ deaths	Relative risk (95% CI)	Adjustment for potential confounders	Comments
North American multicentric study								
Mundt et al. (2000), USA	10 109 white male workers employed in 37 plants ≥ 1 year in jobs that entailed exposure to VCM in 1942–72; mortality follow-up, 1942–95; vital status, 96.8%; cause of death, 99%	JEM	Brain and CNS (ICD-9 191–192)	Job exposed to VC	36	**SMR** 1.4 (1.0–2.0)	Age at first exposure, duration of exposure, year of first exposure	Reference rates: state rates and USA population; p value for likelihood ratio test for equality of survivor functions, controlling for time at risk
				Age at first exposure (years)		**Hazard ratio**		
				< 25	11	1.0		
				25–34	12	0.9 (0.4–2.0)		
				≥ 35	13	2.6 (1.2–5.9) $p = 0.02$		
				Duration of exposure (years)				
				< 5	11	1.0		
				5–9	11	2.0 (0.9–4.7)		
				10–19	5	0.7 (0.2–2.0)		
				≥ 20	9	1.9 (0.8–5.0) $p = 0.09$		

Table 7 (contd)

Name of study Reference, location	Cohort description	Exposure assessment	Type of cancer (ICD code)	Exposure categories	No. of cases/ deaths	Relative risk (95% CI)	Adjustment for potential confounders	Comments
European multicentric study								
Ward et al. (2000, 2001), Italy, Norway, Sweden, United Kingdom	12 700 male workers employed in 19 VCM/PVC plants ≥ 1 year in 1950–85; mortality follow-up, 1955–97; incidence follow-up, 1955–96	Calendar period JEM for 13/19 factories grouped in 22 broad categories; factory-specific JEM with validated exposure estimates (ppm)	Brain and CNS (ICD-9 191–192)	Employed in VC industry (full cohort)	24	**SMR** 0.93 (0.60–1.39)		Reference rates: national
					19	**SIR** 0.91 (0.55–1.42)		Reference incidence rates: national
				VCM production only	0	**SMR** 0.00 (0.00–5.64)	Age, calendar period	
				PVC production only	5	0.96 (0.31–2.25)		
				VCM and PVC production	16	0.93 (0.53–1.51)		
				PVC processing	18	1.10 (0.23–3.22)		
				Latency (years)		**Relative risk**		Poisson regression analysis
				< 16	9	1.00	Age, calendar period	
				16–21	4	0.71 (0.19–2.68)		
				22–26	3	0.71 (0.16–3.29)		
				27–34	6	1.37 (0.33–5.63)		
				≥ 35	2	0.77 (0.11–5.47)		
						Test for linear trend, p= 0.82		
				Duration (years)				
				1–2	5	1.00		
				3–6	6	1.34 (0.41–4.40)		
				7–11	4	0.95 (0.25–3.57)		
				12–18	4	0.96 (0.25–3.69)		
				≥ 19 years	5	1.59 (0.43–5.91)		
						Test for linear trend, p = 0.72		

Table 7 (contd)

Name of study Reference, location	Cohort description	Exposure assessment	Type of cancer (ICD code)	Exposure categories	No. of cases/ deaths	Relative risk (95% CI)	Adjustment for potential confounders	Comments
Ward et al. (2000, 2001) (contd)				*Cumulative exposure (ppm– years)*				
				0–34	3	1.00		
				35–99	3	1.37 (0.28–6.82)		
				100–535	10	3.45 (0.94–12.6)		
				536–2811	2	0.75 (0.12–4.50)		
				≥ 2812	3	1.58 (0.31–8.04)		
						Test for linear trend, p = 0.778		
				Autoclave worker				
				Never	17	1.00		
				Ever	5	1.08 (0.40–2.92)		
				Unknown	2	1.27 (0.29–5.49)		
Other studies								
Weber et al. (1981), Germany	7021 male VCM/PVC production workers from beginning of operation to 1974; mortality follow-up, from beginning of operation to 1974; vital status, > 90%; cause of death, 7–13%	JEM	Brain and CNS (ICD-8 191)	VCM/PVC production and processing	2	**SMR** 1.62 (NR)		Reference rates: national

Table 7 (contd)

Name of study Reference, location	Cohort description	Exposure assessment	Type of cancer (ICD code)	Exposure categories	No. of cases/ deaths	Relative risk (95% CI)	Adjustment for potential confounders	Comments
Smulevich *et al.* (1988), former Soviet Union	3232 VCM/PVC production workers (2195 men, 1037 women) employed for ≥ 1 month in VCM-exposed jobs; mortality follow-up, 1939–77	Exposure data in 1953–66 from JEM	Brain and CNS (ICD-9 191–192)	Estimated area exposure: low, medium and high	4	**SMR** 1.54 (0.41–3.94)		City (Gorki) mean death rates in 1959, 1969 and 1975
Wong, O. *et al.* (2002), Taiwan, China	3293 male workers in 6 PVC polymerization plants exposed to VCM ≥ 1 year in 1950–92; mortality follow-up, 1985–97; vital status 99%	JEM	Brain and CNS (ICD-9 191–192)		2	**SMR** [2.86 (0.57–9.16)]		Reference rates, national; cohort assembled from records of the Labour Insurance Bureau

CI, confidence interval; CNS, central nervous system; ICD, International Classification of Diseases; JEM, job–exposure matrix; NR, not reported; SIR, standardized incidence ratio; SMR, standardized mortality ratio; VC, vinyl chloride significantly increased with time since first exposure of ≥ 35 years (hazard ratio, 2.6; 95% CI, 1.2–5.9). The highest SMR was found for those first exposed before 1950 (SMR, 1.74; 95% CI, 0.97–2.88). Mortality from brain cancer was also in excess among subjects who had worked in plants that began production before 1946 (22 deaths; SMR, 1.77; 95% CI, 1.11–2.68).

(b)   European multicentric study

An update of the European multicentric study found an overall SMR for brain cancer of 0.93 (24 observed deaths; 95% CI, 0.60–1.39); the SIR was 0.91 based on 19 cases (Ward et al., 2000, 2001). No trends in the SMRs were observed with respect to time since first employment, duration of employment, cumulative exposure or calendar period of hire. The risk for brain cancer among those who had ever been autoclave workers was similar to that of those who had never been autoclave workers. Poisson regression analyses of deaths from brain cancer found no significant trends with latency, duration of employment or cumulative exposure to vinyl chloride, although the rate ratio was elevated in the middle-dose category of cumulative dose (relative risk, 3.45; 95% CI, 0.94–12.6).

In the incidence analyses, significant excesses were found for the category of 27–35 years since first employment (eight observed deaths; SMR, 2.67; 95% CI, 1.15–5.27) and in the highest category of duration of employment (six observed deaths; SMR, 2.15; 95% CI, 0.79–4.68), but no apparent trend with cumulative exposure was observed (data not shown).

(c)   Other studies

An SMR of 1.62 (based on two deaths) was reported in the historical cohort study of VCM/PVC production workers in Germany (Weber et al., 1981). The SMRs by duration of exposure of < 12 months, 13–16 months, 61–120 months and > 121 months were 0, 0, 3.50 (one death) and 2.78 (one death), respectively.

An SMR of 1.54 (four observed deaths) was reported in a Russian cohort of more than 3200 VCM/PVC production workers (Smulevich et al., 1988). The SMR was 0.9 for men and 5 for women.

An SMR of 2.86 for brain cancer (based on two deaths) was reported in a cohort in Taiwan, China (Wong, O. et al., 2002).

(d)   Meta-analysis

In the meta-analysis by Boffetta et al. (2003), the meta-SMR for brain cancer calculated from five studies was 1.26 (95% CI, 0.98–1.62). The authors noted that the increase in the meta-SMR was mainly due to the North American multicentric study (Mundt et al., 2000) and that no trend with duration of exposure was found in either of the two large studies (Mundt et al., 2000; Ward et al., 2000).

2.4.2   *Case–control and case–cohort studies*

A case–cohort and matched case–control analysis of brain cancer was conducted at a polymer production plant included in the North American multicentric cohort (Lewis & Rempala, 2003) in which 15 of 36 deaths from brain cancer were identified. The SMR for brain cancer was 2.29 (95% CI, 1.29–3.81) at this facility and 1.12 (95% CI, 0.69–1.71) at all other plants combined (Lewis *et al.*, 2003). Sixteen deaths from brain cancer from 1963 to 2000 were included in the case–cohort and case–control studies. The cases of brain cancer were slightly less likely than other cohort members to have worked in any PVC building (18.8% versus 26.5%, respectively), and slightly more likely to have worked in the building that manufactured nitrile rubber copolymers (31.3% versus 25.9%, respectively). In general, estimates of cumulative exposure to materials used in PVC production among cases of brain cancer were lower than those for other cohort members, while exposures to chemicals used in nitrile rubber production were similar. In the matched case–control analysis, no significant associations were observed between status of brain cancer case and any of the materials used in either PVC or nitrile rubber copolymer production.

2.5   Cancer of the lung and respiratory tract

2.5.1   *Lung cancer*

(a)   Cohort studies (Table 8)

(i)   *North American multicentric study*

In an update of the North American multicentric study (Mundt *et al.*, 2000), there was no evidence of any association between employment with exposure to vinyl chloride and mortality from lung cancer overall (303 deaths; SMR, 0.82; 95% CI, 0.73–0.92), nor was there any pattern of association by year of first exposure or year at which production of vinyl chloride began. The authors noted that regional mortality rates for lung cancer, used as the primary referent rates in the analysis, were higher than those in the USA as a whole. The SMR for lung cancer based on national referent rates was 0.96 (95% CI, 0.86–2.07).

(ii)   *European multicentric study*

An update of the European multicentric study found an overall SMR for lung cancer of 0.95 (272 cases; 95% CI, 0.84–1.07) and an SIR of 0.80 (154 deaths; 95% CI, 0.68–0.94). No association was observed between mortality from lung cancer and exposure to vinyl chloride, as estimated by ranked level of exposure, latency, duration of employment, cumulative exposure to vinyl chloride and ever/never employment as an autoclave worker (Ward *et al.*, 2000, 2001). Non-significant associations were found for time since first employment, production or processing and duration of employment. In Poisson regression

Table 8. Cohort studies of lung cancer in vinyl chloride monomer (VCM) and polyvinyl chloride (PVC) production workers

Name of study Reference, location	Cohort description	Exposure assessment	Type of cancer (ICD code)	Exposure categories	No. of cases/ deaths	Relative risk (95% CI)	Adjustment for potential confounders	Comments
North American multicentric study								
Mundt et al. (2000), USA	10 109 white male workers employed at least ≥ 1 year in jobs that entailed exposure to VCM in 1942–72; mortality follow-up, 1942–95; vital status, 96.8%; cause of death, 99%	JEM	Trachea, bronchus and lung (ICD-9 162)	Job exposed to VC	303	**SMR** (state rates) 0.82 (0.73–0.92) **SMR** (national rates) 0.96 (0.86–2.07)		Reference rates: state rates and USA population
European multicentric study								
Ward et al. (2000, 2001), Italy, Norway, Sweden, United Kingdom	12 700 male workers employed in 19 VCM/PVC plants ≥ 1 year in 1950–85; mortality follow-up, 1955–97; incidence follow-up, 1955–96	Calendar period JEM for 13/19 factories grouped in 22 broad categories; factory-specific JEM with validated exposure estimates (ppm)	Trachea, bronchus and lung (ICD-9 162)	Employed in VC industry (full cohort) VCM production PVC production VCM and PVC production PVC processing	272 154 14 56 184 18	**SMR** 0.95 (0.84–1.07) **SIR** 0.80 (0.68–0.94) **SMR** 1.47 (0.80–2.47) 0.88 (0.67–1.15) 0.91 (0.79–1.05) 1.43 (0.85–2.26)	Age, calendar period	Reference rates: national; incidence rates: national

Table 8 (contd)

Name of study Reference, location	Cohort description	Exposure assessment	Type of cancer (ICD code)	Exposure categories	No. of cases/ deaths	Relative risk (95% CI)	Adjustment for potential confounders	Comments
Ward et al. (2000, 2001) (contd)				*Latency (years)*		**Relative risk**	Age, calendar period	Poisson regression analysis
				< 16	57	1.00		
				16–21	55	0.96 (0.65–1.41)		
				22–26	66	1.21 (0.82–1.78)		
				27–34	54	0.73 (0.48–1.11)		
				≥ 35	40	0.76 (0.47–1.25)		
						Test for linear trend, $p = 0.119$		
				Duration (years)				
				1–2	57	1.00		
				3–6	55	1.12 (0.76–1.64)		
				7–11	66	1.31 (0.91–1.88)		
				12–18	54	0.89 (0.60–1.30)		
				≥ 19 years	40	0.77 (0.52–1.15)		
						Test for linear trend, $p = 0.094$		
				Cumulative exposure (ppm–years)				
				0–34	52	1.00		
				35–99	52	1.11 (0.75–1.62)		
				100–535	55	0.90 (0.62–1.32)		
				536–2811	46	0.85 (0.57–1.27)		
				≥ 2812	43	0.84 (0.56–1.26)		
						Test for linear trend, $p = 0.190$		

Table 8 (contd)

Name of study Reference, location	Cohort description	Exposure assessment	Type of cancer (ICD code)	Exposure categories	No. of cases/ deaths	Relative risk (95% CI)	Adjustment for potential confounders	Comments
Ward et al. (2000, 2001) (contd)				*Autoclave worker*				
				Never	220	1.00		
				Ever	44	0.84 (0.61–1.16)		
				Unknown	8	0.38 (0.19–0.77)		
				Cumulative exposure (ppm–years)				
				Ever employed as packers and baggers				
				0–34	9	1.12 (0.51–2.13)		
				35–99	9	0.99 (0.45–1.88)		
				100–535	14	1.08 (0.59–1.82)		
				536–2811	9	0.85 (0.39–1.60)		
				≥ 2812	10	1.02 (0.49–1.88)		
				Never employed as packers and baggers				
				0–34	43	0.98 (0.71–1.33)		
				35–99	43	1.09 (0.79–1.46)		
				100–535	41	0.83 (0.60–1.13)		
				536–2811	37	0.86 (0.60–1.18)		
				≥ 2812	33	0.87 (0.60–1.23)		
				Only employed as packers and baggers				
				0–34	5	0.88 (0.28–2.04)		
				35–99	6	1.28 (0.47–2.78)		
				100–535	11	1.63 (0.81–2.92)		
				536–2811	4	1.37 (0.37–3.52)		
				≥ 2812	4	3.12 (0.85–8.00)		
						Test for trend χ^2, $p = 0.009$		

Table 8 (contd)

Name of study Reference, location	Cohort description	Exposure assessment	Type of cancer (ICD code)	Exposure categories	No. of cases/ deaths	Relative risk (95% CI)	Adjustment for potential confounders	Comments
Pirastu et al. (2003), Porto Marghera, Italy	1658 male workers employed in 1956–99; mortality follow–up, 1973–99; vital status, 100%; cause of death, 99%	JEMs, job- and time-specific VCM estimates (ppm); ever/never autoclave worker	Lung cancer (ICD-9 162.1–162.9)	Full cohort Only versus never baggers	40 7 7	**SMR** 0.83 (0.64–1.07)[a] 1.73 (0.93–3.21) **SMR** 2.31 (1.15–4.61)[a]	Not adjusted Latency	Reference rates: regional Internal comparison versus never baggers
Other studies								
Thériault & Allard (1981), Québec, Canada	451 male workers exposed to VCM for ≥ 5 years in a polymerization plant, employed in 1948–72; mortality follow-up, 1948–77	Questionnaire to the worker or next of kin on detailed occupational history	Trachea, bronchus and lung (ICD-9 162)	Exposed to VCM	2	**SMR** 0.34 (0.04–1.25)		Reference rates: Canadian population in 1971; comparison population: 870 workers not exposed to VCM for ≥ 5 months
Smulevich et al. (1988), former Soviet Union	3232 VCM/PVC production workers (2195 men, 1037 women) employed for ≥ 1 month in VCM-exposed jobs; mortality follow-up, 1939–77	Exposure data in 1953–66 from JEM	Trachea, bronchus and lung (ICD-9 162)	Estimated area exposure: low, medium and high	17	**SMR** 1.39 (0.81–2.23)		City (Gorki) mean death rates in 1959, 1969 and 1975

Table 8 (contd)

Name of study Reference, location	Cohort description	Exposure assessment	Type of cancer (ICD code)	Exposure categories	No. of cases/ deaths	Relative risk (95% CI)	Adjustment for potential confounders	Comments
Laplanche *et al.* (1992), France	1100 VCM–exposed and 1100 unexposed subjects; matched on age, plant, physician, aged 40–55 years, identified in 1980; mortality and morbidity follow-up, 1980–88	JEM	Trachea, bronchus and lung (ICD-9 162)		6 among exposed; 2 among un-exposed	NR		Prospective study
Wong, O. *et al.* (2002), Taiwan, China	3293 male workers in 6 PVC polymerization plants exposed to VCM ≥ 1 year in 1950–92; mortality follow-up, 1985–97; vital status 99%	JEM	Trachea, bronchus and lung (ICD-9 162)		4	**SMR** 0.59 (0.16-1.52)		Reference rates: national; cohort enumerated from records of the Labour Insurance Bureau

CI, confidence interval; ICD, International Classification of Diseases; JEM, job–exposure matrix; NR, not reported; SIR, standardized incidence ratio; SMR, standardized mortality ratio; VC, vinyl chloride
[a] 90% confidence interval

analyses, non-significant negative trends were observed with increasing cumulative exposure.

A possible association between exposure to PVC dust and lung cancer was suggested by several early studies as well as recent investigations of PVC baggers in a VCM/PVC manufacturing plant in Italy (Pirastu *et al.*, 1998; Mastrangelo *et al.*, 2003). Therefore, packers and baggers were examined separately in the European multicentric cohort study. No trend in risk was observed with increasing cumulative exposure for those who had ever been employed as packers and baggers, among whom 53 deaths from lung cancer occurred (Ward *et al.*, 2000). However, among individuals who only worked as packers and baggers, 30 deaths from lung cancer occurred, and the trend with increasing cumulative exposure was statistically significant.

In the cohort of 1658 vinyl chloride workers in Porto Marghera (Pirastu *et al.*, 2003), an SMR for lung cancer of 1.73 (seven deaths; 90% CI, 0.93–3.21) was observed among 'only baggers'; the SMR for 'only baggers' versus 'never baggers' adjusted for latency was 2.31 (90% CI, 1.15–4.61; $p = 0.047$).

(iii)   *Other studies*

In a Canadian cohort, an SMR of 0.34 (95% CI, 0.04–1.25) was reported for cancer of the lung, trachea or bronchus (Thériault & Allard, 1981).

A study in the former Soviet Union (Smulevich *et al.*, 1988) showed an SMR of 1.39 (17 observed deaths; 95% CI, 0.81–2.23) for lung cancer and a cohort study in France (LaPlanche *et al.*, 1992) reported eight observed deaths from lung cancer but did not include risk estimates.

A study in Taiwan, China, reported an SMR of 0.59 (four observed deaths) for lung cancer (Wong, O. *et al.*, 2002).

(iv)   *Meta-analysis*

The meta-analysis by Boffetta *et al.* (2003) showed a meta-SMR for lung cancer of 0.90 (95% CI, 0.77–1.06) based on five studies.

(b)   *Case–control studies* (Table 9)

In a nested case–control study in Porto Marghera, Italy, risk factors for lung cancer were examined among 38 subjects who had lung cancer and 224 subjects with no history of cancer (Mastrangelo *et al.*, 2003). Although no association was observed between estimated cumulative exposure to VCM and lung cancer, the odds ratio for exposure to PVC dust among baggers with known length of exposure was 5.60 (95% CI, 2.03–16.3). When stratified by duration of work as a bagger, the odds ratio was 2.87 (95% CI, 0.84–8.56) among those who were employed for < 3.6 years and 7.15 (95% CI, 2.55–19.3) among those employed for > 3.6 years. Although the quantity of cigarettes smoked per day was associated with lung cancer, this did not appear to confound the association between lung cancer and work as a bagger.

Table 9. Case-control studies of lung cancer in vinyl chloride monomer (VCM) and polyvinyl chloride (PVC) production workers

Reference, location	Organ site (ICD code)	Characteristics of cases	Characteristics of controls	Exposure assessment	Exposure category	No. of cases/controls	Odds ratio (95% CI)	Adjustment for potential confounders	Comments
Mastrangelo et al. (2003), Italy	Trachea, bronchus and lung (ICD-9 162)	38 histologically confirmed lung cancers	228 with no history of cancer	Facility-specific JEM	*Cumulative exposure to VCM (ppm–years)*			Smoking habits in relation to years of work as a bagger	Italian cohort of 1658 vinyl chloride workers; nested case–control
					≤ 392	16/71	1.00		
					393–1650	13/74	0.78 (0.32–1.87)		
					≥ 1651	9/79	0.51 (0.18–1.31)		
							χ^2 trend $p > 0.01$		
					Circumstances of exposure to PVC dust				
					None	8/87	1.00		
					PVC compounding	8/49	1.78 (0.54–5.78)		
					Baggers (unknown length)	5/55	0.99 (0.24–3.63)		
					Baggers (known length)	17/33	5.60 (2.03–16.3)		
					PVC compounding				
					None	30/175	1.00		
					≤ 8.0 years	4/23	1.10 (0.24–3.28)		
					> 8.0 years	4/26	0.90 (0.21–2.86)		

Table 9 (contd)

Reference, location	Organ site (ICD code)	Characteristics of cases	Characteristics of controls	Exposure assessment	Exposure category	No. of cases/controls	Odds ratio (95% CI)	Adjustment for potential confounders	Comments
Mastrangelo et al. (2003) (contd)					**Baggers**				Nested case–control
					Duration of job				
					None	21/191	1.00		
					< 3.6 years	6/19	2.87 (0.84–8.56)		
					≥ 3.6 years	11/14	7.51 (2.55–19.3)		
					Calendar year of onset				
					None	21/191	1.00		
					Before 1967	10/19	4.79 (1.73–12.5)		
					Since 1967 onwards	7/14	4.55 (1.38–13.6)		
					Age at onset				
					No	21/191	1.00		
					≤ 33 years	6/20	2.73 (0.80–8.07)		
					> 33 years	11/13	7.70 (2.72–21.1)		
					Length of time elapsed from onset of job to end of follow-up or death				
					None	21/191	1.00		
					20 years	12/29	3.76 (1.51–8.99)		
					≤ 20 years	5/4	11.4 (2.21–60.7)		

Table 9 (contd)

Reference, location	Organ site (ICD code)	Characteristics of cases	Characteristics of controls	Exposure assessment	Exposure category	No. of cases/controls	Odds ratio (95% CI)	Adjustment for potential confounders	Comments
Scélo et al. (2004), seven European countries	Trachea, bronchus and lung (ICD-9 162)	2861 lung cancers in 1998–2002	3118 (excluded hospital patients admitted for tobacco-related diseases)	For each job held, local experts assessed intensity and frequency of exposure to vinyl chloride, acrylonitrile and styrene	Never	2822/3098	1.00	Gender, age, tobacco, acrylonitrile, styrene, plastics pyrolysis products, chromium dust	Population-based
					Ever		1.05 (0.68–1.62)		
					Duration (years)				
					None	2794/3062	1.0		
					1–6	18/17	0.74 (0.35–1.56)		
					7–14	15/18	0.86 (0.39–1.90)		
					> 14	34/21	1.56 (0.81–3.03)		
							Test for linear trend, p= 0.119		
					Cumulative exposure (ppm–years)				
					None	2794/3062	1.00		
					0.01–1.75	25/23	0.90 (0.46–1.75)		
					1.76–12.50	24/16	0.96 (0.47–1.98)		
					> 12.50	18/17	1.51 (0.65–3.47)		

CI, confidence interval; ICD, International Classification of Diseases; JEM, job–exposure matrix

In a case–control study from seven European countries (Scélo *et al.*, 2004) that included 2861 cases of lung cancer and 3118 hospital controls, the odds ratio for ever exposure to vinyl chloride was 1.05 (95% CI, 0.68–1.62). A modest non-significant increase in the risk for lung cancer was found in the highest-exposed subgroup.

2.5.2   *Other cancers of the respiratory tract*

With respect to other cancers of the respiratory tract, neither the European nor the North American multicentric cohort studies found any evidence of an excess incidence of or mortality from laryngeal cancer. Mortality from cancer of the pleura was moderately elevated in the update of the European multicentric cohort (nine deaths; SMR, 1.89; 95% CI, 0.86–3.59) (Ward *et al.*, 2000, 2001). In an update of the North American multicentric study (Mundt *et al.*, 2000), an elevated SMR was found for cancer of other parts of the respiratory tract (six deaths; SMR, 1.80; 95% CI, 0.66–3.92).

2.6   Cancer of the lymphatic and haematopoeitic tissues (Table 10)

2.6.1   *North American multicentric study*

In the update of the North American multicentric study, the SMR for cancer of the lymphatic and haematopoeitic tissues was 0.86 (71 observed deaths; 95% CI, 0.67–1.08). The SMR for lymphosarcoma and reticulosarcoma (defined as ICD-9 code 200) was 1.20 (12 deaths; 95% CI, 0.62–2.09). No excesses were reported for other leukaemias or Hodgkin lymphoma (Mundt *et al.*, 2000).

2.6.2   *European multicentric study*

In an update of the European multicentric cohort study, an SMR of 0.94 (62 deaths; 95% CI, 0.72–1.21) was observed for cancers of lymphatic and haematopoeitic tissue; no significant excess was reported in any category of leukaemia or lymphoma. The overall SMR of 1.19 (26 deaths; 95% CI, 0.78–1.75) for non-Hodgkin lymphoma (Ward *et al.*, 2000, 2001) was much lower than that observed in the original study (seven deaths; SMR, 1.70; 95% CI, 0.69–3.71) (Simonato *et al.*, 1991). The SIR for non-Hodgkin lymphoma (ICD-9 code 200 and 202) in the updated study was 0.78 (20 deaths; 95% CI, 0.48–1.21); SIRs reported for other leukaemias and lymphomas were all below 1.00. Among the four countries, Italy had the highest SMR of 1.86 (95% CI, 0.84–3.54) and much of the excess was in the mixed production plants (SMR, 1.52; 95% CI, 0.96–2.27). No significant trends were observed with time since first employment, duration of employment, cumulative exposure or calendar period of hire. In the Poisson regression analyses, there appeared to be some elevation in rate ratios above the baseline category of cumulative dose, but the trend was not statistically significant (data not shown).

Table 10. Cohort studies of lymphohaematopoietic neoplasms in vinyl chloride monomer (VCM) and polyvinyl chloride (PVC) production workers

Name of study Reference, location	Cohort description	Exposure assessment	Type of cancer (ICD code)	Exposure categories	No. of cases/ deaths	Relative risk (95% CI)	Adjustment for potential confounders	Comments
North American multicentric study								
Mundt et al. (2000), USA	10 109 white male workers from 37 plants (race unknown, 6%) employed at least ≥ 1 year in jobs that entailed exposure to VCM in 1942–72; mortality follow-up, 1942–95; vital status, 96.8%; cause of death, 99%	JEM	Lymphohaemato-poeitic (ICD-9 200–208)	Job exposed to VC	71	**SMR** 0.86 (0.67–1.08)		Reference rates: state rates
			Lymphosarcoma or reticulosarcoma (ICD-9 200)		12	1.20 (0.62–2.09)		
			Hodgkin lymphoma (ICD-9 201)		3	0.44 (0.09–1.29)		
			Leukaemia/ aleukaemia (204–208)		31	0.94 (0.64–1.34)		
European multicentric study								
Ward et al. (2000, 2001), Italy, Norway, Sweden, United Kingdom	12 700 male workers employed at 19 VCM/PVC plants ≥ 1 year in 1950–85; mortality follow-up, 1955–97; incidence follow-up 1955–96	Calendar period JEM for 13/19 factories grouped in 22 broad categories; factory-specific JEM with validated exposure estimates (ppm)	Lymphohaemato-poeitic (ICD-9 200–208)	Employed in VC industry (full cohort)	62	**SMR** 0.94 (0.72–1.21)	Age, calendar period	Reference rates and incidence rates: national Poisson regression analysis
			Non-Hodgkin lymphoma (ICD-9 200, 202)		26	1.19 (0.78–1.75)		
			Hodgkin lymphoma (ICD-9 201)		7	1.03 (0.41–2.12)		
			Leukaemia (ICD-9 204–208)		22	0.87 (0.54–1.31)		

Table 10 (contd)

Name of study Reference, location	Cohort description	Exposure assessment	Type of cancer (ICD code)	Exposure categories	No. of cases/ deaths	Relative risk (95% CI)	Adjustment for potential confounders	Comments
Other studies								
Thériault & Allard (1981), Québec, Canada	451 male workers exposed to VCM for ≥ 5 years in a polymerization plant, employed in 1948–72; mortality follow-up, 1948–77	Questionnaire to the worker or next of kin on detailed occupational history	Leukaemia (ICD-9 200–209)	Exposed versus unexposed	1	**SMR** 0.60 (NR)		Reference rates: Canadian population in 1971; comparison population: 870 workers not exposed to VCM for ≥ 5 months
Weber *et al.* (1981), Germany	7021 male VCM/PVC production workers from beginning of operation to 1974; mortality follow-up, from beginning of operation to 1974; vital status, > 90%; cause of death, 7–13%	JEM	Lymphatic and haematopoietic (ICD-8 200–209)	Exposed versus unexposed	15	2.14 (1.12–3.53)		Reference rates: national

Table 10 (contd)

Name of study Reference, location	Cohort description	Exposure assessment	Type of cancer (ICD code)	Exposure categories	No. of cases/ deaths	Relative risk (95% CI)	Adjustment for potential confounders	Comments
Smulevich et al. (1988), former Soviet Union	3232 VCM/PVC production workers (2195 men, 1037 women) employed for ≥ 1 month in VCM-exposed jobs; mortality follow-up, 1939–77	Exposure data in 1953–66 from JEM	Non-Hodgkin lymphoma and multiple myeloma (ICD-9 200, 202, 203)	Estimated area exposure: low, medium and high	5	**SMR** 4.17 ($p < 0.05$)		City (Gorki) mean death rates in 1959, 1969 and 1975
			Leukaemia (ICD-9 204–207)		5	5.00 ($p < 0.05$)		
Wong, O. et al. (2002), Taiwan, China	3293 male workers in 6 PVC polymerization plants exposed to VCM ≥ 1 year in 1950–92; mortality follow-up, 1985–97; vital status, 99%	JEM	Lymphatic and haematopoietic (ICD-9 200–208)		7	**SMR** 2.71 (1.09–5.60)		Reference rates: national; cohort assembled from Bureau of Labour Insurance

CI, confidence interval; ICD, International Classification of Diseases; JEM, job–exposure matrix; NR, not reported; SMR, standardized mortality ratio; VC, vinyl chloride

2.6.3   *Other studies*

Only one death from leukaemia (1.67 expected; SMR, 0.60) was reported in the Canadian study (Thériault & Allard, 1981).

Two independent European studies in Germany (Weber *et al.*, 1981) and the former Soviet Union (Smulevich *et al.*, 1988) have reported significantly increased mortality from neoplasms of the lymphatic and haematopoeitic system (Germany: SMR, 2.14; 95% CI, 1.12–3.53; former Soviet Union: SMR, 4; $p < 0.05$.

A study in Taiwan, China, reported a significant SMR for neoplasms of the lymphatic and haematopoeitic system (seven deaths; SMR, 2.71; 95% CI, 1.09–5.60) (Wong, O. *et al.*, 2002).

2.6.4   *Meta-analysis*

The meta-analysis by Boffetta *et al.* (2003) showed a meta-SMR for neoplasms of the lymphatic and haematopoeitic system of 0.90 (95% CI, 0.75–1.07) based on the two multicentric cohorts. A meta-SMR for all studies was not calculated due to the high degree of heterogeneity between studies.

Non-Hodgkin lymphoma and multiple myeloma (ICD-9 200, 202, 203) were combined in the meta-analysis (Boffetta *et al.*, 2003). SMRs for both the European and North American multicentric cohorts were below 1.00. However, an independent study from the former Soviet Union reported a significantly elevated SMR of 4.17 ($p < 0.05$) for this category of neoplasms (Smulevich *et al.*, 1988). Due to borderline results for tests of heterogeneity, the multicentric cohorts and three independent studies were combined in the meta-analysis to yield a meta-SMR of 1.23 (95% CI, 0.70–2.19).

2.7   **Malignant melanoma and cancer of the skin** (Table 11)

2.7.1   *North American multicentric cohort study*

In the update of the North American cohort (Mundt *et al.*, 2000), no elevation in mortality from skin cancer was observed (12 observed deaths; SMR, 0.64; 95% CI, 0.33–1.12).

2.7.2   *European multicentric cohort study*

An update of the European multicentric study found a non-significantly elevated SMR for malignant melanoma (15 deaths; SMR, 1.60; 95% CI, 0.90–2.65) (Ward *et al.*, 2000, 2001). The analysis of incidence did not show an excess of melanoma (18 observed cases; SIR, 1.06; 95% CI, 0.63–1.68). An excess of mortality from melanoma had been previously noted for the Norwegian cohort and was found to be dose-related (Heldaas *et al.*, 1984, 1987; Langård *et al.*, 2000). In the update of the European multicentric study, the excess in Norway was statistically significant (five deaths; SMR, 6.27; 95% CI, 2.04–14.6) (Ward *et al.*, 2001). An excess of mortality from melanoma was also observed in

Table 11. Cohort studies of malignant melanoma or skin cancer in vinyl chloride monomer (VCM) and polyvinyl chloride (PVC) production workers

Name of study Reference, location	Cohort description	Exposure assessment	Type of cancer (ICD code)	Exposure categories	No. of cases/ deaths	Relative risk (95% CI)	Adjustment for potential confounders	Comments
North American multicentric study								
Mundt et al. (2000), USA	10 109 white male workers in 37 plants (race unknown, 6%) employed at least ≥ 1 year in jobs that entailed exposure to VCM in 1942–72; mortality follow-up, 1942–95; vital status, 96.8%; cause of death, 99%	JEM	Skin (ICD-9 172–173)	Job exposed to VC	12	**SMR** 0.64 (0.33–1.12)		Reference rates: state and USA population
European multicentric study								
Ward et al. (2000, 2001), Italy, Norway, Sweden, United Kingdom	12 700 male workers employed in 19 VCM/PVC plants ≥ 1 year in 1950–85; mortality follow-up, 1955–97; incidence follow-up, 1955–96	Calendar period JEM for 13/19 factories grouped in 22 broad categories; factory-specific JEM with validated exposure estimates (ppm)	Melanoma (ICD-9 172)	Employed in VC industry (full cohort)	15	**SMR** 1.60 (0.90–2.65)		Reference rates and incidence rates: national
					18	**SIR** 1.06 (0.63–1.68)		
				VCM production	1	**SMR** 5.13 (0.13–28.6)	Age, calendar period	
				PVC production	0	(0.00–2.45)		
				VCM and PVC production	13	2.12 (1.13–3.62)		
				PVC processing	1	0.66 (0.02–3.68)		
				Latency (years)		**Relative risk**	Age, calendar period	Poisson regression analysis
				< 16	4	1.00		
				16–21	3	1.06 (0.20–5.61)		
				22–26	1	0.49 (0.04–5.43)		
				27–34	3	1.78 (0.25–12.8)		
				≥ 35	4	4.41 (0.51–38.4)		
						Test for linear trend, $p = 0.193$		

Table 11 (contd)

Name of study Reference, location	Cohort description	Exposure assessment	Type of cancer (ICD code)	Exposure categories	No. of cases/ deaths	Relative risk (95% CI)	Adjustment for potential confounders	Comments
Ward et al. (2000, 2001) (contd)				*Duration (years)*				
				1–2	5	1.00		
				3–6	1	0.22 (0.03–1.85)		
				7–11	1	0.22 (0.03–1.89)		
				12–18	4	0.83 (0.22–3.16)		
				≥ 19	4	1.10 (0.27–4.44)		
						Test for linear trend, p = 0.665		
				Cumulative exposure (ppm–years)				
				35–99	3	1.00		
				100–535	4	2.31 (0.51–10.3)		
				536–2811	4	2.57 (0.57–11.5)		
				≥ 2812	3	2.68 (0.53–13.7)		
						Test for linear trend, p = 0.193		
Other studies								
Smulevich et al. (1988), former Soviet Union	3232 VCM/PVC production workers (2195 men, 1037 women) employed for ≥ 1 month in VCM-exposed jobs; mortality follow-up, 1939–77	Exposure data in 1953–66 from JEM		Estimated area exposure: low, medium and high	1	**SMR** 2.00 (p > 0.05)		City (Gorki) mean death rates in 1959, 1969 and 1975

CI, confidence interval; ICD, International Classification of Diseases; JEM, job–exposure matrix; SIR, standardized incidence ratio; SMR, standardized mortality ratio; VC, vinyl chloride the Italian cohort (four deaths; SMR, 1.96; 95% CI, 0.53–5.01). No association was observed with previous employment as an autoclave cleaner.

2.7.3   *Other cohort studies*

In a study in the former Soviet Union (Smulevich *et al.*, 1988), one case of melanoma skin cancer was reported (SMR, 2.00; $p > 0.05$).

No cases were reported from the other independent studies (Thériault & Allard, 1981; Weber *et al.*, 1981; Laplanche *et al.*, 1992; Wong, O. *et al.*, 2002).

2.7.4   *Meta-analysis*

In the meta-analysis, results for mortality from skin cancer were heterogeneous, with no overall indication of an increased risk (meta-SMR, 1.11; 95% CI, 0.49–2.54) (Boffetta *et al.*, 2003).

2.8   Cancer of the breast

Although concern has been raised about a potential association between exposure to vinyl chloride and the risk for breast cancer, human studies to date are not informative on this issue because of the very small numbers of women included. The analyses of both the European and North American cohorts included only men because of the extremely small number of women available for analysis (59 in the European multicentric cohort and 11 in the North American cohort) (Mundt *et al.*, 2000; Ward *et al.*, 2000, 2001). No deaths from breast cancer were observed in the European multicentric cohort (Ward *et al.*, 2000), with only 0.53 expected, and two deaths were observed in the North American cohort, with 1.05 expected (SMR, 1.90; 95% CI, 0.23–6.87) (Mundt *et al.*, 2000).

2.9   Soft-tissue sarcoma

2.9.1   *North American multicentric cohort study*

In the update of the North American multicentric study (Mundt *et al.*, 2000), the SMR for cancer of connective and soft tissue was 2.70 (12 deaths; 95% CI, 1.39–4.72); significant excesses were observed for those employed for 10–19 years (SMR, 4.77; 95% CI, 1.55–11.1) and for those employed for 20 years or more (SMR, 7.25; 95% CI, 1.97–18.6). SMRs were also significantly increased for first exposure before 1950 (SMR, 3.33; CI, 1.08–7.77) and between 1950 and 1959 (SMR, 4.68; 95% CI, 1.88–9.64). Seven of the 12 cancers were specific soft tissue other than angiosarcomas, and four were angiosarcomas with site not specified.

2.9.2   *European multicentric cohort study*

A total of six soft-tissue sarcomas were observed in the European multicentric study (SMR, 1.89; 95% CI, 0.69–4.11) (Ward *et al.*, 2000, 2001), all of which occurred in the United Kingdom. Three additional soft-tissue sarcomas were identified from the incidence data (one in the United Kingdom and two in Sweden). However, during the review of the best available data for diagnosis to ascertain cases of liver cancer, it became apparent that three of the six deaths coded as tumours of the connective tissue were actually angiosarcomas of the liver, the primary site of which had been miscoded. A Poisson regression analysis was not conducted for the remaining soft-tissue sarcomas due to the small number of cases involved.

2.9.3   *Other cohort studies*

Two deaths from soft-tissue sarcoma were observed in the Canadian cohort (SMR, 5.26) (Thériault & Allard, 1981).

One case of soft-tissue sarcoma was observed in the cohort from the former Soviet Union (SMR, 1.43; *p* > 0.05) (Smulevich *et al.*, 1988)

3.   Studies of Cancer in Experimental Animals

Studies of the carcinogenicity of vinyl chloride following oral, inhalation and/or intratracheal administration, subcutaneous and/or intramuscular administration, intraperitoneal administration and perinatal exposure have been reviewed previously (IARC, 1979, 1987). Those that were found to be adequate and/or reported more fully in later publications are included in this section.

The carcinogenicity of vinyl chloride has been studied intensively and repeatedly by inhalation exposure of experimental animals at a range of concentrations that spanned decimal orders of magnitude. The numerous studies were generally mutually reinforced and consistently yielded hepatic and extrahepatic angiosarcomas in mice, rats and hamsters. Various other malignant neoplasms also occurred at several anatomical sites. However, the reporting of this multitude of data has often been incomplete, and the outcomes of many studies are available only from summary tables in the published literature, in which technical details are given only as footnotes.

3.1   Inhalation exposure

3.1.1   *Mouse*

Groups of 12 male and 12 female NMRI mice, 12 weeks of age, were exposed by inhalation to 50 or 500 ppm [130 or 1300 mg/m^3] vinyl chloride [purity unspecified] on

6 h per day for 5 days per week for either 26 (500 ppm) or 52 (50 ppm) weeks. Two groups of 12 male and 12 female control mice were untreated and were observed for either 26 or 52 weeks. The treatment with 500 ppm vinyl chloride was terminated at week 26 because of poor survival. The incidence of treatment-related tumours in males of the two control groups combined, and low- and high-dose groups, respectively, was: extra-hepatic angiosarcomas, 0/24, 6/12 and 3/12; and lung tumours, 0/24, 9/12 and 12/12. That in females was: extrahepatic angiosarcomas, 0/24, 8/12 and 5/12; and lung tumours, 0/24, 4/12 and 12/12. Mammary carcinomas were observed in 1/24, 1/12 and 4/12 control, low-dose and high-dose females, respectively [no statistical analysis reported] (Holmberg et al., 1976).

Groups of 36 male and 36 female CD-1 mice, 2 months of age, were exposed by inhalation to 0, 50, 250 or 1000 ppm [0, 130, 650 or 2600 mg/m³] vinyl chloride (99.8% pure) in air for 6 h per day on 5 days per week for 52 weeks. Four animals per group were terminated at 1, 2, 3, 6 or 9 months for laboratory tests and gross and histological examination. The incidence of liver angiosarcomas in control, 50-, 250- and 1000-ppm vinyl chloride-treated mice, respectively, was 0/26, 3/29, 7/29 ($p < 0.05$, Fisher's exact test) and 13/33 ($p < 0.05$) males and 0/36, 0/34, 16/34 ($p < 0.05$) and 18/36 [$p < 0.05$] females; that of extrahepatic angiosarcomas was 0/26, 5/29 ($p < 0.05$), 2/29 and 0/33 males and 0/36, 1/34, 3/34 and 9/36 ($p < 0.05$) females, respectively; and that of lung tumours (adenomas) was 1/26, 8/29, 10/29 and 22/33 males and 0/36, 4/34, 12/34 and 26/36 females, respectively. The incidence of mammary tumours (adenocarcinomas and carcinomas) in female mice was 0/36, 9/34, 3/34 and 13/36, respectively [no statistical analysis reported for lung and mammary tumours] (Lee et al., 1978).

Groups of 8–28 male and 8–28 female CD1 mice, 2 months of age, were exposed by whole-body inhalation to 0, 130, 650 or 2600 mg/m³ [0, 340, 1690 or 6760 ppm] vinyl chloride (99.8% pure) for 6 h per day on 5 days per week for 1, 3 or 6 months and were then removed from exposure chambers and observed for an additional 12 months. The incidence of haemangiosarcoma and lung and mammary gland tumours is presented in Table 12. An increased cumulative incidence of haemangiosarcomas and bronchiolo-alveolar lung tumours was seen in male and female mice and an increase in the cumulative incidence of mammary gland adenocarcinomas/carcinomas in females (Hong et al., 1981).

Groups of 30 male and 30 female Swiss mice [data reported for both sexes combined], 11 weeks of age, were exposed by inhalation to 50, 250, 500, 2500, 6000 or 10 000 ppm [130, 650, 1300, 6500, 15 600 or 26 000 mg/m³] vinyl chloride (99.97% pure) on 4 h per day on 5 days per week for 30 weeks. Control animals comprised 150 untreated mice [sex distribution not specified; data reported for both sexes combined]. Animals were observed until 81 weeks, when the experiment (experiment BT4) was terminated. Survival rates of the groups were not reported. The incidence of treatment-related tumours in control and 50-, 250-, 500-, 2500-, 6000- and 10 000-ppm vinyl chloride-treated mice, respectively, was: liver angiosarcomas, 0/150, 1/60, 18/60, 14/60, 16/59, 13/60 and 10/56; extrahepatic angiosarcomas, 1/150, 1/60, 3/60, 7/60, 8/59, 1/60

Table 12. Tumour incidence in CD1 mice exposed by inhalation to vinyl chloride for 1–6 months and observed for an additional 12 months

Tumour type	Tumour incidence/no. examined			
	Concentration (ppm) [mg/m^3]			
	0	50 [130]	250 [650]	1000 [2600]
Males				
1 month				
Liver				
Haemangiosarcoma	0/16	1/16	0/16	0/16
Lung				
Bronchioloalveolar tumour	2/16	3/16	10/16	11/16
3 months				
Liver				
Haemangiosarcoma	0/16	0/16	1/16	1/10
Lung				
Bronchioloalveolar tumour	2/16	7/16	11/16	9/10
6 months				
Liver				
Haemangiosarcoma	0/28	0/8	7/12	5/12
Lung				
Bronchioloalveolar tumour	4/28	2/8	8/12	7/12
Cumulative incidence				
Liver				
Haemangiosarcoma[a]	0/60	1/40	8/44[c]	6/38[c]
Lung				
Bronchioloalveolar tumour[b]	8/60	12/40	29/44[c]	27/38[c]
Females				
1 month				
Liver				
Haemangiosarcoma	0/16	0/16	0/16	0/16
Lung				
Bronchioloalveolar tumour	1/16	0/16	9/16	9/16
Mammary gland				
Adenocarcinoma/carcinoma	1/16	4/16	2/16	0/16
3 months				
Liver				
Haemangiosarcoma	0/16	0/16	3/16	4/10
Lung				
Bronchioloalveolar tumour	0/16	5/16	10/16	7/10
Mammary gland				
Adenocarcinoma/carcinoma	0/16	4/16	6/16	2/10

Table 12 (contd)

Tumour type	Tumour incidence/no. examined			
	Concentration (ppm) [mg/m^3]			
	0	50 [130]	250 [650]	1000 [2600]
6 months				
Liver				
Haemangiosarcoma	1/28	1/8	2/8	8/12
Lung				
Bronchioloalveolar tumour	7/28	1/8	4/8	7/12
Mammary gland				
Adenocarcinoma/carcinoma	3/28	2/8	5/8	4/12
Cumulative incidence				
Liver				
Haemangiosarcoma[a]	1/60	1/40	5/40[c]	12/38[c]
Lung				
Bronchioloalveolar tumour[b]	8/60	6/40	23/40[c]	23/38[c]
Mammary gland				
Adenocarcinoma/carcinoma	4/60	10/40[d]	13/40[d]	6/38[d]

From Hong *et al.* (1981)
[a] Significant dose-related incidence (males and females combined); Cochran-Armitage trend test
[b] Significant non-linearity in dose–incidence curve (males and females combined); Cochran-Armitage trend test
[c] Combined incidence in males and females significantly different from controls ($p < 0.05$, Fisher's exact test)
[d] Incidence in females significantly different from controls ($p < 0.05$, Fisher's exact test)

and 1/56; lung tumours, 15/150, 6/60, 41/60, 50/60, 40/59, 47/60 and 46/56; and mammary carcinomas, 1/150, 12/60, 12/60, 8/60, 8/59, 8/60 and 13/56. A low incidence of skin tumours was also reported [no statistical analysis provided] (Maltoni *et al.*, 1981).

Groups of female Swiss CD-1 mice [initial numbers not specified], 8–9 weeks of age, were exposed by whole-body inhalation to 0 (control) or 130 mg/m^3 [0 or 50 ppm] vinyl chloride (commercial grade) [purity unspecified] for 6 h per day on 5 days per week for 6, 12 or 18 months. Animals were allowed to complete their lifespan and were necropsied when moribund or dead. There was a significant decrease ($p < 0.01$) in survival of the animals treated for 6, 12 and 18 months compared with controls. Statistically significant increases ($p < 0.01$, life-table analysis) in the incidence of haemangiosarcomas (all sites, mainly peritoneal and skin), mammary gland carcinomas and lung carcinomas were observed in all exposure groups. The incidence of haemangiosarcomas (all sites) was: control, 1/71; exposed for 6 months, 29/67; 12 months, 30/47; and 18 months, 20/45. The incidence of mammary gland carcinomas was 2/71, 33/67, 22/47 and 22/45, respectively; and that of lung carcinomas was 9/71, 18/65, 15/47 and 11/45, respectively. In the same study, groups of female Swiss CD-1 mice [initial numbers not specified], 8 or 14 months of age, were exposed by whole-body inhalation to 0 (control) or 130 mg/m^3 [0 or 50 ppm] vinyl chloride for 6 h per day on 5 days per week for 6 or 12 months. Animals were allowed to complete their lifespan and were necropsied when found moribund or dead. Among animals exposed for 6 months beginning at 8 and 14 months of age, statistically significant increases (life-table analysis) in the incidence of haemangiosarcomas (all sites) (control, 1/71; 8 months of age, 11/49, $p < 0.01$; and 14 months of age, 5/53), mammary gland carcinomas (control, 2/71; 8 months of age, 13/49, $p < 0.01$; and 14 months of age, 2/53) and lung carcinomas (control, 9/71; 8 months of age, 13/49, $p < 0.05$; and 14 months of age, 7/53) were observed in the animals exposed beginning at 8 months of age only. Among those exposed for 12 months, statistically significant increases in the incidence of haemangiosarcomas (all sites) (control, 1/71; 8 months of age, 17/46, $p < 0.01$; and 14 months of age, 3/50), mammary gland carcinomas (control, 2/71; 8 months of age, 8/45, $p < 0.01$; and 14 months of age, 0/50) and lung carcinomas (control, 9/71; 8 months of age, 9/46, $p < 0.05$; and 14 months of age, 3/50) were observed in the animals exposed beginning at 8 months of age only (Drew et al., 1983).

Groups of female B6C3F$_1$ mice [initial number not specified], 8–9 weeks of age, were exposed by whole-body inhalation to 0 (control) or 130 mg/m^3 [0 or 5.0 ppm] vinyl chloride (commercial grade) [purity unspecified] for 6 h per day on 5 days per week for 6 or 12 months. Animals were allowed to complete their lifespan and were necropsied when found moribund or dead. There was a significant decrease ($p < 0.01$) in survival of the animals treated for 6 or 12 months compared with controls. Statistically significant increases ($p < 0.01$, life-table analysis) in the incidence of haemangiosarcomas (all sites) and mammary gland tumours were observed in all exposure groups. The incidence of haemangiosarcomas (all sites, mainly peritoneal and subcutis) was: control, 4/69; exposed for 6 months, 46/67; and 12 months, 69/90; that of mammary gland carcinomas was 3/69 (control), 29/67 and 37/90, respectively. In the same study, groups of female B6C3F$_1$ mice [initial number not specified], 8 or 14 months of age, were exposed by whole-body inhalation to 0 (control) or 130 mg/m^3 [0 or 50 ppm] vinyl chloride for 6 h per day on 5 days per week for 6 or 12 months. Animals were allowed complete their lifespan and were necropsied when found moribund or dead. There was a significant decrease ($p < 0.01$) in survival of the treated animals compared with controls. Among the animals exposed for 6 and 12 months, statistically significant increases ($p < 0.01$ except $p < 0.05$ where indicated, life-table analysis) were observed in the incidence of haemangio-sarcomas (all sites) (control, 4/69; 6-month exposures: 8 months of age, 27/42; and 14 months of age, 30/51; 12-month exposures: 8 months of age, 30/48; and 14 months of age, 29/48) and mammary gland carcinomas (control, 3/69; 6-month exposures: 8 months of age, 13/42; and 14 months of age, 4/51, $p < 0.05$; 12-month exposures: 8 months of age, 9/48; and 14 months of age, 4/48) (Drew et al., 1983).

[The Working Group noted that lung tumours were not observed in B6C3F$_1$ mice exposed to vinyl chloride in the studies of Drew et al. (1983), whereas Swiss CD-1 mice, a strain that is more susceptible to the induction of lung tumours, did develop such tumours in these and other studies.]

Groups of 30, 40 or 60 male CD1 mice, 5–6 weeks of age, were exposed by whole-body inhalation to 0, 2.6, 26, 260, 780 or 1560 mg/m³ [0, 1, 10, 100, 300 or 600 ppm] vinyl chloride [purity unspecified] for 6 h per day on 5 days per week for 4 weeks and were then observed for an additional 0, 12 or 40–41 weeks. Surviving animals were killed after each observation period. The study focused on lung tumours. After 12 weeks of exposure, the incidence of pulmonary tumours was 0/18, 0/10, 0/9, 0/6, 6/9 and 8/9 for mice treated with 0 (control), 2.6, 26, 260, 780 and 1560 mg/m³, respectively; after 40–41 weeks of exposure, the incidence was 0/17, 1/9, 3/9, 6/9, 5/7 and 6/7, respectively [no statistical analysis provided] (Suzuki, 1983).

3.1.2   Rat

Groups of 36 male and 36 female CD rats, 2 months of age, were exposed by inhalation to 0, 50, 250 or 1000 ppm [0, 130, 650 or 2600 mg/m³] vinyl chloride (99.8% pure) in air for 6 h per day on 5 days per week for 52 weeks. Four animals per group were terminated at 1, 2, 3, 6 or 9 months for laboratory tests and gross and histological examination. The combined incidence of liver angiosarcomas by increasing level of exposure was 0/35 (control), 0/36, 2/36 and 6/34 in males and 0/35 (control), 0/36, 10/34 ($p < 0.05$, Fisher's exact test) and 15/36 ($p < 0.05$) in females, respectively. Similarly, the incidence of extrahepatic angiosarcomas was 0/35 (control), 1/36, 2/36 and 4/34 in males and 0/35 (control), 1/36, 3/34 and 10/36 ($p < 0.05$) in females, respectively (Lee et al., 1978).

Groups of 62 newly weaned male and female Wistar rats were exposed by whole-body inhalation to 0 or 13 000 mg/m³ [0 or 5000 ppm] vinyl chloride (≥ 99.97% pure) for 7 h per day on 5 days per week for 52 weeks. Ten animals per dose per sex were killed at 4, 13, 26 and 52 weeks. No information on survival was provided. At 52 weeks, an increase in the incidence of angiosarcomas of the liver (males, 3/9; females, 6/10), Zymbal gland squamous-cell carcinomas (males, 3/9; females, 2/10) and carcinomas of the nasal cavity (males, 2/9; females, 5/10) compared with controls (no tumours) was observed [no statistical evaluation provided] (Feron & Kroes, 1979; Feron et al., 1979).

Groups of 110–128 male and 110–128 female Sprague-Dawley rats, 6, 18, 32 or 52 weeks of age, were exposed in chambers by whole-body inhalation to 0 (controls) or 2465 mg/m³ [0 or 940 ppm] vinyl chloride [purity unspecified] for 7 h per day on 5 days per week for 24.5 weeks. An epidemic of pneumonia in exposed rats during the 28th week forced premature conclusion of the study and all surviving rats were killed 43 weeks after the beginning of exposure. Rats killed at 3, 6 or 9 months (interim sacrifice group) were evaluated separately from rats that either died, were killed in poor condition or were killed at the conclusion of the study (non-scheduled sacrifice group). Angiosarcomas, mostly primary tumours in the liver, were highly anaplastic and frequently metastasized to the lung. The incidence of angiosarcomas in vinyl chloride-exposed male rats in the non-scheduled sacrifice group was 0/37, 0/44, 3/45 and 13/55 in rats that were exposed beginning at 6, 18, 32 or 52 weeks of age, respectively. The corresponding incidence of angiosarcomas in exposed females was 2/38, 7/47, 23/49 and 11/54. Only one angiosarcoma occurred in subcutaneous tissues in a control male placed on study at 32 weeks of age (incidence for this control group, 1/86; incidence for all control males, 1/357). The incidence of angiosarcomas in control females was 0/382. Pituitary tumours and mammary tumours occurred in both control and exposed rats at comparable rates. A few rats in the control and exposed groups had Zymbal gland or brain tumours (Groth *et al.*, 1981).

Five groups of 51–93 male random-bred white rats, weighing 160–180 g at the beginning of the experiment, were exposed by whole-body inhalation to 0 (control), 14, 25, 266 or 3690 mg/m^3 [0, 5.4, 9.6, 102 or 1420 ppm] vinyl chloride [purity unspecified] for 4.5 h per day on 5 days per week for 52 weeks and observed until their death, but no longer than 126 weeks. The authors reported the development of angiosarcomas of liver or other sites in rats of the three highest-dose groups (9.3–15.7%). No such tumours were observed in control animals (Kurlyandski *et al.*, 1981).

Groups of 30 male and 30 female Sprague-Dawley rats [data reported for both sexes combined], 12 weeks of age, were exposed by inhalation to 50, 250, 500, 2500, 6000 or 10 000 ppm [130, 650, 1300, 6500, 15 600 or 26 000 mg/m^3] vinyl chloride (99.97% pure) for 4 h per day on 5 days per week for 17 weeks. Control animals comprised 190 untreated rats [data reported for both sexes combined]. Animals were observed until 156 weeks, when the experiment (experiment BT3) was terminated. Survival rates of the groups were not reported. The incidence of tumours was: liver angiosarcomas, 0/190, 0/58, 0/59, 1/60, 1/60, 1/60 and 0/58 in control, 50-, 250-, 500-, 2500-, 6000- and 10 000-ppm vinyl chloride-treated rats, respectively; 'hepatomas', 0/190 (control), 0/58, 0/59, 0/60, 2/60, 1/60 and 1/58, respectively; Zymbal gland carcinomas, 2/190 (control), 0/58, 1/59, 1/60, 7/60, 9/60 and 9/58, respectively; and 'skin epitheliomas', 1/190 (control), 1/58, 0/59, 0/60, 2/60, 5/60 and 5/58, respectively [no statistical analysis reported] (Maltoni *et al.*, 1981).

Groups of 60 male and 60 female Sprague-Dawley rats [data reported for both sexes combined], 13 weeks of age, were exposed by inhalation to 6000 or 10 000 ppm [15 600 or 26 000 mg/m^3] vinyl chloride (99.97% pure) for 4 h per day on 5 days per week for 5 weeks (groups I and II), for 1 h per day on 4 days per week for 25 weeks (groups III and IV) or for 4 h per day once a week for 25 weeks (groups V and VI). Control animals comprised two groups of 120 untreated rats [data reported for both sexes combined]. Animals were observed until 154 weeks, when the experiment (experiment BT10) was terminated. Survival rates of the groups were not reported. The incidence of tumours was: liver angiosarcomas, 0/227, 1/118, 0/120, 1/119, 3/118, 1/119 and 1/120 in controls and groups I, II, III, IV, V and VI, respectively; extrahepatic angiosarcomas, 0/227 (control), 0/118, 0/120, 0/119, 2/118, 0/119 and 1/120, respectively; Zymbal gland carcinomas, 0/227 (control), 9/118, 9/120, 9/119, 5/118, 8/119 and 9/120, respectively; and mammary tumours, 17/227 (control), 13/118, 13/120, 16/119, 11/118, 20/119 and 12/120, respectively. The predominant carcinogenic effect was in the Zymbal gland [no statistical analysis reported] (Maltoni *et al.*, 1981).

Five experiments (BT1, BT2, BT6, BT9, BT15) performed by Maltoni *et al.* (1981) were combined to construct a dose–response table. Groups of 60–300 male and female Sprague-Dawley rats [data reported for both sexes combined], 13–17 weeks of age, were exposed by inhalation to 1, 5, 10, 25, 50, 100, 150, 200, 250, 500, 2500, 6000, 10 000 or 30 000 ppm [2.6, 13, 26, 65, 130, 260, 390, 520, 650, 1300, 6500, 15 600, 26 000 or 78 000 mg/m^3] vinyl chloride (99.97% pure) for 4 h per day on 5 days per week for 52 weeks. Controls comprised 461 untreated rats from four experiments [data reported for both sexes combined]. Animals were observed until 68 (BT6) or 135–147 (BT1, BT2, BT9, BT15) weeks, when the experiments were terminated. Survival rates of the groups were not reported. Selected tumour incidences are presented in Table 13 [no statistical analysis reported] (Maltoni *et al.*, 1981). [The Working Group noted that the clearest dose–response was observed for hepatic angiosarcomas and Zymbal gland carcinomas.]

Groups of 30–40 male (BT7) or 120–130 male [exact numbers not specified] (BT17) Wistar rats, 11–13 weeks of age, were exposed by inhalation to 1, 50, 250, 500, 2500, 6000 or 10 000 ppm [2.6, 130, 650, 1300, 6500, 15 600 or 26 000 mg/m^3] vinyl chloride (99.97% pure) for 4 h per day on 5 days per week for 52 weeks. Control animals comprised 40 (BT7) or 120–130 [exact number not specified] (BT17) untreated rats. Animals were observed until 134 (BT17) or 165 (BT7) weeks, when the experiment was terminated. Survival rates of the groups were not reported. The incidence of selected tumours in order of increasing doses was: liver angiosarcomas, 0/132 (control), 0/99, 0/28, 1/27, 3/28, 3/25, 3/26 and 8/27, respectively; extrahepatic angiosarcomas, 1/132 (control), 3/99, 0/28, 1/27, 0/28, 1/25, 1/26 and 0/27, respectively; 'hepatomas', 0/132 (control), 1/99, 0/28, 0/27, 0/28, 1/25, 2/26 and 0/27, respectively; and Zymbal gland carcinomas, 3/132 (control), 2/99, 0/28, 0/27, 0/28, 0/25, 2/26 and 2/27, respectively [no statistical analysis provided] (Maltoni *et al.*, 1981). [The Working Group noted the lack of a dose–response for extrahepatic angiosarcomas, Zymbal gland carcinomas and hepatomas.]

Groups of 55–112 female Fischer 344 rats, 8–9 weeks of age, were exposed by whole-body inhalation to 0 (control) or 260 mg/m^3 [0 or 100 ppm] vinyl chloride (commercial grade) [purity unspecified] for 6 h per day on 5 days per week for 6, 12, 18 or 24 months. Animals were allowed to complete their lifespan and were necropsied when found moribund or dead. There was a significant decrease ($p < 0.01$) in survival of animals exposed for 1 year or more compared with controls. Statistically significant increases ($p < 0.01$, life-table analysis) were observed in the incidence of liver haemangiosarcomas, haemangiosarcomas (all sites), mammary gland fibroadenomas and liver neoplastic nodules [hepatocellular adenomas] in all exposure groups and of mammary gland adenocarcinomas and hepatocellular carcinomas in the groups exposed for 12, 18 and 24 months. Tumour incidence after 24 months of exposure was: haemangiosarcoma of the liver, 1/112 control versus 19/55 exposed; haemangiosarcoma (all sites), 2/112 control versus 24/55 exposed; fibroadenoma of the mammary gland, 24/112 control versus 26/55 exposed; adenocarcinoma of mammary gland, 5/112 control versus 5/55 exposed; liver neoplastic nodules [hepatocellular adenomas], 4/112 control versus 6/55

Table 13. Tumour incidence in a dose–response study of vinyl chloride administered by inhalation to Sprague-Dawley rats for 52 weeks

Exposure (ppm) [mg/m³]	Experiment	Liver angiosarcomas	Extrahepatic angiosarcomas	Hepatomas	Zymbal gland carcinomas	Mammary tumours	Nephroblastomas[a]	Neuroblastomas[b]
0	BT1, BT2, BT9, BT15	0/461	2/461	0/461	4/461	19/461	0/461	0/461
1 [2.6]	BT15	0/118	0/118	0/118	1/118	15/118	0/118	0/118
5 [13]	BT15	0/119	0/119	0/119	1/119	22/119	0/119	0/119
10 [26]	BT15	1/119	2/119	0/119	2/119	21/119	0/119	0/119
25 [65]	BT15	5/120	0/120	0/120	4/120	17/120	1/120	0/120
50 [130]	BT1	1/60	1/60	0/60	0/60	2/60	1/60	0/60
50 [130]	BT9	14/294	9/294	0/294	9/294	62/294	1/294	0/294
100 [260]	BT2	1/120	0/120	0/120	1/120	4/120	10/120	0/120
150 [390]	BT2	6/119	0/119	0/119	4/119	6/119	11/119	0/119
200 [520]	BT2	12/120	1/120	3/120	4/120	6/120	7/120	0/120
250 [650]	BT1	3/59	2/59	1/59	0/59	2/59	5/59	0/59
500 [1300]	BT1	6/60	1/60	5/60	4/60	1/60	6/60	0/60
2500 [6500]	BT1	13/60	3/60	2/60	2/60	2/60	6/60	4/60
6000 [15 600]	BT1	13/59	3/59	1/59	7/59	0/59	5/59	3/59
10 000 [26 000]	BT1	7/60	3/60	1/60	16/60	3/60	5/60	7/60
30 000 [78 000]	BT6	18/60	1/60	1/60	35/60	2/60	0/60	1/60

From Maltoni et al. (1981)

[a] Primary renal tumours were not necessarily embryonal in morphology.

[b] See Working Group comment on this diagnosis in the text that describes the Maltoni and Cotti (1988) study.

exposed; and hepatocellular carcinoma, 1/112 control versus 9/55 exposed. In the same study, groups of 51–112 female Fischer 344 rats, aged 2, 8, 14 or 20 months, were exposed by whole-body inhalation to 0 (control) or 260 mg/m^3 [100 ppm] vinyl chloride for 6 h per day on 5 days per week for 6 or 12 months. Exposures were initiated when the animals were 2, 8, 14 or 20 months of age for the 6-month exposures and 2, 8 or 14 months of age for the 12-month exposures. Animals were allowed to complete their lifespan and were necropsied when found moribund or dead. The incidence of haemangiosarcomas, and mammary gland and liver tumours is presented in Table 14. For the 6-month exposures, increases were observed in the incidence of liver haemangiosarcomas in one exposure group, of mammary gland fibroadenomas and neoplastic liver nodules [hepatocellular adenomas] in the 2- and 8-month-old groups, respectively, and of hepato-cellular carcinomas in the 8-month-old group. After the 12-month exposures, increases were observed in the incidence of liver haemangiosarcomas, haemangiosarcomas (all sites) and mammary gland fibroadenomas in the 2- and 8-month-old groups and of mammary gland adenocarcinomas, neoplastic liver nodules [hepatocellular adenomas] and hepatocellular carcinomas in the 2-month-old group (Drew *et al.*, 1983).

Table 14. Incidence of tumours in female Fischer 344 rats exposed to 260 mg/m^3 [100 ppm] vinyl chloride by inhalation

Exposure period (months)	Age at start (months)	Haemangiosarcoma		Mammary gland		Liver neoplastic nodules [hepato-cellular adenoma]	Hepato-cellular carcinoma
		Liver	All sites	Fibro-adenoma	Adeno-carcinoma		
0 (control)	–	1/112	2/112	24/112	5/112	4/112	1/112
6	2	4/76[a]	4/76	28/76[a]	6/76	15/75[a]	3/75
6	8	2/52	2/53	23/53[b]	2/53	10/52[a]	6/52[a]
6	14	0/51	0/53	17/53	3/53	2/51	0/51
6	20	0/53	0/53	20/53[b]	2/53	4/53	1/53
12	2	11/55[a]	12/56[a]	28/56[a]	11/56[a]	20/56[a]	4/56[a]
12	8	5/54[a]	5/55[a]	16/55[a]	4/55	4/54	1/54
12	14	2/49	2/50	15/50	0/50	4/49	0/49

Adapted from Drew *et al.* (1983)
[a] Difference from controls, $p < 0.01$ (life-table analysis)
[b] Difference from controls, $p < 0.05$ (life-table analysis)

3.1.3   Hamster

Groups of 30 male Golden hamsters, 11 weeks of age, were exposed by inhalation to 50, 250, 500, 2500, 6000 or 10 000 ppm [30, 650, 1300, 6500, 15 600 or 26 000 mg/m^3] vinyl chloride (99.97% pure) for 4 h per day on 5 days per week for 30 weeks. Control animals comprised 60 untreated male hamsters. Animals were observed until 109 weeks, when the experiment (experiment BT8) was terminated. Survival rates of the groups were not reported. The incidence of treatment-related tumours by increasing dose of exposure was: liver angiosarcomas, 0/60 (control), 0/30, 0/30, 2/30, 0/30, 1/30 and 0/30, respectively; skin epitheliomas, 3/60 (control), 9/30, 3/30, 7/30, 3/30, 1/30 and 7/30, respectively; and forestomach papillomas and acanthomas, 3/60 (control), 3/30, 4/30, 9/30, 17/30, 10/30 and 10/30, respectively. Leukaemia was observed at a similar incidence in control and treated groups (8/60 (control), 6/30, 6/30, 5/30, 9/30, 6/30 and 5/30, respectively), but the authors reported a decrease in the latency period [no statistical analysis provided] (Maltoni *et al.*, 1981).

Groups of female Syrian golden hamsters [initial numbers not specified], 8–9 weeks of age, were exposed by whole-body inhalation to 0 or 520 mg/m^3 [0 or 200 ppm] vinyl chloride (commercial grade) [purity unspecified] or 6 h per day on 5 days per week for 6, 12 or 18 months. Animals were allowed to complete their lifespan and were necropsied when found moribund or dead. There was a significant decrease ($p < 0.01$) in survival of all exposed animals compared with controls. Statistically significant increases (see Table 15) were observed in the incidence of mammary gland carcinomas and stomach adenomas in all exposure groups and of haemangiosarcomas (all sites) in the groups exposed for 6 and 12 months. A significant increase in the incidence of skin carcinomas was also seen in the 12-month exposure group. In the same study, groups of female Syrian golden hamsters, 2, 8, 14 or 20 months of age (Groups I, II, III and IV, respectively) [initial numbers not specified], were exposed by whole-body inhalation to 0 or 520 mg/m^3 [0 or

Table 15.   Incidence of tumours in female Syrian golden hamsters exposed to 520 mg/m^3 [200 ppm] vinyl chloride by inhalation

Exposure period (months)	Age at first exposure	Haemangiosarcoma (all sites)[a]	Mammary gland carcinoma	Stomach adenoma	Skin carcinoma
0 (control)	–	0/143	0/143	5/138	0/133
6	8 weeks	13/88[b]	28/87 [b]	23/88[b]	2/80
12	8 weeks	4/52 [b]	31/52 [b]	3/50[c]	9/48[b]
18	8 weeks	2/103	47/102[b]	20/101[b]	3/90
6	8 months	3/53 [c]	2/52[c]	15/53[b]	0/49
6	14 months	0/50	0/50	6/49[c]	0/46
6	20 months	0/52	1/52	0/52	0/50
12	2 months	4/52 [b]	31/52[b]	3/50[c]	2/80
12	8 months	1/44	6/44 [b]	10/44[b]	0/38
12	14 months	0/43	0/42	3/41	0/30

Modified from Drew *et al.* (1983)
[a] These tumours occurred primarily in the skin, spleen and liver.
[b] Difference from controls, $p < 0.01$ (life-table analysis)
[c] Difference from controls, $p < 0.05$ (life-table analysis)

200 ppm] vinyl chloride for 6 h per day on 5 days per week for 6 or 12 months. Exposures were initiated when the animals were 2, 8, 14 or 20 months of age for the 6-month exposures and 2, 8 or 14 months of age for the 12-month exposures. Animals were allowed to complete their lifespan and were necropsied when found moribund or dead. There was a significant decrease ($p < 0.01$) in the survival of animals that were exposed early in life for 12 months compared with controls. In some of the 6-month and 12-month exposure groups (see Table 15), statistically significant increases were observed in the incidence of stomach adenomas, haemangiosarcomas (all sites) and mammary gland carcinomas (Drew *et al.*, 1983).

[The Working Group noted the successful induction of hepatic angiosarcomas in three species (rats, mice and hamsters) exposed to vinyl chloride by inhalation.]

3.2   Oral administration

Rat

Groups of 40 male and 40 female Sprague-Dawley rats [data reported only for both sexes combined], 13 weeks of age, were administered 3.3, 17 or 50 mg/kg bw vinyl chloride (99.97% pure) in olive oil by gastric intubation four or five times a week for 52 weeks. Control rats comprised 40 males and 40 females [data reported for both sexes combined] that were treated with olive oil alone. Animals were observed until 136 weeks, when the experiment (experiment BT11) was terminated. Survival rates of the groups were not reported. The incidence of treatment-related tumours in control and 3.3-, 17- and 50-mg/kg bw vinyl chloride-treated rats, respectively, was: liver angiosarcomas, 0/80, 0/80, 10/80 and 17/80; extrahepatic angiosarcomas, 0/80, 2/80, 0/80 and 2/80; and primary renal tumours ('nephroblastomas'), 0/80, 0/80, 3/80 and 2/80 [no statistical analysis reported] (Maltoni *et al.*, 1981).

Groups of 75 male and 75 female Sprague-Dawley rats [data reported only for both sexes combined], 10 weeks of age, were administered 0.03, 0.3 or 1 mg/kg bw vinyl chloride (99.97% pure) in olive oil by gastric intubation four or five times a week for 52–59 weeks. Controls comprised 75 males and 75 females [data reported for both sexes combined] that were treated with olive oil alone. Animals were observed until 136 weeks, when the experiment (experiment BT27) was terminated. Survival rates of the groups were not reported. The incidence of several tumours was increased in the treated groups. The incidence in control and 0.03-, 0.3- and 1-mg/kg bw vinyl chloride-treated rats, respectively, was: hepatic angiosarcomas, 0/150, 0/150, 1/148 and 3/149; extrahepatic angiosarcomas, 0/150, 0/150, 0/148 and 1/149; hepatomas [not otherwise specified], 0/150, 0/150, 1/148 and 1/149; Zymbal gland carcinomas, 1/50, 0/150, 0/148, 5/149; and mammary tumours, 7/150, 14/150, 4/148 and 12/149 [no statistical analysis reported] (Maltoni *et al.*, 1981).

Groups of 60–80 male and 60–80 female Wistar rats, 5 weeks of age, were fed diets that contained 0, 1, 3 or 10% of 4000 ppm vinyl chloride ($\geq$ 99.97% pure) in a PVC powder (vehicle) (which resulted in calculated daily doses of 0, 1.7, 5.0 or 14 mg/kg bw vinyl chloride, respectively) during a 4-h feeding period each day on 7 days per week. Animals were treated for a total of 135 (males) or 144 (females) weeks, after which the experiment was terminated. Survival of males at the end of the study was 14/60 control, 20/60 low-dose, 0/60 intermediate-dose and 0/60 high-dose animals; for females, survival was 19/60 control, 5/60 low-dose, 0/60 intermediate-dose and 0/60 high-dose animals. Neoplastic responses included a significantly increased incidence ($p < 0.05$, χ^2 test) of liver haemangiosarcomas and lung angiosarcomas in high- and mid-dose males and high-dose females, of hepatocellular carcinomas in high-dose males and high- and mid-dose females and of neoplastic liver nodules (hepatocellular adenomas) in high- and mid-dose males and females. The incidence of hepatocellular carcinomas was 0/55 control, 1/58 low-dose, 2/56 mid-dose and 8/59 high-dose males and 0/57 control, 4/58 low-dose, 19/59 mid-dose and 29/57 high-dose females; that of liver haemangiosarcomas was 0/55 control, 0/58 low-dose, 6/56 mid-dose and 27/59 high-dose males and 0/57 control, 0/58 low-dose, 2/59 mid-dose and 9/57 high-dose females; and that of neoplastic nodules (hepatocellular adenomas) was 0/55 control, 1/58 low-dose, 7/56 mid-dose and 23/59 high-dose males and 2/57 control, 26/58 low-dose, 39/54 mid-dose and 44/57 high-dose females (Feron *et al.*, 1981).

As in the previous experiment, groups of 50–100 male and 50–100 female Wistar rats [age unspecified] were fed diets similar to those described in Feron *et al.* (1981) that resulted in calculated daily doses of 0, 0.014, 0.13 and 1.3 mg/kg bw vinyl chloride ($\geq$ 99.97% pure), respectively, during a daily 4–6-h feeding period on 7 days per week. Animals were treated for a total of 149 (males) or 150 (females) weeks, after which the experiment was terminated. Survival of males at the end of the study was 20/100 control, 20/100 low-dose, 18/100 intermediate-dose and 8/50 high-dose animals; for females, survival was 24/100 control, 23/100 low-dose, 26/100 intermediate-dose and 5/50 ($p < 0.05$) high-dose animals. Neoplastic responses included a significantly increased incidence of hepatocellular carcinomas in high-dose males and of liver neoplastic nodules (hepatocellular adenomas) in high-dose females ($p < 0.05$). The incidence of hepato-cellular carcinoma was 0/99 control, 0/99 low-dose, 0/99 mid-dose and 3/49 high-dose males and 1/98 control, 0/100 low-dose, 1/96 mid-dose and 3/49 high-dose females; that of neoplastic nodules (hepatocellular adenomas) was 0/99 control, 0/99 low-dose, 0/99 mid-dose and 1/49 high-dose males and 0/98 control, 1/100 low-dose, 1/96 mid-dose and 9/49 high-dose females; and that of liver haemangiosarcomas was 0/99 control, 0/99 low-dose, 0/99 mid-dose and 1/49 high-dose males and 0/98 control, 0/100 low-dose, 0/96 mid-dose and 2/49 high-dose females (Til *et al.*, 1991).

3.3   Subcutaneous injection

Rat

Groups of 35 male and 40 female Sprague-Dawley rats, 21 weeks of age, were administered a single subcutaneous injection of 4.25 mg vinyl chloride (99.97% pure) in 1 mL olive oil. Control animals comprised 35 male and 40 female rats that were treated with olive oil alone (1 mL). Animals were followed until 145 weeks, when the experiment [BT13] was terminated. Survival rates of the groups were not reported. No hepatic or extrahepatic angiosarcomas were observed. Tumour incidence was reported for both sexes combined. Mammary tumours were observed in 1/75 vinyl chloride-treated rats and 3/75 controls. Nephroblastomas were observed in 1/75 treated rats and 0/75 controls. No other tumour types were reported in vinyl chloride-treated animals (Maltoni *et al.*, 1981).

3.4   Intraperitoneal injection

Rat

Groups of 30 male and 30 female Sprague-Dawley rats [data reported for both sexes combined], 17 weeks of age, were administered 4.25 mg vinyl chloride (99.97% pure) in 1 mL olive oil by intraperitoneal injection once, twice, three times or four times at 2-month intervals. Control animals comprised 60 rats that were treated with olive oil alone (1 mL) [number of treatments not reported; data reported for both sexes combined]. Animals were followed until 144 weeks, when the experiment (BT12) was terminated. Survival rates of the groups were not reported. No liver angiosarcomas were observed. Extrahepatic angiosarcomas were observed in 0/55 controls, and 0/55, 1/56, 1/53 and 0/56 rats treated with vinyl chloride once, twice, three times or four times, respectively; mammary tumours were observed in 0/55 controls, and 2/55, 3/56, 1/53, and 1/56 rats treated with vinyl chloride once, twice, three times or four times, respectively [no statistical analysis reported] (Maltoni *et al.*, 1981).

3.5   Transplacental administration

Rat

Groups of 30–54 pregnant female Sprague-Dawley rats, 19 weeks of age, were exposed by inhalation to 6000 or 10 000 ppm [15 600 or 26 000 mg/m^3] vinyl chloride (99.97% pure) for 4 h per day for 7 days, from days 12 to 18 of pregnancy (experiment BT5). Both dams and offspring were observed until the experiment was terminated at 143 weeks, without further exposure to vinyl chloride [the Working Group noted the lack of control groups]. Survival rates of the various groups were not reported. No hepatic or extrahepatic angiosarcomas or hepatomas were observed in either dams or offspring. Tumours appeared at several sites in offspring, including extrahepatic angioma (1/32 low-dose, 0/51 high-dose), kidney tumours (0/32 low-dose, 3/51 high-dose), Zymbal gland carcinomas (3/32 low-dose, 5/51 high-dose), skin epitheliomas (1/32 low-dose, 0/51 high-dose), forestomach papillomas and achanthomas (1/32 low-dose, 1/51 high-dose) and mammary gland tumours (2/32 low-dose, 1/51 high-dose). No tumours occurred at these sites in low-dose dams. One Zymbal gland carcinoma was seen in a high-dose dam (1/30) (Maltoni *et al.*, 1981). [The Working Group considered that, despite the lack of controls, this study provides some evidence of the transplacental carcinogenicity of vinyl chloride.]

3.6   Perinatal exposure

Rat

Male and female Sprague-Dawley rats (breeders), 21 weeks of age, were exposed by inhalation together with their newborn offspring to 6000 or 10 000 ppm [15 600 or 26 000 mg/m^3] vinyl chloride (99.97% pure) on 4 h per day on 5 days per week for 5 weeks. Offspring [data reported for both sexes combined] included 44 rats in the high-dose and 42 in the low-dose group. All vinyl chloride-treated rats were followed until 124 weeks, when the experiment (experiment BT14) was terminated [the Working Group noted the lack of controls]. Survival rates of the groups were not reported. In rats treated perinatally, the incidence of hepatic angiosarcomas was 17/42 and 15/44 in 6000- and 10 000-ppm vinyl chloride-treated animals, respectively. Other tumours that occurred in low-dose and high-dose groups, respectively, were liver angiomas (1/42, 0/44), extra-hepatic angiosarcomas (1/42, 0/44), extrahepatic angiomas (1/42, 3/44), 'hepatomas' (20/42, 20/44), Zymbal gland carcinomas (2/42, 1/44), skin epitheliomas (2/42, 1/44) and mammary tumours (1/42, 0/44). No tumours were reported in breeders at the sites where tumours occurred in offspring (Maltoni *et al.*, 1981).

Male and female Sprague-Dawley rats (breeders), 13 weeks of age, were exposed by inhalation to 0 (controls) or 2500 ppm [6500 mg/m^3] vinyl chloride (99.97% pure) for 4 h per day on 5 days per week for an initial 7-week period during which 54 exposed females and 60 control females became pregnant and delivered young. Exposed dams then con-tinued to receive vinyl chloride by inhalation for 7 h per day on 5 days per week for an additional 69 weeks. Offspring [details of delivery and perinatal husbandry not given] were exposed with their dams pre- and postnatally during the initial 7-week exposure period, and were then either exposed similarly to their dams for 7 h per day on 5 days per week for a further 69 weeks (63 males, 64 females; Group I) or for a shorter 8-week period (60 males, 60 females; Group II). Control offspring were 158 males and 149 females. Hepatocarcinomas occurred in 5/54 exposed female breeders and 0/60 control breeders, in 27/64 male and 38/63 female Group I offspring, in 42/60 male and 43/60 female Group II offspring and in 1/158 control male and 0/149 control female offspring. Angiosarcomas [origin not specified; presumably hepatic] occurred in 27/54 exposed female breeders, in 36/64 male and 46/63 female Group I offspring and 24/60 male and 28/60 female Group II offspring. No angiosarcomas were seen in 60 control breeders or in 158 male and 149 female control offspring. Latencies for both hepatocellular carcinomas and angiosarcomas averaged approximately 52 weeks in Group I offspring and approximately 80 weeks in Group II offspring. Tumours in the brain described as 'neuroblastomas' were seen in vinyl chloride-exposed rats only: 32/54 female breeders, 31/64 male and 27/63 female Group I offspring and 7/60 male and 11/60 female Group II offspring (Maltoni & Cotti, 1988). [The Working Group noted that these latter neoplasms occurred at a high frequency in vinyl chloride-exposed adult rats which is unprecedented for primary brain tumours in bioassays; that this diagnosis has not been established in other bioassays of vinyl chloride or other chemicals; and that the photomicrographs and the preferential location of the tumours in the anterior frontal lobes support the alternative diagnosis of an origin in the metabolically active olfactory neuroepithelium of the posterior nasal cavity (aesthesioneuroepithelioma).]

3.7   Carcinogenicity of metabolites

Mouse

Local tumours (mainly fibrosarcomas) were observed in 15/28 male, 12/24 female and 0/30 control male XVIInc/Z mice, 8–10 weeks of age, following 32 subcutaneous injections of 0 (controls) or 0.1 mg chloroethylene oxide [purity unspecified] over 42 weeks (the experiment was terminated 36.5 weeks post-exposure). Chloroethylene oxide increased the incidence of skin papillomas and carcinomas in male XVIInc/Z mice in a classical initiation–promotion experiment (chloroethylene oxide was used as an initiator and 12-O-tetradecanoylphorbol-13-acetate [TPA] as a promoter) (skin papilloma, 18/28 versus 4/28 TPA controls; skin carcinoma, 5/28 versus 0/28 TPA controls), whereas chloroacetaldehyde [purity unspecified]did not produce such tumours under comparable conditions (Zajdela *et al.*, 1980).

Chloroacetaldehyde ($\geq$ 95% pure with no identifiable impurities) slightly increased the incidence of hepatocellular tumours (10/26 versus 3/20 controls [not significant]) in male $B6C3F_1$ mice when administered orally in the drinking-water at a mean daily ingested dose of 17 mg/kg bw per day for 104 weeks (Daniel *et al.*, 1992).

3.8   Co-exposure with modifying agents

Rat

Groups of 80 male Sprague-Dawley rats [age not specified] were used in a 2 × 2 factorial design and were exposed by whole-body inhalation to 1500 mg/m^3 [577 ppm] vinyl chloride (99.9% pure) for 4 h per day on 5 days per week for 12 months and were then held for an additional 18 months. Animals were kept until spontaneous death or were killed at the end of the 18-month post-exposure observation period. Additional groups were exposed to vinyl chloride and ingested 5% ethanol in water (v/v), were exposed to filtered air and ethanol or were exposed to filtered air alone. Ingestion of 5% ethanol was begun 4 weeks before inhalation of vinyl chloride and continued for life or until termination of the study 30 months after the first vinyl chloride exposure. No information on survival was provided. The incidence of hepatocellular carcinomas was: 1/80 control, 8/80 ethanol-treated, 35/80 vinyl chloride-treated and 48/80 vinyl chloride plus ethanol-treated rats; that of liver angiosarcomas was: 0/80 control, 0/80 ethanol-treated, 18/80 vinyl chloride-treated and 40/80 vinyl chloride plus ethanol-treated rats; that of pituitary tumours was: 8/80 control, 26/80 ethanol-treated, 19/80 vinyl chloride-treated and 12/80 vinyl chloride plus ethanol-treated; and that of lymphosarcomas was 2/80 control, 4/80 ethanol-treated, 6/80 vinyl chloride-treated and 11/80 vinyl chloride plus ethanol-treated rats. The authors stated that these results indicate that ethanol potentiates the carcinogenicity of vinyl chloride (Radike *et al.*, 1981). [The Working Group noted that isocaloric and isonutrient intakes were not controlled in either the treated or control groups.]

4.   Mechanistic and Other Relevant Data

4.1   Absorption, distribution, metabolism and excretion

4.1.1   *Humans*

No data on absorption, distribution, metabolism or elimination of vinyl chloride in humans were presented in the previous review (IARC, 1979). Since that time, a number of studies have contributed to the understanding of the inhalation pharmacokinetics of vinyl chloride in humans.

Pulmonary absorption of vinyl chloride in humans appeared to be rapid and the percentage absorbed was independent of the concentration inhaled. Krajewski *et al.* (1980; cited in ATSDR, 2006) reported that adult male volunteers exposed for 6 h to 2.9, 5.8, 11.6 or 23.1 ppm [7.5, 15, 30 or 60 mg/m^3] by gas mask retained on average approximately 42% of inhaled vinyl chloride. Pulmonary uptake is determined in part by the blood:air partition coefficient, which is 1.16 for vinyl chloride (Gargas *et al.*, 1989). No data were available on human tissue:blood partition coefficients or tissue concentrations of vinyl chloride in exposed humans. However, calculations based on the assumption of an identical solubility of vinyl chloride in rodent and human tissues indicate that the tissue:blood partition coefficients of vinyl chloride would be twofold greater in humans (Clewell *et al.*, 2001), as a consequence of the twofold lower blood:air partition coefficient of vinyl chloride in humans compared with rats and mice.

Vinyl chloride is primarily and rapidly metabolized in the liver, and this metabolism is saturable (Bolt, 2005). The proposed metabolic pathways for vinyl chloride are presented in Figure 1. The first step in the metabolism of vinyl chloride is oxidation, which is predominantly mediated by human cytochrome P450 (CYP) 2E1, to form the highly reactive chloroethylene oxide, which can spontaneously rearrange to chloro-acetaldehyde (Barbin *et al.*, 1975). Both metabolites can bind with proteins, DNA and RNA and form etheno-adducts; chloroethylene oxide is the most reactive with nucleotides

Figure 1. Proposed metabolic pathways for vinyl chloride

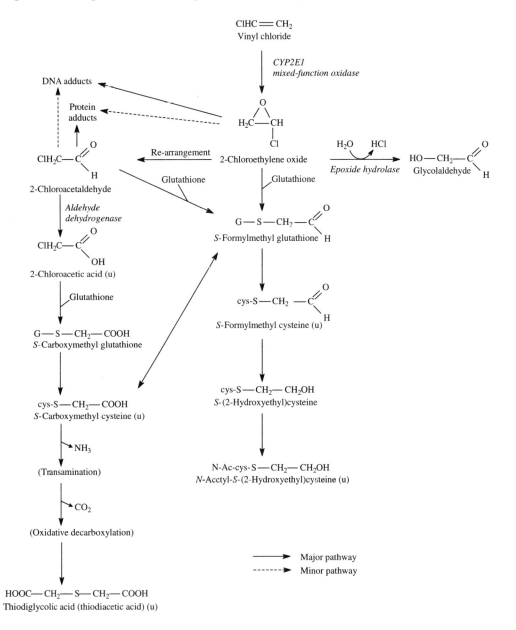

From Barbin *et al.* (1975); Plugge & Safe (1977); Green & Hathway (1977); Guengerich & Watanabe (1979); Guengerich *et al.* (1979); Bolt *et al.* (1980); adapted from ATSDR (2006)
CYP, cytochrome P450; (u), excreted in urine

(Guengerich *et al.*, 1979). Conjugation of chloroethylene oxide and chloroacetaldehyde with glutathione (GSH) eventually leads to the major urinary metabolites *N*-acetyl-*S*-(2-hydroxyethyl)cysteine and thiodiglycolic acid. Chloroethylene oxide and chloro-acetaldehyde can also be detoxified to glycolaldehyde by microsomal epoxide hydrolase (mEH) and to the urinary metabolite chloroacetic acid by aldehyde dehydrogenase 2 (ALDH2), respectively (Guengerich & Watanabe, 1979; ASTDR, 2006).

A number of in-vitro studies that used purified human CYP2E1 and liver microsomes confirmed that vinyl chloride is activated mainly by CYP2E1 (reviewed in WHO, 1999). In hepatic postmitochondrial fractions, Sabadie *et al.* (1980) found significant interindividual variability in the metabolism of vinyl chloride, although the average activity in human samples was comparable with that in rat samples.

The main routes of elimination of vinyl chloride and its metabolites are exhalation and urinary excretion, respectively. Accordingly, thiodiglycolic acid has been reported to be the major metabolite of vinyl chloride detected in the urine of exposed workers (Cheng *et al.*, 2001). Urinary levels of thiodiglycolic acid were correlated with levels of vinyl chloride in the air at concentrations of > 5 ppm (ATSDR, 2006). In contrast, exhalation of unmetabolized vinyl chloride has been reported to occur in humans at low levels (Müller *et al.*, 1978; Krajewski *et al.*, 1980; Pleil & Lindstrom, 1997). For example, the mean concentration in expired air of humans exposed for 6 h to air that contained 6.8–23.1 ppm [15–60 mg/m^3] vinyl chloride ranged from 0.21 to 1.11 ppm [0.54–2.84 mg/m^3], which represented 3.6 and 4.73% of the inhaled amounts, respectively (Krajewski *et al,.* 1980).

4.1.2 *Experimental systems*

The absorption, distribution, metabolism and elimination of vinyl chloride in rats and mice have been reviewed (IARC, 1979; WHO, 1999; ATSDR, 2006). The following section summarizes the salient features of the studies reviewed in IARC (1979) as well as significant new information on the metabolism and pharmacokinetics of vinyl chloride in animals.

Animal data have demonstrated that pulmonary and gastrointestinal absorption of vinyl chloride occurs readily and rapidly. On the contrary, dermal absorption of airborne vinyl chloride is probably not significant. In monkeys, Hefner *et al.* (1975a) reported that only 0.023–0.031% of the total available vinyl chloride was absorbed by the dermal route, whereas absorption in rats was virtually complete following single oral doses (44–92 mg/kg bw) of vinyl chloride in aqueous solution (Withey, 1976). When rats were exposed to initial concentrations of < 260 mg/m^3 [100 ppm], about 40% of inhaled [^{14}C]vinyl chloride was absorbed by the lung (Bolt *et al.*, 1976).

The tissue:blood partition coefficients (which determine the volume of distribution) of vinyl chloride range from 0.4 (muscle) to 10 (fat) in male rats (Barton *et al.*, 1995). The fat:air partition coefficient for vinyl chloride, reported by several authors, tended to be higher in female than in male rats (WHO, 1999). Bolt *et al.* (1976) reported that, following inhalation exposure to [^{14}C]vinyl chloride, several tissues (brain, liver, spleen, kidney, adipose tissue and muscle) contained radioactivity, and that the highest levels were found in liver and kidney. Ungvary *et al.* (1978) reported that vinyl chloride was present in fetal blood and amniotic fluid following exposure of pregnant rats on gestation day 18 to ~2000–13 000 ppm [5500–33 000 mg/m³] (2.5-h exposures), which indicates that vinyl chloride crossed the placental barrier.

Osterman-Golkar *et al.* (1977) reported the alkylation of cysteine and histidine of haemoglobin and small amounts of alkylated histidine in proteins from the testis mice exposed to [¹⁴C]vinyl chloride.

The metabolism of vinyl chloride to chloroethylene oxide, the probable carcinogenic metabolite, appears to be a saturable, dose-dependent process that occurs in the liver predominantly through the CYP system (Reynolds *et al.*, 1975; Ivanetich *et al.*, 1977; Barbin & Bartsch, 1989; Lilly *et al.*, 1998; Bolt, 2005). CYP2E1 appears to account for all metabolic activity in rat liver microsomes, with a maximum velocity (V_{max}) of 4674 pmol/mg protein/min and a Michaelis-Menten constant (K_m) of 7.42 µmol/L (El Ghissassi *et al.*, 1998). Since CYP2E1 has been demonstrated to be present in several other tissues at low levels (compared with the liver), it is reasonable to anticipate that extrahepatic metabolism of systemically available vinyl chloride occurs

Inhibitors of CYP, such as 3-bromophenyl-4(5)-imidazole or 6-nitro-1,2,3-benzothiadiazole, reduced the metabolism of vinyl chloride *in vivo* (Bolt *et al.*, 1976). Chloroethylene oxide, which has a half-life of 1.6 min in aqueous solution at neutral pH (Barbin *et al.*, 1975), rearranges to chloroacetaldehyde (Bonse *et al.*, 1975), conjugates with GSH and can be hydrolysed by EH to glycolaldehyde (WHO, 1999). Chloro-acetaldehyde combines directly or enzymatically via glutathione-*S*-transferase (GST) with GSH to form *S*-formylmethyl glutathione, which is excreted as *N*-acetyl-*S*-(2-hydroxy-ethyl)cysteine (Green & Hathway, 1977) (Figure 1). Chloroacetaldehyde can be oxidized to chloroacetic acid, which is either excreted as such or bound to GSH to form *S*-carboxy-methyl glutathione, which, upon further enzymic degradation, is excreted as thiodi-glycolic acid (thiodiacetic acid) (Plugge & Safe, 1977).

Chloroacetic acid was metabolized in rats to two major urinary metabolites, *S*-carboxymethyl cysteine and thiodiacetic acid (Yllner, 1971). *N*-Acetyl-*S*-(2-hydroxy-ethyl)cysteine (a major metabolite) (Watanabe *et al.*, 1976a,b; Green & Hathway, 1977), *S*-(carboxymethyl)cysteine and *N*-acetyl-*S*-vinyl cysteine have been shown to be metab-olites of vinyl chloride in rats after oral administration (Green & Hathway, 1977) and *N*-acetyl-*S*-(2-hydroxyethyl)cysteine after inhalation (Watanabe *et al.*, 1976b); *S*-(2-chloroethyl)cysteine was also identified after oral administration of vinyl chloride to rats (Green & Hathway, 1975). As thiodiglycolic acid was obtained as a common metab-olite in rats dosed separately with chloroacetaldehyde, chloroacetic acid or *S*-(carboxy-methyl)cysteine, the identification of the same *S*-containing metabolite from vinyl chloride-treated animals gives further support to the hypothesis that chloroethylene oxide or chloroacetaldehyde are formed and react with GSH (Green & Hathway, 1977).

Following oral administration of [^{14}C]vinyl chloride, [^{14}C]carbon dioxide (Green & Hathway, 1975; Watanabe *et al.*, 1976a), ^{14}C-labelled urea and glutamic acid were identified as minor metabolites (Green & Hathway, 1975).

Saturation of the metabolism of vinyl chloride (Gehring *et al.*, 1978; Filser & Bolt, 1979) appears to occur at an inhalation concentration of above 200 ppm [518.6 mg/m^3] in rhesus monkeys (Buchter *et al.*, 1980) and 250 ppm [648 mg/m^3] in rats (Bolt *et al.*, 1977; Filser & Bolt, 1979). The plateau of incidence of hepatic angiosarcoma in rat carcinogenicity bioassays is also observed at above 250 ppm (reviewed in Bolt, 2005).

ATSDR (2006) summarized the kinetic constants obtained *in vivo* in male Sprague-Dawley rats (V_{max}, 58 µmol/h/kg; K_m, 1 µM) and rhesus monkeys (V_{max}, 50 µmol/h/kg) (based on Buchter *et al.*, 1980; Barton *et al.*, 1995). The V_{max} of 50 µmol/h/kg in rhesus monkeys was suggested to be a closer approximation of metabolism in humans than the value of 110 µmol/h/kg estimated for rats by Filser and Bolt (1979) (ATSDR, 2006). Although vinyl chloride has not been associated with the induction of CYP, several authors reported the destruction of CYP protein following exposures to vinyl chloride (WHO, 1999). However, Watanabe *et al.* (1978a) reported that the rate of elimination of vinyl chloride was not altered during repeated exposures (5 days per week for 7 weeks) compared with single inhalation exposure (~13 000 mg/m^3 [5000 ppm]).

Urinary excretion of polar metabolites is the predominant process of elimination at low concentrations of exposure, and very small amounts are expired in air as unchanged vinyl chloride (Hefner *et al.*, 1975b). Following exposure of male rats by inhalation to 26 mg/m^3 [10 ppm] [^{14}C]vinyl chloride for 6 h, urinary ^{14}C activity and expired vinyl chloride comprised 68 and 2%, respectively, of the recovered radioactivity; after exposure to 2600 mg/m^3 [1000 ppm] [^{14}C]vinyl chloride, the proportion of radioactivity in the urine was lower and that expired as vinyl chloride was higher, and represented 56 and 12%, respectively (Watanabe *et al.*, 1976b). Following a single oral administration of 0.05, 1 or 100 mg/kg bw [^{14}C]vinyl chloride to male rats, excretion in the urine was 68, 59 and 11%, respectively; [^{14}C]carbon dioxide in expired air accounted for 9, 13 and 3%, respectively; pulmonary elimination of unchanged vinyl chloride represented only 1–3% of the lower dose and 67% of the higher dose (Watanabe *et al.*, 1976a). These data are consistent with the fact that, once metabolic saturation is attained, the elimination of vinyl chloride occurs via other routes, mainly exhalation of the parent chemical. The route of elimination also depends upon the route of administration; urinary excretion is favoured following oral or intraperitoneal administration, which indicates a first-pass effect due to metabolism in the liver (reviewed in Clewell *et al.*, 2001).

Several investigators have observed the binding of non-volatile metabolites of [^{14}C]vinyl chloride to liver macromolecules, both *in vitro* and in rats exposed by inhalation (Kappus *et al.* 1976; Watanabe *et al.*, 1978a,b; Guengerich & Watanabe, 1979; Guengerich *et al.*, 1979; Bolt *et al.*, 1980; Guengerich *et al.*, 1981; Barton *et al.*, 1995). Jedrychowski *et al.* (1984) reported a decrease in non-protein sulfhydryl concentration in rats exposed to high concentrations of vinyl chloride, and Kappus *et al.* (1975) and Laib and Bolt (1977) reported binding of vinyl chloride to RNA *in vitro* and *in vivo*. In single-exposure experiments at various concentrations, the extent of macromolecular binding increased proportionately to the amount of vinyl chloride metabolized and disproportionately to the exposure concentration (Watanabe *et al.*, 1978b).

4.1.3   *Toxicokinetic models*

The data on absorption, distribution, metabolism and excretion of vinyl chloride have been analysed with the use of empirical and physiologically based compartmental models (Gehring *et al.*, 1978; Chen & Blancato, 1989; Clewell *et al.*, 1995; Reitz *et al.*, 1996; Clewell *et al.*, 2001). These models indicate that vinyl chloride is rapidly absorbed by the inhalation and oral routes and is distributed to all tissues; the adipose tissues show the greatest affinity. The physiologically based pharmacokinetic models developed by Chen and Blancato (1989), Clewell *et al.* (1995, 2001) and Reitz *et al.* (1996) permit the prediction of the pharmacokinetics, GSH depletion and the amount of vinyl chloride metabolized in animals and/or humans exposed to various concentrations by different routes and schedules. However, these models do not currently permit the simulation of the time course of the formation and persistence of DNA adducts in target tissues.

4.2   Genetic and related effects

Since the last review of vinyl chloride (IARC, 1979), a large amount of data on vinyl chloride has been produced and reviewed (WHO, 1999). Only the more recent data that are relevant to the comprehension of vinyl chloride-induced carcinogenicity are reported in this section.

4.2.1   *Humans*

(a)   *DNA adducts*

In vitro, both chloroethylene oxide, the biologically reactive intermediate of vinyl chloride that is formed in the liver, and its rearrangement product, chloroacetaldehyde, can form etheno adducts with nucleic acid bases. Chloroethylene oxide has, however, greater reactivity and it was shown *in vitro* to be the main entity that gives rise to etheno adducts (Guengerich, 1992). The reaction of 2-chloroethylene oxide with nucleic acid bases yields the N-7-(2-oxoethyl)guanine adduct (7-OEG) and four etheno adducts— $1,N^6$-ethenoadenine (εA), $3,N^4$-ethenocytosine (εC), $N^2,3$-ethenoguanine (N^2,3-εG) and $1,N^2$-ethenoguanine ($1,N^2$-εG) (Figure 2) (Ciroussel *et al.*, 1990; Guengerich, 1992). Another adduct, formed by chloroethylene oxide, 5,6,7,9-tetrahydro-7-hydroxy-9-oxoimidazo[1,2-*a*]purine (HO-ethanoG), has also been identified *in vitro* (Müller *et al.*, 1996).

Data on the occurrence and persistence of DNA adducts in tissues of humans exposed to vinyl chloride are lacking. Only one study that used immunoaffinity purification of the etheno adducts and subsequent ^{32}P-postlabelling reported levels of 14.1 εA and 8.1 εC per

10^9 parent bases in non-neoplastic liver tissue of a vinyl chloride-exposed patient with hepatocellular carcinoma (Nair *et al.*, 1995). These adducts can also result from lipid peroxidation (El Ghissassi *et al.*, 1995) and their level can be quite high (in the range of ≤ 0.5–$40\ \varepsilon A$ and εC per 10^9 parent bases in liver DNA samples from patients with unknown exposure) (Bartsch & Nair, 2000a,b).

Figure 2. Reactive metabolites and main nucleic acid adducts of vinyl chloride identified *in vitro* and *in vivo*

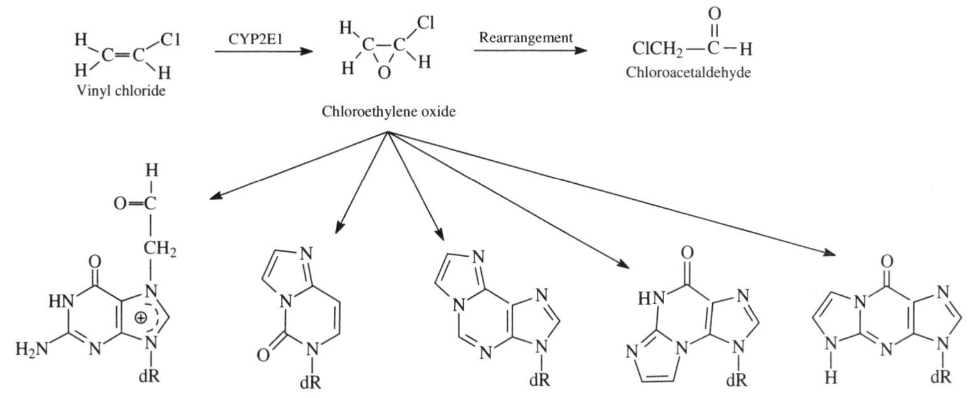

N-7-(2-Oxoethyl)guanine adduct   3,N^4-Ethenocytosine adduct   1,N^6-Ethenoadenine adduct N^2,3-Ethenoguanine adduct   1,N^2-Ethenoguanine adduct
(7-OEG)   (εC)   (εA)   (N^2,3-εG)   (1,N^2-εG)

Adapted from Ciroussel *et al.* (1990)
CYP, cytochrome P450

(b)   *Mutations and other related effects*

(i)   *Mutated p21[ras] and p53 proteins in the blood of vinyl chloride-exposed workers*

Mutated p21[ras] and p53 proteins in the blood of vinyl chloride-exposed workers may reflect the mutagenic effects of vinyl chloride. A G→A transition at the second base of codon 13 of the Ki-*ras* gene was found in four liver angiosarcomas that were associated with occupational exposure to vinyl chloride (Marion *et al.*, 1991). The resulting Asp13p21[ras] protein was also detected in the serum of these four patients by immuno-histochemistry using a monoclonal antibody specific for the Asp13p21[ras] protein (De Vivo *et al.*, 1994). The presence of the mutant RAS protein in the blood correlates with the mutated *ras* gene in the tumour (Table 16).

Several studies showed a high concentration of the Asp13p21[ras] mutant protein in the sera of workers who had been heavily exposed to vinyl chloride whereas all unexposed controls showed negative results. In addition, these studies found a significant dose–

Table 16. Ki-*ras* and *p53* Gene analysis of vinyl chloride-related liver angio-sarcoma (ASL) and detection of mutated p21^{ras} and p53 proteins and anti-p53 antibodies in the serum from the same patients

	Ki-*ras* 2 Gene			*p53* Gene		
	Tissue		Serum	Tissue	Serum	
	DNA GGC$_{13}$→GAC$_{13}$	Asp13p21^{ras}	Asp13p21^{ras}	DNA	Mutant p53 protein	Anti-p53 antibodies
ASL1	+	+	+	ATC→TTC	+	–^{a}
ASL2	+	+	+	AGG→TGG	+	++
ASL3	+	+	+	–	–	–
ASL4	+	+	+	–	–	–
ASL5^b	–	–		CAT→CTT	±	+
ASL6	–	–	–	NR	–	++

From Marion (1998)
NR, not reported; +, positive; –, negative; ±, equivocal; ++, strongly positive
^{a} Patient with abnormal immunological response
^{b} Fibroblastic cell line established from a liver angiosarcoma

response relationship between exposure to vinyl chloride and the detection of Asp13p21^{ras} mutant protein in the sera of exposed workers (Tables 17 and 18).

Mutated p53 proteins and/or anti-p53 antibodies were also found in the blood of vinyl chloride-exposed patients. In a pilot study, Trivers *et al.* (1995) analysed 148 serum samples from 92 vinyl chloride-exposed workers from factories in France and industrial plants in Kentucky, USA. Serum anti-p53 antibodies were found in five of 15 workers who had liver angiosarcoma (33%), two of whom had confirmed mutated *p53* gene (Hollstein *et al.*, 1994), and in four (5%) of 77 workers with no clinical evidence of cancer. Two of 26 workers who had clinical symptoms of vinyl chloride toxicity had antibodies that were detectable by enzyme immunoassays. No antibodies were detected in the two workers who had hepatocellular carcinoma or in seven of eight workers who had liver angiomas. In two liver angiosarcoma patients, anti-p53 antibodies were detected 4 months and 11 years, respectively, before the diagnosis of cancer and one patient had anti-p53 antibodies before and after surgery. Anti-p53 antibodies were thought to be the result of earlier antigenic presentation to the immune system, through accumulation of the mutated protein.

The main purpose of these studies was to determine whether the expression of serum biomarkers was indeed related to exposure to vinyl chloride. The finding of a significant dose–response relationship strongly supports this hypothesis and confirms that *RAS* gene mutations are involved in the onset of liver angiosarcoma induced by vinyl chloride and that mutant p21^{ras} plays a key role in the development of vinyl chloride-induced liver

Table 17. Dose–response relationship between the detection of Asp13p21^{ras} protein in blood and exposure to vinyl chloride (VC)

References	Cohort description	Exposure assessment	Exposure categories	No. of Asp13p21-positive	Odds ratio (95% CI) (adjusted)	Adjustment for potential confounders
De Vivo et al. (1994)	60 male workers heavily exposed to VC (at least 1 year before 1974 or 5 years of total exposure); average exposure, 19.5 years with an average of 12.2 years before 1974; 5 ASL, 1 HCC, 9 liver angiomas, 45 subjects with no liver lesion	Estimates of VC based on years worked with VC: total years worked and years worked before 1974	Years of total exposure 0 (n = 28) < 10 (n = 10) 10–19 (n = 22) 20–29 (n = 20) ≥ 30 (n = 8)	0 4 11 13 6	1.0 37 56 104 168 χ^2 for linear trend = 24.986; $p < 10^{-5}$	None
Li et al. (1998a)	225 men randomly selected among the job categories involving exposure to VC; average exposure level, 3735 ppm–years (range, 4–46 702 ppm–years): 42.2% with a history of having smoked cigarettes, 25.3% with regular daily alcoholic beverage consumption	VC exposure levels were attributed to each subject on the basis of the job, using estimated values assigned to the various jobs[a]	0 (n = 111) ≤ 500 ppm–years (n = 54) 501–2500 ppm–years (n = 62) 2501–5000 ppm–years (n = 51) > 5000 ppm–years (n = 58)	4 13 19 18 26	1.0 10.18 (2.94–35.25) 13.61 (4.26–43.46) 15.43 (4.83–49.28) 21.55 (6.99–66.44) $p < 0.0001$	Age, smoking, alcoholic beverage consumption
Luo et al. (1998)	117 randomly selected workers including 7 with liver tumours (angiomas); average exposure, 2734.9 ± 4299.9 ppm–months (range, 5.4–34 521 ppm–months)	Estimated accumulated ppm–months	No exposure (n = 18) > 1000 ppm–months (n = 69) ≤ 1000 ppm–months (n = 48)	0 10 4	1.0 2.65 (0.42–16.8) 1.64 (0.17–15.8) χ^2 for linear trend = 3.92; $p = 0.048$	Age, alcoholic beverage consumption, smoking, hepatitis C and HBV infection

ASL, liver angiosarcoma; CI, confidence interval; HBV, hepatitis B virus; HCC, hepatocellular carcinoma
[a] Estimates of VC exposure in ppm–years were based on years of a given job category weighted by the presumed level of exposure as defined by the exposure matrix of Heldaas et al. (1984)

Table 18. Prevalence of Asp13p21^{ras} mutant protein in blood samples of vinyl chloride-exposed workers

Reference	Mean exposure to vinyl chloride	No. of subjects tested	Asp13p21-positive (%)
De Vivo *et al.* (1994)	19.5 years, 12.2 years before 1974	60, including 5 ASL and 1 HCC	56.6 (0 in controls)
Li *et al.* (1998a)	2735 ppm–years (range, 4–46 702 ppm–years)	225	33.8 (3.7 in controls)
Luo *et al.* (1998)	2734.9 ppm–months (range, 5.4–34 521 ppm–months)	117	12 (0 in controls)

ASL, liver angiosarcoma; HCC, hepatocellular carcinoma

angiosarcoma (Table 17). A similar relationship was found between the presence of mutated p53 in blood and exposure to vinyl chloride (Tables 19 and 20).

Anti-p53 antibodies have also been tested as a possible biomarker of exposure to vinyl chloride. The occurrence of anti-p53 antibodies in the blood of vinyl chloride-exposed workers seems to be related to the level of exposure with a threshold [~1000 ppm–years]. Below this threshold, this effect is not detected (Table 21).

When two markers, Asp13p21^{ras} and mutated p53, were tested against exposure to vinyl chloride, each biomarker alone demonstrated a highly statistically significant trend with exposure ($p < 0.0001$). Similarly, a highly statistically significant increase was observed in the serum concentration of one or both of the biomarkers with increasing exposure (Table 22).

(ii)   *Cytogenetic studies of vinyl chloride-exposed workers*

Studies on the genotoxicity of vinyl chloride, including studies of chromosomal aberrations, micronucleus formation and sister chromatid exchange, have recently been reviewed (WHO, 1999). There was a clear relationship between the incidence of chromo-somal aberrations and exposure concentration, although exposure concentration and duration of exposure were only estimated. Lesser or no effects were seen when the expo-sure was reduced to levels < 5 ppm [< 13 mg/m^3].

The frequency of sister chromatid exchange increased with the level of exposure to vinyl chloride, and sister chromatid exchange was generally not detected in the blood of workers exposed to levels < 5 ppm [< 13 mg/m^3]. A recent study conducted to investigate the genotoxicity of vinyl chloride at low levels confirmed the absence of sister chromatid exchange in the blood of workers exposed to vinyl chloride levels of approximately 1 ppm [2.59 mg/m^3] (Cheng *et al.*, 2000).

DNA single-strand breaks measured in the alkaline comet assay were thought to occur by transformation of apurinic sites that resulted from repair of vinyl chloride–etheno

Table 19. Dose–response relationship between detection of mutant p53 protein in blood and occupational exposure to vinyl chloride (VC)

Reference, location	Cohort description	Exposure assessment	Exposure categories	No of mutant p53-positive	Odds ratio (95% CI) (adjusted)	Adjustment for potential confounders
Smith et al. (1998), France	225 men randomly selected among job categories that involved exposure to VC; average VC exposure level, 3735 ppm–years (range, 4–46 702 ppm–years)	VC exposure levels were attributed to each subject on the basis of the job, using estimated values assigned to the various jobs[a]	0 (n = 111)	9	1	Age, smoking status, alcoholic beverage consumption
			≤ 500 ppm–years (n = 54)	16	4.16 (1.63–10.64)	
			501–2500 ppm–years (n = 62)	21	5.76 (2.39–13.85)	
			2501–5000 ppm–years (n = 51)	24	10.24 (4.20–24.95)	
			> 5000 ppm–years (n = 58)	30	13.26 (5.52–31.88)	
					p < 0.0001	

CI, confidence interval
[a] Estimates of VC exposure in ppm–years were based on years of a given job category weighted by the presumed level of exposure as defined by the exposure matrix of Heldaas et al. (1984)

Table 20. Prevalence of mutant p53 and anti-p53 antibody-positive blood samples in vinyl chloride-exposed workers

Reference	Mean cumulative exposure to vinyl chloride	No of subjects tested	Mutant p53-positive (%)	Anti-p53 antibody-positive (%)
Smith *et al.* (1998)	3735 ppm–years (range, 4–46 702 ppm–years)	225	40.4 (8 in controls)	–
Luo *et al.* (1999)	1341 ± 3148 ppm–months (range, 0–34 521 ppm–months)	251	11 (2.8 in controls)	3.6 (2.3 in controls)
Mocci & Nettuno (2006)	484 ppm–years (range, 4–2823 ppm–years)	151	2 (0 in controls)	3.3 (0 in controls)

adducts through base-excision repair by glycosylase. The level of DNA single-strand breaks was found to be significantly higher in workers exposed to levels of vinyl chloride > 5 ppm [13 mg/m³] than in workers exposed to levels < 5 ppm (Lei *et al.*, 2004).

      (iii)   *Mutations at the hypoxanthine guanine phosphoribosyl transferase (HPRT) locus*

With the *HPRT* lymphocyte clonal assay, it is possible to determine the mutation frequency of the *HPRT* gene and to characterize its mutant spectra. Mutagenesis induced in the lymphocytes of PVC production workers was measured by selecting resistant mutant T cells in a medium that contained 6-thioguanine. Exposed workers and controls had similar mutation frequencies. However, great differences occurred in the spectrum of mutants. In particular, the percentage of large deletions in the exposed group was much higher (21%) than in unexposed controls (11%) (Hüttner & Holzapfel, 1996). The mutant frequency of *HPRT* in T lymphocytes of 29 individuals accidentally exposed to levels of vinyl chloride between 1 and 8 ppm [2.6–20.7 mg/m³] was measured after the accident and in a follow-up study 2 years later. A statistically significantly higher cloning efficiency was observed in the exposed population after the accident (68.1 versus 50.7% in the controls; $p = 0.007$, Mann-Whitney test). However, no significant difference in the mutant frequency could be found between the exposed population and controls ($3.28 \pm 1.84 \times 10^{-6}$ versus $3.01 \pm 2.38 \times 10^{-6}$) (Becker *et al.*, 2001).

4.2.2   *Experimental systems*

      (a)   *DNA adducts*

Studies on the formation of DNA adducts in animals have recently been reviewed (WHO, 1999). New data are summarized in Table 23.

Table 21. Dose–response relationship between detection of mutant p53 protein and anti-p53 antibody in blood and occupational exposure to vinyl chloride (VC)

Reference, location	Cohort description	Exposure assessment	Exposure categories	No of mutant p53-positive	Odds ratio (95% CI) (adjusted)	No. of total p53 responses (mutant or antibody)	Odds ratio (95% CI) (adjusted)	Adjustment for potential confounders	Comments
Luo et al. (1999), Taiwan, China	251 workers including 7 with liver tumours (assumed to be angiomas); average cumulative exposure, 1341 ± 3148 ppm–months (range, 0–34 521 ppm–months)	Estimated accumulated ppm–months	0 (n = 36)	1	1	2	1	Age, smoking, alcoholic beverage consumption	Significant dose–response relationship between plasma total p53 protein overexpression and cumulative VC exposure concentration
			Low exposure ≤ 480 ppm–months (n = 156)	14	1.6 (0.21–12.54) χ^2 for linear trend = 1.37; $p = 0.24$	19	1.49 (0.24–9.2) χ^2 for linear trend = 0.95; $p = 0.33$		
			High exposure > 480 ppm–months (n = 95)	11	3.5 (0.54–22.5)	14	2.5 (0.5–12.14)		
Mocci & Nettuno (2006), Italy	151 male workers; mean cumulative exposure, 484 ± 725 ppm–years (range, 4–2823 ppm–years)	VC exposure levels before 1983 were attributed to each subject on the basis of the job, using estimated values assigned to the various jobs	0 (n = 136)	0		0		Age, smoking, alcoholic beverage consumption	Trend for increasing serum positivity for p53 antibodies with increasing level of VC exposure; logistic regression using mutant p53 antigen or p53 antibodies adjusted for smoking, alcoholic beverage consumption and age shows cumulative VC exposure as only significant predictor ($p = 0.03$ and 0.005)
			1–100 ppm–years (n = 86)	0		0			
			101–1000 ppm–years (n = 35)	0		1	1		
			1001–2000 ppm–years (n = 18)	1		1	2		
			> 2000 ppm–years (n = 12)	2		3	11.33 χ^2 for linear trend = 5.6; $p = 0.02$		

CI, confidence interval

Table 22. Dose–response relationship between detection of Asp13p21[ras] protein and/or mutated p53 protein in blood of vinyl chloride (VC)-exposed workers

Reference, location	Cohort description	Exposure assessment	Exposure categories	One marker positive	Both markers positive	Odds ratio (95% CI) (adjusted)	Adjustment for potential confounders	Comments
Li et al. (1998b), France	172 exposed men randomly selected among job categories that involved VC exposure employed since 1950; average VC exposure level, 4107 ppm–years (range, 4–46 702 ppm–years)	VC exposure levels were attributed to each subject on the basis of the job, using estimated values assigned to the various jobs[a]	0 (n = 43) ≤ 500 ppm–years (n = 42) 501–2500 ppm–years (n = 45) 2501–5000 ppm–years (n = 31) > 5000 ppm–years (n = 54)	5 21 21 19 22	0 1 4 6 17	1 11.1 (3.3–37.5) 12.8 (4.1–40.2) 29.9 (9.0–99.1) 31.2 (10.4–94.2) $p < 0.0001$	Age, smoking, alcoholic beverage consumption	Each biomarker alone demonstrated a highly statistically significant trend with exposure ($p < 0.0001$). Similarly, highly statistically significant increasing likelihood of seropositivity for one or both of the biomarkers with increasing exposure
Luo et al. (2003), Taiwan, China	251 workers (7 with liver tumours assumed to be angiomas); average cumulative exposure, 112 ± 262 ppm–years (range, 0–2877 ppm–years)	Estimated accumulated ppm–months	0 (n = 44) 0–10 ppm–years (n = 71) 10–40 ppm–years (n = 77) > 40 ppm–years (n = 95)	2 12 13 29	0 1 1 0	1 2 18 (0.09–54.8) 2.01 (0.08–50.5) –		Significant linear trend between exposure concentration and one oncoprotein over-expression

CI, confidence interval

[a] Estimates of VC exposure in ppm–years were based on years of a given job category weighted by the presumed level of exposure as defined by the exposure matrix of Heldaas et al. (1984)

Table 23. Formation of DNA adducts in rats exposed to vinyl chloride (VC)

Strain, sex, age	Treatment	Organs investigated	Alkylated bases/10^8 unmodified bases in DNA		Comments	Reference
			Background levels	After vinyl chloride exposure		
Sprague-Dawley, male, 6 weeks	1300 mg/m³ [500 ppm], 4 h/d, 5 d/wk for 8 wks	Liver, lung, kidney, circulating lymphocytes, brain, spleen testis	εA: mean value from 0.043 in the liver to 35 in brain εC: mean value from 0.062 in the liver to 20.4 in brain	εA: 4.1 ± 1.5 in liver, lung, lymphocytes and testis; no increase in kidney and spleen εC: 7.8 ± 1.2 in liver, kidney, lymphocytes and spleen No significant increase in brain for either etheno adduct	Levels of VC-induced and endogenous adducts were not higher in the liver, the major target organ of VC, than in other tissues	Barbin (1999)
Sprague-Dawley, female, 10 days	600 ppm [139 mg/m³], 4 h/d, 5 d	Liver	NR	εA: (immunohistochemical levels) 1.5 times higher in VC-exposed rats than in controls	After VC exposure, staining for εA was higher in both parenchymal cells and non-parenchymal cells. Significantly elevated adduct levels persisted in the liver of VC-exposed rats 14 days after cessation of exposure	Yang et al. (2000)
Fischer 344	0, 10, 100, 1100 ppm [0, 26, 259, 2858 mg/m³], 6 h/d, 5 d/wk, 1 or 4 wks	Liver	N^2,3-εG: 9 ± 0.4	N^2,3-εG: 10 ppm VC, 5 d: 20 ± 5.0 10 ppm VC, 20 d: 53 ± 1.1 100 ppm VC, 5 d: 68 ± 9 100 ppm VC, 20 d: 228 ± 18	After 10 ppm VC exposure, respectively 2.2- and 5.9-fold increase in N^2,3-εG compared with the amount of endogenous N^2,3-εG	Swenberg et al. (2000)
Sprague-Dawley, male, 11 weeks	0 and 1100 ppm [2858 mg/m³], 6 h/d, 5 d/wk, 1 or 4 wks	Liver	NR	N^2,3-εG: 20 d, 80.6 ± 2.58 1,N^2-εG: below the detection limit of 15 fmol		Morinello et al. (2001)

Table 23 (contd)

Strain, sex, age	Treatment	Organs investigated	Alkylated bases/10^8 unmodified bases in DNA — Background levels	Alkylated bases/10^8 unmodified bases in DNA — After vinyl chloride exposure	Comments	Reference
Adult study Sprague-Dawley, male, 11 weeks *Weanling study* 40 pups weaned at day 25	Whole-body inhalation: 0 and 1100 ppm [2852 mg/m³], 6 h/d, 5 d/wk, 1 or 4 wks	Liver, brain	*Adult study* $N^2,3$-**εG**: ~ 5 in liver and brain *Weanling study* $N^2,3$-**εG**: ~ 1.5 in liver and brain	*Adult study* $N^2,3$-**εG**: 11) ± 20 in liver after 20 d exposure *Weanling study* $N^2,3$-**εG**: 97 ± 5.0 in liver after 5 d exposure; 4.4 ± 1.1 in brain after 5 d exposure	*Adult study* No increase after 5 d exposure in liver; no increase observed in brain *Weanling study* Levels of $N^2,3$-εG in wealings after 5 d exposure similar to those in adults exposed for 4 wks; small but statistically significant increase of $N^2,3$-εG in brain	Morinello *et al.* (2002a)
Adult study Sprague-Dawley, male, 11 weeks *Weanling study* 40 pups weaned at day 25	Whole-body inhalation: 0, 10, 100, 1100 ppm [0, 26, 259, 2852 mg/m³], 6 h/d, 5 d/wk, 1 or 4 wks	Liver, hepatocytes (HEP) and non-parenchymal cells (NPC)	*Adult study* $N^2,3$-**εG**: ~ 5 in HEP; ~ 9 in NPC *Weanling study* $N^2,3$-**εG**: ~1.6 in HEP; ~ 4.9 in NPC	*Adult study* $N^2,3$-**εG**: ~35 in HEP and NPC after 5 d exposure to 100 ppm; 110 ± 1 and 71 ± 1.1 in HEP and NPC, respectively: after 20 d exposure to 100 ppm *Weanling study* $N^2,3$-**εG**: 90 ± 0.7 and 43 ± 0.5 in HEP and NPC, respectively, after 5 d exposure to 100 ppm	Linear increase from 0 to 100 ppm and plateau between 100 and 1100 ppm In contrast to adults, difference in adducts concentration detected between the HEP and NPC populations from the weanlings	Morinello *et al.* (2002b)

d, day; **εA**: 1,N^6-ethenoadenine; **εC**: 3,N^4-ethenocytosine; $N^2,3$-**εG**: $N^2,3$-ethenoguanine; **1,N^2-εG**: 1,N^2-ethenoguanine; NR, not reported; wk, week

The DNA adducts εA and εC have been found in various organs in rats after inhalation exposure to vinyl chloride. 7-OEG was shown to be the major DNA adduct formed *in vivo* and was found in greater amounts in young animals (Swenberg *et al.*, 2000). However, 7-OEG has a short half-life of about 62 h while etheno adducts were more persistent. For example, N^2,3-εG has a half-life of about 30 days (Fedtke *et al.*, 1990). Of the etheno adducts, N^2,3-εG was present in greatest amounts in tissues of exposed animals (10–100-fold greater than other etheno adducts).

After exposure of rats to 500 ppm [1300 mg/m^3] vinyl chloride for 8 weeks, the level of εA was increased significantly above background in the liver, lung, lymphocytes and testis. The level of εC was also increased significantly in the liver, kidney, lymphocytes and spleen. No significant increase was found in brain for either ethano adducts (Guichard *et al.*, 1996; Barbin, 1999). When adult rats were exposed to 1100 ppm [2858 mg/m^3] vinyl chloride for 1 or 4 weeks, there was a significant increase in the level of N^2,3-εG in hepatocytes, but not in the brain. In contrast to adults, there was a small, statistically significant increase in N^2,3-εG in the brain of weanling animals exposed for 5 days. In addition, in weanlings, the concentration of N^2,3-εG in hepatocytes was significantly greater than that measured in non-parenchymal cells after exposures to 10 and 100 ppm [26 and 259 mg/m^3] vinyl chloride (Morinello *et al.*, 2002a). These differential responses between weanlings and adults may contribute to the particular susceptibility of young rats to vinyl chloride-induced neuroblastomas and hepatocarcinomas (Maltoni & Cotti, 1988).

In adult rats, N^2,3-εG was clearly induced in both hepatocytes and non-parenchymal cells after exposure to vinyl chloride for 1 or 4 weeks, with a linear increase at exposure concentrations from 0 to 100 ppm [259 mg/m^3] and a plateau at levels of 100–1100 ppm [259–2852 mg/m^3]. There was no significant difference in N^2,3-εG adduct levels, nor in the rate of repair between hepatocytes and non-parenchymal cells (Morinello *et al.*, 2002b), which confirms the earlier observation of Yang *et al.* (2000) (see also Table 23).

(b)   *Mutations and other related effects* (see Table 24)

Genotoxicity studies on vinyl chloride *in vitro* and *in vivo* have recently been reviewed (WHO, 1999). The genotoxicity of vinyl chloride has been clearly demonstrated in several in-vitro systems. Vinyl chloride vapour induced reverse mutation in various strains of *Salmonella typhymurium*. In aqueous or alcoholic solutions, vinyl chloride induced mutations in *Escherichia coli*, *Saccharomyces cerevisiae* and *Schizosaccharomyces pombe*. It was also mutagenic in the recessive lethal test in *Drosophila melanogaster,* but not in the dominant lethal test in mice. It induced DNA strand breaks, sister chromatid exchange, micronucleus formation and chromosomal aberrations in rodents. *In vitro*, a higher mutagenic response was obtained in the presence of an exogenous metabolic activation system from rat liver.

Table 24. Genetic and related effects of vinyl chloride

Test system	Result[a] Without exogenous metabolic system	Result[a] With exogenous metabolic system	Dose[b] (LED or HID)	Reference
Salmonella typhimurium TA100, TA1535, reverse mutation	+	+	200 000 ppm/48 h	McCann et al. (1975)
Salmonella typhimurium TA100, TA1535, reverse mutation	+	+	1000 ppm	Shimada et al. (1985)
Salmonella typhimurium TA1530, TA1535, G-46, reverse mutation	+	+	2000 ppm/48 h	Bartsch et al. (1975)
Salmonella typhimurium TA1530, reverse mutation	+	+	2–20% in air	de Meester et al. (1980)
Salmonella typhimurium TA1535, reverse mutation	–	+	110 000 ppm	Rannug et al. (1974)
Salmonella typhimurium TA1536, TA1537, TA1538, reverse mutation	(+)	(+)	200 000 ppm	Rannug et al. (1974)
Salmonella typhimurium TA1538, G-46, reverse mutation	–	–	200 000 ppm	Bartsch et al. (1975)
Salmonella typhimurium TA1537, TA1538, TA98, reverse mutation	+		100 000 ppm	Shimada et al. (1985)
Escherichia coli K12, gene mutation	+		10.5 mM (medium)	Greim et al. (1975)
Schizosaccharomyces pombe P1, SP.198, gene mutation	+	+	16–48 mM (medium)	Loprieno et al. (1976)
Drosophila melanogaster male Berlin K, sex-linked recessive lethal mutation	+		850 ppm/2 d or 30 ppm/17 d	Verburgt & Vogel (1977)
Drosophila melanogaster male Karnäs, sex-linked recessive lethal mutation	+		10 000 ppm/3 h	Magnusson & Ramel (1978)
Drosophila melanogaster male Berlin K, dominant lethal test	–		30 000 ppm/2 d	Verburgt & Vogel (1977)
Drosophila melanogaster male Berlin K, aneuploidy (sex chromosome loss)	–		30 000 ppm/2 d	Verburgt & Vogel (1977)
Drosophila melanogaster male Berlin K, aneuploidy (sex chromosome loss)	+		48 500 ppm	Ballering et al. (1996)
Host-mediated assay, forward mutation, *Schizosaccharomyces pombe* SP.198 in Swiss mice	+		74 mg/kg bw po	Loprieno et al. (1976)
Host-mediated assay, gene conversion, *Saccharomyces cerevisiae* in male Wistar rats	+		10 000 ppm/24 h	Eckardt et al. (1981)
DNA single-strand breaks, female NMR mice *in vivo*	+		500 ppm, 6 h/d × 5	Walles & Holmberg (1984)
Mouse spot test, pregnant female C57BL mice	–		4600 ppm/5 h	Peter & Ungváry (1980)
Sister chromatid exchange, male and female Chinese hamsters *in vivo*	+		12 500 ppm/6 h	Basler & Röhrborn (1980)
Micronucleus formation, male CBA mice *in vivo*	+		50 000 ppm/4 h	Jenssen & Ramel (1980)
Micronucleus formation, male and female C57BL/6J mouse bone-marrow cells *in vivo*	+		50 000 ppm/6 h	Richardson et al. (1983)

Table 24 (contd)

Test system	Result[a] Without exogenous metabolic system	With exogenous metabolic system	Dose[b] (LED or HID)	Reference
Chromosomal aberrations, male and female Chinese hamster bone-marrow cells *in vivo*	+		25 000 ppm/24 h	Basler & Röhrborn (1980)
Chromosomal aberrations, male Wistar rat bone-marrow cells *in vivo*	+		1500 ppm, 6 h/d × 5	Anderson & Richardson (1981)
Dominant lethal test, male CD-1 mice *in vivo*	−		30 000 ppm, 6 h/d × 5	Anderson *et al.* (1976, 1977)
Dominant lethal test, male CD-1 mice *in vivo*	−		10 000 ppm, 4 h/d × 5	Himeno *et al.* (1983)
Dominant lethal test, male CD-1 mice *in vivo*	−		5000 ppm, 4 h/d, 5 d/wk × 10	Himeno *et al.* (1983)
Dominant lethal test, male CD rats *in vivo*	−		1000 ppm, 6 h/d × 5	Short *et al.* (1977)

[a] +, positive; (+), weak positive; −, negative
[b] LED, lowest effective dose; HID, highest ineffective dose; d, day; po, orally; wk, week

4.2.3   *Mutagenic or promutagenic properties of DNA adducts formed by vinyl chloride metabolites*

The major DNA adduct 7-OEG lacks miscoding properties (Barbin *et al.*, 1985). In contrast, promutagenic properties have been shown for the etheno and related exocyclic DNA adducts, ϵA, ϵC, N^2,3-ϵG, and HO-ethanoG that involve mainly base-pair substitution mutations (WHO, 1999; see Table 25)

Various assays have been designed to explore the mutagenic properties of DNA adducts, which have been incorporated into oligonucleotides or into site-specific vectors and used in experiments of misincorporation. Vector plasmids have also been treated with 2-chloroethyleneoxide or 2-chloroacetaldehyde and propagated in *E. coli* or mammalian cells. The more significant and recent studies are listed in Table 25. The mechanism by which adducts cause mutations still remains unclear. At least two vinyl chloride-induced DNA adducts, HO-ethanoG and 1, N^2-ϵG have been shown to block replication with many different polymerases, thereby causing base misincorporation (Langouët *et al.*, 1997, 1998; Guengerich *et al.*, 1999). The misincorporation events appear to be clearly dependent on the individual mechanisms of DNA polymerases (Choi *et al.*, 2006). Mutation frequencies induced by etheno adducts may also depend on the system used since ϵA was shown to be highly miscoding in COS7 simian kidney cells, in contrast to the findings in *E. coli* (Pandaya & Moriya, 1996). [Clearly, the patterns of base substitution vary among the different systems used and cannot be extrapolated easily to predict mutations in human tumour tissue.]

4.2.4   *Alterations in oncogenes and suppressor-genes in tumours*

(a)   *RAS genes*

Carcinogens are believed to alter genes that are involved in cell proliferation and differentiation. The *RAS* genes, Ha-*ras*, Ki-*ras* and N-*ras*, are members of a family of genes that code for closely homologous proteins that are termed p21[ras] and function as signal-switch molecules in the cell. *RAS* genes activated by point mutations are found in a wide variety of human cancers. In a study of mutations of *RAS* oncogenes at codons 12, 13 and 61 in angiosarcomas of the liver of vinyl chloride-exposed workers, five of six tumours were found to contain a G→A transition at the second base of codon 13 (GGC→GAC) of the Ki-*ras*-2 gene (Marion *et al.*, 1991). This mutation leads to substitution of glycine by aspartic acid at amino acid residue 13 in the encoded p21[ras] protein. In another series, eight of 15 tumours contained a mutated Ki-*ras* gene, either at codon 12 or at codon 13. In five cases, the mutation led to substitution of glycine by aspartic acid. Two mutations were also found in non-neoplastic tissue (Weihrauch *et al.*, 2002a).

In studies of hepatocellular carcinomas of vinyl chloride-exposed workers, three tumours were found to contain mutations at codon 12 in the first exon of the Ki-*ras*-2 gene due to a G→A transition in two tumours (GGT→GAT) and to a G→T transversion

Table 25. Miscoding specificities of etheno bases

Method	Etheno base tested	Incorporation opposite the lesion	Mutation	Comments	Reference
Incorporation of etheno bases into oligodeoxynucleotides and used as templates with the Klenow fragment of *Escherichia coli* DNA polymerase I	εC	A, T	CG→TA CG→AT	εC facilitates translesional synthesis	Zhang *et al.* (1995)
Incorporation of etheno bases into oligodeoxynucleotides and used as templates with various polymerases	1,N^2-εG	A, G	GC→AT (2%) GC→TA (0.74%) GC→AT (0.71%) GC→TA (0.71%)	Both adducts strongly blocked replication with all polymerases tested.	Langouët *et al.* (1997, 1998)
	HO-ethanoG	A, G			
Incorporation of 1,N^2-εG into oligodeoxynucleotides and used as templates with translesion human DNA polymerases	1,N^2-εG	G		Incorporation events are determined by the individual mechanisms of DNA polymerases.	Choi *et al.* (2006)
Incorporation of 1,N^2-εG at a single site in a pCNheIA vector integrated in the chromosomes, CHO cells	1,N^2-εG	G	Various mutations mainly GC→AT		Akasaka & Guengerich (1999)
Incorporation of HO-ethanoG in the single-stranded vector pMS2, COS7 simian kidney cell line	HO-ethanoG		GC→TA (11 mutations) GC→CG (2 mutations) GC→AT (1 mutation)		Fernandes *et al.* (2005)
Single-stranded vector pMS2 containing a single εA residue; propagated in 5 strains of *E. coli* and in COS7 simian kidney cell line	εA	G > T > C	AT→GC (63%) AT→TA (6%) AT→CG (1%)	εA highly miscoding in COS cells (frequency of mutations 70%) in contrast to results for *E. coli*	Pandya & Moriya (1996)
supF Gene in vector plasmid pMY189 treated with CAA, human fibroblast W138-VA13 cells	εC and N^2,3-εG as possible adducts		GC→AT (53.8%) GC→TA (29.5%) GC→CG (6.4%)	71% of mutations were single base mutations	Matsuda *et al.* (1995)

εA, 1,N^6-ethenoadenine; εC, 3,N^4-ethenocytosine; N^2,3-εG, N^2,3-ethenoguanine; 1,N^2-εG, 1,N^2-ethenoguanine; CAA, chloroacetaldehyde; CHO, Chinese hamster ovary; HO-ethanoG, 5,6,7,9,-tetrahydro-7-hydroxy-9-oxoimidazol[1,2-*a*]purine

in one tumour (GGT→TGT). In addition, one tumour contained a mutation due to a
G→T transversion at the second base of codon 12 (GGT→GTT) in neoplastic tissue and
a G→A transition at the second base of codon 12 in non-neoplastic tissue (GGT→GAT).
One tumour contained a mutation at the first base of codon 13 (G→T transversion,
GGC→TGC) in neoplastic tissue and a G→A transition at the second base of codon 13 in
non-neoplastic tissue (GGC→GAC). In one case, the wild-type Ki-*ras*-2 gene was detected in neoplastic tissue while a codon 13 mutation was found in non-neoplastic cirrhotic
tissue (GGC→CAT) (Weinrauch *et al.*, 2001a). In the same study, 20 hepatocellular
carcinomas from a control group and associated with hepatitis B or C virus infection or
alcoholic beverage consumption were also analysed. Ki-*ras*-2 mutations were found in
three cases, two of which were attributed to HBV infection (GGT→GTT and GGC→GAC)
and one to hepatitis C virus infection (GGT→TGT) (Weihrauch *et al.*, 2001a,b).

No mutations were found in the Ki-*ras* gene in vinyl chloride-induced liver angiosarcoma or hepatocellular carcinoma in rats. One mutation was found at codon 13 of
N-*ras* in a liver angiosarcoma (G→A, GGC→GAC). However, mutations that involved
the second base of codon 61 of the Ha-*ras* gene and were due to A→T transversions
(CAA→CTA) were found in five of eight hepatocellular carcinomas (Froment *et al.*,
1994; Boivin-Angèle *et al.*, 2000a) (Table 26).

(b)   *p53*

The *p53* gene is a tumour-suppressor gene at the crossroads of many cellular
pathways that involve cell cycle control, DNA repair, DNA replication, apoptosis and
senescence. The majority of cancer-related mutations in *p53* cluster in several regions of
the gene that determine the protein structure and that have been highly conserved through
evolution. These regions occur in the sequence-specific DNA-binding core domain of the
protein between amino acid residues 102 and 292. The mutations found in malignancies
could result in substitution of amino acid residues in these regions that are critical for p53
function (Cho *et al.*, 1994; Brandt-Rauf *et al.*, 1996).

A comparison of the mutation spectra in the *p53* gene in vinyl chloride-associated
liver tumours in humans and rats is detailed in Table 27.

Five liver tumours (four liver angiosarcomas and one hepatocellular carcinoma) from
workers who were heavily exposed to vinyl chloride were investigated for mutations in
the *p53* gene in exons 5 to 8. Two A→T missense mutations were found in a highly
conserved domain: one at codon 249 (AGG→TGG, *Arg* to *Trp*) and one at codon 255
(ATC→TTC, *Ile* to *Phe*) each in the tumour but not in the normal cells of two of the liver
angiosarcoma patients, of whom both were smokers (Hollstein *et al.*, 1994). A third
mutation, also due to an A→T transversion, was found at codon 179 (CAT→CTT, *His* to
Leu) in a fibroblastic cell line established from a liver angiosarcoma from a vinyl
chloride-exposed patient (Boivin-Angèle *et al.*, 2000b). Such mutations are uncommon in
human cancers (2.7% of a total of 5085 cancers; Hollstein *et al.*, 1996). Futhermore, *p53* gene
mutations are uncommon in sporadic (non-vinyl chloride-induced) liver angiosarcomas

Table 26. Comparison of the mutation spectra in *ras* proto-oncogenes in vinyl chloride-associated liver tumours in humans and rats

Tumour origin	Gene involved	Codon	No. of mutations/ no. of tumours	No. of base-pair changes/codon change	Reference
Human ASL	Ki-*ras*-2	13	5/6	5 G→A/GGC→GAC	Marion *et al.* (1991)
Human ASL	Ki-*ras*-2	12	5/8	3/5 G→A/GGT→GAT	Weihrauch *et al.* (2002a)
		13	3/8	2/5 G→T/GGT→GTT, GGT→TGT	
				2/3 G→A/GGC→GAC, GGC→CAT	
		12		1/3 G→T/GGC→TGC	
				1/2 G→T/GGT→TGT (non-neoplastic tissue)	
				1/2 G→A/GGT→GAT (non-neoplastic tissue)	
Human HCC	Ki-*ras*-2	12	4/12	2 G→A/GGT→GAT	Weihrauch *et al.* (2001a)
				G→T/GGT→TGT	
				G→T/GGT→GTT (with GGT→GAT in the non-neoplastic tissue)	
		13	1/12	G→T/GGC→TGC (with GGC→GAC in the non-neoplastic tissue)	
				G→A/GGC→CAT non-neoplastic tissue	
Rat ASL	Ki-*ras*-2 N-*ras* A	12, 13, and 61	0/11	None	Froment *et al.* (1994); Boivin-Angèle *et al.* (2000a)
		13	2/11	G→A/GGC→GAC	
		36		A→T/ATA→CTA	
Rat HCC	Ha-*ras*	61	5/8	5 A→T/CAA→CTA	Froment *et al.* (1994); Boivin-Angèle *et al.* (2000a)

ASL, liver angiosarcoma; HCC, hepatocellular carcinoma

Table 27. Comparison of the mutation spectra in the *p53* gene in vinyl chloride-associated liver tumours in humans and rats

Tumour origin	No. of mutations/no. of tumours	Codon (exon)	No. of base-pair changes/ codon change	References
Human ASL	2/4		2 A→T/	Hollstein *et al.* (1994)
		249 (7)	AGG→TGG	
		255 (7)	ATC→TTC	
Human ASL	6/17	131 (5)	1 A→T/AAC→ATC	Weihrauch *et al.* (2002b)
		248 (7)	1 G→A/CGG→CAG	
		282 (8)	1 C→T/CGG→TGG	
		342 (10)	1 C→T/CGA→TGA	
		200 (6)	del-2	
		216 (6)	del-3	
Human fibroblastic cell line from an ASL	1/1	179 (5)	1 A→T/CAT→CTT	Boivin-Angèle *et al.* (2000b)
Human HCC	11/18	130 (5)	1 T→G/CTC→CGC	Weihrauch *et al.* (2000)
		175 (5)	1 C→A/CAC→AAC	
		282 (8)	1 C→T/CGG→TGG	
		179 (5)	1 A→T/CAT→CTT	
		193 (6)	1 A→C/CAT→CCT	
		246 (7)	1 A→G/ATG→GTG	
			3 G→A/	
		245 (7)	GGC→GAC	
		248 (7)	CGG→CAG	
		273 (8)	CGT→CAT	
		226 (6)	1 G→C/GGC→GCC	
		236 (7)	del(-3)	
Rat ASL	11/25		4 A→T/	Barbin *et al.* (1997)
		160 (5)	ATC→TTC	
		235 (7)	ATG→TTG	
		253 (7)	ATC→TTC	
		253 (7)	ATC→TTC	
		235 (7)	1 A→C/ATG→CTG	
			2 A→G/	
		203 (6)	TAT→TGT	
		203 (6)	TAT→TGT	
			2 G→A/	
		152 (5)	GGT→AGT	
		246 (7)	CGC→CAC	
		147 (5)	1 C→T/TCC→TCT	
		235 (7)	1 T→G/ATG→AGG	
		177–181 (5)	del(-12)	
Rat HCC	1/8	283 (8)	1 A→T/GAG→GTG	Barbin *et al.* (1997)

ASL, liver angiosarcoma; HCC, hepatocellular carcinoma

(2/21 cases, 9%; Soini *et al.*, 1995), which supports the evidence that links exposure to vinyl chloride with liver angiosarcoma that contains *p53* mutations due to A→T transversions.

In another series, six mutations were found in 17 vinyl chloride-induced liver angiosarcomas (four point mutations and two deletions); only one mutation was due to an A→T transversion (codon 131, AAC→ATC) (Weihrauch *et al.*, 2002b).

Eighteen hepatocellular carcinomas from vinyl chloride-exposed workers were analysed for mutations in the *p53* gene in exons 5–9. In this series, 11 of 18 hepatocellular carcinomas exhibited a *p53* gene mutation, with five transversions and five transitions. Five of the 11 mutations (codons 175, 245, 248, 273 and 282) affected CpG dinu-cleotides, three of which (codons 175, 248, 273) were also found in hepatocellular carcinomas induced by alcoholic beverage consumption and viral or autoimmune cir-rhosis, which led the authors to conclude that the *p53* mutations in their series might be due to spontaneous processes such as deamination of 5-methylcytosine (Weihrauch *et al.*, 2000). In studies of both liver angiosarcoma and hepatocellular carcinoma, no *p53* mutations were found in the surrounding non-neoplastic tissue.

Mutations in the *p53* gene were also found in 11 of 25 (44%) liver angiosarcomas induced by vinyl chloride in Sprague-Dawley rats and in one of eight hepatocellular carcinomas (Barbin *et al.*, 1997). Five mutations involved an A→T transversion as seen in human vinyl chloride-induced liver angiosarcoma. The A→T transversion in the first base of codon 253 in two rat liver angiosarcomas was equivalent to the transversion observed in codon 255 in one human liver angiosarcoma associated with exposure to vinyl chloride (Hollstein *et al.*, 1994) (Table 27).

4.3   Mechanisms of carcinogenesis

Many key events in the pathway of vinyl chloride-induced hepatocarcinogenesis have been established. These include (*a*) metabolic activation (to chloroethylene oxide), (*b*) DNA binding of the reactive metabolites (characteristic exocyclic etheno-adducts, (*c*) promutagenicity of these adducts that lead to G→A and A→T transitions and (*d*) effects of such mutations on proto-oncogenes/tumour-suppressor genes at the gene and gene product levels, with tumorigenesis as the final outcome (Bolt, 2005).

Vinyl chloride has been demonstrated to be a genotoxic carcinogen in animal and human studies (Block, 1974; Creech & Johnson, 1974; Lee & Harry, 1974; Maltoni *et al.*, 1974, 1981). It is absorbed rapidly after inhalation and oral exposure (Bolt, 1978), and is metabolized (activated) mainly by CYP2E1 to 2-chloroethylene oxide which spon-taneously rearranges to 2-chloroacetaldehyde. 2-Chloroethylene oxide and 2-chloro-acetaldehyde can be transported intercellularly from parenchymal cells to non-paren-chymal cells in the liver (Kuchenmeister *et al.*, 1996). The primary detoxification reaction of the two reactive metabolites is conjugation with GSH catalysed by GST; the conjugation products are then excreted in urine (reviewed in WHO, 1999).

Both 2-chloroethylene oxide and 2-chloroacetaldehyde can form DNA adducts. Five DNA adducts are formed by 2-chloroethylene oxide or 2-chloroacetaldehyde (Cheng *et al.*, 1991; Basu *et al.*, 1993). These include the major adduct, 7-OEG, and four cyclic etheno adducts (1,N^2-εG, εC, εA and N^2,3-εG). These etheno adducts generate mainly base-pair substitution mutations and specific mutations in cancer-related genes (i.e. *RAS* oncogenes, *p53* tumour-suppressor genes). The major reaction product of 2-chloro-ethylene oxide is 7-OEG, but 2-chloroacetaldehyde does not form this adduct. 7-OEG does not exhibit promutagenic properties whereas εA, εC, N^2,3-εG and 1,N^2-εG do. εA, εC and N^2,3-εG have demonstrated miscoding potential *in vitro* and *in vivo* (Singer *et al.*, 1987; Cheng *et al.*, 1991; Mroczkowska & Kusmierek, 1991; Singer *et al.*, 1991; Basu *et al.*, 1993) and others have shown that εA causes A→G transitions and A→T trans-versions, εC causes C→A transversions and C→T transitions and εG causes G→A transitions (reviewed in Bolt, 2005; see Table 25). These changes were consistent with the mutations of *p53* and *RAS* genes observed in tumours from vinyl chloride-exposed humans and rats (Tables 26 and 27).

Etheno adducts appear to have long persistence and are repaired by glycolases (Gros *et al.*, 2004). In addition to the DNA adducts produced by vinyl chloride, a physiological background of endogenously produced etheno adducts is possibly the product of oxi-dative stress and lipid peroxidation (Bartsch & Nair, 2000a,b; De Bont & van Larebeke, 2004; Bolt, 2005).

The induction of extrahepatic tumours by vinyl chloride has been established experi-mentally, but the mechanism for this extrahepatic tumour formation, e.g. in the brain or lung, is not well elucidated (Bolt, 2005).

While the data overall suggest that etheno adducts are probably involved in the initiation of hepatocarcinogenesis by vinyl chloride, some factors have yet to be explained. These include observed tissue and cell specificity and variability in various biomarkers such as mutant p53 protein and anti-p53 antibodies in vinyl chloride-exposed workers with tumours (Trivers *et al.*, 1995; Brand-Rauf *et al.*, 1996). One source for this variability might be explained by differences in genetic polymorphisms of genes that encode for enzymes involved in vinyl chloride metabolism and for proteins involved in DNA repair (Li *et al.*, 2003a).

4.4   Susceptibility

4.4.1   *Genetic polymorphisms and enzyme induction*

The enzymes that are involved in vinyl chloride activation and detoxification, i.e. CYP2E1, ALDH2, GST and mEH (Figure 1), are known to have polymorphic variants with altered activity. Polymorphisms of each of these enzymes may modulate the metabolism of vinyl chloride, the levels of 2-chloroethylene oxide and 2-chloro-acetaldehyde and hence the frequency and nature of vinyl chloride-induced mutations.

For example, individuals who have high-activity variants of CYP2E1 and/or low-activity variants of ALDH2 or GST enzymes may have elevated levels of chloroethylene oxide and chloroacetaldehyde and increased DNA damage.

Among the many CYP2E1 polymorphisms described, *c1* and *c2* alleles have been identified in the 5-regulatory region of the gene. According to in-vitro studies that investigated gene transcription and enzyme activity, workers who have at least one *c2* allele may have higher CYP2E1 activity than the homozygous *c1c1*, although this was not clearly confirmed *in vivo*. The frequency of the rare *c2* allele is 24–30% for Asian populations, 2–3% for Caucasians, 0.3–7% for African-Americans, 15% for Mexican Americans and 18% for Chinese (Province of Taiwan) (Danko & Chaschin, 2005). The levels of CYP2E1 vary in human populations and have been shown in addition to be induced by repetitive alcoholic beverage consumption and exposure to other agents (Lieber & DeCarli, 1970; Roberts *et al.*, 1995; Mastrangelo *et al.*, 2004).

GSTs are encoded by a supergene family that is divided, on the basis of the chromosomal location and sequence homology, into four classes; Alpha, Mu, Pi and Theta (Lo & Li-Osman, 2007). Approximately half of the Caucasian population has no GSTM1-1 enzyme because of a homozygous deletion of the *GSTM1* gene. The other half is either heterozygous or homozygously normal. The frequency of the *GSTM1* null-null genotype is similar in Asians but lower in African-Americans (~ 27%) (Parl, 2005).

Genotypic differences are also frequent for the *GSTT1* gene. The *GSTT1$^{-/-}$* genotype is more common in Asians, at frequencies that range from 47 to 64%, whereas this homozygous null genotype is found only in 20% of Caucasians (Parl, 2005).

There is a structural polymorphism at amino acid position 487 of the *ALDH2* gene. A substitution of lysine for glutamic acid results from a transition of G (allele 1) to A (allele 2). The *ALDH2* alleles that encode the active and inactive subunits are termed *ALDH2*1* and *ALDH2*2*, respectively (Farres *et al.*, 1994). The dominant-negative mutant allele, *ALDH2*2*, is extremely rare in Caucasians, but is widely present in Mongoloids (28–45%; Goedde *et al.*, 1992).

Polymorphisms in genes that encode for the proteins that are involved in DNA-repair processes, such as XRCC1 (X-ray cross-complementing group 1) and XPD (xeroderma pigmentosum group D), may also modulate the occurrence of vinyl chloride-induced mutations. The XRCC1 protein is responsible for the repair of DNA lesions that are caused by alkylating agents. Etheno adducts produced by vinyl chloride are normally removed by the base-excision repair pathway which contains several proteins that are coordinated by XRCC1. Three polymorphisms have been identified at codon 194 (*Arg* to *Trp*), 280 (*Arg* to *His*) and 399 at codon 10 (*Arg* to *Gln*, termed *Gln* phenotype) for XRCC1 (Lindahl & Wood, 1999; Goode *et al.*, 2002).

The XPD protein is an adenosine triphosphate-dependent 5'-3' helicase involved in nucleotide excision repair. Several polymorphisms have also been described for the *XPD* gene (Lindahl & Wood, 1999; Goode *et al.*, 2002).

Few studies have investigated vinyl chloride-induced alterations at the chromosome level (sister chromatid exchange) and at the gene level (*RAS* and *p53* point mutations) in vinyl chloride-exposed workers with various polymorphisms. In a study from Taiwan, China, *CYP2E1c1c2/c2c2*, *ALDH2 1-2/2-2* and *XRCC1 Gln-Gln* polymorphisms appeared to be weak susceptibility factors for the frequency of sister chromatid exchange in relation to exposure to vinyl chloride, but not *GSTT1* or *GSTM1* genes (Table 28). *CYP2E1 c2c2* was also associated with a higher risk for p53 protein overexpression in the plasma of vinyl chloride-exposed workers (adjusted odds ratio, 9.8; 95% CI, 1.2–81.6), and this increased risk was also associated with *GSTT1* non-null (odds ratio, 2.4; 95% CI, 0.8–7.6) or *ALDH2 1-2/2-2* (odds ratio, 1.6; 95% CI, 0.5–4.6), particularly in the low-exposure group (≤ 40 ppm–years) (Wong, R.H. *et al.*, 2002). These authors suggested that frequency of sister chromatid exchange reflects recent exposure to vinyl chloride, while *p53* gene mutations reflect cumulative exposure to vinyl chloride. However, *CYP2E1 c1/c2* genotype compared with the wild-type *c1/c1* genotype appeared to contribute only slightly to the occurrence of mutant p21^{ras} or p53 proteins in French vinyl chloride-exposed workers (Li *et al.*, 2003b).

In contrast, a joint effect of the *XRCC1* codon 399 polymorphism and cumulative exposure to vinyl chloride on the occurrence of the p53 biomarker was observed (Li *et al.*, 2003a). While *GSTM1*, *GSTT1* and *GSTP1* polymorphisms were not found to be associated with an increased occurrence of mutant p53, a significant trend for the prevalence of p53 biomarkers was observed when the combined effects of *GSTM1*, *GSTT1* and *XRCC1* were analysed. The *GSTM1* and *GSTT1* null genotypes appeared to modify the effect of *XRCC1* codon 399 genotype on p53 biomarker status, possibly in a synergistic fashion (Table 29) (Li *et al.*, 2005a). All *XRCC1* codon 194, 280 and 399 polymorphisms also had an effect on the occurrence of the p53 biomarker (Table 30), but not on that of the p21^{ras} biomarker in the blood of vinyl chloride-exposed workers (Li *et al.*, 2006). In contrast, the *mEH* genotype has no effect on p21^{ras} or p53 biomarkers of vinyl chloride-induced mutagenic damage and may not be involved as a major detoxification enzyme in the metabolism of vinyl chloride in humans (Li *et al.*, 2005b). A follow-up of these studies has recently reported the analysis of a cohort of 597 French vinyl chloride-exposed workers. The presence of biomarkers for mutant p21^{ras} and mutant *p53* was found to be highly significantly associated with cumulative exposure to vinyl chloride (*p* for trend < 0.0001). The *CYP2E1* variant *c2* allele was significantly associated with the presence of either or both mutant biomarkers even after controlling for potential confounders including cumulative exposure to vinyl chloride (odds ratio, 2.3; 95% CI, 1.2–4.1), and the effects of the *c2* allele and vinyl chloride exposure were approximately additive. *GSTT1* null status was found to have an increased but not significant association with the presence of either or both biomarkers after controlling for confounders (odds ratio, 1.3; 95% CI, 0.8–2.0) (Schindler *et al.*, 2007).

The effects of polymorphisms of the DNA repair gene *XPD* on DNA damage in lymphocytes were studied in vinyl chloride-exposed workers in China using the comet assay. The study compared workers with ≥ 5 damaged cells per 100 cells studied with workers with no DNA damage who were matched for age, gender, cumulative exposure to VCM and worksite. Three *XPD* polymorphisms were investigated: *Ile199Met, Asp312Asn*

Table 28. Association between frequency of sister chromatid exchange and different polymorphisms (multiple regression model for frequencies of sister chromatid exchange per cell)

Reference	Cohort description	Exposure assessment	Exposure categories	One marker positive	Regression coefficient/SE	p value
Wong et al. (1998)	44 men with 4–36 years' exposure to VC, from 3 PVC plants; study based on predetermined VC exposure levels and smoking status; mean age, 45.1 ± 1.4 years; current smokers, 55.6%	A TWA exposure to VC assigned to each category of job based on monitored air levels of VC	High VC exposure group > 1 ppm (n = 28) Low VC exposure < 1 ppm (n = 16)	Smoking status, yes versus no VC exposure, high versus low CYP2E1 c1c2/c2c2 versus c1c1 ALDH2 1-2/2-2 versus 1-1 GSTM1 non-null versus null GSTT1 non-null versus null	0.85/0.31 0.64/0.34 0.50/0.33 0.63/0.31 −0.41/0.31 0.27/0.30	< 0.01 0.06 0.14 0.05 0.19 0.38
Wong et al. (2003b)	61 men, 29 controls	A TWA exposure to VC assigned to each category of job based on monitored air levels of VC	Controls (n = 29) High VC exposure > 1 ppm (n = 32) Low VC exposure < 1 ppm (n = 29)	Smoking status, yes versus no Alcohol drinking, yes versus no High VC exposure versus controls Low VC exposure versus controls XRCC1 exon 10: Gln-Gln versus Arg-Arg/Arg-Gln CYP2E1 c2c2 versus c1c1/c1c2 ALDH2 1-2/2-2 versus 1-1 GSTT1 null versus non null	0.56/0.26 −0.21/0.33 1.00/0.46 0.60/0.42 1.09/0.49 1.54/0.72 0.44/0.25 0.12/0.25	0.03 0.52 0.03 0.16 0.03 0.04 0.08 0.63

ALDH2, aldehyde dehydrogenase 2; CYP, cytochrome P450; GST, glutathione-S-transferase; PVC, polyvinyl chloride; SE, standard error; TWA, time-weighted average ; VC, vinyl chloride; XRCC1, X-ray cross-complementing group 1

Table 29. Association between *XRCC1/GSTM1/GSTT1* polymorphisms and mutant p53 in vinyl chloride (VC) workers

Reference	Cohort description	Exposure assessment	*XRCC1* codon 399/*GSTM1* or *GSTT1* genotypes	Exposure categories (in ppm-years)	No. positive mutant p53 biomarker (%)	Adjusted odds ratio (95% CI)[a]
Li *et al.* (2003a)	211 VC-exposed workers; average age, 56 years (range, 35–74 years); current smokers, 39%; current drinkers, 20%	Average cumulative exposure, 5871 ppm-years (range, 6–46 702 ppm-years): VC exposure levels were attributed to each subject on the basis of the job, using estimated values assigned to the various jobs[b]	*Arg-Arg*	≤1000 (n = 24); 1001–4000 (n = 31); >4000 (n = 31)	6 (25); 12 (39); 11 (35)	1.00; 2.19 (0.65–7.40); 1.96 (0.56–6.80)
			Arg-Gln	≤1000 (n = 26); 1001–4000 (n = 25); >4000 (n = 39)	10 (38); 9 (36); 23 (59)	1.90 (0.55–6.52); 1.89 (0.53–6.69); 5.43 (1.57–18.83)
			Gln-Gln	≤1000 (n = 11); 1001–4000 (n = 14); >4000 (n = 10)	5 (45); 10 (71); 8 (80)	2.50 (0.54–11.51); 8.84 (1.87–41.70); 12.17 (1.88–78.67); *p* for trend = 0.0004
Li *et al.* (2005a)	Same cohort as Li *et al.* (2003a)	Same as Li *et al.* (2003a)	*Arg-Arg*/both wild types (n = 31); *Arg-Arg*/either null (n = 47); *Arg-Arg*/ both null (n = 8); *Arg-Gln-Gln*/both wild types (n = 50); *Arg-Gln+Gln-Gln*/either null (n = 68); *Arg-Gln+Gln-Gln*/both null (n = 7)	NR	8 (26); 18 (38); 3 (38); 25 (50); 35 (51); 5 (71)	1; 1.8 (0.7–5.0); 1.8 (0.3–9.3); 2.9 (1.1–7.8); 3.2 (1.2–8.3); 8.4 (1.3–54.0); *p* for trend = 0.00037

CI, confidence interval; GST, glutathione-*S*-transferase; NR, not reported; XRCC1, X-ray cross-complementing group 1
[a] Adjusted for age, smoking, alcoholic beverage consumption and cumulative VC exposure
[b] Estimates of VC exposure in ppm-years based on years of a given job category weighted by the presumed ppm level of exposure as defined by the exposure matrix of Heldaas *et al.* (1984)

Table 30. Association between *XRCC1* codons 194, 280 and 399 polymorphisms and mutant p53 in vinyl chloride (VC) workers

Reference	Cohort description	Exposure assessment	*XRCC1* codons 194, 28 and 399	Mutant p53 biomarker		Adjusted odds ratio (95% CI)[a]
				+	−	
Li *et al.* (2006)	211 VC-exposed workers; average age, 56 years (range, 35–74 years); current smokers, 39%; current drinkers, 20%	Average cumulative exposure, 5871 ppm–years (range, 6–46 702 ppm–years); VC exposure levels were attributed to each subject on the basis of the job, using estimated values assigned to the various jobs[b]	All wild type	21 (34%)	41 (66%)	1
			One variant allele	41 (43%)	55 (57%)	1.5 (0.8–3.0)
			Two variant alleles	32 (60%)	21 (40%)	3.1 (1.4–6.7)
						p for trend = 0.005

CI, confidence interval; XRCC1, X-ray cross-complementing group 1
[a] Adjusted for age, smoking, alcoholic beverage consumption and cumulative exposure to VC
[b] Estimates of VC exposure in ppm–years based on years of a given job category weighted by the presumed ppm level of exposure as defined by the exposure matrix of Heldaas *et al.* (1984)

and *Lys751Gln*. Using univariate analysis, it was shown that only the *XPD751 Lys/Gln* and *Gln/Gln* genotypes were significantly associated with DNA damage (odds ratio, 2.21; 95% CI, 1.01–5.13; *p* < 0.05). After adjusting for the effects of smoking, alcoholic beverage consumption, liver damage and polymophisms of the DNA repair gene, and using the group with low exposure to vinyl chloride and the *XPD312 Asp/Asp* genotype as a reference, it was found that workers with high exposure and the *XPD312 Asp/Asn* and *Asn/Asn* genotypes had a significantly reduced risk for DNA damage (odds ratio, 0.33; 95% CI, 0.11–0.95) (Zhu *et al.*, 2005b).

These results suggest possible interactions between polymorphisms in the metabolic pathway of vinyl chloride and/or in the DNA repair processes and exposure to vinyl chloride that could contribute to the variable susceptibility to the mutagenic effects of vinyl chloride in exposed populations and might shed some light on the mechanism of tumour formation in humans.

4.4.2   Age

After results were published to indicate that hepatocytes of young, postnatal rats are much more susceptible than those of adult rats to the carcinogenic effect of vinyl chloride (Maltoni *et al.*, 1981; see Section 3), several investigations began to characterize the potentially susceptible period and the underlying mechanisms.

Laib *et al.* (1985a) investigated the age-dependence of the induction of preneoplastic enzyme-altered hepatic foci. Male and female Wistar rats were exposed to 2000 ppm [5186 mg/m³] vinyl chloride either transplacentally or immediately (1 day) after birth for a period of 5, 11, 17, 47 or 83 days, or from age 7 days or 21 days until death. Adenosine triphosphatase-deficient foci were increased compared with control rats after newborn exposures of 11 days or more, although foci area did not further increase after 17 days. Transplacental exposure and exposures before day 5 did not increase adenosine triphosphatase-deficient foci.

In accompanying studies, Laib *et al.* (1985b) also investigated the effects of a range of lower concentrations administered early in life. Wistar rats were exposed to 10, 40, 70, 150, 500 or 2000 ppm [26, 104, 182, 389, 1300 or 5186 mg/m³] vinyl chloride for 10 weeks beginning at 1 day of age, and Wistar and Sprague–Dawley rats were exposed to 2.5, 5, 10, 20, 40 or 80 ppm [6.5, 13, 26, 52, 104 or 208 mg/m³] vinyl chloride for 3 weeks beginning at 3 days of age. In each case, a linear relationship was observed between the concentration of vinyl chloride and the percentage of foci area induced, with no obvious threshold for the induction of preneoplastic foci.

Ciroussel *et al.* (1990) measured the levels of εA and εC adducts in DNA from several target organs. Rats were exposed to 500 ppm [1300 mg/m³] vinyl chloride for 2 weeks beginning at 7 days or 13 weeks of age. Both εA and εC adducts were detected in the liver, lungs and brain (but not kidneys) of rats that were 7 days old when first exposed. In rats that were 13 weeks old when first exposed, only liver DNA was analysed and levels of each adduct were one-sixth of those observed in the younger rats.

Fedtke *et al.* (1990) investigated the formation and persistence of the DNA adducts 7-OEG and N^2,3-εG. Lactating Sprague–Dawley rats and their 10-day-old offspring were exposed to 600 ppm [1560 mg/m^3] vinyl chloride for 4 h per day for 5 days. In the neonatal rats, concentrations of both DNA adducts were highest in the liver, followed by kidney and lung. No adducts were found in the brain or spleen. DNA adducts were detected only in the liver and lung of the dams. Concentrations of DNA adducts in the liver and lung were fourfold higher in the neonatal rats than in the dams.

Morinello *et al.* (2002a) studied the exposure–response relationship of N^2,3-εG adducts over a range of dose levels. Adult Sprague-Dawley rats were exposed to 0, 10, 100 or 1100 ppm [0, 26, 260 or 2852 mg/m^3] vinyl chloride for 1 or 4 weeks, and weanlings were similarly exposed for 5 days. The exposure–response relationship was linear from 0 to 100 ppm, then did not increase further. Compared with adult rats, two- to threefold higher concentrations of $N2$,3-εG adduct were measured in hepatocytes in the weanlings.

5. Summary of Data Reported

5.1 Exposure data

Vinyl chloride is a gas that is produced predominantly by breaking down ethylene dichloride into smaller molecules. Production of vinyl chloride by the initial acetylene-based process is still carried out in China. More than 95% of vinyl chloride is used for the production of polyvinyl chloride resin, which in turn is mainly used to produce plastic piping and other plastic items. Vinyl chloride is also used in the manufacture of chlorinated solvents. Production of vinyl chloride monomer is increasing. In 2005, production in Asia had outgrown that in both western Europe and North America. An increasing number of workers worldwide are exposed to vinyl chloride monomer during either its production, the manufacture of polyvinyl chloride or polyvinyl chloride processing. Since the late 1970s when the closed-loop polymerization process was introduced, the concentrations to which workers are exposed have decreased substantially in North America and western Europe. Levels before that time had been higher than 100 mg/m^3. In low- and medium-resource countries, older technologies have continued to be used and therefore high exposures probably occur. Exposures in polyvinyl chloride processing plants are usually considerably lower than those in vinyl chloride monomer/polyvinyl chloride production; in western Europe and North America, current exposure levels are generally below 1 mg/m^3. Concentrations of vinyl chloride monomer in ambient air are normally below 0.01 mg/m^3, but higher concentrations have been measured in the vicinity of vinyl chloride/polyvinyl chloride production plants.

5.2   Cancer in humans

Epidemiological evidence for the carcinogenicity of vinyl chloride in humans derives principally from two large, multicentric cohort studies, one of which was carried out in the USA and the other in Europe. These investigations focused on plants that manufactured vinyl chloride monomer, polyvinyl chloride or polyvinyl chloride products. Additional information is provided by several smaller cohort studies.

Both of the multicentric cohort studies found a substantial increase in the relative risk for angiosarcoma of the liver, a tumour that is extremely rare in the general population, in exposed workers. In both studies, the risk for liver angiosarcoma increased strongly with duration of exposure to vinyl chloride. In the European study, there was also a clear trend of higher risk with increasing cumulative exposure. Multiple cases of liver angiosarcoma were also reported in two smaller cohort studies. Overall, these findings constitute compelling evidence that vinyl chloride causes angiosarcoma of the liver.

Assessment of whether vinyl chloride also causes hepatocellular carcinoma is complicated because many studies do not have histological or other definitive clinical information to discriminate hepatocellular carcinoma from angiosarcoma of the liver and/or secondary neoplasms. However, in an internal analysis of the European multicentric cohort, the risk for hepatocellular carcinoma increased significantly and substantially with cumulative exposure to vinyl chloride, based on nine confirmed cases. Another analysis of a single Italian plant with extended follow-up that was included in the European multicentric study included 12 confirmed hepatocellular carcinomas. The maximal overlap between these two analyses was four cases, since only four hepatocellular carcinomas from Italy were included in the multicentric cohort. In this subcohort, the incidence of hepatocellular carcinoma again increased significantly with cumulative exposure to vinyl chloride. Together with the observation that vinyl chloride increases the risk for liver cirrhosis, which is a known risk factor for hepatocellular carcinoma, these findings provide convincing evidence that vinyl chloride causes hepatocellular carcinoma as well as angiosarcoma of the liver.

There was suggestive evidence that the risk for hepatocellular carcinoma from vinyl chloride is substantially higher among workers who are infected with hepatitis virus or report high levels of alcoholic beverage consumption.

Among vinyl chloride workers overall, there was no evidence of an increased risk for lung cancer. However, in polyvinyl chloride packers and baggers, the risk for lung cancer increased significantly with cumulative exposure to vinyl chloride. These workers are known to have had concomitant exposure to polyvinyl chloride dust, and the study did not allow attribution of the association to a specific agent or combination of agents.

Among the other cancer sites, suggestive evidence was found for malignant neoplasms of connective and soft tissue. This derived from the multicentric study in North America, in which a nearly threefold statistically significant overall increase in incidence was observed that persisted after the exclusion of four angiosarcomas for which the site was unknown. The risk was higher for workers with longer duration of employment (i.e. 10–19 and ≥ 20 years). These findings were not supported by the European multi-centric study, in which too few cases of connective tissue neoplasms were observed for an evaluation of exposure–response.

The Working Group did not find strong epidemiological evidence for associations of exposure to vinyl chloride with cancers of the brain or lymphatic and haematopoeitic tissue or melanoma. Although the associations found for these cancers in specific studies may reflect true increases in risk, the findings were inconsistent between studies, no clear exposure–response relationships were found in the European multicentric study and, for several of the sites, the numbers of observed and expected cases were small. No conclusion could be reached for breast cancer since the studies included too few women.

5.3   Cancer in experimental animals

The carcinogenicity of vinyl chloride has been studied intensively and repeatedly in experimental animals. The numerous studies are generally mutually reinforced. This wealth of data has generally been incompletely reported, however, and the outcomes of many experiments in the published studies are available only from summary tables, in which technical details are given only as footnotes.

Vinyl chloride was tested by inhalation exposure in seven studies in mice, in nine studies in rats and in two studies in hamsters. Male and female animals were treated in all three species, although some experiments were carried out only in one sex. Vinyl chloride induced hepatic angiosarcomas in three studies in mice and in eight studies in rats; a positive dose–response was observed for hepatic angiosarcomas in mice and rats over a wide range of exposures. It induced angiosarcomas (all sites) in four studies in mice, in three studies in rats and in one study in hamsters. Extrahepatic angiosarcomas related to treatment with vinyl chloride were observed in three studies in mice and two studies in rats. Vinyl chloride increased the incidence of mammary tumours in six studies in mice, in three studies in rats and in one study in hamsters. Exposure to vinyl chloride increased the incidence of skin tumours in one study in rats and in two studies in hamsters, and increased the incidence of Zymbal gland carcinomas in four studies in rats, with a dose–response pattern in one experiment. Vinyl chloride increased the incidence of lung tumours in six studies in mice, induced renal tumours and tumours of the nasal cavity in one study in rats, increased the incidence of hepatocellular carcinomas in two studies in rats and increased the incidence of glandular stomach tumours in one study in hamsters.

In one study in rats, combined oral administration of ethanol and inhalation exposure to vinyl chloride caused more liver tumours (including angiosarcomas and hepatocellular carcinomas) than exposure to vinyl chloride alone.

Vinyl chloride was tested by oral administration in four studies in male and female rats. It induced hepatic angiosarcomas in all studies, extrahepatic angiosarcomas in one study and hepatocellular carcinomas in two studies. When vinyl chloride was tested by subcutaneous injection and by intraperitoneal injection in single studies in rats, no hepatic angiosarcomas were induced.

The transplacental carcinogenicity of vinyl chloride was evaluated in one study in the offspring of rats exposed by inhalation during pregnancy. A low but significant incidence of tumours was observed in exposed offspring at sites that included the kidney, Zymbal gland and several others. However, no angiosarcomas or liver-cell tumours developed in the offspring.

Vinyl chloride was tested by perinatal inhalation exposure in two studies in rats. In one study, rats were exposed transplacentally, neonatally and during adulthood. Treatment with vinyl chloride induced hepatic angiosarcomas and hepatocellular carcinomas. Rats also demonstrated high incidences of tumours that were probably of olfactory neuroepithelial origin, but which were formerly reported as cerebral neuroblastomas in some studies. In a second study, rats were exposed to vinyl chloride for 5 weeks only beginning at birth. Hepatic angiosarcomas and 'hepatomas' occurred at a high incidence in the offspring, but not in the dams that were co-exposed with the offspring.

Chloroethylene oxide, a chemically reactive metabolite of vinyl chloride, was tested for carcinogenicity in a single study in mice by subcutaneous injection and in an initiation–promotion protocol on the skin. It caused fibrosarcomas at the site of subcutaneous injection and increased the incidence of squamous-cell papillomas and carcinomas of the skin at the site of application.

5.4   Mechanistic and other relevant data

Pulmonary absorption of vinyl chloride in humans appears to be rapid, and the percentage that is absorbed (about 40%) is independent of the concentration inhaled. Vinyl chloride is oxidized to highly reactive chloroethylene oxide, which rearranges to chloroacetaldehyde. The initial oxidation is predominantly mediated by cytochrome P450 2E1, an enzyme that is induced by ethanol among other agents. In rats, the metabolism of vinyl chloride is saturable at an inhalation concentration of 250 ppm [~650 mg/m^3], at which the incidence of hepatic angiosarcoma in these animals has been reported to plateau. The rate of vinyl chloride metabolism in humans is approximately 50 μmol/h/kg. The rate of elimination of vinyl chloride does not appear to be altered during repeated compared with single inhalation exposures.

Following metabolic activation of vinyl chloride in rats, the two metabolites, chloroethylene oxide and chloroacetaldehyde, react with nucleic acid bases to form adducts. These include the major adduct N7-(2-oxoethyl)guanine, four etheno adducts and 5,6,7,9-tetrahydro-7-hydroxy-9-oxoimidazol[1,2-a]purine, as identified in $vitro$ and in rats in $vivo$. In rats exposed to vinyl chloride, increased levels of etheno adducts have been found in different organs, such as the liver, lung and kidney, and in lymphocytes but not in the brain. Young animals are particularly prone to the formation and persistence of vinyl chloride-induced adducts. In rats, adducts have been found equally in non-parenchymal liver cells and in hepatocytes. In humans, etheno adducts are formed by lipid peroxidation; there is, however, a paucity of data on the occurrence of such adducts in vinyl chloride-exposed humans. The mechanism that leads to base misincorporation following adduct formation is still unclear.

Vinyl chloride is mutagenic, usually in the presence of metabolic activation, in various assays with bacteria, yeast or mammalian cells and is clastogenic in in-vivo and in-vitro systems. It induces unscheduled DNA synthesis and increases the frequency of sister chromatid exchange in rat and human cells. Exposure to vinyl chloride has been associated with an increase in the frequency of chromosomal aberrations, micronucleus formation and sister chromatid exchange in humans.

Ki-*ras* gene mutations are associated with vinyl chloride-induced angiosarcoma in humans but not in rats. In half of the cases, Ki-*ras* mutations lead to the incorporation of aspartate instead of glycine. Ki-*ras* mutations were also found to a lesser extend in vinyl-chloride induced hepatocellular carcinomas. A specific Ha-*ras* gene mutation (CAA61CTA) was found vinyl chloride-induced hepatocarcinomas in rats. A mutated *p53* gene was found in approximately half of the angiosarcomas in humans and rats that resulted from exposure to vinyl chloride. The *p53* mutations in both species are often due to A→T transversions.

The presence of mutated p21^{ras} and p53 proteins in the blood of a high proportion of workers exposed to vinyl chloride and the positive correlation between the occurrence of the mutated proteins and cumulative exposure to vinyl chloride suggest that the mutation is an early event.

In humans, genetic polymorphisms in genes that encode the enzymes involved in the metabolism of vinyl chloride (*CYP2E1*, *GSTT1*, *GSTM1*, *ALDH2*) and in DNA repair (*XRCC1*) modulate the DNA damage induced by vinyl chloride.

6. Evaluation and Rationale

6.1 Carcinogenicity in humans

There is *sufficient evidence* in humans for the carcinogenicity of vinyl chloride. Vinyl chloride causes angiosarcomas of the liver and hepatocellular carcinomas.

6.2 Carcinogenicity in experimental animals

There is *sufficient evidence* in experimental animals for the carcinogenicity of vinyl chloride.

There is *sufficient evidence* in experimental animals for the carcinogenicity of chloroethylene oxide.

6.3 Overall evaluation

Vinyl chloride is *carcinogenic to humans (Group 1)*.

7.   References

ACGIH (2001) Vinyl chloride, Cincinnati, OH, American Conference of Government Industrial Hygienists

ACGIH® Worldwide (2005) *Documentation of the TLVs® and BEIs® with Other Worldwide Occupational Exposure Values — 2005 CD-ROM*, Cincinnati, OH, American Conference of Government Industrial Hygienists

Akasaka, S. & Guengerich, F.P. (1999) Mutagenicity of site-specifically located 1,N²-etheno-guanine in Chinese hamster ovary cell chromosomal DNA. *Chem. Res. Toxicol.*, **12**, 501–507

Anderson, D. & Richardson, C.R. (1981) Issues relevant to the assessment of chemically induced chromosome damage in vivo and their relationship to chemical mutagenesis. *Mutat. Res.*, **90**, 261–272

Anderson, D., Hodge, M.C. & Purchase, I.F. (1976) Vinyl chloride: Dominant lethal studies in male CD-1 mice. *Mutat. Res.*, **40**, 359–370

Anderson, D., Hodge, M.C. & Purchase, I.F. (1977) Dominant lethal studies with the halogenated olefins vinyl chloride and vinylidene dichloride in male CD-1 mice. *Environ. Health Perspect.*, **21**, 71–78

Anghelescu, F., Otoiu, M., Dobrinescu, E., Hagi-Paraschiv-Dossios, L., Dobrinescu, G. & Ganea, V. (1969) Clinico-pathogenic considerations on Raynaud's phenomenon in the employees of the vinyl polychloride industry. *Med. intern.*, **21**, 473–482

ATSDR (Agency for Toxic Substances and Disease Registry) (2006) *Toxicological Profile on Vinyl Chloride*, Atlanta, GA, Centers for Disease Control and Prevention. [available at http://www.atsdr.cdc.gov/toxprofiles/phs20.html]

Ballering, L.A., Nivard, M.J. & Vogel, E.W. (1996) Characterization by two-endpoint comparisons of the genetic toxicity profiles of vinyl chloride and related etheno-adduct forming carcinogens in Drosophila. *Carcinogenesis,* **17**, 1083–1092

Bao, Y.S., Jiang, H. & Liu, J. (1988) [The effects of vinyl chloride on pregnancy parturition and fetal development among female workers.] *Chin. J. prev. Med.*, **22**, 343–346 (in Chinese)

Barbin, A. (1999) Role of etheno DNA adducts in carcinogenesis induced by vinyl chloride in rats. In: Singer, B. & Bartsch, H., eds, *Exocyclic DNA Adducts in Mutagenesis and Carcinogenesis* (IARC Scientific Publications No. 150), Lyon, IARC, pp. 303–313

Barbin, A. & Bartsch, H. (1989) Nucleophilic selectivity as a determinant of carcinogenic potency (TD50) in rodents: A comparison of mono- and bi-functional alkylating agents and vinyl chloride metabolites. *Mutat Res.*, **215**, 95–106

Barbin, A., Bresil, H., Croisy, A., Jacquignon, P., Malaveille, C., Montesano, R. & Bartsch, H. (1975) Liver-microsome-mediated formation of alkylating agents from vinyl bromide and vinyl chloride. *Biochem. biophys. Res. Commun.*, **67**, 596–603

Barbin, A., Laib, R.J. & Bartsch, H. (1985) Lack of miscoding properties of 7-(2-oxoethyl)guanine, the major vinyl chloride-DNA adduct. *Cancer Res.*, **45**, 2440–2444

Barbin, A., Froment, O., Boivin, S., Marion, M.J., Belpoggi, F., Maltoni, C. & Montesano, R. (1997) p53 Gene mutation pattern in rat liver tumors induced by vinyl chloride. *Cancer Res.*, **57**, 1695–1698

Baretta, E.D., Stewart, R.D. & Mutchler, J.E. (1969) Monitoring exposures to vinyl chloride vapor: breath analysis and continuous air sampling. *Am. ind. Hyg. Assoc. J.*, **30**, 537–544

Barnes, A.W. (1976) Vinyl chloride and the production of PVC. *Proc. R. Soc. Med.*, **69**, 277–281

Barton, H.A., Creech, J.R., Godin, C.S., Randall, G.M. & Seckel, C.S. (1995) Chloroethylene mixtures: Pharmacokinetic modeling and in vitro metabolism of vinyl chloride, trichloroethylene, and trans-1,2-dichloroethylene in rat. *Toxicol. appl. Pharmacol.*, **130**, 237–247

Bartsch, H. & Nair, J. (2000a) New DNA-based biomarkers for oxidative stress and cancer chemoprevention studies. *Eur. J. Cancer*, **36**, 1229–1234

Bartsch, H. & Nair, J. (2000b) Ultrasensitive and specific detection methods for exocyclic DNA adducts: Markers for lipid peroxidation and oxidative stress. *Toxicology*, **153**, 105–114

Bartsch, H., Malaveille, C. & Montesano, R. (1975) Human, rat and mouse liver-mediated mutagenicity of vinyl chloride in S. typhimurium strains. *Int. J. Cancer*, **15**, 429–437

Basler, A. & Röhrborn, G. (1980) Vinyl chloride: An example for evaluating mutagenic effects in mammals in vivo after exposure to inhalation. *Arch. Toxicol.*, **45**, 1–7

Basu, A.K., Wood, M.L., Niedernhofer, L.J., Ramos, L.A. & Essigmann, J.M. (1993) Mutagenic and genotoxic effects of three vinyl chloride-induced DNA lesions: $1,N^6$-Ethenoadenine, $3,N^4$-ethenocytosine, and 4-amino-5-(imidazol-2-yl)imidazole. *Biochemistry*, **32**, 12793–12801

Baxter, P.J. (1981) The British hepatic angiosarcoma register. *Environ. Health Perspect.*, **41**, 115–116

Becker, R., Nikolova, T., Wolff, I., Lovell, D., Huttner, E. & Foth, H. (2001) Frequency of HPRT mutants in humans exposed to vinyl chloride via an environmental accident. *Mutat. Res.*, **494**, 87–96

BIA (German Professional Associations' Institute for Occupational Safety) (1996) [Report on the Occupational Exposure to Cancer-inducing Substances], Sankt Augustin, Professional Association Office (HVBG), pp. 1–68 (in German)

Block, J.B. (1974) Angiosarcoma of the liver following vinyl chloride exposure. *J. Am. med. Assoc.*, **229**, 53–54

Boffetta, P., Matisane, L., Mundt, K.A., & Dell, L.D. (2003) Meta-analysis of studies of occupational exposure to vinyl chloride in relation to cancer mortality. *Scand. J. Work Environ. Health*, **29**, 220–229

Boivin-Angèle, S., Lefrancois, L., Froment, O., Spiethoff, A., Bogdanffy, M.S., Wegener, K., Wesch, H., Barbin, A., Bancel, B., Trepo, C., Bartsch, H., Swenberg, J. & Marion, M.J. (2000a) Ras gene mutations in vinyl chloride-induced liver tumours are carcinogen-specific but vary with cell type and species. *Int. J. Cancer*, **85**, 223–227

Boivin-Angèle, S., Pedron, S., Bertrand, S., Desmouliere, A., Martel-Planche, G., Lefrancois, L., Bancel, B., Trepo, C. & Marion, M.J. (2000) Establishment and characterization of a spontaneously immortalized myofibroblast cell line derived from a human liver angiosarcoma. *J. Hepatol.*, **33**, 290–300

Bol'shakov, A.M. (1969) [Working conditions in the production of synthetic leather.] In: *Proceedings of a Conference on Hygienic Problems in Manufacture and Use of Polymer Materials*, Moscow, Moscovic Research Institute of Hygiene, pp. 47–52 [*Chem. Abstr.*, **75**, 143701p] (in Russian)

Bolt, H.M. (1978) Pharmacokinetics of vinyl chloride. *Gen. Pharmacol.*, **9**, 91–95

Bolt, H.M. (2005) Vinyl chloride — A classical industrial toxicant of new interest. *Crit. Rev. Toxicol.*, **35**, 307–323

Bolt, H.M., Kappus, H., Buchter, A. & Bolt, W. (1976) Disposition of $(1,2-^{14}C)$ vinyl chloride in the rat. *Arch. Toxicol.*, **35**, 153–162

Bolt, H.M., Laib, R.J., Kappus, H. & Buchter, A. (1977) Pharmacokinetics of vinyl chloride in the rat. *Toxicology*, **7**, 179–188

Bolt, H.M., Filser, J.G., Laib, R.J. & Ottenwalder, H. (1980) Binding kinetics of vinyl chloride and vinyl bromide at very low doses. *Arch. Toxicol.*, **Suppl. 3**, 129–142

Bond, G.G., McLaren, E.A., Sabel, F.L., Bodner, K.M., Lipps, T.E. & Cook, R.R. (1990) Liver and biliary tract cancer among chemical worker. *Am. J. ind. Med.*, **18**, 19–24

Bonse, G., Urban, T., Reichert, D. & Henschler, D. (1975) Chemical reactivity, metabolic oxirane formation and biological reactivity of chlorinated ethylenes in the isolated perfused rat liver preparation. *Biochem. Pharmacol.*, **24**, 1829–1834

Boraiko, C. & Batt, J. (2005) Evaluation of employee exposure to organic tin compounds used as stabilizers at PVC processing facilities. *J. occup. environ. Hyg.*, **2**, 73–76

Borruso, A.V. (2006) *CEH Product Review. Vinyl chloride Monomer (VCM). Chemical Economics Handbook*, Zürich, SRI Consulting

Brandt-Rauf, P.W., Chen, J.M., Marion, M.J., Smith, S.J., Luo, J.C., Carney, W. & Pincus, M.R. (1996) Conformational effects in the p53 protein of mutations induced during chemical carcinogenesis: Molecular dynamic and immunologic analyses. *J. Protein Chem.*, **15**, 367–375

Buchter, A., Filser, J.G., Peter, H. & Bolt, H.M. (1980) Pharmacokinetics of vinyl chloride in the rhesus monkey. *Toxicol. Lett.*, **6**, 33–36

Byren, D., Engholm, G., Englund, A. & Westerholm, P. (1976) Mortality and cancer morbidity in a group of Swedish VCM and PCV production workers. *Environ. Health Perspect.*, **17**, 167–170

Casula, D., Cherchi, P., Spiga, G. & Spinazzola, A. (1977) [Environmental dust in a plant for the production of polyvinyl chloride.] *Ann. Ist. super. Sanita*, **13**, 189–198 (in Italian)

CDC (Centers for Disease Control and Prevention) (1997) Epidemiologic notes and reports of angiosarcoma of the liver among PVC workers — Kentucky. *Morbid. Mortal. wkly Rep.*, **46**, 97–101

Charvet, P., Cun, C. & Leroy, P. (2000) Vinyl chloride analysis with solid phase microextraction (SPME)/GC/MS applied to analysis in materials and aqueous samples. *Analysis*, **28**, 980–987

Chen, C.W. & Blancato, J.N. (1989) Incorporation of biological information in cancer risk assessment: Example — Vinyl chloride. *Cell Biol. Toxicol.*, **5**, 417–444

Cheng, K.C., Preston, B.D., Cahill, D.S., Dosanjh, M.K., Singer, B. & Loeb, L.A. (1991) The vinyl chloride DNA derivative N^2,3-ethenoguanine produces G–A transitions in *Escherichia coli*. *Proc. natl. Acad. Sci. USA*, **88**, 9974–9978

Cheng, T.J., Chou, P.Y., Huang, M.L., Du, C.L., Wong, R.H. & Chen, P.C. (2000) Increased lymphocyte sister chromatid exchange frequency in workers with exposure to low level of ethylene dichloride. *Mutat. Res.*, **470**, 109–114

Cheng, T.J., Huang, Y.F. & Ma, Y.C. (2001) Urinary thiodiglycolic acid levels for vinyl chloride monomer-exposed polyvinyl chloride workers. *J. occup. environ. Med.*, **43**, 934–938

Chiazze, L., Jr & Ference L.D. (1981) Mortality among PVC-fabricating employees. *Environ. Health Perspect.*, **41**, 137–143

Cho, Y., Gorina, S., Jeffrey, P.D. & Pavletich, N.P. (1994) Crystal structure of a p53 tumor suppressor–DNA complex: Understanding tumorigenic mutations. *Science*, **265**, 346–355

Choi, J.Y., Zang, H., Angel, K.C., Kozekov, I.D., Goodenough, A.K., Rizzo, C.J. & Guengerich, F.P. (2006) Translesion synthesis across 1,N^2-ethenoguanine by human DNA polymerases. *Chem. Res. Toxicol.*, **19**, 879–886

Ciroussel, F., Barbin, A., Eberle, G. & Bartsch, H. (1990) Investigations on the relationship between DNA ethenobase adduct levels in several organs of vinyl chloride-exposed rats and cancer susceptibility. *Biochem. Pharmacol.*, **39**, 1109–1113

Clewell, H.J., Gentry, P.R., Gearhart, J.M., Allen, B.C. & Andersen, M.E. (1995) Considering pharmacokinetic and mechanistic information in cancer risk assessments for environmental contaminants: Examples with vinyl chloride and trichloroethylene. *Chemosphere*, **31**, 2561–2578

Clewell, H.J., Gentry, P.R., Gearhart, J.M., Allen, B.C. & Andersen, M.E. (2001) Comparison of cancer risk estimates for vinyl chloride using animal and human data with a PBPK model. *Sci. total Environ.*, **274**, 37–66

Coenen, W. (1986) [Concentration of carcinogenic substances at the workplace: An analysis of results from the BIA data bank.] *Berufsgen. inform. Arb. Sicherh. Unfallvers.*, **1**, 1–5 (in German)

Cooper, W.C. (1981) Epidemiological study of vinyl chloride workers, mortality through December 1972. *Environ. Health Perspect.*, **41**, 101–106

Cowfer, J.A. & Gorensek, M.B. (2006) Vinyl chloride. In: *Kirk-Othmer Encyclopedia of Chemical Technology*, New York, John Wiley & Sons, pp. 1–31 (on line)

Creech, J.L., Jr & Johnson, M.N. (1974) Angiosarcoma of liver in the manufacture of polyvinyl chloride. *J. occup. Med.*, **16**, 150–151

Daniel, F.B., DeAngelo, A.B., Stober, J.A., Olson, G.R. & Page, N.P. (1992) Hepatocarcinogenicity of chloral hydrate, 2-chloroacetaldehyde, and dichloroacetic acid in the male B6C3F1 mouse. *Fundam. appl. Toxicol.*, **19**, 159–168

Danko, I.M. & Chaschin, N.A. (2005) Association of CYP2E1 gene polymorphism with predisposition to cancer development. *Exp. Oncol.*, **27**, 248–256

De Bont, R. & van Larebeke, N. (2004) Endogenous DNA damage in humans: A review of quantitative data. *Mutagenesis*, **19**, 169–185

De Jong, G., van Sittert, N.J. & Natarajan, A.T. (1988) Cytogenetic monitoring of industrial populations potentially exposed to genotoxic chemicals and of control populations. *Mutat. Res.*, **204**, 451–464

Department of Labor (1989) *Vinyl Chloride, Chemical Sampling*, Washington DC, Occupational Safety and Health Administration [available at: http://www.osha.gov/dts/sltc/methods/organic/org075/org 075.html; accessed 11.12.2007]

De Vivo, I., Marion, M.J., Smith, S.J., Carney, W.P. & Brandt-Rauf, P.W. (1994) Mutant c-Ki-ras p21 protein in chemical carcinogenesis in humans exposed to vinyl chloride. *Cancer Causes Control*, **5**, 273–278

Dietz, A., Langbeing, G. & Permatter, W. (1985) [Vinyl chloride-induced hepatocellular carcinoma] *Klin. Wochenschr.*, **63**, 325–331 (in German)

Dimmick, W.F. (1981) EPA programs of vinyl chloride monitoring in ambient air. *Environ. Health Perspect.*, **41**, 203–206

Dobecki, M. & Romaniwicz, B. (1993) [Occupational exposure to toxic substances during the production of vinyl chloride and chlorinated organic solvents.] *Med. Prac.*, **44**, 99–102 (in Polish)

Dow Chemical Company (2007) [available at http://www.dow.com/productsafety/finder/vcm.htm; accessed May 21, 2007]

Drew, R.T., Boorman, G.A., Haseman, J.K., McConnell, E.E., Busey, W.M. & Moore, J.A. (1983) The effect of age and exposure duration on cancer induction by a known carcinogen in rats, mice and hamsters. *Toxicol. appl. Pharmacol.*, **68**, 120–130

Du, C.L. & Wang, J.D. (1998) Increased morbidity odds ratio of primary liver cancer and cirrhosis of the liver among vinyl chloride monomer workers. *Occup. environ. Med.*, **55**, 528–532

Du, C.L., Chan, C.C. & Wang, J.D. (1996) Comparison of personal and area sampling strategies in assessing workers' exposure to vinyl chloride monomer. *Bull. environ. Contam. Toxicol.*, **56**, 534–542

Du, C.L., Chan, C.C. & Wang, J.D. (2001) [Development of a job exposure matrix model for polyvinyl chloride workers.] *Inst. occup. Saf. Health J.*, **9**, 151–166 (in Chinese with English abstract)

Eckardt, F., Muliawan, H., de Ruiter, N. & Kappus, H. (1981) Rat hepatic vinyl chloride metabolites induce gene conversion in the yeast strain D7RAD in vitro and in vivo. *Mutat. Res.*, **91**, 381–390

Egan, H., Squirrell, D.C.M. & Thain, W., eds (1978) *Environmental Carcinogens, Selected Methods of Analysis*, Vol. 2, *Methods for the Measurement of Vinyl Chloride in Poly(vinyl Chloride), Air, Water and Foodstuffs* (IARC Scientific Publications No. 22), IARC, Lyon

El Ghissassi, F., Barbin, A., Nair, J. & Bartsch, H. (1995) Formation of $1,N^6$-ethenoadenine and $3,N^1$-ethenocytosine by lipid peroxidation products and nucleic acid bases. *Chem. Res. Toxicol.*, **8**, 278–283

El Ghissassi, F., Barbin, A. & Bartsch, H. (1998) Metabolic activation of vinyl chloride by rat liver microsomes: Low-dose kinetics and involvement of cytochrome P450 2E1. *Biochem. Pharmacol.*, **55**, 1445–1452

Environmental Protection Agency (1975) *Scientific and Technical Assessment Report on Vinyl Chloride and Polyvinyl Chloride* (EPA-600/6-75-004), Springfield, VA, National Technical Information Service, pp. 7–42

Environmental Protection Agency (1999) *Method TO-14. Compendium of Methods for the Determination of Toxic Organic Compounds in Ambient Air*, 2nd Ed., *Compendium Method TO-14A Determination of Volatile Organic Compounds (VOCs) in Ambient Air Using Specially Prepared Canisters with Subsequent Analysis by Gas Chromatography*, Washington DC

European Commission (1978) Council Directive of 30 January 1978 on the approximation of the laws of the Member States relating to materials and articles which contain vinyl chloride monomer and are intended to come into contact with foodstuffs (78/142/EEC). *Off. J. Eur. Union*, **L44**, pp. 15–17

European Commission (2003) *Integrated Pollution Prevention and Control (IPPC). Reference Document on Best Available Techniques in the Large Volume Organic Chemical Industry*, Luxembourg

Evans, D.M.D., Jones, W.W. & Kung, I.T.M. (1983) Angiosarcoma and hepatocellular carcinoma in vinyl chloride workers. *Histopathology*, **7**, 377–388

Farres, J., Wang, X., Takahashi, K., Cunningham, S.J., Wang, T.T. & Weiner, H. (1994) Effects of changing glutamate 487 to lysine in rat and human liver mitochondrial aldehyde dehydrogenase. A model to study human (Oriental type) class 2 aldehyde dehydrogenase. *J. biol. Chem.*, **269**, 13854–13860

Fedtke, N., Boucheron, J.A., Walker, V.E. & Swenberg, J.A. (1990) Vinyl chloride-induced DNA adducts. II: Formation and persistence of 7-(2'-oxoethyl)guanine and N^2,3-ethenoguanine in rat tissue DNA. *Carcinogenesis*, **11**, 1287–1292

Fernandes, P.H., Kanuri, M., Nechev, L.V., Harris, T.M. & Lloyd, R.S. (2005) Mammalian cell mutagenesis of the DNA adducts of vinyl chloride and crotonaldehyde. *Environ. mol. Mutag.*, **45**, 455–459

Feron, V.J. & Kroes, R. (1979) One-year time-sequence inhalation toxicity study of vinyl chloride in rats. II. Morphological changes in the respiratory tract, ceruminous gland, brain, kidneys, heart and spleen. *Toxicology*, **13**, 131–141

Feron, V.J., Spit, B.J., Immel, H.R. & Kroes, R. (1979) One-year time-sequence inhalation toxicity study of vinyl chloride in rats: III. Morphological changes in the liver. *Toxicology*, **13**, 143–154

Feron, V.J., Hendriksen, C.F.M., Speek, A.J., Til, H.P. & Spit, B.J. (1981) Lifespan oral toxicity study of vinyl chloride in rats. *Food Cosmet. Toxicol.*, **19**, 317–333

Filatova, V.S. & Gronsberg, E.S. (1957) [Sanitary–hygienic conditions of work in the production of polychlorvinylic tar and measures of improvement.] *Gig. Sanit.*, **22**, 38–42 (in Russian)

Filser, J.G. & Bolt, H.M. (1979) Pharmacokinetics of halogenated ethylenes in rats. *Arch. Toxicol.*, **42**, 123–136

Fleig, I. & Thiess, A.M. (1974) [Chromosome tests in vinyl chloride exposed workers.] *Arbeitsmed. Sozialmed. Präventivmed.*, **12**, 280–283 (in German)

Forman, D., Bennett, B., Stafford, J. & Doll, R. (1985) Exposure to vinyl chloride and angiosarcoma of the liver: A report of the register of cases. *Br. J. ind. Med.*, **42**, 750–753

Fox, A.J. & Collier, P.F. (1977) Mortality experience of workers exposed to vinyl chloride monomer in the manufacture of polyvinyl chloride in Great Britain. *Br. J. ind. Med.*, **34**, 1–10

Frentzel-Beyme, R., Schmitz, T. & Thiess, A.M. (1978) [Mortality study of VC-/PVC workers at BASF company, Ludwigshafen am Rhein.] *Arbeitsmed. Sozialmed. Präventivmed.*, 218–228 (in German)

Froment, O., Boivin, S., Barbin, A., Bancel, B., Trepo, C. & Marion, M.J. (1994) Mutagenesis of ras proto-oncogenes in rat liver tumors induced by vinyl chloride. *Cancer Res.*, **54**, 5340–5345

Fucic, A., Horvat, D. & Dimitrovic, B. (1990) Localization of breaks induced by vinyl chloride in the human chromosomes of lymphocytes. *Mutat. Res.*, **243**, 95–99

Gáliková, E., Tomíková, K., Zigová, A., Mesko, D., Buchancová, J., Petrisková, J., L'uptáková, M., Ja, M. & Karaffová, N. (1994) [General health of workers in the Nováky chemical works exposed to vinyl chloride.] *Prac. Lék.*, **46**, 251–256 (in Czech)

Gargas, M.L., Burgess, R.J., Voisard, D.E., Cason, G.H. & Andersen, M.E. (1989) Partition coefficients of low-molecular-weight volatile chemicals in various liquids and tissues. *Toxicol. appl. Pharmacol.*, **98**, 87–99

Gehring, P.J., Watanabe, P.G. & Park, C.N. (1978) Resolution of dose-response toxicity data for chemicals requiring metabolic activation: Example — Vinyl chloride. *Toxicol. appl. Pharmacol.*, **44**, 581–591

Gennaro, V., Ceppi, M. & Montanaro, F. (2003) Reanalysis of mortality in a petrochemical plant producing vinyl chloride and polyvinyl chloride. *Epidemiol. Prev.*, **27**, 221–225

German Environmental Office (1978) [Air contamination with vinyl chloride (VC) from PVC-products.] *Umweltbundes. Ber.*, **5**, 1–23 (in German)

Goedde, H.W., Agarwal, D.P., Fritze, G., Meier-Tackmann, D., Singh, S., Beckmann, G., Bhatia, K., Chen, L.Z., Fang, B., Lisker, R., Paik, Y.K., Rothhammer, F., Saha, N., Segal, B., Srivastava, L.M. & Czeizel, A. (1992) Distribution of ADH_2 and ALDH2 genotypes in different populations. *Hum. Genet.*, **88**, 344–346

Gokel, J.M., Liebezeit, E. & Eder, M. (1976) Hemangiosarcoma and hepatocellular carcinoma of the liver following vinyl chloride exposure. A report of two cases. *Virchows Arch.*, **372**, 195–203

Goode, E.L., Ulrich, C.M. & Potter, J.D. (2002) Polymorphisms in DNA repair genes and associations with cancer risk. *Cancer Epidemiol. Biomarkers Prev.*, **11**, 1513–1530

Grasselli, J.G. & Ritchey, W.M., eds (1975) *CRC Atlas of Spectral Data and Physical Constants for Organic Compounds*, 2nd Ed., Vol. III, Cleveland, OH, Chemical Rubber Co., p. 279

Green, T. & Hathway, D.E. (1975) The biological fate in rats of vinyl chloride in relation to its oncogenicity. *Chem.-biol. Interact.*, **11**, 545–562

Green, T. & Hathway, D.E. (1977) The chemistry and biogenesis of the S-containing metabolites of vinyl chloride in rats. *Chem.-biol. Interact.*, **17**, 137–150

Greim, H., Bonse, G., Radwan, Z., Reichert, D. & Henschler, D. (1975) Mutagenicity in vitro and potential carcinogenicity of chlorinated ethylenes as a function of metabolic oxirane formation. *Biochem. Pharmacol.*, **24**, 2013–2017

Gros, L., Maksimenko, A.V., Privezentzev, C.V., Laval, J. & Saparbaev, M.K. (2004) Hijacking of the human alkyl-N-purine–DNA glycosylase by $3,N^4$-ethenocytosine, a lipid peroxidation-induced DNA adduct. *J. biol. Chem.*, **279**, 17723–17730

Groth, D.H., Coate, W.B., Ulland, B.M. & Hornung, R.W. (1981) Effects of aging on the induction of angiosarcoma. *Environ. Health Perspect.*, **41**, 53–57

Guengerich, F.P. (1992) Roles of the vinyl chloride oxidation products 1-chlorooxirane and 2-chloroacetaldehyde in the in vitro formation of etheno adducts of nucleic acid bases. *Chem. Res. Toxicol.*, **5**, 2–5

Guengerich, F.P. & Watanabe, P.G. (1979) Metabolism of [^{14}C]- and [^{36}C]-labeled vinyl chloride in vivo and in vitro. *Biochem. Pharmacol.*, **28**, 589–596

Guengerich, F.P., Crawford, W.M., Jr & Watanabe, P.G. (1979) Activation of vinyl chloride to covalently bound metabolites: Roles of 2-chloroethylene oxide and 2-chloroacetaldehyde. *Biochemistry*, **18**, 5177–5182

Guengerich, F.P., Mason, P.S., Stott, W.T., Fox, T.R. & Watanabe, P.G. (1981) Roles of 2-haloethylene oxides and 2-haloacetaldehydes derived from vinyl bromide and vinyl chloride in irreversible binding to protein and DNA. *Cancer Res.*, **41**, 4391–4398

Guengerich, F.P., Langouet, S., Mican, A.N., Akasaka, S., Muller, M. & Persmark, M. (1999) Formation of etheno adducts and their effects on DNA polymerases. In: Singer, B. & Bartsch, H., eds, *Exocyclic DNA Adducts in Mutagenesis and Carcinogenesis* (IARC Scientific Publications No. **150**), Lyon, IARC, pp. 137–145

Guichard, Y., El Ghissassi, F., Nair, J., Bartsch, H. & Barbin, A. (1996) Formation and accumulation of DNA ethenobases in adult Sprague-Dawley rats exposed to vinyl chloride. *Carcinogenesis*, **17**, 1553–1559

Hagmar, L., Akesson, B., Nielsen, J., Andersson, C., Linden, K., Attewell, R. & Moller, T. (1990) Mortality and cancer morbidity in workers exposed to low levels of vinyl chloride monomer at a polyvinylchloride processing plant. *Am. J. ind. Med.*, **17**, 553–565

Haguenoer, J.M., Frimat, P., Cantineau, A., Pollard, F. & Bobowski, R. (1979) [The risks linked to vinyl chloride (VCM) and their prevention in a polymerization factory.] *Arch. Mal. prof. Méd. Trav. Séc. soc.*, **40**, 1115–1130 (in French)

Hansteen, I.L., Hillestad, L., Thiis-Evensen, E. & Heldaas, S.S. (1978) Effects of vinyl chloride in man: A cytogenetic follow-up study. *Mutat. Res.*, **51**, 271–278

Hefner, R.E., Jr, Watanabe, P.G. & Gehring, P.J. (1975a) Preliminary studies on the fate of inhaled vinyl chloride monomer (VCM) in rats. *Environ. Health Perspect.*, **11**, 85–95

Hefner, R.E., Jr, Watanabe, P.G. & Gehring, P.J. (1975b) Percutaneous absorption of vinyl chloride. *Toxicol. appl. Pharmacol.*, **34**, 529–532

Heger, M., Müller, G. & Norpoth, K. (1981) [Investigations on the correlation between vinyl chloride (=VCM)-uptake and excretion of its metabolites by 15 VCM-exposed workers.] *Int. Arch. occup. environ. Health*, **48**, 205–210 (in German)

Heldaas, S.S., Langard, S.L. & Andersen, A. (1984) Incidence of cancer among vinyl chloride and polyvinyl chloride workers. *Br. J. ind. Med.*, **41**, 25–30

Heldaas, S.S., Andersen, A.A. & Langard, S. (1987) Incidence of cancer among vinyl chloride and polyvinyl chloride workers: Further evidence for an association with malignant melanoma. *Br. J. ind. Med.*, **44**, 278–280

Himeno, S., Okuda, H. & Suzuki, T. (1983) Lack of dominant lethal effects in male CD-1 mice after short-term and long-term exposures to vinyl chloride monomer. *Toxicol. Lett.*, **16**, 47–53

Ho, S.F., Phoon, W.H., Gan, S.L. & Chan, Y.K. (1991) Persistent liver dysfunction among workers at a vinyl chloride monomer polymerization plant. *J. soc. occup. Med.*, **41**, 10–16

Hoffmann, D., Patrianakos, C., Brunnemann, K.D. & Gori, G.B. (1976) Chromatographic determination of vinyl chloride in tobacco smoke. *Anal. Chem.*, **48**, 47–50

Hollstein, M., Marion, M.J., Lehman, T., Welsh, J., Harris, C.C., Martel-Planche, G., Kusters, I. & Montesano, R. (1994) p53 Mutations at A:T base pairs in angiosarcomas of vinyl chloride-exposed factory workers. *Carcinogenesis*, **15**, 1–3

Hollstein, M., Shomer, B., Greenblatt, M., Soussi, T., Hovig, E., Montesano, R. & Harris, C.C. (1996) Somatic point mutations in the p53 gene of human tumors and cell lines: Updated compilation. *Nucleic Acids Res.*, **24**, 141–146

Holm, L., Westlin, A. & Holmberg, B. (1982) Technical control measures in the prevention of occupational cancer. An example from the PVC industry. In: *Proceedings of the International Symposium on Prevention of Occupational Cancer*, Geneva, International Labour Office, pp. 538–546

Holmberg, B., Kronevi, T. & Winell, M. (1976) The pathology of vinyl chloride exposed mice. *Acta vet. scand.*, **17**, 328–342

Hong, C.B., Winston, J.M., Thornburg, L.P., Lee, C.C. & Woods, J.S. (1981) Follow-up study on the carcinogenicity of vinyl chloride and vinylidene chloride in rats and mice: Tumor incidence and mortality subsequent to exposure. *J. Toxicol. environ. Health*, **7**, 909–924

Hozo, I., Andelinovic, S., Ljutic, D., Miric, D., Bojic, L. & Gasperic, I. (1996) Vinyl chloride monomer exposure by the plastic industry workers — Basic condition for liver angiosarcoma appearance. *Med. Arhiv*, **50**, 9–14

Hozo, I., Andelinovic, S., Ljutic, D., Bojic, L., Miric, D. & Giunio, L. (1997) Two new cases of liver angiosarcoma: History and perspectives of liver angiosarcoma among plastic industry workers. *Toxicol. ind. Health*, **13**, 639–647

Hrivnak, L., Rozinova, Z., Korony, S. & Fabianova, E. (1990) Cytogenetic analysis of peripheral blood lymphocytes in workers exposed to vinyl chloride. *Mutat. Res.*, **240**, 83–85

Huang, M. (1996) [Epidemiological investigation on occupational malignant tumor in workers exposed to vinyl chloride.] In: *Ministry of Public Health of China, National Epidemiological Study on Eight Occupational Cancers (1982–84)*, Beijing, Ministry of Public Health of China, pp. 86–98 (in Chinese)

Hüttner, E. & Holzapfel, B. (1996) HPRT mutant frequencies and detection of large deletions by multiplex-PCR in human lymphocytes of vinyl chloride exposed and non-exposed populations. *Toxicol. Lett.*, **88**, 175–183

IARC (1974) *IARC Monographs on the Evaluation of Carcinogenic Risk of Chemicals to Man*, Vol. 7, *Some Anti-thyroid and Related Substances, Nitrofurans and Industrial Chemicals*, Lyon, pp. 291–318

IARC (1979) *IARC Monographs on the Evaluation of the Carcinogenic Risk of Chemicals to Humans*, Vol. 19, *Some Monomers, Plastic and Synthetic Elastomers and Acrolein*, Lyon, pp. 377–438

IARC (1987) *IARC Monographs on the Evaluation of Carcinogenic Risks to Humans*, Suppl. 7, *Overall Evaluations of Carcinogenicity: An Updating of* IARC Monographs *Volumes 1 to 42*, Lyon, pp. 373–376

IARC (1995) *IARC Monographs on the Evaluation of Carcinogenic Risks to Humans*, Vol. 63, *Dry Cleaning, Some Chlorinated Solvents and Other Industrial Chemicals*, Lyon, pp. 443–465

IARC (1999) *IARC Monographs on the Evaluation of Carcinogenic Risks to Humans*, Vol. 71, *Re-evaluation of Some Organic Chemicals, Hydrazine and Hydrogen Peroxide*, Lyon

IARC (2002) *IARC Monographs on the Evaluation of Carcinogenic Risks to Humans*, Vol. 82, *Some Traditional Herbal Medicines, Some Mycotoxins, Naphthalene and Styrene*, Lyon, pp. 437–550

IARC (2004) *IARC Monographs on the Evaluation of Carcinogenic Risks to Humans*, Vol. 83, *Tobacco Smoke and Involuntary Smoking*, Lyon

IPCS-CEC (2000) *International Chemical Safety Cards, Vinyl Chloride ICSC 0082*, Geneva, World Health Organization

Ivanetich, K.M., Aronson, I. & Katz, I.D. (1977) The interaction of vinyl chloride with rat hepatic microsomal cytochrome P-450 in vitro. *Biochem. biophys. Res. Commun.*, **74**, 1411–1418

Jedrychowski, R.A., Sokal, J.A. & Chmielnicka, J. (1984) Influence of exposure mode on vinyl chloride action. *Arch. Toxicol.*, **55**, 195–198

Jenssen, D. & Ramel, C. (1980) The micronucleus test as part of a short-term mutagenicity test program for the prediction of carcinogenicity evaluated by 143 agents tested. *Mutat. Res.*, **75**, 191–202

Jones, R.D., Smith, D.M. & Thomas, P.G. (1988) A mortality study of vinyl chloride monomer workers employed in the United Kingdom in 1940–1974. *Scand. J. Work Environ. Health*, **14**, 153–160

Kappus, H., Bold, H.M., Buchter, A. & Bolt, W. (1975) Rat liver microsomes catalyse covalent binding of 14C-vinyl chloride to macromolecules. *Nature*, **257**, 134–135

Kappus, H., Bolt, H.M., Buchter, A. & Bolt, W. (1976) Liver microsomal uptake of (^{14}C)vinyl chloride and transformation to protein alkylating metabolites in vitro. *Toxicol. appl. Pharmacol.*, **37**, 461–471

Kauppinen, T., Toikkanen, J., Pedersen, D., Young, R., Ahrens, W., Boffetta, P., Hansen, J., Kromhout, H., Maqueda Blasco, J., Mirabelli, D., de la Orden-Rivera, V., Pannett, B., Plato, N., Savela, A., Vincent, R. & Kogevinas, M. (2000) Occupational exposure to carcinogens in the European Union. *Occup. environ. Med.*, **57**, 10–18 [Data partially available on the CAREX web site: http://www.ttl.fi/Internet/English/Organization/Collaboration/Carex/Eur_union.htm]

Koischwitz, V.D., Lelbach, W.R., Lackner, K. & Hermanuntz, D. (1981) [Vinyl chloride-induced angiosarcoma of the liver and hepato-cellular carcinoma.] *Fortschr. Rontgenstr.*, **134**, 283–290 (in German)

Krajewski, J., Dobecki, M. & Gromiec, J. (1980) Retention of vinyl chloride in the human lung. *Br. J. ind. Med.*, **37**, 373–374

Krishnan, A.V., Stathis, P., Permuth, S.F., Tokes, L. & Feldman, D. (1993) Bisphenol-A: An estrogenic substance is released from polycarbonate flasks during autoclaving. *Endocrinology*, **132**, 2279–2286

Kuchenmeister, F., Wang, M., Klein, R.G. & Schmezer, P. (1996) Transport of reactive metabolites of procarcinogens between different liver cell types, as demonstrated by the single cell microgel electrophoresis assay. *Toxicol. Lett.*, **88**, 29–34

Kurlyandski, B.A., Stovbur, N.N. & Turusov, V.S. (1981) [About hygienic regimentation of vinyl chloride.] *Gig. Sanit.*, **3**, 74–75 (in Russian).

Laib, R.J. & Bolt, H.M. (1977) Alkylation of RNA by vinyl chloride metabolites in vitro and in vivo: Formation of 1-N^6-etheno-adenosine. *Toxicology*, **8**, 185–195

Laib, R.J., Klein, K.P. & Bolt, H.M. (1985a) The rat liver foci bioassay: I. Age-dependence of induction by vinyl chloride of ATPase-deficient foci. *Carcinogenesis*, **6**, 65–68

Laib, R.J., Pellio, T., Wunschel, U.M., Zimmermann, N. & Bolt, H.M. (1985b) The rat liver foci bioassay: II. Investigations on the dose-dependent induction of ATPase-deficient foci by vinyl chloride at very low doses. *Carcinogenesis*, **6**, 69–72

Langård, S., Rosenberg, J., Andersen, A. & Heldaas, S.S. (2000) Incidence of cancer among workers exposed to vinyl chloride in polyvinyl chloride manufacture. *Occup. environ. Med.*, **57**, 65–68

Langouët, S., Muller, M. & Guengerich, F.P. (1997) Misincorporation of dNTPs opposite 1,N^2-ethenoguanine and 5,6,7,9-tetrahydro-7-hydroxy-9-oxoimidazo[1,2-a]purine in oligo-nucleotides by Escherichia coli polymerases I exo- and II exo-, T7 polymerase exo-, human immunodeficiency virus-1 reverse transcriptase, and rat polymerase beta. *Biochemistry*, **36**, 6069–6079

Langouët, S., Mican, A.N., Muller, M., Fink, S.P., Marnett, L.J., Muhle, S.A. & Guengerich, F.P. (1998) Misincorporation of nucleotides opposite five-membered exocyclic ring guanine derivatives by escherichia coli polymerases in vitro and in vivo: 1,N^2-Ethenoguanine, 5,6,7,9-tetrahydro-9-oxoimidazo[1, 2-a]purine, and 5,6,7,9-tetrahydro-7-hydroxy-9-oxoimidazo[1, 2-a]purine. *Biochemistry*, **37**, 5184–5193

Laplanche, A., Clavel-Chapelon, F., Contassot, J.C. & Lanouziere, C. (1992) Exposure to vinyl chloride monomer, results of a cohort study after a seven year follow-up. *Br. J. ind. Med.*, **49**, 134–137

Laramy, R.E. (1977) Analytical chemistry of vinyl chloride—A survey. *Am. Lab.*, **December**, pp. 17–27

Lee, F.I. & Harry, D.S. (1974) Angiosarcoma of the liver in a vinyl-chloride worker. *Lancet*, **i**, 1316–1318

Lee, C.C., Bhandari, J.C., Winston, J.M., House, W.B., Dixon, R.L. & Woods, J.S. (1978) Carcinogenicity of vinyl chloride and vinylidene chloride. *J. Toxicol. environ. Health*, **4**, 15–30

Lei, Y.C., Yang, H.T., Ma, Y.C., Huang, M.F., Chang, W.P. & Cheng, T.J. (2004) DNA single
strand breaks in peripheral lymphocytes associated with urinary thiodiglycolic acid levels in
polyvinyl chloride workers. *Mutat. Res.*, **561**, 119–126

Lelbach, W.K. (1996) A 25-year follow-up study of heavily exposed vinyl chloride workers in
Germany. *Am. J. ind. Med.*, **29**, 446–458

Lewis, R. & Rempala, G. (2003) A case–cohort study of angiosarcoma of the liver and brain cancer
at a polymer production plant. *J. occup. environ. Med.*, **45**, 538–545

Lewis, R., Rempala, G., Dell, L.D. & Mundt, K.A. (2003) Vinyl chloride and liver and brain cancer at polymer production plant in Louisville, Kentucky. *J. occup. environ. Med.*, **45**, 533–537

Li, Y., Asherova, M., Marion, M.J. & Brandt-Rauf, P.W. (1998a) Mutant oncoprotein biomarkers
in chemical carcinogenesis. In: Mendelsohn, M.L., Mohr, L.C. & Peeters, J.P., eds., *Biomarkers: Medical and Workplace Applications*, Washington DC, Joseph Henri Press, pp. 345–
353.

Li, Y., Marion, M.J., Asherova, M., Coulibaly, D., Smith, S.J., Do, T., Carney, W.P. & Brandt-
Rauf, P.W. (1998b) Mutant p21ras in vinyl chloride exposed workers. *Biomarkers*, **3**, 433–439

Li, Y., Marion, M.J., Rundle, A. & Brandt-Rauf, P.W. (2003a) A common polymorphism in
XRCC1 as a biomarker of susceptibility for chemically induced genetic damage. *Biomarkers*,
8, 408–414

Li, Y., Marion, M.J., Ho, R., Cheng, T.J., Coulibaly, D., Rosal, R. & Brandt-Rauf, P.W. (2003b)
Polymorphisms for vinyl chloride metabolism in French vinyl chloride workers. *Int. J. occup.
Med. environ. Health*, **16**, 55–59

Li, Y., Zhou, M., Marion, M.J., Lee, S. & Brandt-Rauf, P.W. (2005a) Polymorphisms in
glutathione S-transferases in French vinyl chloride workers. *Biomarkers*, **10**, 72–79

Li, Y., Lee, S., Marion, M.J. & Brandt-Rauf, P.W. (2005b) Polymorphisms of microsomal epoxide
hydrolase in French vinyl chloride workers. *Int. J. occup. Med. environ. Health*, **18**, 133–138

Li, Y., Marion, M.J., Zipprich, J., Freyer, G., Santella, R.M., Kanki, C. & Brandt-Rauf, P.W.
(2006) The role of XRCC1 polymorphisms in base excision repair of etheno-DNA adducts in
French vinyl chloride workers. *Int. J. occup. Med. environ. Health*, **19**, 45–52

Lide, D.R., ed. (2005) *CRC Handbook of Chemistry and Physics*, 86th Ed., Boca Raton, FL, CRC
Press. pp. 3–100

Lieber, C.S. & DeCarli, L.M. (1970) Hepatic microsomal ethanol-oxidizing system. In vitro
characteristics and adaptive properties in vivo. *J. biol. Chem.*, **245**, 2505–2512

Lilly, P.D., Thornton-Manning, J.R., Gargas, M.L., Clewell, H.J. & Andersen, M.E. (1998) Kinetic
characterization of CYP2E1 inhibition in vivo and in vitro by the chloroethylenes. *Arch.
Toxicol.*, **72**, 609–621

Lindahl, T. & Wood, R.D. (1999) Quality control by DNA repair. *Science*, **286**, 1897–1905

Lo, H.W. & Li-Osman, F. (2007) Genetic polymorphism and function of glutathione S-transferases
in tumor drug resistance. *Curr. Opin. Pharmacol.*, **7**, 367–374

Loprieno, N., Barale, R., Baroncelli, S., Bauer, C., Bronzetti, G., Cammellini, A., Cercignani, G.,
Corsi, C., Gervasi, G., Leporini, C., Nieri, R., Rossi, A.M., Stretti, G. & Turchi, G. (1976)
Evaluation of the genetic effects induced by vinyl chloride monomer (VCM) under
mammalian metabolic activation: Studies in vitro and in vivo. *Mutat. Res.*, **40**, 85–96

Lundberg, I., Gustavsson, A., Holmberg, B., Molina, G. & Westerholm, P. (1993) Mortality and cancer incidence among PVC-processing workers in Sweden. *Am. J. ind. Med.*, **23**, 313–319

Luo, J.C., Liu, H.T., Cheng, T.J., Du, C.L. & Wang, J.D. (1998) Plasma Asp13-Ki-ras oncoprotein expression in vinyl chloride monomer workers in Taiwan. *J. occup. environ. Med.*, **40**, 1053–1058

Luo, J.C.J., Liu, H.T., Cheng, T.J., Du, C.L. & Wang, J.D. (1999) Plasma p53 protein and anti-p53 antibody expression in vinyl chloride monomer workers in Taiwan. *J. occup. environ. Med.*, **41**, 521–526

Luo, J.C., Cheng, T.J., Du, C.L. & Wang, J.D. (2003) Molecular epidemiology of plasma oncoproteins in vinyl chloride monomer workers in Taiwan. *Cancer Detect. Prev.*, **27**, 94–101

Magnusson, J. & Ramel, C. (1978) Mutagenic effects of vinyl chloride on Drosophila melanogaster with and without pretreatment with sodium phenobarbiturate. *Mutat. Res.*, **57**, 307–312

Makita, O., Ono, K., Sakurai, T., Tanigawa H., Ando Y., Yamashita, K., Yoshimatsu, M. & Takahashi, M. (1997) A case of hepatocellular carcinoma related with exposure to vinyl chloride monomers. *NSG Zasshi*, **94**, 215–219

Maltoni, C. & Cotti, G. (1988) Carcinogenicity of vinyl chloride in Sprague-Dawley rats after prenatal and postnatal exposure. *Ann. N.Y. Acad. Sci.*, **534**, 145–159

Maltoni, C., Lefemine, G., Chieco, P. & Carretti, D. (1974) Vinyl chloride carcinogenesis: Current results and perspectives. *Med. Lav.*, **65**, 421–444

Maltoni, C., Lefemine, G., Ciliberti, A., Cotti, G. & Caretti, D. (1981) Carcinogenicity bioassays of vinyl chloride monomer: A model of risk assessment on an experimental basis. *Environ. Health Perspect.*, **41**, 3–29

Marion, M.J. (1998) Critical genes as early warning signs: Example of vinyl chloride. *Toxicol. Lett.*, **102–103**, 603–607

Marion, M.J., Froment, O. & Trepo, C. (1991) Activation of Ki-ras gene by point mutation in human liver angiosarcoma associated with vinyl chloride exposure. *Mol. Carcinog.*, **4**, 450–454

Mastrangelo, G., Fedeli, U., Fadda, E., Milan, G., Turato, A. & Pavanello, S. (2003) Lung cancer risk in workers exposed to poly(vinyl chloride) dust: A nested case–referent study. *Occup. environ. Med.*, **60**, 423–428

Mastrangelo, G., Fedeli, U., Fadda, E., Valentini, F., Agnesi, R., Magarotto, G., Marchi, T., Buda, A., Pinzani, M. & Martines, D. (2004) Increased risk of hepatocellular carcinoma and liver cirrhosis in vinyl chloride workers: Synergistic effect of occupational exposure with alcohol intake. *Environ. Health Perspect.*, **112**, 1188–1192

Matsuda, T., Yagi, T., Kawanishi, M., Matsui, S. & Takebe, H. (1995) Molecular analysis of mutations induced by 2-chloroacetaldehyde, the ultimate carcinogenic form of vinyl chloride, in human cells using shuttle vectors. *Carcinogenesis*, **16**, 2389–2394

McCann, J., Simmon, V., Streitwieser, D. & Ames, B.N. (1975) Mutagenicity of chloro-acetaldehyde, a possible metabolic product of 1,2-dichloroethane (ethylene dichloride), chloro-ethanol (ethylene chlorohydrin), vinyl chloride, and cyclophosphamide. *Proc. natl Acad. Sci. USA*, **72**, 3190–3193

de Meester C., van Duverger, B.M., Lambotte-Vandepaer, M., Roberfroid, M., Poncelet, F. & Mercier, M. (1980) Mutagenicity of vinyl chloride in the Ames test: Possible artifacts related to experimental conditions. *Mutat. Res.*, **77**, 175–179

Mocci, F. & Nettuno, M. (2006) Plasma mutant-p53 protein and anti-p53 antibody as a marker: An experience in vinyl chloride workers in Italy. *J. occup. environ. Med.*, **48**, 158–164

Molina, G., Holmberg, B., Elofsson, S., Holmlund, L., Moosing, R. & Westerholm, P. (1981) Mortality and cancer rates among workers in the Swedish PVC processing industry. *Environ. Health Perspect.*, **41**, 145–151

Morinello, E.J., Ham, A.J., Ranasinghe, A., Sangaiah, R. & Swenberg, J.A. (2001) Simultaneous quantitation of N^2,3-ethenoguanine and 1,N^2,3-ethenoguanine with an immunoaffinity/gas chromatography/high-resolution mass spectrometry assay. *Chem. Res. Toxicol.*, **14**, 327–334

Morinello, E.J., Koc, H., Ranasinghe, A. & Swenberg, J.A. (2002a) Differential induction of N^2,3-ethenoguanine in rat brain and liver after exposure to vinyl chloride. *Cancer Res.*, **62**, 5183–5188

Morinello, E.J., Ham, A.J., Ranasinghe, A., Nakamura, J., Upton, P.B. & Swenberg, J.A. (2002b) Molecular dosimetry and repair of N^2,3-ethenoguanine in rats exposed to vinyl chloride. *Cancer Res.*, **62**, 5189–5195

Mroczkowska, M.M. & Kusmierek, J.T. (1991) Miscoding potential of N^2,3-ethenoguanine studied in an Escherichia coli DNA-dependent RNA polymerase in vitro system and possible role of this adduct in vinyl chloride-induced mutagenesis. *Mutagenesis*, **6**, 385–390

Müller, G., Norpoth, K., Kusters, E., Herweg, K. & Versin, E. (1978) Determination of thio-diglycolic acid in urine specimens of vinyl chloride exposed workers. *Int. Arch. occup. environ. Health*, **41**, 199–205

Müller, M., Belas, F., Ueno, H. & Guengerich, F.P. (1996) Development of a mass spectrometric assay for 5,6,7,9-tetrahydro-7-hydroxy-9-oximidazo[1,2-alpha] purine in DNA modified by 2-chloro-oxirane. *Adv. exp. Med. Biol.*, **387**, 31–36

Mundt, K.A., Dell, L.D., Austin, R.P., Luippold, R.S., Noess, R. & Bigelow, C. (2000) Historical cohort study of 10109 men in the North American vinyl chloride industry, 1942–72, update of cancer mortality to 31 December 1995. *Occup. environ. Med.*, **57**, 774–781

Murdoch, I.A. & Hammond, A.R. (1977) A practical method for the measurement of vinyl chloride monomer (VCM) in air. *Ann. occup. Hyg.*, **20**, 55–61

Nair, J., Barbin, A., Guichard, Y. & Bartsch, H. (1995) 1,N^6-Ethenodeoxyadenosine and 3,N^4-ethenodeoxycytine in liver DNA from humans and untreated rodents detected by immunoaffinity/32P-postlabeling. *Carcinogenesis*, **16**, 613–617

National Library of Medicine (2007) *Toxic Chemical Release Inventory (TRI) Data Banks*, Bethesda, MD

Nelson, N.A., Robins, T.G., Garrison, R.P., Schuman, M. & White, R.F. (1993) Historical characterization of exposure to mixed solvents for an epidemiologic study of automotive assembly plant workers. *Appl. occup. environ. Hyg.*, **8**, 693–702

NOES (1997) *National Occupational Exposure Survey (1981–1983)*, Cincinnati, OH, National Institute for Occupational Safety and Health [available at: http://www.cdc.gov/noes/noes2/76445occ.html; accessed 11.11.07]

O'Neil, M.J., ed. (2006) *Merck Index*, 14th Ed., Whitehouse Station, NJ, Merck, pp. 1719–1720

Orusev, T., Popovski, P., Bauer, S. & Nikolova, K. (1976) Occupational risk in the production of poly(vinyl)chloride. *God. Zb. Med. Fak. Skopje*, **22**, 33–38

Osterman-Golkar, S., Hultmark, D., Segerback, D., Calleman, C.J., Gothe, R., Ehrenberg, L. & Wachtmeister, C.A. (1976) Alkylation of DNA and proteins in mice exposed to vinyl chloride. *Biochem. biophys. Res. Commun.*, **76**, 259–266

Ott, M.G., Langner, R.R. & Holder, B.H. (1975) Vinyl chloride exposure in a controlled industrial environment. A long-term mortality experience in 594 employees. *Arch. environ. Health*, **30**, 333–339

Pandya, G.A. & Moriya, M. (1996) 1,N^6-Ethenodeoxyadenosine, a DNA adduct highly mutagenic in mammalian cells. *Biochemistry*, **35**, 11487–11492

Parl, F.F. (2005) Glutathione S-transferase genotypes and cancer risk. *Cancer Lett.*, **221**, 123–129

Peter, S. & Ungváry, G. (1980) Lack of mutagenic effect of vinyl chloride monomer in the mammalian spot test. *Mutat. Res.*, **77**, 193–196

Pirastu, R., Comba, P., Reggiani, A., Foa', V., Masina, C. & Maltoni, C. (1990) Mortality from liver disease among Italian vinyl chloride monomer/polyvinyl chloride manufactures. *Am. J. ind. Med.*, **17**, 155–161

Pirastu, R., Bellis, S., Bruno, C., Maltoni, C., Masina, A. & Reggiani, A. (1991) [The mortality among the workers of vinyl chloride in Italy.] *Med. Lav.*, **82**, 388–423 (in Italian)

Pirastu, R., Bruno, C., De Santis, M., & Comba, P. (1998) [An epidemiological study of workers exposed to vinyl chloride in the plants of Ferrara, Rosignano and Ravenna.] *Epidemiol. Prev.*, **22**, 226–236 (in Italian)

Pirastu, R., Baccini, M., Biggeri, A. & Comba, P. (2003) [Epidemiological study of workers exposed to vinyl chloride in a Porto Marghera factory: Mortality update.] *Epidemiol. Prev.*, **27**, 161–172 (in Italian)

Pleil, J.D. & Lindstrom, A.B. (1997) Exhaled human breath measurement method for assessing exposure to halogenated volatile organic compounds. *Clin. Chem.*, **43**, 723–730

Plugge, H. & Safe, S. (1977) Vinyl chloride metabolism — A review. *Chemosphere*, **6**, 309–325

Radike, M.J., Stemmer, K.L. & Bingham, E. (1981) Effect of ethanol on vinyl chloride carcinogenesis. *Environ. Health Perspect.*, **41**, 59–62

Rannug, U., Johansson, A., Ramel, C. & Wachtmeister, C.A. (1974) The mutagenicity of vinyl chloride after metabolic activation. *Ambio*, **3**, 194–197

Rashad, M.M., El-Belbessy, S.F., Hussein, N.G., Helmey, M.H. & El-Toukhy, M.A. (1994) Effect on some enzyme activities of occupational exposure to vinyl chloride monomer for five consecutive years. *Med. Sci. Res.*, **22**, 289–290

Reitz, R.H., Gargas, M.L., Andersen, M.E., Provan, W.M. & Green, T.L. (1996) Predicting cancer risk from vinyl chloride exposure with a physiologically based pharmacokinetic model. *Toxicol. appl. Pharmacol.*, **137**, 253–267

Reynolds, E.S., Moslen, M.T., Szabo, S. & Jaeger, R.J. (1975) Vinyl chloride-induced deactivation of cytochrome P-450 and other components of the liver mixed function oxidase system: An in vivo study. *Res. Commun. Chem. Pathol. Pharmacol.*, **12**, 685–694

Richardson, C.R., Styles, J.A. & Bennett, I.P. (1983) Activity of vinyl chloride monomer in the mouse micronucleus assay. *Mutat. Res.*, **122**, 139–142

Roberts, B.J., Song, B.J., Soh, Y., Park, S.S. & Shoaf, S.E. (1995) Ethanol induces CYP2E1 by protein stabilization. Role of ubiquitin conjugation in the rapid degradation of CYP2E1. *J. biol. Chem.*, **270**, 29632–29635

Rowe, V.K. (1975) Experience in industrial exposure control. *Ann. N.Y. Acad. Sci.*, **246**, 306–310

Saalo, A., Soosaar, A., Vuorela, R. & Kauppinen, T. (2006) [ASA 2004], Helsinki, Finnish Institute of Occupational Health [available at: http://www.ttl.fi/NR/rdonlyres/5A54A452-7350-4255-8DF3-AF632D9D2775/0/ASA_2004.pdf] (in Finnish)

Sabadie, N., Malaveille, C., Camus, A.M. & Bartsch, H. (1980) Comparison of the hydroxylation of benzo(a)pyrene with the metabolism of vinyl chloride, N-nitrosomorpholine, and N-nitroso-N'-methylpiperazine to mutagens by human and rat liver microsomal fractions. *Cancer Res.*, **40**, 119–126

Saurin, J.C., Tanière, P., Mion, F., Jacob, P., Partensky, C., Paliard, P. & Berger, F. (1997) Primary hepatocellular carcinoma in workers exposed to vinyl chloride. *Cancer*, **79**, 1671–1677

Scélo, G., Constantinescu, V., Csiki, I., Zaridze, D., Szeszenia-Dabrowska, N., Rudnai, P., Lissowska, J., Fabiánová, E., Cassidy, A., Slamova, A., Foretova, L., Janout, V., Fevotte, J., Fletcher, T., 't Mannetje, A., Brennan, P. & Boffetta, P. (2004) Occupational exposure to vinyl chloride, acrylonitrile and styrene and lung cancer risk (Europe). *Cancer Causes Control*, **15**, 445–452

Schindler, J., Li, Y., Marion, M.J., Paroly, A. & Brandt-Rauf, P.W. (2007) The effect of genetic polymorphisms in the vinyl chloride metabolic pathway on mutagenic risk. *J. hum. Genet.*, **52**, 448–455

Shimada, T., Swanson, A.F., Leber, P. & Williams, G.M. (1985) Activities of chlorinated ethane and ethylene compounds in the Salmonella/rat microsome mutagenesis and rat hepatocyte/-DNA repair assays under vapor phase exposure conditions. *Cell Biol. Toxicol.*, **1**, 159–179

Short, R.D., Minor, J.L., Winston, J.M. & Lee, C.C. (1977) A dominant lethal study in male rats after repeated exposures to vinyl chloride or vinylidene chloride. *J. Toxicol. environ. Health*, **3**, 965–968

SIDS (Screening Information Dataset) (2001) *Initial Assessment Report Vinyl Chloride*, Bern, UNEP Publications

Simonato, L., L'Abbé, K.A., Andersen, A., Belli, S., Comba, P., Engholm, G., Ferro, G., Hagmar, L., Langård, S., Lundberg, I., Pirastu, R., Thomas, P., Winkelmann, R. & Saracci, R. (1991) A collaborative study of cancer incidence and mortality among vinyl chloride workers. *Scand. J. Work Environ. Health*, **17**, 159–169

Singer, B., Spengler, S.J., Chavez, F. & Kusmierek, J.T. (1987) The vinyl chloride-derived nucleoside, N^2,3-ethenoguanosine, is a highly efficient mutagen in transcription. *Carcinogenesis*, **8**, 745–747

Singer, B., Kusmierek, J.T., Folkman, W., Chavez, F. & Dosanjh, M.K. (1991) Evidence for the mutagenic potential of the vinyl chloride induced adduct, N^2,3-etheno-deoxyguanosine, using a site-directed kinetic assay. *Carcinogenesis*, **12**, 745–747

Smith, S.J., Li, Y., Whitley, R., Marion, M.J., Partilo, S., Carney, W.P. & Brandt-Rauf, P.W. (1998) Molecular epidemiology of p53 protein mutations in workers exposed to vinyl chloride. *Am. J. Epidemiol.*, **147**, 302–308

Smulevich, V.B., Fedotova, I.V. & Filatova, V.S. (1988) Increasing evidence of the risk of cancer in workers exposed to vinyl chloride. *Br. J. ind. Med.*, **45**, 93–97

Soini, Y., Welsh, J.A., Ishak, K.G. & Bennett, W.P. (1995) p53 Mutations in primary hepatic angiosarcomas not associated with vinyl chloride exposure. *Carcinogenesis*, **16**, 2879–2881

Solionova, L.G., Smulevich, V.B., Turbin, E.V., Krivosheyeva, L.V. & Plotnikov, J.V. (1992) Carcinogens in rubber production in the Soviet Union. *Scand. J. Work Environ. Health*, **18**, 120–123

Studniarek, M., Durski, K., Liniecki, J., Brykalski, D., Poznanska, A. & Gluszcz, M. (1989) Effects of vinyl chloride on liver function of exposed workers, evaluated by measurements of plasma clearance of the 99mTc-N-2,4-dimethylacetanilido-iminoiacetate complex. *J. appl. Toxicol.*, **9**, 213–218

Summers, J.W. (2006) Vinyl chloride polymers. In: *Kirk-Othmer Encyclopedia of Chemical Technology*, John Wiley & Sons, pp. 1–41 (on line)

Suzuki, Y. (1983) Neoplastic effect of vinyl chloride in mouse lung — Lower doses and short-term exposure. *Environ. Res.*, **32**, 91–103

Swenberg, J.A., Ham, A., Koc, H., Morinello, E., Ranasinghe, A., Tretyakova, N., Upton, P.B. & Wu, K. (2000) DNA adducts: Effects of low exposure to ethylene oxide, vinyl chloride and butadiene. *Mutat. Res.*, **464**, 77–86

Tabershaw, I.R. & Gaffey, W.R. (1974) Mortality study of workers in the manufacture of vinyl chloride and its polymers. *J. occup. Med.*, **16**, 509–518

Tariff Commission (1928) *Census of Dyes and of Other Synthetic Organic Chemicals, 1927* (Tariff Information Series No. 37), Washington DC, US Government Printing Office, p. 139

Tarkowski, S., Wisniewska-Knypl, J.M., Klimczak, J., Dramiński, W. & Wróblewska, K. (1980) Urinary excretion of thiodiglycollic acid and hepatic content of free thiols in rats at different levels of exposure to vinyl chloride. *J. Hyg. Epidemiol. Microbiol. Immunol.*, **24**, 253–261

Thériault, G. & Allard, P. (1981) Cancer mortality of a group of Canadian workers exposed to vinyl chloride monomer. *J. occup. Med.*, **23**, 671–676

Thriene, B., Benkwitz, F., Willer, H., Neske, P. & Bilsing, H. (2000) [The chemical accident in Schönebeck — An assessment of health and environment risks.] *Gesundheitswesen*, **62**, 34–38 (in German)

Til, H.P., Feron, V.J. & Immel, H.R. (1991) Lifetime (149-week) oral carcinogenicity study of vinyl chloride in rats. *Food chem. Toxicol.*, **29**, 713–718

Trivers, G.E., Cawley, H.L., DeBenedetti, V.M.G, Hollstein, M., Marion, M.J., Bennett, W.P., Hoover, M.L., Prives, C.C., Tamburro, C.C. & Harris, C.C. (1995) Anti-p53 antibodies in sera of workers occupationally exposed to vinyl chloride. *J. natl Cancer Inst.*, **87**, 1400–1407

Ungvary, G., Hudak, A., Tatrai, E., Lorincz, M. & Folly, G. (1978) Effects of vinyl chloride exposure alone and in combination with trypan blue applied systematically during all thirds of pregnancy on the fetuses of CFY rats. *Toxicology*, **11**, 45–54

Verburgt, F.G. & Vogel, E. (1977) Vinyl chloride mutagenesis in Drosophila melanogaster. *Mutat. Res.*, **48**, 327–336

Viinanen, R. (1993) *Monitoring Results of VC in a PVC plant in 1981–1993* (Research Report No. 93025T), Porvoo, Neste Environmental and Industrial Hygiene Institute

Walles, S.A. & Holmberg, B. (1984) Induction of single-strand breaks in DNA of mice after inhalation of vinyl chloride. *Cancer Lett.*, **25**, 13–18

Ward, E., Boffetta, P., Andersen, A., Colin, D., Comba, P., Deddens, J.A., De Santis, M., Engholò, G., Hagmar, L., Langard, S., Lundberg, I., Mcelvenny, D., Pirastu, R., Sali, D. & Simonato, L. (2000) *Update of the Follow-up of Mortality and Cancer Incidence among European Workers Employed in the Vinyl Chloride Industry* (IARC Internal Report No. 00/001), Lyon, IARC

Ward, E., Boffetta, P., Andersen, A., Colin, D., Comba, P., Deddens, J.A., De Santis, M., Engholò, G., Hagmar, L., Langard, S., Lundberg, I., Mcelvenny, D., Pirastu, R., Sali, D. & Simonato, L. (2001) Update of the follow-up of mortality and cancer incidence among European workers employed in the vinyl chloride industry. *Epidemiology*, **12**, 710–718

Watanabe, P.G., McGowan, G.R. & Gehring, P.J. (1976a) Fate of (^{14}C)vinyl chloride after single oral administration in rats. *Toxicol. appl. Pharmacol.*, **36**, 339–352

Watanabe, P.G., McGowan, G.R., Madrid, E.O. & Gehring, P.J. (1976b) Fate of [^{14}C]vinyl chloride following inhalation exposure in rats. *Toxicol. appl. Pharmacol.*, **37**, 49–59

Watanabe, P.G., Zempel, J.A., & Gehring, P.J. (1978a) Comparison of the fate of vinyl chloride following single and repeated exposure in rats. *Toxicol appl. Pharmacol.*, **44**, 391–399

Watanabe, P.G., Zempel, J.A., Pegg, D.G. & Gehring, P.J. (1978b) Hepatic macromolecular binding following exposure to vinyl chloride. *Toxicol. appl. Pharmacol.*, **44**, 571–579

Weber, H., Reinl, W. & Greiser, E. (1981) German investigations on morbidity and mortality of workers exposed to vinyl chloride. *Environ. Health Perspect.*, **41**, 95–99

Weihrauch, M., Lehnert, G., Kockerling, F., Wittekind, C. & Tannapfel, A. (2000) p53 Mutation pattern in hepatocellular carcinoma in workers exposed to vinyl chloride. *Cancer*, **88**, 1030–1036

Weihrauch, M., Benick, M., Lehner, G., Wittekind, M., Bader, M., Wrbitzk, R. & Tannapfel, A. (2001a) High prevalence of K-ras-2 mutations in hepatocellular carcinomas in workers exposed to vinyl chloride. *Int. Arch. occup. environ. Health*, **74**, 405–410

Weihrauch, M., Benicke, M., Lehnert, G., Wittekind, C., Wrbitzky, R. & Tannapfel, A. (2001b) Frequent k-ras-2 mutations and p16^{INK4A} methylation in hepatocellular carcinomas in workers exposed to vinyl chloride. *Br. J. Cancer*, **84**, 982–989

Weihrauch, M., Bader, M., Lehnert, G., Koch, B., Wittekind, C., Wrbitzky, R. & Tannapfel, A. (2002a) Mutation analysis of K-ras-2 in liver angiosarcoma and adjacent nonneoplastic liver tissue from patients occupationally exposed to vinyl chloride. *Environ. mol. Mutag.*, **40**, 36–40

Weihrauch, M., Markwarth, A., Lehnert, G., Wittekind, C., Wrbitzky, R. & Tannapfel, A. (2002b) Abnormalities of the ARF-p53 pathway in primary angiosarcomas of the liver. *Hum. Pathol.*, **33**, 884–892

WHO (1999) *Vinyl Chloride* (Environmental Health Criteria 215), Geneva, World Health Organization

Withey, J.R. (1976) Pharmacodynamics and uptake of vinyl chloride monomer administered by various routes to rats. *J. Toxicol. environ. Health*, **1**, 381–394

Wong, O., Whorton, M.D., Foliart, D.E. & Ragland, D. (1991) An industry-wide epidemiologic study of vinyl chloride workers, 1942–1982. *Am. J. ind. Med.*, **20**, 317–334

Wong, R.H., Wang, J.D., Hsieh, L.L., Du, C.L. & Cheng, T.J. (1998) Effects on sister chromatid exchange frequency of aldehyde dehydrogenase 2 genotype and smoking in vinyl chloride workers. *Mutat. Res.*, **420**, 99–107

Wong, O., Chen, P.C., Du, L.C., Wang, J.D. & Cheng, T.J. (2002) An increased standardized mortality ratio for liver cancer among polyvinyl chloride workers in Taiwan. *Occup. environ. Med.*, **59**, 405–409

Wong, R.H., Du, C.L., Wang, J.D., Chan, C.C., Luo, J.C. & Cheng, T.J. (2002) XRCC1 and CYP2E1 polymorphisms as susceptibility factors of plasma mutant p53 protein and anti-p53 antibody expression in vinyl chloride monomer-exposed polyvinyl chloride workers. *Cancer Epidemiol. Biomarkers Prev.*, **11**, 475–482

Wong, R.H., Chen, P.C., Wang, J.D., Du, C.L. & Cheng, T.J. (2003a) Interaction of vinyl choride monomer exposure and hepatitis B viral infection on liver cancer. *J. occup. environ. Med.*, **45**, 379–383

Wong, R.H., Wang, J.D., Hsieh, L.L. & Cheng, T.J. (2003b) XRCC1, CYP2E1 and ALDH2 genetic polymorphisms and sister chromatid exchange frequency alterations amongst vinyl chloride monomer-exposed polyvinyl chloride workers. *Arch. Toxicol.*, **77**, 433–440

Yang, Y., Nair, J., Barbin, A. & Bartsch, H. (2000) Immunohistochemical detection of 1,N[6]-ethenodeoxyadenosine, a promutagenic DNA adduct, in liver of rats exposed to vinyl chloride or an iron overload. *Carcinogenesis*, **21**, 777–781

Yllner, S. (1971) Metabolism of chloroacetate-1-^{14}C in the mouse. *Acta pharmacol. toxicol.*, **30**, 69–80

Zajdela, F., Croisy, A., Barbin, A., Malaveille, C., Tomatis, L. & Bartsch, H. (1980) Carcinogenicity of chloroethylene oxide, an ultimate reactive metabolite of vinyl chloride, and bis(chloromethyl)ether after subcutaneous administration and in initiation–promotion experiments in mice. *Cancer Res.*, **40**, 352–356

Zhang, W., Johnson, F., Grollman, A.P. & Shibutani, S. (1995) Miscoding by the exocyclic and related DNA adducts 3,N[4]-etheno-2'-deoxycytidine, 3,N[4]-ethano-2'-deoxycytidine, and 3-(2-hydroxyethyl)-2'-deoxyuridine. *Chem. Res. Toxicol.*, **8**, 157–163

Zhu, S.M., Ren, X.F., Wan, J.X. & Xia, Z.L. (2005a) Evaluation in vinyl chloride monomer (VCM)-exposed workers and the relationship between liver lesions and gene polymorphisms of metabolic enzymes. *World J. Gastroenterol.*, **11**, 5821–5827

Zhu, S., Wang, A. & Xia, Z. (2005b) Polymorphisms of DNA repair gene XPD and DNA damage of workers exposed to vinylchloride monomer. *Int. J. Hyg. environ. Health*, **208**, 383–390

VINYL BROMIDE

This substance was considered by previous Working Groups in February 1978 (IARC, 1979), June 1985 (IARC, 1986), March 1987 (IARC, 1987) and February 1998 (IARC, 1999). Since that time, new data have become available, and these have been incorporated into the monograph and taken into consideration in the present evaluation.

1.   Exposure Data

1.1   Chemical and physical data

1.1.1   *Nomenclature*

From IARC (1999) and IPCS-CEC (2002)
Chem. Abstr. Services Reg. No.: 593-60-2
Chem. Abstr. Name: Bromoethene
IUPAC Systematic Name: Bromoethylene
RTECS No.: KU8400000
UN TDG No.: 1085
EC Index No.: 602-024-00-2
EINECS No.: 209-800-6

1.1.2   *Structural and molecular formulae and relative molecular mass*

$$H_2C=CHBr$$

C_2H_3Br Relative molecular mass: 106.96

1.1.3   *Chemical and physical properties of the pure substance*

From IPCS-CEC (2002) and Lide (2005), unless otherwise specified
(a)   *Description*: Colourless gas with a characteristic pungent odour; colourless liquid under pressure
(b)   *Boiling-point*: 15.8 °C

(c)   *Melting-point:* –139.5 °C
(d)   *Density*: 1.522 at 20 °C
(e)   *Solubility*: Insoluble in water; soluble in ethanol, ether, acetone, benzene and chloroform
(f)   *Vapour pressure*: 119 kPa at 20 °C
(g)   *Explosive limits*: Upper, 15%; lower, 9% by volume (National Library of Medicine, 1998)
(h)   *Relative vapor density (air = 1)*: 3.7
(i)   *Relative density (water = 1)*: 1.49
(j)   *Flash-point*: Flammable gas
(k)   *Auto-ignition temperature*: 530 °C
(l)   *Octanol/water partition coefficient*: log P_{ow}, 1.57
(m)   *Conversion factor*: mg/m^3 = 4.37 × ppm[1]

1.1.4   Technical impurities

According to Ethyl Corporation (1980), hydroquinone methyl ether is used as an inhibitor (175–225 mg/kg) in vinyl bromide. Water (max. 100 mg/kg) and non-volatile matter (max. 500 mg/kg including the inhibitor) represent the major impurities.

1.1.5   Analysis

The Occupational Safety and Health Administration (1979) in the USA has developed a method (OSHA Method 8) to measure vinyl bromide with a detection limit of 0.2 ppm.

1.2   Production and use

1.2.1   Production

Vinyl bromide can be produced by the catalytic addition of hydrogen bromide to acetylene in the presence of mercury and copper halide catalysts or by partial dehydro-bromination of ethylene dibromide with alcoholic potassium hydroxide (Ramey & Lini, 1971).

The Hazardous Substance Database indicated only one manufacturer of vinyl bromide in the USA in 2002 (National Toxicology Program, 2005). One plant in China reported a production capacity of 500 million tonnes per year in 2006 (Loyal Gain, 2006).

---

[1] Calculated from mg/m^3 = (molecular weight/24.45) × ppm, assuming normal temperature (25 °C) and pressure (101.3 kPa)

1.2.2   Use

According to a notice in the Federal Register (Anon., 2002), vinyl bromide has been used predominantly in polymers in the production of fabrics and fabric blends that are used in nightwear (mostly for children) and home furnishings, in leather and fabricated metal products and in the production of pharmaceuticals and fumigants. Current applications of vinyl bromide include its use as an intermediate in the synthesis of pharmaceutical products, as a component of fire extinguishers in blends with compounds that contain fluorine, as a monomer in the formation of copolymers that possess flame-retardant properties and as a starting material for the preparation of vinylmagnesium bromide, which is a component of variety of other polymers (Far Research, 2000). According to the Chinese manufacturer Loyal Gain (2006), vinyl bromide is also used in the pharmaceutical industry in the production of the coenzyme Q_{10} and in the synthesis of organic bromo compounds.

1.3   Occurrence

1.3.1   Natural occurrence

Vinyl bromide is not known to occur naturally in the environment.

1.3.2   Occupational exposure

Vinyl bromide has been available commercially since 1968. Occupational exposure may occur during the production of vinyl bromide and its polymers. According to the 1981–83 National Occupational Exposure Survey (NOES, 2002), approximately 1822 workers in the USA were potentially exposed to vinyl bromide (see General Remarks). Exposure to vinyl bromide was considered by CAREX but did not yield many exposed individuals (Kauppinen et al., 2000). Other estimates of the number of workers exposed to vinyl bromide in Europe are available only from the Finnish Register of Occupational Exposure to Carcinogens which reported one individual who was notified as having been exposed to vinyl bromide in 2004 (Saalo et al., 2006).

Median 8-h time-weighted average exposures at a vinyl bromide manufacturing plant ranged from 0.4 to 27.5 mg/m^3, depending on the job and area surveyed. Personal air samples showed that a plant operator was exposed to 0.4–1.7 mg/m^3, a laboratory technician to 1.3–2.2 mg/m^3 and two loading crewmen to 5.2 and 27.5 (1-h samples) mg/m^3 (Bales, 1978; Oser, 1980).

1.3.3   Environmental occurrence

Vinyl bromide may form in the air as a degradation product of 1,2-dibromoethane (IARC, 1999). It may also be released into the environment from facilities that manufacture or use vinyl bromide as a flame retardant for acrylic fibres. Vinyl bromide has been qualitatively identified in ambient air samples (National Library of Medicine, 1998).

1.4   Regulations and guidelines

No international guidelines for vinyl bromide in drinking-water have been established (WHO, 2006). Many countries, regions or organizations have established guideline values for vinyl bromide in the workplace (Table 1).

Table 1.   Guidelines for levels of vinyl bromide in the workplace

Country/region or Organization	TWA	STEL	Carcinogenicity[a]	Notes
Australia	5		2	
Belgium	5			
Canada				
Alberta	0.5			Schedule 2
British Columbia	5		2[a]	ALARA substance
Ontario	0.5			
Quebec	5		A2	
Finland	1			
Ireland	0.5		Ca2	
Malaysia	0.5			
Netherlands	5			
New Zealand	5		A2	
Norway	1		Ca	
South Africa (DOL-RL)	5			
Spain	0.5		Ca2	
USA				
NIOSH (REL)			Ca	LFC
ACGIH	0.5		A2	

From ACGIH® Worldwide (2005)
ACGIH, American Conference of Governmental Industrial Hygienists; ALARA, as low as reasonably achievable; DOL-RL, Department of Labour - recommended limit; LFC, lowest feasible concentration; NIOSH, National Institute of Occupational Safety and Health; REL, recommended exposure limit; STEL, short-term exposure limit; TWA, time-weighted average
[a] 2, probable human carcinogen; 2[a], considered to be carcinogenic to humans; A2, suspected human carcinogen; Ca2, suspected human carcinogen; Ca, potential cancer-causing agent

The United Nations Committee on Transport of Dangerous Goods had classified vinyl bromide as Hazard class 2.1. (IPCS-CEC, 2002; UNTDG, 2005).

The classification expert group of the European Union (REACH) classified vinyl bromide as F+ (extremely flammable), T (toxic), with R (risk) phrases of 45 (causes cancer) and 12 (extremely flammable) and S (safety) phrases of 53 (avoid exposure) and 45 (show label where possible; if you feel unwell, seek medical advice) (IPCS-CEC, 2002; ECB, 2004).

2. Studies of Cancer in Humans

No data were available to the Working Group.

3. Studies of Cancer in Experimental Animals

3.1 Inhalation exposure

Rat

Groups of 120 male and 120 female Sprague-Dawley rats, approximately 9–10 weeks of age, were exposed by inhalation to approximately 44, 220, 1100 or 5500 mg/m^3 ± 5% [10, 50, 250 or 1250 ppm ± 5%] vinyl bromide (purity ≥ 99.9%) for 6 h per day on 5 days per week for 104 weeks. A group of 144 males and 144 females served as untreated controls. The animals in the highest-dose group were killed at 72 weeks because of 50–60% mortality. Statistical significance was assessed by the χ^2 test. Tumour incidences in rats exposed to vinyl bromide are summarized in Table 2. Treatment-related increases in the incidence of liver angiosarcomas were observed in all exposed groups: males — 0/144 controls, 7/120 at 10 ppm ($p < 0.025$), 36/120 at 50 ppm ($p < 0.001$), 61/120 at 250 ppm ($p < 0.001$) and 43/120 at 1250 ppm ($p < 0.001$); females — 1/144, 10/120, 50/120, 61/120 and 41/120, respectively ($p < 0.01$ for all exposed groups). An increased incidence of Zymbal gland squamous-cell carcinomas also occurred in both sexes of exposed rats: males — 2/142 controls, 1/99 at 10 ppm, 1/112 at 50 ppm, 13/114 at 250 ppm ($p < 0.005$) and 35/116 at 1250 ppm ($p < 0.005$); females — 0/139, 0/99, 3/113, 2/119 and 11/114 ($p < 0.001$), respectively. Hepatic neoplastic nodules [hepatocellular adenomas] and hepatocellular carcinomas were also observed, the incidence of which was significantly increased in some but not all treatment groups. The incidence of benign and malignant hepatocellular liver tumours combined as 4/143 control, and 5/103, 10/119, 13/120 ($p < 0.025$) and 5/119 males treated with successively higher exposure levels; and 7/142 control, and 18/101 ($p < 0.005$), 12/113, 21/118 ($p < 0.005$) and 9/112 females, respectively. Failure of the highest dose to increase the incidence of hepatocellular tumours was most probably a consequence of the reduced survival and early termination of these animals. No exposure-related increased incidence of brain tumours was observed (Benya *et al.*, 1982).

Table 2.   Tumour incidence in rats exposed to vinyl bromide by inhalation for up to 104 weeks

Tumour type	Rats with tumour/no. examined				
	Concentration (ppm) [mg/m³]				
	0	10 [44]	50 [220]	250 [1100]	1250 [5500]
Males					
Liver					
Angiosarcoma	0/144	7/120[a]	36/120[b]	61/120[b]	43/120[b]
Neoplastic nodules and hepatocellular carcinoma	4/143	5/103	10/119	13/120[a]	5/119
Hepatocellular carcinoma	3/143	1/103	7/119	9/120	3/119
Zymbal gland					
Squamous-cell carcinoma	2/142	1/99	1/112	13/114	35/116[c]
Females					
Liver					
Angiosarcoma	1/144	10/120[d]	50/120[b]	61/120[b]	41/120[b]
Neoplastic nodules and hepatocellular carcinoma	7/142	18/101[c]	12/113	21/118[c]	9/112
Hepatocellular carcinoma	4/142	6/101	3/113	11/118[e]	4/112
Zymbal gland					
Squamous-cell carcinoma	0/139	0/99	3/113	2/119	11/114[b]

Adapted from Benya *et al.* (1982)
Statistical evaluation by χ^2 test
[a] $p < 0.025$
[b] $p < 0.001$
[c] $p < 0.005$
[d] $p < 0.01$
[e] $p < 0.05$

3.2   Dermal exposure

Mouse

A group of 30 female ICR/Ha Swiss mice [age unspecified] received dermal applications of 15 mg vinyl bromide [purity unspecified] in 0.1 mL acetone three times a week for 60 weeks. No skin tumours were observed. In a two-stage skin carcinogenesis study, groups of 30 female ICR/Ha Swiss mice received a single dermal application of 15 mg vinyl bromide in 0.1 mL acetone, followed by thrice-weekly applications of 2.5 µg of 12-*O*- tetradecanoylphorbol-13-acetate (TPA) in 0.1 mL acetone for 60 weeks. Additional groups of mice received TPA alone or no treatment. One of 30 mice treated with vinyl bromide followed by TPA had a skin papilloma at 412 days, and one of 30 mice treated with TPA alone had a skin carcinoma at 44 days. No tumours were found in 160 untreated mice. Systemic carcinogenesis was not assessed (Van Duuren, 1977). [The Working Group noted that the volatility of vinyl bromide would have led to very low doses in these studies of dermal application.]

3.3   Subcutaneous administration

Mouse

Groups of 30 female ICR/Ha Swiss mice [age unspecified] received weekly subcutaneous injections of 0 or 25 mg vinyl bromide [purity unspecified] in 0.05 mL trioctanoin for 48 weeks and were observed for up to 420 days. No tumours were reported in vinyl bromide-treated mice or in vehicle or in 60 untreated controls. Systemic carcinogenesis was not assessed (Van Duuren, 1977).

4.   Mechanistic and Other Relevant Data

4.1   Absorption, distribution, metabolism and excretion

4.1.1   *Humans*

No data were available to the Working Group.

4.1.2   *Experimental systems*

The limited available data on absorption, distribution, metabolism and excretion of vinyl bromide in experimental systems have been reviewed previously (IARC, 1986, 1999). The following section summarizes the salient features of the studies that were reviewed at that time, as well as significant new information on the metabolism and pharmacokinetics of vinyl bromide in experimental animals.

Vinyl bromide is readily absorbed upon inhalation by rats (IARC, 1986). The blood:air partition coefficient of vinyl bromide in rats is 4.05, which is about 2.5-fold and fivefold greater than the values for vinyl chloride and vinyl fluoride, respectively (Cantoreggi & Keller, 1997). Similarly, the tissue solubility (particularly the affinity for adipose tissues) and the volume of distribution of vinyl bromide are greater than those for vinyl chloride and vinyl fluoride (Cantoreggi & Keller, 1997).

Vinyl bromide is metabolized in a similar manner to vinyl chloride and vinyl fluoride, and it is a substrate for human cytochrome P450 (CYP) 2E1. Guengerich *et al.* (1991) reported that the rate of metabolism of vinyl bromide was identical to that of vinyl chloride (0.027 nmol/min.nmol CYP), using purified human liver CYP2E1. In this study, the in-vitro formation of $1,N^6$-ethenoadenosine that resulted from bromoethylene oxide was also demonstrated (Guengerich *et al.*, 1991). Bromoethylene oxide can be deactivated by epoxide hydrolase and glutathione-*S*-transferases, or can re-arrange to bromoacetaldehyde (National Toxicology Program, 1999).

The metabolism of vinyl bromide in rats is saturable at exposure concentrations greater than 235 mg/m^3 [55 ppm] (Filser & Bolt, 1979). Following inhalation of vinyl bromide by rats, rabbits and monkeys, plasma levels of non-volatile bromide increased with duration of exposure, and were formed more rapidly in hepatic CYP-induced rats (IARC, 1986).

In rats, the conversion of vinyl bromide to reactive metabolites occurs primarily in hepatocytes. Irreversible binding of such metabolites to proteins and RNA has been established with rat liver microsomes *in vitro* as well as in rats *in vivo* (Bolt *et al.*, 1980). These metabolites can also alkylate the CYP prosthetic group of phenobarbital-treated rat liver microsomes. Further, the exposure of rats to high concentrations of vinyl bromide has been shown to cause a decrease in hepatic CYP (IARC, 1986).

4.2   Genetic and related effects

4.2.1   *Humans*

No data were available to the Working Group.

4.2.2   *Experimental systems*

(a)   *DNA adducts*

Vinyl bromide metabolites bind covalently to DNA and proteins; 2-bromoethylene oxide is the major DNA-binding moiety and 2-bromoacetaldehyde is the major protein-binding metabolite (Guengerich *et al.*, 1981). The major adduct that results from exposure to vinyl bromide is *N*-7-(2-oxoethyl)guanosine (Bolt *et al.*, 1981). Bromoacetaldehyde and bromoethylene oxide can react with adenine or cytosine bases to produce the cyclic etheno adducts 1,*N*^{6}-ethenoadenosine and 3,*N*^{4}-ethenocytosine, which can cause mis-coding by modifying base-pairing sites (Bolt, 1988). Cyclic etheno adducts have a longer half-life than *N*-7-(2-oxoethyl)guanine and, therefore, may have a greater potential to accumulate with long-term exposure (Swenberg *et al.*, 1992).

(b)   *Mutations and other related effects*

Vinyl bromide has been shown to be mutagenic in *Salmonella typhimurium* (Lijinsky & Andrews, 1980) and in a recessive lethal mutation test with post-meiotic male germ cells of *Drosophila melanogaster* (Ballering *et al.* 1996). Two GC→AT transitions, five GC→TA and four AT→TA transversions were observed (Ballering *et al.*, 1997; Nivard & Vogel, 1999).

The comet assay was used to assess the genotoxicity of vinyl bromide in the stomach, liver, kidney, bladder, lung, brain and bone marrow of male CD-1 mice. The compound (at 2000 mg/kg bw) induced statistically significant DNA damage in all organs except the bone marrow (Sasaki *et al.*, 1998).

4.3 Mechanisms of carcinogenesis

The metabolism of vinyl bromide is similar to that of vinyl chloride and vinyl fluoride. Vinyl bromide is metabolized to bromoethylene oxide and bromoacetaldehyde by human CYP2E1. In-vitro studies have shown that these intermediates, in the presence of adenosine, form $1,N^6$-ethenoadenosine. The same promutagenic adduct is formed with chloroethylene oxide, the primary intermediate of vinyl chloride metabolism. It is one of the adducts that are implicated in the mutagenicity and carcinogenicity of vinyl chloride.

5. Summary of Data Reported

5.1 Exposure data

Vinyl bromide is a flammable gas that is produced in a limited number of countries. It is used predominantly for the manufacture of polyvinyl bromide and to a smaller extent as a flame retardant in a large variety of industrial and consumer products. Workers may be exposed during the manufacture of vinyl bromide monomer and during production of the polymer.

5.2 Cancer in humans

No data were available to the Working Group.

5.3 Cancer in experimental animals

In a study of inhalation exposure in both sexes of rats, vinyl bromide caused a significant increase in the incidence of angiosarcomas of the liver, hepatocellular adenomas and carcinomas, and squamous-cell carcinomas of the Zymbal gland.

In limited studies in female mice, vinyl bromide neither induced nor initiated skin tumours after dermal application and did not cause injection-site tumours after repeated subcutaneous injection.

5.4 Mechanistic and other relevant data

Vinyl bromide is readily absorbed upon inhalation. It is a substrate for human cytochrome P450 2E1 and is metabolized by this enzyme in a manner similar to that of vinyl chloride and vinyl fluoride. A study in rats has shown that the metabolism of vinyl bromide is saturable at exposure concentrations greater than 55 ppm (~240 mg/m^3).

Bromoethylene oxide and bromoacetaldehyde are known metabolites of vinyl bromide that can form DNA adducts that are similar to those formed by metabolites of vinyl chloride. These include *N*7-(2-oxoethyl)guanosine (the major adduct) and the cyclic adducts, ethenodeoxyadenosine and ethenodeoxycytidine, which can cause miscoding by modifying base-pairing sites. Vinyl bromide caused DNA damage in mice treated *in vivo*, and has been shown to be mutagenic in bacteria and in *Drosophila*.

6.   Evaluation and Rationale

6.1   Carcinogenicity in humans

There is *inadequate evidence* in humans for the carcinogenicity of vinyl bromide.

6.2   Carcinogenicity in experimental animals

There is *sufficient evidence* in experimental animals for the carcinogenicity of vinyl bromide.

6.3   Overall evaluation

Vinyl bromide is *probably carcinogenic to humans (Group 2A)*.

6.4   Rationale

In making the overall evaluation, the Working Group took into consideration the fact that all available studies showed a consistently parallel response between vinyl bromide and vinyl chloride. In addition, both vinyl chloride and vinyl bromide are activated via a human cytochrome P450 2E1-dependent pathway to their corresponding epoxides. For both vinyl chloride and vinyl bromide, the covalent binding of these compounds to nucleosides/DNA yields pro-mutagenic etheno adducts. The weight of positive evidence for both compounds was also noted among the studies for genotoxicity, although the number and variety of tests for vinyl bromide were fewer. For practical purposes, vinyl bromide should be considered to act similarly to the human carcinogen, vinyl chloride.

7.   References

ACGIH® Worldwide (2005) *Documentation of the TLVs® and BEIs® with Other Worldwide Occupational Exposure Values — 2005 CD-ROM*, Cincinnati, OH, American Conference of Government Industrial Hygienists

Anon. (2002) Notices pages. *Fed. Regist.*, **67**, 77283–77285

Bales (1978) *Vinyl Fluoride and Vinyl Bromide Industrial Hygiene Survey Report* (DHEW (NIOSH) Pub. No. 79-111; US NTIS PS80-190150), Cincinnati, OH, National Institute for Occupational Safety and Health

Ballering, L.A., Nivard, M.J. & Vogel, E.W. (1996) Characterization by two-endpoint comparisons of the genetic toxicity profiles of vinyl chloride and related etheno-adduct forming carcinogens in Drosophila. *Carcinogenesis*, **17**, 1083–1092

Ballering, L.A., Nivard, M.J. & Vogel, E.W. (1997) Preferential formation of deletions following in vivo exposure of postmeiotic Drosophila germ cells to the DNA etheno-adduct-forming carcinogen vinyl carbamate. *Environ. mol. Mutag.*, **30**, 321–329

Benya, T.J., Busey, W.M., Dorato, M.A. & Berteau, P.E. (1982) Inhalation carcinogenicity bioassay of vinyl bromide in rats. *Toxicol. appl. Pharmacol.*, **64**, 367–379

Bolt, H.M. (1988) Roles of etheno-DNA adducts in tumorigenicity of olefins. *Crit. Rev. Toxicol.*, **18**, 299–309

Bolt, H.M., Filser, J.G., Laib, R.J. & Ottenwalder, H. (1980) Binding kinetics of vinyl chloride and vinyl bromide at very low doses. *Arch. Toxicol.*, **Suppl**. **3**, 129–142

Bolt, H.M., Filser, J.G. & Laib, R.J. (1981) Covalent binding of haloethylenes. *Adv. exp. Med. Biol.*, **136**, 667–683

Cantoreggi, S. & Keller, D.A. (1997) Pharmacokinetics and metabolism of vinyl fluoride in vivo and in vitro. *Toxicol. appl. Pharmacol.*, **143**, 130–139

ECB (2004) *Annex I to Directive 67/548/EEC on Classification and Labelling of Dangerous Substances, Classification and Labelling*, European Chemicals Bureau [available at: http://ecb.jrc.it/classification-labelling/search-classlab; accessed 14.10.2007]

Ethyl Corporation (1980) *Ethyl Bromide* (Technical Bulletin IC-74), Baton Rouge, LA

Far Research (2000) *Product Profile — Vinyl Bromide, CAS 593-60-2*, Palm Bay, FL, USA

Filser, J.G. & Bolt, H.M. (1979) Pharmacokinetics of halogenated ethylenes in rats. *Arch. Toxicol.*, **42**, 123–136

Guengerich, F.P., Mason, P.S., Stott, W.T., Fox, T.R. & Watanabe, P.G. (1981) Roles of 2-halo-ethylene oxides and 2-haloacetaldehydes derived from vinyl bromide and vinyl chloride in irreversible binding to protein and DNA. *Cancer Res.*, **41**, 4391–4398

Guengerich, F.P., Kim, D.H. & Iwasaki, M. (1991) Role of human cytochrome P-450 IIE1 in the oxidation of many low molecular weight cancer suspects. *Chem. Res. Toxicol.*, **4**, 168–179

IARC (1979) *IARC Monographs on the Evaluation of the Carcinogenic Risk of Chemicals to Humans*, Vol. 19, *Some Monomers, Plastics and Synthetic Elastomers, and Acrolein*, Lyon, pp. 367–375

IARC (1986) *IARC Monographs on the Evaluation of the Carcinogenic Risk of Chemicals to Humans*, Vol. 39, *Some Chemicals Used in Plastics and Elastomers*, Lyon, pp. 133–145

IARC (1987) *IARC Monographs on the Evaluation of Carcinogenic Risks to Humans*, Suppl. 7, *Overall Evaluations of Carcinogenicity: An Updating of* IARC Monographs *Volumes 1 to 42*, Lyon, p. 73

IARC (1999) *IARC Monographs on the Evaluation of Carcinogenic Risks to Humans*, Vol. 71, *Re-evaluation of Some Organic Chemicals, Hydrazine and Hydrogen Peroxide*, Lyon, pp. 923–928

IPCS-CEC (2002) *International Chemical Safety Cards, Vinyl Bromide ICSC 0597*, Geneva, World Health Organization

Kauppinen, T., Toikkanen, J., Pedersen, D., Young, R., Ahrens, W., Boffetta, P., Hansen, J., Kromhout, H., Maqueda Blasco, J., Mirabelli, D., de la Orden-Rivera, V., Pannett, B., Plato, N., Savela, A., Vincent, R. & Kogevinas, M. (2000) Occupational exposure to carcinogens in the European Union. *Occup. environ. Med.*, **57**, 10–18

Lide, D.R., ed. (2005) *CRC Handbook of Chemistry and Physics*, 86th Ed., Boca Raton, FL, CRC Press

Lijinsky, W. & Andrews, A.W. (1980) Mutagenicity of vinyl compounds in Salmonella typhimurium. *Teratog. Carcinog. Mutag.*, **1**, 259–267

Loyal Gain (2006) *Loyal Gain Enterprise Limited, Products, Organic Chemicals* [available at: http://www.loyalgain.cn/product/Organic.htm; accessed 14.10.2007]

National Library of Medicine (1998) *Hazardous Substances Data Bank (HSDB) Database*, Bethesda, MD [Record No. 1030]

National Toxicology Program (1999) *Report on Carcinogens, Background Documents for Vinyl Bromide*, Research Triangle Park, NC

National Toxicology Program (2005) *Report on Carcinogens*, 11th Ed., Research Triangle Park, NC [available at http://ntp.niehs.nih.gov/ntp/roc/eleventh/profiles/s185viny.pdf, accessed 14.10.2007]

Nivard, M.J. & Vogel, E.W. (1999) Genetic effects of exocyclic DNA adducts in vivo: Heritable genetic damage in comparison with loss of heterozygosity in somatic cells. In: Singer, B. & Bartsch, H., eds, *Exocyclic DNA Adducts in Mutagenesis and Carcinogenesis* (IARC Scientific Publications No.150), 335–349

NOES (2002) *National Occupational Exposure Survey 1981-83*, National Institute for Occupational Safety and Health, Cincinnati, OH [available at http://www.cdc.gov/noes/noes2/84575occ.html, accessed 14.10.2007]

Occupational Safety and Health Administration (1979) *Vinyl Bromide, Organic, Method 8.* [available at http://www.osha.gov/dts/sltc/methods/organic/org008/org008.html, accessed 17.10.2007]

Oser, J.L. (1980) Extent of industrial exposure to epichlorohydrin, vinyl fluoride, vinyl bromide and ethylene dibromide. *Am. ind. Hyg. Assoc. J.*, **41**, 463–468

Ramey, K.C. & Lini, D.C. (1971) Vinyl bromide polymers. In: Bikales, N.M., ed., *Encyclopedia of Polymer Science and Technology*, Vol. 14, New York, Wiley Interscience, pp. 273–281

Saalo, A., Soosaar, A., Vuorela, R. & Kauppinen, T. (2006) [ASA 2004], Helsinki, Finnish Institute of Occupational Health [available at: http://www.ttl.fi/NR/rdonlyres/5A54A452-7350-4255-8DF3-AF632D9D2775/0/ASA 2004.pdf] (in Finnish)

Sasaki, Y.F., Saga, A., Akasaka, M., Ishibashi, S., Yoshida, K., Su, Y.Q., Matsusaka, N. & Tsuda, S. (1998) Detection of in vivo genotoxicity of haloalkanes and haloalkenes carcinogenic to rodents by the alkaline single cell gel electrophoresis (comet) assay in multiple mouse organs. *Mutat Res.*, **419**, 13–20

Swenberg, J.A., Fedtke, N., Ciroussel, F., Barbin, A. & Bartsch, H. (1992) Etheno adducts formed in DNA of vinyl chloride-exposed rats are highly persistent in liver. *Carcinogenesis*, **13**, 727–729

UNTDG (United Nations Committee on Transport of Dangerous Goods) (2005) *Guide 116 – Gases – Flammable (Unstable)*, New York, pp. 196–197

Van Duuren, B.L. (1977) Chemical structure, reactivity, and carcinogenicity of halohydrocarbons. *Environ. Health Perspect.*, **21**, 17–23

WHO (2006) *Guidelines for Drinking Water Quality*, Vol. 1, *Recommendations*, First addendum to 3rd Ed., Geneva

VINYL FLUORIDE

This substance was considered by a previous Working Group in February 1995 (IARC, 1995). Since that time, new data have become available, and these have been incorporated into the monograph and taken into consideration in the present evaluation.

1. Exposure Data

1.1 Chemical and physical data

1.1.1 *Nomenclature*

From IARC (1995) and IPCS-CEC (1997)
Chem. Abstr. Serv. Reg. No.: 75-02-5
Chem. Abstr. Name: Fluoroethene
IUPAC Systematic Name: Fluoroethylene
Synonyms: 1-Fluoroethene; 1-fluoroethylene; monofluoroethene; monofluoroethylene
RTECS No.: YZ7351000
UN TDG No.: 1860 (stabilized)
EINECS No.: 200-832-6

1.1.2 *Structural and molecular formulae and relative molecular mass*

$$ \begin{array}{ccc} H & & H \\ \diagdown & & \diagup \\ & C=C & \\ \diagup & & \diagdown \\ H & & F \end{array} $$

C2H3F   Relative molecular mass: 46.04

1.1.3 *Chemical and physical properties of the pure substance*

From IARC (1995), IPCS-CEC (1997), Ebnesajjad (2001) and Lide (2005), unless otherwise specified

(a) *Description*: Compressed liquefied gas with characteristic odour; may travel along the ground; distant ignition possible

(b) *Boiling-point*: –72.2 °C

(c) *Melting-point*: –160.5 °C

(d) *Spectroscopy data*: Infrared (prism [30864]; grating [48458P]) and mass [15] spectral data have been reported.

(e) *Solubility*: Slightly soluble in water (15.4 g/L at 6.9 MPa)

(f) *Vapour pressure*: 370 psi [2.553 MPa] at 21 °C

(g) *Relative vapour density (air = 1)*: 1.6

(h) *Reactivity*: Reacts with alkali and alkaline earth metals, powdered aluminium, zinc and beryllium.

(i) *Density:* 0.636 at 21 °C

(j) *Stability in water:* The HYDROWIN Program (v1.67) cannot estimate a hydrolysis rate constant for this chemical structure; volatilization is a major fate process for vinyl fluoride in water; volatilization half-lives of 2 and 23.5 h have been estimated for a model river (1 m deep) and a model pond (2 m deep), respectively (Lyman *et al.*, 1990).

(k) *Octanol/water partition coefficient:* log P_{ow}, 1.19 (Meylan & Howard, 1995)

(l) *Flash-point:* Flammable gas

(m) *Auto-ignition temperature:* 385 °C

(n) *Explosive limits (vol. %) in air:* 2.6–21.7

(o) *Chemical danger:* The substance may polymerize freely; it decomposes on heating to produce hydrogen fluoride.

(p) *Conversion factor:* mg/m^3 = 1.88 × ppm[1]

1.1.4   *Technical products and impurities*

Vinyl fluoride is available commercially at a purity of 99.9%; 0.1% *d*-limonene (see IARC, 1993) is added as a stabilizer (IARC, 1995).

1.1.5   *Analysis*

Vinyl fluoride has been determined in workplace air collected in poly(tetra-fluoroethylene) bags and analysed by gas chromatography (Oser, 1980). Non-specific methods that involve fluorescence spectrophotometry and chemiluminescence have been reported (Quickert *et al.*, 1975; Sutton *et al.*, 1979).

---

[1] Calculated from: mg/m^3 = (relative molecular mass/24.45) × ppm, assuming normal temperature (25 °C) and pressure (101.3 kPa)

1.2   Production and use

1.2.1   *Production*

Vinyl fluoride was first prepared by the reaction of 1,1-difluoro-2-bromoethane with zinc. Most approaches to vinyl fluoride synthesis have employed reactions of acetylene with hydrogen fluoride either directly or utilizing catalysts. Other routes have involved ethylene and hydrogen fluoride, pyrolysis of 1,1-difluoroethane and fluorochloroethanes, reaction of 1,1-difluoroethane with acetylene and halogen exchange of vinyl chloride with hydrogen fluoride (Siegmund *et al.*, 1988; Ebnesajjad, 2001).

Use of vinyl fluoride in the Member States of the European Union in 1991 was estimated to be about 3600 tonnes (Environmental Chemicals Data and Information Network, 1993). In 1994, vinyl fluoride was produced by one company each in Japan and the USA (Chemical Information Services, 1994). Annual production in the USA was above one million pounds [454 000 kg] in 1990 and approximately 3.3 millions pounds [1.5 million kg] in 2001 (National Toxicology Program, 2005).

1.2.2   *Use*

Since the 1960s, vinyl fluoride has mainly been used in the production of polyvinyl fluoride (PVF) and other fluoropolymers. PVF homopolymers and copolymers have excellent resistance to degradation by sunlight, chemical attack, water absorption and solvents, and have a high solar energy transmittance rate. These properties have resulted in the utilization of PVF film and coating in outdoor and indoor functional and decorative applications. These films have found use where thermal stability, outdoor durability, stain resistance, adherence and release properties are required (Ebnesajjad, 2001).

PVF is converted to a thin film by plasticized melt extrusion and is sold under the trade marks Tedlar PVF film and Dalvor. The growing market for solar panels has increased the demand for photovoltaic materials such as Tedlar and has forced the manu-facturer to boost its production of vinyl fluoride (Dupont, 2007).

1.3   Occurrence

1.3.1   *Natural occurrence*

Vinyl fluoride is not known to occur as a natural product.

1.3.2   *Occupational exposure*

No estimates of the number of workers exposed to vinyl fluoride are available.

The concentration of vinyl fluoride in air was determined at a manufacturing and at a polymerization plant in the USA. The concentrations in eight samples taken at the manufacturing plant were generally < 2 ppm [3.76 mg/m^3], but a level of 21 ppm

[39.5 mg/m^3] was reported in one personal sample. The concentrations in seven personal samples taken in the polymerization plant were 1–4 ppm [1.88–7.52 mg/m^3] and those in four general area samples were 1–5 ppm [1.88–9.4 mg/m^3] (Oser, 1980).

1.3.3 *Environmental exposure*

No data were available to the Working Group on environmental exposure to vinyl fluoride.

1.4   Regulations and guidelines

Table 1 presents the few guidelines that are available for the workplace in various countries, regions or organizations.

Table 1.   Guidelines for levels of vinyl fluoride in the workplace

Country/region or Organizations	TWA (ppm)	STEL (ppm)	Carcinogenicity	Notes
Canada				
Alberta	1			
Ontario	1			
Ireland	1			
Japan-JSOH			2A	
New Zealand			A2	
USA				
NIOSH REL	1	5 (ceiling)		
ACGIH TLV	1		A2	

From ACGIH® Worldwide (2005)
2A/A2, suspected human carcinogen; ACGIH, American Conference of Governmental Industrial Hygienists; JSOH, Japanese Society of Occupational Health; NIOSH, National Institute of Occupational Safety and Health; REL, recommended exposure limit; STEL, short-term exposure limit; TLV, threshold limit value; TWA, time-weighted average

2.   Studies of Cancer in Humans

No data were available to the Working Group.

3. Studies of Cancer in Experimental Animals

3.1 Inhalation exposure

3.1.1 *Mouse*

Groups of 80 or 81 male and 80 or 81 female Crl:CD-1(ICR)BR mice, approximately 47 days of age, were exposed by inhalation to 0, 25, 250 or 2500 ppm [0, 47, 470 or 4700 mg/m³] vinyl fluoride (purity > 99.94%) for 6 h per day on 5 days per week for up to 18 months. Animals in the 250- and 2500-ppm groups were killed when survival of the groups reached approximately 25% (after 375 and 450 days for high-dose males and females and 412 and 459 days for mid-dose males and females, respectively). Surviving control and low-dose mice of each sex were killed at the scheduled termination of the study at 18 months. The survival rates for the control and low-dose groups were 58% and 22%, respectively, for both sexes. All organs of control and high-dose animals were examined microscopically; only nose, lungs, liver, kidneys, gross lesions and target organs of animals in all other groups underwent microscopic evaluation. The mice were evaluated after necropsy at intervals of 0–6 and 7–18 months. Statistical analyses of the overall tumour incidence were not conducted because of the varying durations of exposure to vinyl fluoride. An early, significant increase in the incidence of lung tumours (bronchioalveolar adenomas) was observed in males in the 250- and 2500-ppm groups and in females in the 2500-ppm group that were killed at 6 months ($p < 0.05$). The overall incidence of primary lung tumours (alveolar-bronchiolar adenomas and adeno-carcinomas) in males was 11/81 controls, 45/80 at 25 ppm, 52/80 at 250 ppm and 56/81 at 2500 ppm and that in females was 9/81 (controls), 24/80 at 25 ppm, 47/80 at 250 ppm and 53/81 at 2500 ppm. Hepatic angiosarcomas occurred in 1/81 control, 16/80 low-dose, 42/80 mid-dose and 42/81 high-dose males and in 0/81 control, 13/81 low-dose, 25/80 mid-dose and 32/81 high-dose females. Mammary gland adenocarcinomas were seen only in female mice that were necropsied between 7 and 18 months of observation and occurred in 0/62 controls and 22/60, 20/65 and 19/64 animals exposed to 25, 250 and 250 ppm, respectively. Two fibroadenomas and one mammary adenoma also occurred in the high-dose group. The incidence of Harderian gland adenomas was increased in both sexes of exposed animals that survived beyond 6 months. The incidence in males was 3/66 controls and 13/68, 12/66 and 31/62 mice exposed to 25, 250 and 2500 ppm, respectively; in females, the incidence was 1/64 controls and 7/61, 6/66 and 12/66 mice exposed to increasing concentrations of vinyl fluoride, respectively. No carcinomas of the Harderian gland were seen. The overall (aggregate) incidence of tumours in the lungs, liver (haemangiosarcomas and hepatocellular tumours), Harderian gland and mammary gland is summarized in Table 2. Although the incidence of hepatocellular adenomas was not dose-dependent, the decreased tumour latency, increased multiplicity and associated increase in putatively preneoplastic basophilic foci led to the conclusion that the tumours observed in males in the 25 ppm-treated group were related to exposure to vinyl fluoride (Bogdanffy *et al.*, 1995).

Table 2. Incidence of primary tumours of the liver, lung, mammary gland and Harderian gland in mice exposed to vinyl fluoride by inhalation for up to 18 months

Tumour type	Tumour-bearing mice/no. examined			
	Concentration (ppm) [mg/m³]			
	0	25 [47]	250 [470]	2500 [4700]
Males				
Liver				
Haemangiosarcoma	1/81	16/80	42/80	42/81
Hepatocellular adenoma	7/81	15/80	5/80	3/81
Hepatocellular carcinoma	2/81	2/80	1/80	0/81
Lung				
Primary lung tumour	11/81	45/80	52/80	56/81
Bronchioalveolar adenoma	11/81	45/80	52/80	56/81
Bronchioalveolar adenocarcinoma	1/81	1/80	4/80	4/81
Harderian gland adenoma	3/81	13/80	12/80	31/81
Females				
Liver				
Haemangiosarcoma	0/81	13/80	25/80	32/81
Hepatocellular adenoma	0/81	0/81	1/80	0/81
Lung				
Primary lung tumour	9/81	24/80	47/80	53/81
Bronchioalveolar adenoma	9/81	24/80	47/80	53/81
Bronchioalveolar adenocarcinoma	0/81	1/80	1/80	3/81
Mammary gland				
Adenocarcinoma	0/81	22/81	20/80	19/81
Harderian gland adenoma	1/81	7/81	6/80	12/81

From Bogdanffy *et al.* (1995)

3.1.2   *Rat*

Groups of 95 male and 95 female Sprague-Dawley (Crl:CD®BR) rats, approximately 40 days of age, were exposed by inhalation to 0, 25, 250 or 2500 ppm [0, 47, 470 or 4700 mg/m³] vinyl fluoride (purity > 99.94%) for 6 h per day on 5 days per week for up to 2 years. Ten rats per group were killed on test days 275 and 276 for interim examination. Because of high mortality, rats in the 250- and 2500-ppm groups were killed when the percentage of surviving animals in each group reached approximately 25% (657 days and 586 days for all surviving animals in the 250-and 2500-ppm groups, respectively). All surviving control and low-dose animals were killed at the scheduled termination of the study (2 years). The survival rates for control and low-dose groups at the end of the study were 25% and 20% (males) and 25% and 15% (females), respectively. The rats were evaluated after necropsy at intervals of 0–12, 13–18 and 19–24 months. Statistical analyses of the overall tumour incidence were not conducted because of the varying durations of exposure to vinyl fluoride. An early appearance of liver and Zymbal gland tumours was observed at the 12-month evaluation. Exposure of the rats to vinyl fluoride for up to 2 years caused an increase in the incidence of haemangiosarcomas of the liver and Zymbal gland carcinomas in males and females and hepatocellular adenomas and carcinomas in females. The overall incidence of tumours in rats exposed to vinyl fluoride for up to 2 years is summarized in Table 3 (Bogdanffy *et al.*, 1995).

Table 3. Incidence of primary tumours of the liver and Zymbal gland in rats exposed to vinyl fluoride by inhalation for up to 2 years

Tumour type	Tumour-bearing rats/no. examined			
	Concentration (ppm) [mg/m^3]			
	0	25 [47]	250 [470]	2500 [4700]
Males				
Liver				
Haemangiosarcoma	0/80	5/80	30/80	20/80
Hepatocellular adenoma	1/80	4/80	4/80	4/80
Hepatocellular carcinoma	4/80	6/80	6/80	3/80
Zymbal gland				
Carcinoma, sebaceous/squamous-cell	0/80	2/80	3/80	11/80
Females				
Liver				
Haemangiosarcoma	0/80	8/80	19/80	15/80
Hepatocellular adenoma	0/80	4/80	9/80	5/80
Hepatocellular carcinoma	0/80	0/80	0/80	3/80
Zymbal gland				
Carcinoma, sebaceous/squamous-cell	0/80	0/80	1/80	12/80

From Bogdanffy *et al.* (1995)

4. Mechanistic and Other Relevant Data

4.1 Absorption, distribution, metabolism and excretion

4.1.1 *Humans*

No data were available to the Working Group.

4.1.2   *Experimental systems*

The limited available data on the absorption, distribution, metabolism and excretion of vinyl fluoride in experimental systems have been reviewed previously (IARC, 1995). The following section summarizes the salient features of the studies reviewed at that time, as well as significant new information on the metabolism and pharmacokinetics of vinyl fluoride in experimental animals.

Vinyl fluoride is readily absorbed after inhalation (Filser & Bolt, 1979, 1981). The very low solubility of vinyl fluoride in tissues and blood suggests that it rapidly equilibrates within the body during inhalation exposures. The low blood:air and tissue:air partition coefficients (0.54–1.82 in rats) indicate a low volume of distribution for vinyl fluoride. Moreover, a fat:blood partition coefficient of 2.4 for this chemical indicates that it is unlikely to be stored to a significant extent in the adipose tissues (Cantoreggi & Keller, 1997).

The metabolic pathways of vinyl fluoride are thought to be similar to those of vinyl chloride and vinyl bromide (National Toxicology Program, 1999). The initial oxidation of vinyl fluoride results in the formation of fluoroethylene oxide and is probably mediated by cytochrome P450 (CYP) 2E1, as indicated by the inhibition of the metabolism of vinyl fluoride by 4-methylpyrazole (Cantoreggi & Keller, 1997). Vinyl fluoride, similarly to vinyl chloride, is shown to mediate in-vitro nicotinamide adenine dinucleotide phosphate-dependent inactivation of CYP (Ortiz de Montellano *et al.*, 1982).

In-vitro studies with human liver microsomes indicated that the apparent affinity for the metabolism of vinyl fluoride (Michaelis-Menten constant, 0.5 μM) and the maximum velocity (0.57–3.3 nmol/h/mg protein) were in the same range as those found in rodents (Cantoreggi & Keller 1997). However, considerable interindividual variation in maximum velocity (sixfold) was observed in 10 human samples (Cantoreggi & Keller, 1997).

The saturation of vinyl fluoride metabolism occurs at about 75 ppm [143 mg/m^3] in rats (Filser & Bolt, 1979). Both in-vitro and in-vivo metabolism studies indicated that the rate of metabolism of vinyl fluoride is about three times greater in mice than in rats (3.5 versus 1.1 nmol/h/mg protein) (Cantoreggi & Keller, 1997). Pharmacokinetic data also indicate that the rate of biotransformation of vinyl fluoride in rats is about one-fifth that of vinyl chloride (Filser & Bolt, 1979). Administration of vinyl fluoride to rats results in increased exhalation of acetone, which implies an inhibition of Krebs cycle by the fluoroacetate that results from vinyl fluoride metabolism (Filser *et al.*, 1982).

Fluoride appears to be a metabolite of vinyl fluoride since it is found in the urine of rats 6 days after exposure. The concentrations of fluoride in the urine of rats were found to be increased 45 and 90 days after exposure by inhalation to 200 or 2000 ppm [382 or 3820 mg/m^3] vinyl fluoride for 6 h per day on 5 days per week for about 90 days. A plateau was observed at about 2000 ppm [3820 mg/m^3], which suggests saturation of vinyl fluoride metabolism (Bogdanffy *et al.*, 1990). When rats and mice were exposed to 0, 25, 250 or 2500 ppm [0, 47, 470 or 4700 mg/m^3] vinyl fluoride for 18 months, a plateau of urinary excretion of fluoride was seen at ≥ 250 ppm (Bogdanffy *et al.*, 1995).

4.2   Genetic and related effects

4.2.1   *Humans*

No data were available to the Working Group.

4.2.1   *Experimental systems*

(a)   *DNA adducts*

Vinyl fluoride metabolites form covalent DNA adducts that are similar to those formed by metabolites of vinyl chloride. These include $N7$-(2′-oxoethyl)guanine (7-OEG), N^2,3-ethenoguanine (N^2,3-εG), 1,N^6-ethenoadenine and 3,N^4-ethenocytosine. Target cell populations for angiosarcomas in vinyl fluoride-exposed rats are non-parenchymal cells, which contain more N^2,3-εG than hepatocytes and have lower expression of the associated DNA-repair enzyme N-methylpurine–DNA glycosylase (Swenberg et al., 1999; Holt et al., 2000). Other vinyl fluoride-induced DNA adducts were not measured in these animals.

During a 2-year study, rats and mice were exposed by whole-body inhalation to 0, 25, 250 or 2500 ppm [0, 47, 470 or 4700 mg/m^3] vinyl fluoride for 6 h per day on 5 days per week. Tissues were collected after 12 months for detection of 7-OEG and εG adducts in liver DNA. Similarly to vinyl chloride, a supralinear response was observed for εG as well as 7-OEG due to saturation of metabolic activation. The number of 7-OEG adducts in preweanling rats was two to three times greater than that in adults. Exposure for 12 months to 25 ppm vinyl fluoride caused a 2.5-fold increase in εG in mice and a 3.5-fold increase in rats compared with controls. In mice, a linear relationship between the incidence of angiosarcomas and the number of εG adducts was observed, while rats showed a sublinear relationship between 250 and 2500 ppm due to an increase in cell proliferation. Hepatocytes and non-parenchymal cells were isolated: non-parenchymal cells contain little or no CYP2E1; however, after 4 weeks of exposure, non-parenchymal cells contained 1.2 ± 0.9 pmol εG/μmol guanine while hepatocytes contained 0.4 pmol εG/μmol guanine which was due to a lower expression of N-methylpurine–DNA glycosylase (a DNA-repair enzyme) in non-parenchymal cells (Swenberg et al., 1999).

(b)   *Mutations and other related effects*

Vinyl fluoride is mutagenic in *Salmonella typhimurium*, Chinese hamster ovary cells and *Drosophila melanogaster* and induces micronucleus formation in the bone-marrow cells of female mice *in vivo* (IARC, 1995).

Ten rat and 10 mouse liver angiosarcomas from the 2-year study of Bogdanffy et al. (1995) were analysed for the presence of point mutations in Ki-*ras* exon 1 and Ha-*ras* exon 2 by polymerase chain reaction, single-strand conformational polymorphism and sequencing. No specific hot-spot mutation could be identified, although some samples displayed a shifted band of low intensity in the single-strand conformational poly-morphism analysis (Boivin-Angèle *et al.*, 2000).

4.3   Mechanisms of carcinogenesis

The metabolism of vinyl fluoride is thought to be similar to that of vinyl chloride and vinyl bromide, and occurs at similar rates in human, rat and mouse livers (Cantoreggi & Keller, 1997). Vinyl fluoride is probably activated by CYP2E1 to 2-fluoroethylene oxide, which rearranges to 2-fluoroacetadehyde (Holt *et al.*, 2000). Exposure of mice and rats to vinyl fluoride results in the formation of $N^2$3-εG, one of the promutagenic adducts that may be implicated in the mutagenicity and carcinogenicity of vinyl chloride.

5.   Summary of Data Reported

5.1   Exposure data

Vinyl fluoride is a flammable gas that is produced in a limited number of countries. It is used predominantly for the production of polyvinyl fluoride and other fluoride poly-mers. The use of vinyl fluoride is increasing. Workers may be exposed during the manu-facture of vinyl fluoride monomer and during production of the polymers.

5.2   Cancer in humans

No data were available to the Working Group.

5.3   Cancer in experimental animals

Vinyl fluoride was tested by inhalation in one study in rats and one study in mice. It increased the incidence of haemangiosarcomas in both sexes of mice and rats. Vinyl fluoride also increased the incidence of tumours of the lung and Harderian gland ade-nomas in male and female mice and mammary gland tumours in female mice, and that of Zymbal gland carcinomas in male and female rats and of hepatocellular neoplasms in female rats.

5.4   Mechanistic and other relevant data

Vinyl fluoride is readily absorbed after inhalation. The metabolic pathways of vinyl fluoride are thought to be similar to those of vinyl chloride and vinyl bromide. The initial oxidation results in formation of fluoroethylene oxide, a reaction that is probably medi-ated by cytochrome P450 2E1. In-vitro studies indicate that the rate of vinyl fluoride metabolism in human liver microsomes is comparable with that in rodent cells. Pharmacokinetic data indicate that the metabolism of vinyl fluoride is saturated at about 75 ppm (~140 mg/m³) in rats.

Fluoroethylene oxide and fluoroacetaldehyde are metabolites of vinyl fluoride that can form DNA adducts that are similar to those formed by metabolites of vinyl chloride. These include N7-(2-oxoethyl)guanosine and the cyclic adducts ethenodeoxyguanosine, ethenodeoxyadenosine and ethenodeoxycytidine, which can cause miscoding by modifying base-pairing sites. N7-(2-Oxoethyl)guanosine and ethenodeoxyguanosine adducts were found in the liver of rats and mice after 1 year of exposure to vinyl fluoride. In addition, a correlation between the amount of the ethenodeoxyguanosine adducts and the incidence of vinyl fluoride-induced angiosarcomas was observed in both species.

Vinyl fluoride was shown to be mutagenic in bacteria, Chinese hamster ovary cells and *Drosophila*.

6.   Evaluation and Rationale

6.1   Carcinogenicity in humans

There is *inadequate evidence* in humans for the carcinogenicity of vinyl fluoride.

6.2   Carcinogenicity in experimental animals

There is *sufficient evidence* in experimental animals for the carcinogenicity of vinyl fluoride.

6.3   Overall evaluation

Vinyl fluoride is *probably carcinogenic to humans (Group 2A)*.

6.4   Rationale

In making the overall evaluation, the Working Group took into consideration the fact that all available studies showed a consistently parallel response between vinyl fluoride and vinyl chloride. In addition, both vinyl chloride and vinyl fluoride are activated via a cytochrome P450 2E1-dependent pathway to their corresponding epoxides. For both vinyl chloride and vinyl fluoride, the covalent binding of these compounds to DNA yields promutagenic etheno adducts. The weight of positive evidence for both compounds was also noted among the studies for genotoxicity, although the number and variety of tests for vinyl fluoride were fewer. For practical purposes, vinyl fluoride should be considered to act similarly to the human carcinogen, vinyl chloride.

7.   References

ACGIH® Worldwide (2005) *Documentation of the TLVs® and BEIs® with Other Worldwide Occupational Exposure Values — 2005 CD-ROM*, Cincinnati, OH, American Conference of Government Industrial Hygienists

Bogdanffy, M.S., Kee, C.R., Kelly, D.P., Carakostas, M.C. & Sykes, G.P. (1990) Subchronic inhalation study with vinyl fluoride: Effects on hepatic cell proliferation and urinary fluoride excretion. *Fundam. appl. Toxicol.*, **15**, 394–406

Bogdanffy, M.S., Makovec, G.T. & Frame, S.R. (1995) Inhalation oncogenicity bioassay in rats and mice with vinyl fluoride. *Fundam. appl. Toxicol.*, **26**, 223–238

Boivin-Angèle, S., Lefrancois, L., Froment, O., Spiethoff, A., Bogdanffy, M.S., Wegener, K., Wesch, H., Barbin, A., Bancel, B., Trepo, C., Bartsch, H., Swenberg, J. & Marion, M.J. (2000) Ras gene mutations in vinyl chloride-induced liver tumours are carcinogen-specific but vary with cell type and species. *Int. J. Cancer*, **85**, 223–227

Cantoreggi, S. & Keller, D.A. (1997) Pharmacokinetics and metabolism of vinyl fluoride in vivo and in vitro. *Toxicol. appl. Pharmacol.*, **143**, 130–139

Chemical Information Services (1994) *Directory of World Chemical Producers 1995/1996 Standard Edition*, Dallas, TX, p. 706

Dupont (2007) [available at: http://www2.dupont.com/Photovoltaic/en_US/index.html]

Ebnesajjad, S. (2001) Poly(vinyl fluoride). In: *Kirk-Othmer Encyclopedia of Chemical Technology*, New York, John Wiley & Sons (online)

Environmental Chemicals Data and Information Network (1993) *Fluoroethene*, Ispra, JRC-CEC (last update: 02.09.1993)

Filser, J.G. & Bolt, H.M. (1979) Pharmacokinetics of halogenated ethylenes in rats. *Arch. Toxicol.*, **42**, 123–136

Filser, J.G. & Bolt, H.M. (1981) Inhalation pharmacokinetics based on gas uptake studies. I. Improvement of kinetic models. *Arch. Toxicol.*, **47**, 279–292

Filser, J.G., Jung, P. & Bolt, H.M. (1982) Increased acetone exhalation induced by metabolites of halogenated C1 and C2 compounds. *Arch. Toxicol.*, **49**, 107–116

Holt, S., Roy, G., Mitra, S., Upton, P.B., Bogdanffy, M.S. & Swenberg, J.A. (2000) Deficiency of N-methylpurine–DNA-glycosylase expression in nonparenchymal cells, the target cell for vinyl chloride and vinyl fluoride. *Mutat Res.*, **460**, 105–115

IARC (1993) *IARC Monographs on the Evaluation of Carcinogenic Risks to Humans*, Vol. 56, *Some Naturally Occurring Substances: Food Items and Constituents, Heterocyclic Aromatic Amines and Mycotoxins*, Lyon, pp. 135–162

IARC (1995) *IARC Monographs on the Evaluation of Carcinogenic Risks to Humans*, Vol. 63, *Dry Cleaning, Some Chlorinated Solvents and Other Industrial Chemicals*, Lyon

IPCS-CEC (1997) *International Chemical Safety Cards, Vinyl Fluoride ICSC 0598*, Geneva, World Health Organization

Lide, D.R., ed. (2005) *CRC Handbook of Chemistry and Physics*, 86th Ed., Boca Raton, FL, CRC Press, p. 3–260

Lyman, W.J., Reehl, W.F. & Rosenblatt, D.H. (1990) *Handbook of Chemical Property Estimation Methods*, Washington DC, American Chemical Society, p. 15-15–15-29

Meylan, W.M. & Howard, P.H. (1995) Atom/fragment contribution method for estimating octanol–water partition coefficients. *J. pharm. Sci.*, **84**, 83–92

National Toxicology Program (1999) *Report on Carcinogens: Background Documents for Vinyl Fluoride*, Research Triangle Park, NC

National Toxicology Program (2005) *Report of Carcinogens,* 11th Ed., Research Triangle Park, NC [available at http://ntp.niehs.nih.gov/ntp/roc/eleventh/profiles/s188viny.pdf, accessed 08.01.2008]

Ortiz de Montellano, P.R., Kunze, K.L., Beilan, H.S. & Wheeler, C. (1982) Destruction of cytochrome P-450 by vinyl fluoride, fluroxene, and acetylene. Evidence for a radical intermediate in olefin oxidation. *Biochemistry*, **21**, 1331–1339

Oser, J.L. (1980) Extent of industrial exposure to epichlorohydrin, vinyl fluoride, vinyl bromide and ethylene dibromide. *Am. ind. Hyg. Assoc. J.*, **41**, 463–468

Quickert, N., Findlay, W.J. & Monkman, J.L. (1975) Modification of a chemiluminescent ozone monitor for the measurement of gaseous unsaturated hydrocarbons. *Sci. total Environ.*, **3**, 323–328

Sutton, D.G., Westberg, K.R. & Melzer, J.E. (1979) Chemiluminescence detector based on active nitrogen for gas chromatography of hydrocarbons. *Anal. Chem.*, **51**, 1399–1401

Swenberg, J.A., Bogdanffy, M.S., Ham, A., Holt, S., Kim, A., Morinello, E.J., Ranasinghe, A., Scheller, N. & Upton, P.B. (1999) Formation and repair of DNA adducts in vinyl chloride- and vinyl fluoride-induced carcinogenesis. In: Singer, B. & Bartsch, H., eds, *Exocyclic DNA Adducts in Mutagenesis and Carcinogenesis* (IARC Scientific Publications No. 150), Lyon, IARC, pp. 29–43

LIST OF ABBREVIATIONS

εA	1,N^6-ethenoadenine adduct
A1	N^3-(2-hydroxy-3-buten-1-yl)adenine adduct
A2	N^3-(1-hydroxy-3-buten-2-yl)adenine adduct
ACGIH	American Conference of Government Industrial Hygienists
ADH	alcohol dehydrogenase
AGT	O^6-alkylguanine–DNA alkyltransferase
ALARA	as low as reasonably achieved
ALDH	aldehyde dehydrogenase
AML	acute myelogenous leukaemia
ASL	angiosarcoma of the liver
ASTM	American Society for Testing and Materials
ATSDR	Agency for Toxic Substances and Disease Registry
BD	butadiene
BDT	N^6-(2,3,4-trihydroxybutyl)-2′-deoxyadenosyl
bw	body weight
εC	3,N^4-ethenocytosine adduct
CA	chromosomal abberations
CD	circular dichroism
CDC	Centers for Disease Control and Prevention
CERM	cumulative exposure rank months
CI	confidence interval
CLL	chronic lymphocytic leukaemia
CMAI	Chemical Marketing Associates International
CML	chronic myelogenous leukaemia
CNS	central nervous system
CONCAWE	Conservation of Clean Air and Water in Europe
CT	computed tomography
CYP	cytochrome P450
DEB	diepoxybutane
dG	deoxyguanine
dGMP	desoxyguanosine monophosphate
DHB	4-(N-acetyl-L-cystein-S-yl)-1,2-dihydroxybutane

DHBMA	1,2-dihydroxybutyl mercapturic acid
DMDTC	dimethyldithiocarbamate
DMF	dimethylformamide
dsDNA	double-stranded DNA
DOL CL	Department of Labour – ceiling limits
dTTP	deoxythymidine triphosphate
EB	epoxybutene
EBD	epoxybutane diol
ECD	electron capture detection
ECETOC	European Centre of Ecotoxicology and Toxicology of Chemicals
EH	epoxide hydrolase
Ephx	epoxide hydrolase gene
exp.	expected
F	female
FAB	positive ion fast atom bombardment
FID	flame ionization detection
FISH	fluorescence in-situ hybridization
$1,N^2$-εG	$1,N^2$-ethenoguanine adduct
$N^2,3$-εG	$N^2,3$-ethenoguanine adduct
G	guanosine
G1	N7-(2-hydroxy-3-buten-1-yl)guanine adduct
G2	N7-(1-hydroxy-3-buten-2-yl)guanine adduct
G3	N7-(1,3,4-trihydroxybut-2-yl)guanine adduct
G4	N7-(2,3,4-trihydroxybut-1-yl)guanine adduct
GC	gas chromatography
GSH	glutathione
GST	glutathione-S-transferase
HB	4-(N-acetyl-L-cystein-S-yl)-1-hydroxy-2-butanone
HBsAg	hepatitis B virus surface antigen
HBV	hepatitis B virus
HCC	hepatocellular carcinoma
3-HEA	N3-(2-hydroxyethyl)adenine adduct
3-HEdU	N3-(2-hydroxyethyl)-2′-deoxyuridine adduct
7-HEG	N7-(2-hydroxyethyl)guanine adduct
O^6-HEG	O^6-(2-hydroxyethyl)guanine
HEMA	N-acetyl-S-(2-hydroxyethyl)cysteine; S-(2-hydroxyethyl)mercapturic acid
HEP	liver hepatocytes
HMVK	hydroxymethylvinyl ketone
HO-ethanoG	5,6,7,9-tetrahydro-7-hydroxy-9-oxoimidazo[1,2-a]purine
HPLC	high-performance liquid chromatography

HPRT	human hypoxanthine-guanine phosphoribosyl transferase gene
Hprt	rodent hypoxanthine-guanine phosphoribosyl transferase gene
ICD	International Classification of Diseases
IDLH	immediate danger to life or health
IL	interleukin
JEM	job–exposure matrix
JSOH	Japanese Society of Occupational Health
K_m	Michaelis-Menten constant
K_{oc}	organic carbon partition coefficient
LC	liquid chromatography
LC/MS	liquid chromatography in combination with tandem mass spectrometry
LFC	lowest feasible concentration
LH	lymphohaemopoietic
LOD	limit of detection
M	male
MAC	maximum acceptable concentration; maximum allowed concentration
MAK	maximum allowed concentration
mEH	microsomal epoxide hydrolase
MHBMA	monohydroxy-3-butenyl mercapturic acid
MHbVal	*N*-(2-hydroxy-3-butenyl)valine
MI (or M-I or M1)	1,2-dihydroxybutyl mercapturic acid
MII (or M-II or M2)	monohydroxy-3-butenyl mercapturic acid
MN	micronuclei
MS	mass spectrometry
NADPH	nicotinamide adenine dinucleotide phosphate
ND	not detected
NHL	non-Hodgkin lymphoma
NI	no information
NIOSH	National Institute of Occupational Safety and Health
NMR	nuclear magnetic resonance
NOES	National Occupational Exposure Survey
NPC	non-parenchymal cells
NR	not reported
NS	not significant
7-OEG	*N*7-(2-oxoethyl)guanine adduct
PCR	polymerase chain reaction
PEL	permissible exposure limit
P_{ow}	octanol/water partition coefficient
PVC	polyvinyl chloride

PVF	polyvinyl fluoride
PyrVal	N,N-(2,3-dihydroxy-1,4-butadiyl)valine
REL	recommended exposure limit
SBR	styrene–butadiene rubber
SCE	sister chromatid exchange
SD	standard deviation
SE	standard error
SEER	Surveillance, Epidemiology and End Result
SIDS	Screening Information Dataset
SIM	single-ion monitoring
SIR	standardized incidence ratio
SMR	standardized mortality ratio
SPME	solid-phase microextraction
STEL	short-term exposure limit
ssDNA	single-stranded DNA
THBG	trihydroxybutylguanine
THbVal	N-(2,3,4-trihydroxybutyl) valine
TK	human thymidine kinase gene
Tk	rodent thymidine kinase gene
TLV	threshold limit value
TPA	12-*O*-tetradecanoylphorbol-13-acetate
TRK	technical guidance concentration
TWA	time-weighted average
UV	ultraviolet
VC	vinyl chloride
VCM	vinyl chloride monomer
V_{max}	maximum velocity
XPD	xeroderma pigmentosum group D
XRCC1	X-ray cross-complementing group

CUMULATIVE CROSS INDEX TO *IARC MONOGRAPHS ON THE EVALUATION OF CARCINOGENIC RISKS TO HUMANS*

The volume, page and year of publication are given. References to corrigenda are given in parentheses.

A

A-α-C	*40*, 245 (1986); *Suppl. 7*, 56 (1987)
Acetaldehyde	*36*, 101 (1985) (*corr. 42*, 263); *Suppl. 7*, 77 (1987); *71*, 319 (1999)
Acetaldehyde formylmethylhydrazone (*see* Gyromitrin)	
Acetamide	*7*, 197 (1974); *Suppl. 7*, 56, 389 (1987); *71*, 1211 (1999)
Acetaminophen (*see* Paracetamol)	
Aciclovir	*76*, 47 (2000)
Acid mists (*see* Sulfuric acid and other strong inorganic acids, occupational exposures to mists and vapours from)	
Acridine orange	*16*, 145 (1978); *Suppl. 7*, 56 (1987)
Acriflavinium chloride	*13*, 31 (1977); *Suppl. 7*, 56 (1987)
Acrolein	*19*, 479 (1979); *36*, 133 (1985); *Suppl. 7*, 78 (1987); *63*, 337 (1995) (*corr. 65*, 549)
Acrylamide	*39*, 41 (1986); *Suppl. 7*, 56 (1987); *60*, 389 (1994)
Acrylic acid	*19*, 47 (1979); *Suppl. 7*, 56 (1987); *71*, 1223 (1999)
Acrylic fibres	*19*, 86 (1979); *Suppl. 7*, 56 (1987)
Acrylonitrile	*19*, 73 (1979); *Suppl. 7*, 79 (1987); *71*, 43 (1999)
Acrylonitrile-butadiene-styrene copolymers	*19*, 91 (1979); *Suppl. 7*, 56 (1987)
Actinolite (*see* Asbestos)	
Actinomycin D (*see also* Actinomycins)	*Suppl. 7*, 80 (1987)
Actinomycins	*10*, 29 (1976) (*corr. 42*, 255)
Adriamycin	*10*, 43 (1976); *Suppl. 7*, 82 (1987)
AF-2	*31*, 47 (1983); *Suppl. 7*, 56 (1987)
Aflatoxins	*1*, 145 (1972) (*corr. 42*, 251); *10*, 51 (1976); *Suppl. 7*, 83 (1987); *56*, 245 (1993); *82*, 171 (2002)
Aflatoxin B₁ (*see* Aflatoxins)	
Aflatoxin B₂ (*see* Aflatoxins)	
Aflatoxin G₁ (*see* Aflatoxins)	
Aflatoxin G₂ (*see* Aflatoxins)	
Aflatoxin M₁ (*see* Aflatoxins)	
Agaritine	*31*, 63 (1983); *Suppl. 7*, 56 (1987)
Alcohol drinking	*44* (1988)

Aldicarb	*53*, 93 (1991)
Aldrin	*5*, 25 (1974); *Suppl. 7*, 88 (1987)
Allyl chloride	*36*, 39 (1985); *Suppl. 7*, 56 (1987); *71*, 1231 (1999)
Allyl isothiocyanate	*36*, 55 (1985); *Suppl. 7*, 56 (1987); *73*, 37 (1999)
Allyl isovalerate	*36*, 69 (1985); *Suppl. 7*, 56 (1987); *71*, 1241 (1999)
Aluminium production	*34*, 37 (1984); *Suppl. 7*, 89 (1987)
Amaranth	*8*, 41 (1975); *Suppl. 7*, 56 (1987)
5-Aminoacenaphthene	*16*, 243 (1978); *Suppl. 7*, 56 (1987)
2-Aminoanthraquinone	*27*, 191 (1982); *Suppl. 7*, 56 (1987)
para-Aminoazobenzene	*8*, 53 (1975); *Suppl. 7*, 56, 390 (1987)
ortho-Aminoazotoluene	*8*, 61 (1975) (*corr. 42*, 254); *Suppl. 7*, 56 (1987)
para-Aminobenzoic acid	*16*, 249 (1978); *Suppl. 7*, 56 (1987)
4-Aminobiphenyl	*1*, 74 (1972) (*corr. 42*, 251); *Suppl. 7*, 91 (1987)
2-Amino-3,4-dimethylimidazo[4,5-*f*]quinoline (*see* MeIQ)	
2-Amino-3,8-dimethylimidazo[4,5-*f*]quinoxaline (*see* MeIQx)	
3-Amino-1,4-dimethyl-5*H*-pyrido[4,3-*b*]indole (*see* Trp-P-1)	
2-Aminodipyrido[1,2-*a*:3′,2′-*d*]imidazole (*see* Glu-P-2)	
1-Amino-2-methylanthraquinone	*27*, 199 (1982); *Suppl. 7*, 57 (1987)
2-Amino-3-methylimidazo[4,5-*f*]quinoline (*see* IQ)	
2-Amino-6-methyldipyrido[1,2-*a*:3′,2′-*d*]imidazole (*see* Glu-P-1)	
2-Amino-1-methyl-6-phenylimidazo[4,5-*b*]pyridine (*see* PhIP)	
2-Amino-3-methyl-9*H*-pyrido[2,3-*b*]indole (*see* MeA-α-C)	
3-Amino-1-methyl-5*H*-pyrido[4,3-*b*]indole (*see* Trp-P-2)	
2-Amino-5-(5-nitro-2-furyl)-1,3,4-thiadiazole	*7*, 143 (1974); *Suppl. 7*, 57 (1987)
2-Amino-4-nitrophenol	*57*, 167 (1993)
2-Amino-5-nitrophenol	*57*, 177 (1993)
4-Amino-2-nitrophenol	*16*, 43 (1978); *Suppl. 7*, 57 (1987)
2-Amino-5-nitrothiazole	*31*, 71 (1983); *Suppl. 7*, 57 (1987)
2-Amino-9*H*-pyrido[2,3-*b*]indole (see A-α-C)	
11-Aminoundecanoic acid	*39*, 239 (1986); *Suppl. 7*, 57 (1987)
Amitrole	*7*, 31 (1974); *41*, 293 (1986) (*corr. 52*, 513; *Suppl. 7*, 92 (1987); *79*, 381 (2001)
Ammonium potassium selenide (*see* Selenium and selenium compounds)	
Amorphous silica (*see also* Silica)	*42*, 39 (1987); *Suppl. 7*, 341 (1987); *68*, 41 (1997) (*corr. 81*, 383)
Amosite (*see* Asbestos)	
Ampicillin	*50*, 153 (1990)
Amsacrine	*76*, 317 (2000)
Anabolic steroids (*see* Androgenic (anabolic) steroids)	
Anaesthetics, volatile	*11*, 285 (1976); *Suppl. 7*, 93 (1987)
Analgesic mixtures containing phenacetin (*see also* Phenacetin)	*Suppl. 7*, 310 (1987)
Androgenic (anabolic) steroids	*Suppl. 7*, 96 (1987)
Angelicin and some synthetic derivatives (*see also* Angelicins)	*40*, 291 (1986)
Angelicin plus ultraviolet radiation (*see also* Angelicin and some synthetic derivatives)	*Suppl. 7*, 57 (1987)
Angelicins	*Suppl. 7*, 57 (1987)

BCNU (*see* Bischloroethyl nitrosourea)

Benz[*a*]acridine | 32, 123 (1983); *Suppl.* 7, 58 (1987)
Benz[*c*]acridine | 3, 241 (1973); 32, 129 (1983); *Suppl.* 7, 58 (1987)

Benzal chloride (*see also* α-Chlorinated toluenes and benzoyl chloride) | 29, 65 (1982); *Suppl.* 7, 148 (1987); 71, 453 (1999)

Benz[*a*]anthracene | 3, 45 (1973); 32, 135 (1983); *Suppl.* 7, 58 (1987)

Benzene | 7, 203 (1974) (*corr.* 42, 254); 29, 93, 391 (1982); *Suppl.* 7, 120 (1987)

Benzidine | 1, 80 (1972); 29, 149, 391 (1982); *Suppl.* 7, 123 (1987)

Benzidine-based dyes | *Suppl.* 7, 125 (1987)
Benzo[*b*]fluoranthene | 3, 69 (1973); 32, 147 (1983); *Suppl.* 7, 58 (1987)

Benzo[*j*]fluoranthene | 3, 82 (1973); 32, 155 (1983); *Suppl.* 7, 58 (1987)

Benzo[*k*]fluoranthene | 32, 163 (1983); *Suppl.* 7, 58 (1987)
Benzo[*ghi*]fluoranthene | 32, 171 (1983); *Suppl.* 7, 58 (1987)
Benzo[*a*]fluorene | 32, 177 (1983); *Suppl.* 7, 58 (1987)
Benzo[*b*]fluorene | 32, 183 (1983); *Suppl.* 7, 58 (1987)
Benzo[*c*]fluorene | 32, 189 (1983); *Suppl.* 7, 58 (1987)
Benzofuran | 63, 431 (1995)
Benzo[*ghi*]perylene | 32, 195 (1983); *Suppl.* 7, 58 (1987)
Benzo[*c*]phenanthrene | 32, 205 (1983); *Suppl.* 7, 58 (1987)
Benzo[*a*]pyrene | 3, 91 (1973); 32, 211 (1983) (*corr.* 68, 477); *Suppl.* 7, 58 (1987)
Benzo[*e*]pyrene | 3, 137 (1973); 32, 225 (1983); *Suppl.* 7, 58 (1987)

1,4-Benzoquinone (*see para*-Quinone)
1,4-Benzoquinone dioxime | 29, 185 (1982); *Suppl.* 7, 58 (1987); 71, 1251 (1999)

Benzotrichloride (*see also* α-Chlorinated toluenes and benzoyl chloride) | 29, 73 (1982); *Suppl.* 7, 148 (1987); 71, 453 (1999)

Benzoyl chloride (*see also* α-Chlorinated toluenes and benzoyl chloride) | 29, 83 (1982) (*corr.* 42, 261); *Suppl.* 7, 126 (1987); 71, 453 (1999)

Benzoyl peroxide | 36, 267 (1985); *Suppl.* 7, 58 (1987); 71, 345 (1999)

Benzyl acetate | 40, 109 (1986); *Suppl.* 7, 58 (1987); 71, 1255 (1999)

Benzyl chloride (see also α-Chlorinated toluenes and benzoyl chloride) | 11, 217 (1976) (*corr.* 42, 256); 29, 49 (1982); *Suppl.* 7, 148 (1987); 71, 453 (1999)

Benzyl violet 4B | 16, 153 (1978); *Suppl.* 7, 58 (1987)
Bertrandite (*see* Beryllium and beryllium compounds)
Beryllium and beryllium compounds | 1, 17 (1972); 23, 143 (1980) (*corr.* 42, 260); *Suppl.* 7, 127 (1987); 58, 41 (1993)

Beryllium acetate (*see* Beryllium and beryllium compounds)
Beryllium acetate, basic (*see* Beryllium and beryllium compounds)
Beryllium-aluminium alloy (*see* Beryllium and beryllium compounds)
Beryllium carbonate (*see* Beryllium and beryllium compounds)

1-*tert*-Butoxypropan-2-ol	*88*, 415 (2006)
n-Butyl acrylate	*39*, 67 (1986); *Suppl. 7*, 59 (1987); *71*, 359 (1999)
Butylated hydroxyanisole	*40*, 123 (1986); *Suppl. 7*, 59 (1987)
Butylated hydroxytoluene	*40*, 161 (1986); *Suppl. 7*, 59 (1987)
Butyl benzyl phthalate	*29*, 193 (1982) (*corr. 42*, 261); *Suppl. 7*, 59 (1987); *73*, 115 (1999)
β-Butyrolactone	*11*, 225 (1976); *Suppl. 7*, 59 (1987); *71*, 1317 (1999)
γ-Butyrolactone	*11*, 231 (1976); *Suppl. 7*, 59 (1987); *71*, 367 (1999)

C

Cabinet-making (*see* Furniture and cabinet-making)	
Cadmium acetate (*see* Cadmium and cadmium compounds)	
Cadmium and cadmium compounds	*2*, 74 (1973); *11*, 39 (1976) (*corr. 42*, 255); *Suppl. 7*, 139 (1987); *58*, 119 (1993)
Cadmium chloride (*see* Cadmium and cadmium compounds)	
Cadmium oxide (*see* Cadmium and cadmium compounds)	
Cadmium sulfate (*see* Cadmium and cadmium compounds)	
Cadmium sulfide (*see* Cadmium and cadmium compounds)	
Caffeic acid	*56*, 115 (1993)
Caffeine	*51*, 291 (1991)
Calcium arsenate (*see* Arsenic in drinking-water)	
Calcium chromate (*see* Chromium and chromium compounds)	
Calcium cyclamate (*see* Cyclamates)	
Calcium saccharin (*see* Saccharin)	
Cantharidin	*10*, 79 (1976); *Suppl. 7*, 59 (1987)
Caprolactam	*19*, 115 (1979) (*corr. 42*, 258); *39*, 247 (1986) (*corr. 42*, 264); *Suppl. 7*, 59, 390 (1987); *71*, 383 (1999)
Captafol	*53*, 353 (1991)
Captan	*30*, 295 (1983); *Suppl. 7*, 59 (1987)
Carbaryl	*12*, 37 (1976); *Suppl. 7*, 59 (1987)
Carbazole	*32*, 239 (1983); *Suppl. 7*, 59 (1987); *71*, 1319 (1999)
3-Carbethoxypsoralen	*40*, 317 (1986); *Suppl. 7*, 59 (1987)
Carbon black	*3*, 22 (1973); *33*, 35 (1984); *Suppl.7*, 142 (1987); *65*, 149 (1996)
Carbon tetrachloride	*1*, 53 (1972); *20*, 371 (1979); *Suppl. 7*, 143 (1987); *71*, 401 (1999)
Carmoisine	*8*, 83 (1975); *Suppl. 7*, 59 (1987)
Carpentry and joinery	*25*, 139 (1981); *Suppl. 7*, 378 (1987)
Carrageenan	*10*, 181 (1976) (*corr. 42*, 255); *31*, 79 (1983); *Suppl. 7*, 59 (1987)
Cassia occidentalis (*see* Traditional herbal medicines)	

Crystalline silica (*see also* Silica)	*42*, 39 (1987); *Suppl. 7*, 341 (1987); *68*, 41 (1997) (*corr. 81*, 383)
Cycasin (*see also* Methylazoxymethanol)	*1*, 157 (1972) (*corr. 42*, 251); *10*, 121 (1976); *Suppl. 7*, 61 (1987)
Cyclamates	*22*, 55 (1980); *Suppl. 7*, 178 (1987); *73*, 195 (1999)
Cyclamic acid (*see* Cyclamates)	
Cyclochlorotine	*10*, 139 (1976); *Suppl. 7*, 61 (1987)
Cyclohexanone	*47*, 157 (1989); *71*, 1359 (1999)
Cyclohexylamine (*see* Cyclamates)	
Cyclopenta[*cd*]pyrene	*32*, 269 (1983); *Suppl. 7*, 61 (1987)
Cyclopropane (*see* Anaesthetics, volatile)	
Cyclophosphamide	*9*, 135 (1975); *26*, 165 (1981); *Suppl. 7*, 182 (1987)
Cyproterone acetate	*72*, 49 (1999)

D

2,4-D (*see also* Chlorophenoxy herbicides; Chlorophenoxy herbicides, occupational exposures to)	*15*, 111 (1977)
Dacarbazine	*26*, 203 (1981); *Suppl. 7*, 184 (1987)
Dantron	*50*, 265 (1990) (*corr. 59*, 257)
D&C Red No. 9	*8*, 107 (1975); *Suppl. 7*, 61 (1987); *57*, 203 (1993)
Dapsone	*24*, 59 (1980); *Suppl. 7*, 185 (1987)
Daunomycin	*10*, 145 (1976); *Suppl. 7*, 61 (1987)
DDD (*see* DDT)	
DDE (*see* DDT)	
DDT	*5*, 83 (1974) (*corr. 42*, 253); *Suppl. 7*, 186 (1987); *53*, 179 (1991)
Decabromodiphenyl oxide	*48*, 73 (1990); *71*, 1365 (1999)
Deltamethrin	*53*, 251 (1991)
Deoxynivalenol (*see* Toxins derived from *Fusarium graminearum*, *F. culmorum* and *F. crookwellense*)	
Diacetylaminoazotoluene	*8*, 113 (1975); *Suppl. 7*, 61 (1987)
N,N'-Diacetylbenzidine	*16*, 293 (1978); *Suppl. 7*, 61 (1987)
Diallate	*12*, 69 (1976); *30*, 235 (1983); *Suppl. 7*, 61 (1987)
2,4-Diaminoanisole and its salts	*16*, 51 (1978); *27*, 103 (1982); *Suppl. 7*, 61 (1987); *79*, 619 (2001)
4,4'-Diaminodiphenyl ether	*16*, 301 (1978); *29*, 203 (1982); *Suppl. 7*, 61 (1987)
1,2-Diamino-4-nitrobenzene	*16*, 63 (1978); *Suppl. 7*, 61 (1987)
1,4-Diamino-2-nitrobenzene	*16*, 73 (1978); *Suppl. 7*, 61 (1987); *57*, 185 (1993)
2,6-Diamino-3-(phenylazo)pyridine (*see* Phenazopyridine hydrochloride)	
2,4-Diaminotoluene (*see* also Toluene diisocyanates)	*16*, 83 (1978); *Suppl. 7*, 61 (1987)
2,5-Diaminotoluene (*see* also Toluene diisocyanates)	*16*, 97 (1978); *Suppl. 7*, 61 (1987)
ortho-Dianisidine (*see* 3,3'-Dimethoxybenzidine)	
Diatomaceous earth, uncalcined (*see* Amorphous silica)	

2,4-Dichlorophenol (*see* Chlorophenols; Chlorophenols,
   occupational exposures to; Polychlorophenols and their sodium salts)
(2,4-Dichlorophenoxy)acetic acid (*see* 2,4-D)
2,6-Dichloro-*para*-phenylenediamine   *39*, 325 (1986); *Suppl. 7*, 62 (1987)
1,2-Dichloropropane   *41*, 131 (1986); *Suppl. 7*, 62
          (1987); *71*, 1393 (1999)
1,3-Dichloropropene (technical-grade)   *41*, 113 (1986); *Suppl. 7*, 195
          (1987); *71*, 933 (1999)
Dichlorvos   *20*, 97 (1979); *Suppl. 7*, 62 (1987);
          53, 267 (1991)
Dicofol   *30*, 87 (1983); *Suppl. 7*, 62 (1987)
Dicyclohexylamine (*see* Cyclamates)
Didanosine   *76*, 153 (2000)
Dieldrin   *5*, 125 (1974); *Suppl. 7*, 196 (1987)
Dienoestrol (*see also* Nonsteroidal oestrogens)   *21*, 161 (1979); *Suppl. 7*, 278
          (1987)
Diepoxybutane (*see* also 1,3-Butadiene)   *11*, 115 (1976) (*corr. 42*, 255);
          Suppl. 7, 62 (1987); *71*, 109 (1999)
Diesel and gasoline engine exhausts   *46*, 41 (1989)
Diesel fuels   *45*, 219 (1989) (*corr. 47*, 505)
Diethanolamine   *77*, 349 (2000)
Diethyl ether (*see* Anaesthetics, volatile)
Di(2-ethylhexyl) adipate   *29*, 257 (1982); *Suppl. 7*, 62
          (1987); *77*, 149 (2000)
Di(2-ethylhexyl) phthalate   *29*, 269 (1982) (*corr. 42*, 261);
          Suppl. 7, 62 (1987); *77*, 41 (2000)
1,2-Diethylhydrazine   *4*, 153 (1974); *Suppl. 7*, 62 (1987);
          71, 1401 (1999)
Diethylstilboestrol   *6*, 55 (1974); *21*, 173 (1979)
          (*corr. 42*, 259); *Suppl. 7*, 273
          (1987)
Diethylstilboestrol dipropionate (*see* Diethylstilboestrol)
Diethyl sulfate   *4*, 277 (1974); *Suppl. 7*, 198
          (1987); *54*, 213 (1992); *71*, 1405
          (1999)
N,N'-Diethylthiourea   *79*, 649 (2001)
Diglycidyl resorcinol ether   *11*, 125 (1976); *36*, 181 (1985);
          Suppl. 7, 62 (1987); *71*, 1417
          (1999)
Dihydrosafrole   *1*, 170 (1972); *10*, 233 (1976)
          Suppl. 7, 62 (1987)
1,8-Dihydroxyanthraquinone (*see* Dantron)
Dihydroxybenzenes (*see* Catechol; Hydroquinone; Resorcinol)
1,3-Dihydroxy-2-hydroxymethylanthraquinone   *82*, 129 (2002)
Dihydroxymethylfuratrizine   *24*, 77 (1980); *Suppl. 7*, 62 (1987)
Diisopropyl sulfate   *54*, 229 (1992); *71*, 1421 (1999)
Dimethisterone (*see also* Progestins; Sequential oral contraceptives)   *6*, 167 (1974); *21*, 377 (1979))
Dimethoxane   *15*, 177 (1977); *Suppl. 7*, 62 (1987)
3,3'-Dimethoxybenzidine   *4*, 41 (1974); *Suppl. 7*, 198 (1987)
3,3'-Dimethoxybenzidine-4,4'-diisocyanate   *39*, 279 (1986); *Suppl. 7*, 62 (1987)
para-Dimethylaminoazobenzene   *8*, 125 (1975); *Suppl. 7*, 62 (1987)
para-Dimethylaminoazobenzenediazo sodium sulfonate   *8*, 147 (1975); *Suppl. 7*, 62 (1987)
trans-2-[(Dimethylamino)methylimino]-5-[2-(5-nitro-2-furyl)-   *7*, 147 (1974) (*corr. 42*, 253);
   vinyl]-1,3,4-oxadiazole   *Suppl. 7*, 62 (1987)

Epichlorohydrin   *11*, 131 (1976) (*corr. 42*, 256);
                                                                    Suppl. 7, 202 (1987); *71*, 603
                                                                    (1999)
1,2-Epoxybutane   *47*, 217 (1989); *71*, 629 (1999)
1-Epoxyethyl-3,4-epoxycyclohexane (*see* 4-Vinylcyclohexene diepoxide)
3,4-Epoxy-6-methylcyclohexylmethyl 3,4-epoxy-6-methyl-   *11*, 147 (1976); *Suppl. 7*, 63
   cyclohexane carboxylate   (1987); *71*, 1441 (1999)
cis-9,10-Epoxystearic acid   *11*, 153 (1976); *Suppl. 7*, 63
                                                                    (1987); *71*, 1443 (1999)

Epstein-Barr virus   *70*, 47 (1997)
d-Equilenin   *72*, 399 (1999)
Equilin   *72*, 399 (1999)
Erionite   *42*, 225 (1987); *Suppl. 7*, 203
                                                                    (1987)

Estazolam   *66*, 105 (1996)
Ethinyloestradiol   *6*, 77 (1974); *21*, 233 (1979);
                                                                    Suppl. 7, 286 (1987); *72*, 49 (1999)

Ethionamide   *13*, 83 (1977); *Suppl. 7*, 63 (1987)
Ethyl acrylate   *19*, 57 (1979); *39*, 81 (1986);
                                                                    Suppl. 7, 63 (1987); *71*, 1447
                                                                    (1999)

Ethylbenzene   *77*, 227 (2000)
Ethylene   *19*, 157 (1979); *Suppl. 7*, 63
                                                                    (1987); *60*, 45 (1994); *71*, 1447
                                                                    (1999)

Ethylene dibromide   *15*, 195 (1977); *Suppl. 7*, 204
                                                                    (1987); *71*, 641 (1999)
Ethylene oxide   *11*, 157 (1976); *36*, 189 (1985)
                                                                    (*corr. 42*, 263); *Suppl. 7*, 205
                                                                    (1987); *60*, 73 (1994); *97*, 185
                                                                    (2008)

Ethylene sulfide   *11*, 257 (1976); *Suppl. 7*, 63 (1987)
Ethylenethiourea   *7*, 45 (1974); *Suppl. 7*, 207 (1987);
                                                                    79, 659 (2001)

2-Ethylhexyl acrylate   *60*, 475 (1994)
Ethyl methanesulfonate   *7*, 245 (1974); *Suppl. 7*, 63 (1987)
N-Ethyl-*N*-nitrosourea   *1*, 135 (1972); *17*, 191 (1978);
                                                                    Suppl. 7, 63 (1987)

Ethyl selenac (*see also* Selenium and selenium compounds)   *12*, 107 (1976); *Suppl. 7*, 63 (1987)
Ethyl tellurac   *12*, 115 (1976); *Suppl. 7*, 63 (1987)
Ethynodiol diacetate   *6*, 173 (1974); *21*, 387 (1979);
                                                                    Suppl. 7, 292 (1987); *72*, 49
                                                                    (1999)

Etoposide   *76*, 177 (2000)
Eugenol   *36*, 75 (1985); *Suppl. 7*, 63 (1987)
Evans blue   *8*, 151 (1975); *Suppl. 7*, 63 (1987)
Extremely low-frequency electric fields   *80* (2002)
Extremely low-frequency magnetic fields   *80* (2002)

F

Fast Green FCF   *16*, 187 (1978); *Suppl. 7*, 63 (1987)
Fenvalerate   *53*, 309 (1991)

G

Glycidaldehyde	*11*, 175 (1976); *Suppl. 7*, 64 (1987); *71*, 1459 (1999)
Glycidol	*77*, 469 (2000)
Glycidyl ethers	*47*, 237 (1989); *71*, 1285, 1417, 1525, 1539 (1999)
Glycidyl oleate	*11*, 183 (1976); *Suppl. 7*, 64 (1987)
Glycidyl stearate	*11*, 187 (1976); *Suppl. 7*, 64 (1987)
Griseofulvin	*10*, 153 (1976); *Suppl. 7*, 64, 391 (1987); *79*, 289 (2001)
Guinea Green B	*16*, 199 (1978); *Suppl. 7*, 64 (1987)
Gyromitrin	*31*, 163 (1983); *Suppl. 7*, 64, 391 (1987)

H

Haematite	*1*, 29 (1972); *Suppl. 7*, 216 (1987)
Haematite and ferric oxide	*Suppl. 7*, 216 (1987)
Haematite mining, underground, with exposure to radon	*1*, 29 (1972); *Suppl. 7*, 216 (1987)
Hairdressers and barbers (occupational exposure as)	*57*, 43 (1993)
Hair dyes, epidemiology of	*16*, 29 (1978); *27*, 307 (1982)
Halogenated acetonitriles	*52*, 269 (1991); *71*, 1325, 1369, 1375, 1533 (1999)
Halothane (*see* Anaesthetics, volatile)	
HC Blue No. 1	*57*, 129 (1993)
HC Blue No. 2	*57*, 143 (1993)
α-HCH (*see* Hexachlorocyclohexanes)	
β-HCH (*see* Hexachlorocyclohexanes)	
γ-HCH (*see* Hexachlorocyclohexanes)	
HC Red No. 3	*57*, 153 (1993)
HC Yellow No. 4	*57*, 159 (1993)
Heating oils (*see* Fuel oils)	
Helicobacter pylori (infection with)	*61*, 177 (1994)
Hepatitis B virus	*59*, 45 (1994)
Hepatitis C virus	*59*, 165 (1994)
Hepatitis D virus	*59*, 223 (1994)
Heptachlor (*see also* Chlordane/Heptachlor)	*5*, 173 (1974); *20*, 129 (1979)
Hexachlorobenzene	*20*, 155 (1979); *Suppl. 7*, 219 (1987); *79*, 493 (2001)
Hexachlorobutadiene	*20*, 179 (1979); *Suppl. 7*, 64 (1987); *73*, 277 (1999)
Hexachlorocyclohexanes	*5*, 47 (1974); *20*, 195 (1979) (*corr. 42*, 258); *Suppl. 7*, 220 (1987)
Hexachlorocyclohexane, technical-grade (*see* Hexachlorocyclohexanes)	
Hexachloroethane	*20*, 467 (1979); *Suppl. 7*, 64 (1987); *73*, 295 (1999)
Hexachlorophene	*20*, 241 (1979); *Suppl. 7*, 64 (1987)
Hexamethylphosphoramide	*15*, 211 (1977); *Suppl. 7*, 64 (1987); *71*, 1465 (1999)
Hexoestrol (*see also* Nonsteroidal oestrogens)	*Suppl. 7*, 279 (1987)
Hormonal contraceptives, progestogens only	*72*, 339 (1999)
Human herpesvirus 8	*70*, 375 (1997)
Human immunodeficiency viruses	*67*, 31 (1996)

M

Mestranol	6, 87 (1974); 21, 257 (1979) (corr. 42, 259); Suppl. 7, 288 (1987); 72, 49 (1999)
Metabisulfites (see Sulfur dioxide and some sulfites, bisulfites and metabisulfites)	
Metallic mercury (see Mercury and mercury compounds)	
Methanearsonic acid, disodium salt (see Arsenic and arsenic compounds)	
Methanearsonic acid, monosodium salt (see Arsenic and arsenic compounds)	
Methimazole	79, 53 (2001)
Methotrexate	26, 267 (1981); Suppl. 7, 241 (1987)
Methoxsalen (see 8-Methoxypsoralen)	
Methoxychlor	5, 193 (1974); 20, 259 (1979); Suppl. 7, 66 (1987)
Methoxyflurane (see Anaesthetics, volatile)	
5-Methoxypsoralen	40, 327 (1986); Suppl. 7, 242 (1987)
8-Methoxypsoralen (see also 8-Methoxypsoralen plus ultraviolet radiation)	24, 101 (1980)
8-Methoxypsoralen plus ultraviolet radiation	Suppl. 7, 243 (1987)
Methyl acrylate	19, 52 (1979); 39, 99 (1986); Suppl. 7, 66 (1987); 71, 1489 (1999)
5-Methylangelicin plus ultraviolet radiation (see also Angelicin and some synthetic derivatives)	Suppl. 7, 57 (1987)
2-Methylaziridine	9, 61 (1975); Suppl. 7, 66 (1987); 71, 1497 (1999)
Methylazoxymethanol acetate (see also Cycasin)	1, 164 (1972); 10, 131 (1976); Suppl. 7, 66 (1987)
Methyl bromide	41, 187 (1986) (corr. 45, 283); Suppl. 7, 245 (1987); 71, 721 (1999)
Methyl tert-butyl ether	73, 339 (1999)
Methyl carbamate	12, 151 (1976); Suppl. 7, 66 (1987)
Methyl-CCNU (see 1-(2-Chloroethyl)-3-(4-methylcyclohexyl)-1-nitrosourea)	
Methyl chloride	41, 161 (1986); Suppl. 7, 246 (1987); 71, 737 (1999)
1-, 2-, 3-, 4-, 5- and 6-Methylchrysenes	32, 379 (1983); Suppl. 7, 66 (1987)
N-Methyl-N,4-dinitrosoaniline	1, 141 (1972); Suppl. 7, 66 (1987)
4,4′-Methylene bis(2-chloroaniline)	4, 65 (1974) (corr. 42, 252); Suppl. 7, 246 (1987); 57, 271 (1993)
4,4′-Methylene bis(N,N-dimethyl)benzenamine	27, 119 (1982); Suppl. 7, 66 (1987)
4,4′-Methylene bis(2-methylaniline)	4, 73 (1974); Suppl. 7, 248 (1987)
4,4′-Methylenedianiline	4, 79 (1974) (corr. 42, 252); 39, 347 (1986); Suppl. 7, 66 (1987)
4,4′-Methylenediphenyl diisocyanate	19, 314 (1979); Suppl. 7, 66 (1987); 71, 1049 (1999)
2-Methylfluoranthene	32, 399 (1983); Suppl. 7, 66 (1987)
3-Methylfluoranthene	32, 399 (1983); Suppl. 7, 66 (1987)
Methylglyoxal	51, 443 (1991)

Mustard gas	*9*, 181 (1975) (*corr. 42*, 254); *Suppl. 7*, 259 (1987)
Myleran (*see* 1,4-Butanediol dimethanesulfonate)	

N

Nafenopin	*24*, 125 (1980); *Suppl. 7*, 67 (1987)
Naphthalcnc	*82*, 367 (2002)
1,5-Naphthalenediamine	*27*, 127 (1982); *Suppl. 7*, 67 (1987)
1,5-Naphthalene diisocyanate	*19*, 311 (1979); *Suppl. 7*, 67 (1987); *71*, 1515 (1999)
1-Naphthylamine	*4*, 87 (1974) (*corr. 42*, 253); *Suppl. 7*, 260 (1987)
2-Naphthylamine	*4*, 97 (1974); *Suppl. 7*, 261 (1987)
1-Naphthylthiourea	*30*, 347 (1983); *Suppl. 7*, 263 (1987)
Neutrons	*75*, 361 (2000)
Nickel acetate (*see* Nickel and nickel compounds)	
Nickel ammonium sulfate (*see* Nickel and nickel compounds)	
Nickel and nickel compounds (*see* also Implants, surgical)	*2*, 126 (1973) (*corr. 42*, 252); *11*, 75 (1976); *Suppl. 7*, 264 (1987) (*corr. 45*, 283); *49*, 257 (1990) (*corr. 67*, 395)
Nickel carbonate (*see* Nickel and nickel compounds)	
Nickel carbonyl (*see* Nickel and nickel compounds)	
Nickel chloride (*see* Nickel and nickel compounds)	
Nickel-gallium alloy (*see* Nickel and nickel compounds)	
Nickel hydroxide (*see* Nickel and nickel compounds)	
Nickelocene (*see* Nickel and nickel compounds)	
Nickel oxide (*see* Nickel and nickel compounds)	
Nickel subsulfide (*see* Nickel and nickel compounds)	
Nickel sulfate (*see* Nickel and nickel compounds)	
Niridazole	*13*, 123 (1977); *Suppl. 7*, 67 (1987)
Nithiazide	*31*, 179 (1983); *Suppl. 7*, 67 (1987)
Nitrilotriacetic acid and its salts	*48*, 181 (1990); *73*, 385 (1999)
5-Nitroacenaphthene	*16*, 319 (1978); *Suppl. 7*, 67 (1987)
5-Nitro-*ortho*-anisidine	*27*, 133 (1982); *Suppl. 7*, 67 (1987)
2-Nitroanisole	*65*, 369 (1996)
9-Nitroanthracene	*33*, 179 (1984); *Suppl. 7*, 67 (1987)
7-Nitrobenz[*a*]anthracene	*46*, 247 (1989)
Nitrobenzene	*65*, 381 (1996)
6-Nitrobenzo[*a*]pyrene	*33*, 187 (1984); *Suppl. 7*, 67 (1987); *46*, 255 (1989)
4-Nitrobiphenyl	*4*, 113 (1974); *Suppl. 7*, 67 (1987)
6-Nitrochrysene	*33*, 195 (1984); *Suppl. 7*, 67 (1987); *46*, 267 (1989)
Nitrofen (technical-grade)	*30*, 271 (1983); *Suppl. 7*, 67 (1987)
3-Nitrofluoranthene	*33*, 201 (1984); *Suppl. 7*, 67 (1987)
2-Nitrofluorene	*46*, 277 (1989)
Nitrofural	*7*, 171 (1974); *Suppl. 7*, 67 (1987); *50*, 195 (1990)
5-Nitro-2-furaldehyde semicarbazone (*see* Nitrofural)	
Nitrofurantoin	*50*, 211 (1990)
Nitrofurazone (*see* Nitrofural)	

N′-Nitrosonornicotine (NNN)	*17*, 281 (1978); *37*, 241 (1985); *Suppl. 7*, 68 (1987); *89*, 419 (2007)
N-Nitrosopiperidine	*17*, 287 (1978); *Suppl. 7*, 68 (1987)
N-Nitrosoproline	*17*, 303 (1978); *Suppl. 7*, 68 (1987)
N-Nitrosopyrrolidine	*17*, 313 (1978); *Suppl. 7*, 68 (1987)
N-Nitrososarcosine	*17*, 327 (1978); *Suppl. 7*, 68 (1987)
Nitrosoureas, chloroethyl (*see* Chloroethyl nitrosoureas)	
5-Nitro-*ortho*-toluidine	*48*, 169 (1990)
2-Nitrotoluene	*65*, 409 (1996)
3-Nitrotoluene	*65*, 409 (1996)
4-Nitrotoluene	*65*, 409 (1996)
Nitrous oxide (*see* Anaesthetics, volatile)	
Nitrovin	*31*, 185 (1983); *Suppl. 7*, 68 (1987)
Nivalenol (*see* Toxins derived from *Fusarium graminearum*, *F. culmorum* and *F. crookwellense*)	
NNK (*see* 4-(*N*-Nitrosomethylamino)-1-(3-pyridyl)-1-butanone)	
NNN (*see N*′-Nitrosonornicotine)	
Nonsteroidal oestrogens	*Suppl. 7*, 273 (1987)
Norethisterone	*6*, 179 (1974); *21*, 461 (1979); *Suppl. 7*, 294 (1987); *72*, 49 (1999)
Norethisterone acetate	*72*, 49 (1999)
Norethynodrel	*6*, 191 (1974); *21*, 461 (1979) (*corr. 42*, 259); *Suppl. 7*, 295 (1987); *72*, 49 (1999)
Norgestrel	*6*, 201 (1974); *21*, 479 (1979); *Suppl. 7*, 295 (1987); *72*, 49 (1999)
Nylon 6	*19*, 120 (1979); *Suppl. 7*, 68 (1987)

O

Ochratoxin A	*10*, 191 (1976); *31*, 191 (1983) (*corr. 42*, 262); *Suppl. 7*, 271 (1987); *56*, 489 (1993)
Oestradiol	*6*, 99 (1974); *21*, 279 (1979); *Suppl. 7*, 284 (1987); *72*, 399 (1999)
Oestradiol-17β (*see* Oestradiol)	
Oestradiol 3-benzoate (*see* Oestradiol)	
Oestradiol dipropionate (*see* Oestradiol)	
Oestradiol mustard	*9*, 217 (1975); *Suppl. 7*, 68 (1987)
Oestradiol valerate (*see* Oestradiol)	
Oestriol	*6*, 117 (1974); *21*, 327 (1979); *Suppl. 7*, 285 (1987); *72*, 399 (1999)
Oestrogen replacement therapy (*see* Post-menopausal oestrogen therapy)	
Oestrogens (*see* Oestrogens, progestins and combinations)	
Oestrogens, conjugated (*see* Conjugated oestrogens)	
Oestrogens, nonsteroidal (*see* Nonsteroidal oestrogens)	
Oestrogens, progestins (progestogens) and combinations	*6* (1974); *21* (1979); *Suppl. 7*, 272 (1987); *72*, 49, 339, 399, 531 (1999)

Phenobarbital and its sodium salt	*13*, 157 (1977); *Suppl. 7*, 313 (1987); *79*, 161 (2001)
Phenol	*47*, 263 (1989) (*corr. 50*, 385); *71*, 749 (1999)
Phenolphthalein	*76*, 387 (2000)
Phenoxyacetic acid herbicides (*see* Chlorophenoxy herbicides)	
Phenoxybenzamine hydrochloride	*9*, 223 (1975); *24*, 185 (1980); *Suppl. 7*, 70 (1987)
Phenylbutazone	*13*, 183 (1977); *Suppl. 7*, 316 (1987)
meta-Phenylenediamine	*16*, 111 (1978); *Suppl. 7*, 70 (1987)
para-Phenylenediamine	*16*, 125 (1978); *Suppl. 7*, 70 (1987)
Phenyl glycidyl ether (*see also* Glycidyl ethers)	*71*, 1525 (1999)
N-Phenyl-2-naphthylamine	*16*, 325 (1978) (*corr. 42*, 257); *Suppl. 7*, 318 (1987)
ortho-Phenylphenol	*30*, 329 (1983); *Suppl. 7*, 70 (1987); *73*, 451 (1999)
Phenytoin	*13*, 201 (1977); *Suppl. 7*, 319 (1987); *66*, 175 (1996)
Phillipsite (*see* Zeolites)	
PhIP	*56*, 229 (1993)
Pickled vegetables	*56*, 83 (1993)
Picloram	*53*, 481 (1991)
Piperazine oestrone sulfate (*see* Conjugated oestrogens)	
Piperonyl butoxide	*30*, 183 (1983); *Suppl. 7*, 70 (1987)
Pitches, coal-tar (*see* Coal-tar pitches)	
Polyacrylic acid	*19*, 62 (1979); *Suppl. 7*, 70 (1987)
Polybrominated biphenyls	*18*, 107 (1978); *41*, 261 (1986); *Suppl. 7*, 321 (1987)
Polychlorinated biphenyls	*7*, 261 (1974); *18*, 43 (1978) (*corr. 42*, 258); *Suppl. 7*, 322 (1987)
Polychlorinated camphenes (*see* Toxaphene)	
Polychlorinated dibenzo-*para*-dioxins (other than 2,3,7,8-tetrachlorodibenzodioxin)	*69*, 33 (1997)
Polychlorinated dibenzofurans	*69*, 345 (1997)
Polychlorophenols and their sodium salts	*71*, 769 (1999)
Polychloroprene	*19*, 141 (1979); *Suppl. 7*, 70 (1987)
Polyethylene (*see also* Implants, surgical)	*19*, 164 (1979); *Suppl. 7*, 70 (1987)
Poly(glycolic acid) (*see* Implants, surgical)	
Polymethylene polyphenyl isocyanate (*see also* 4,4′-Methylenediphenyl diisocyanate)	*19*, 314 (1979); *Suppl. 7*, 70 (1987)
Polymethyl methacrylate (*see also* Implants, surgical)	*19*, 195 (1979); *Suppl. 7*, 70 (1987)
Polyoestradiol phosphate (*see* Oestradiol-17β)	
Polypropylene (*see also* Implants, surgical)	*19*, 218 (1979); *Suppl. 7*, 70 (1987)
Polystyrene (*see also* Implants, surgical)	*19*, 245 (1979); *Suppl. 7*, 70 (1987)
Polytetrafluoroethylene (*see also* Implants, surgical)	*19*, 288 (1979); *Suppl. 7*, 70 (1987)
Polyurethane foams (*see also* Implants, surgical)	*19*, 320 (1979); *Suppl. 7*, 70 (1987)
Polyvinyl acetate (*see also* Implants, surgical)	*19*, 346 (1979); *Suppl. 7*, 70 (1987)
Polyvinyl alcohol (*see also* Implants, surgical)	*19*, 351 (1979); *Suppl. 7*, 70 (1987)
Polyvinyl chloride (*see also* Implants, surgical)	*7*, 306 (1974); *19*, 402 (1979); *Suppl. 7*, 70 (1987)
Polyvinyl pyrrolidone	*19*, 463 (1979); *Suppl. 7*, 70 (1987); *71*, 1181 (1999)

Q

Quartz (*see* Crystalline silica)

Quercetin (*see also* Bracken fern)   *31*, 213 (1983); *Suppl. 7*, 71
                                                       (1987); *73*, 497 (1999)

para-Quinone   *15*, 255 (1977); *Suppl. 7*, 71
                                                       (1987); *71*, 1245 (1999)

Quintozene   *5*, 211 (1974); *Suppl. 7*, 71 (1987)

R

Radiation (*see* gamma-radiation, neutrons, ultraviolet radiation,
      X-radiation)

Radionuclides, internally deposited   *78* (2001)

Radon   *43*, 173 (1988) (*corr. 45*, 283)

Refractory ceramic fibres (*see* Man-made vitreous fibres)

Reserpine   *10*, 217 (1976); *24*, 211 (1980)
                                                       (*corr. 42*, 260); *Suppl. 7*, 330
                                                       (1987)

Resorcinol   *15*, 155 (1977); *Suppl. 7*, 71
                                                       (1987); *71*, 1119 (1990)

Retrorsine   *10*, 303 (1976); *Suppl. 7*, 71 (1987)

Rhodamine B   *16*, 221 (1978); *Suppl. 7*, 71 (1987)

Rhodamine 6G   *16*, 233 (1978); *Suppl. 7*, 71 (1987)

Riddelliine   *10*, 313 (1976); *Suppl. 7*, 71
                                                       (1987); *82*, 153 (2002)

Rifampicin   *24*, 243 (1980); *Suppl. 7*, 71 (1987)

Ripazepam   *66*, 157 (1996)

Rock (stone) wool (*see* Man-made vitreous fibres)

Rubber industry   *28* (1982) (*corr. 42*, 261); *Suppl. 7*,
                                                       332 (1987)

Rubia tinctorum (*see also* Madder root, Traditional herbal medicines)   *82*, 129 (2002)

Rugulosin   *40*, 99 (1986); *Suppl. 7*, 71 (1987)

S

Saccharated iron oxide   *2*, 161 (1973); *Suppl. 7*, 71 (1987)

Saccharin and its salts   *22*, 111 (1980) (*corr. 42*, 259);
                                                       Suppl. 7, 334 (1987); *73*, 517 (1999)

Safrole   *1*, 169 (1972); *10*, 231 (1976);
                                                       Suppl. 7, 71 (1987)

Salted fish   *56*, 41 (1993)

Sawmill industry (including logging) (*see* Lumber and
      sawmill industry (including logging))

Scarlet Red   *8*, 217 (1975); *Suppl. 7*, 71 (1987)

Schistosoma haematobium (infection with)   *61*, 45 (1994)

Schistosoma japonicum (infection with)   *61*, 45 (1994)

Schistosoma mansoni (infection with)   *61*, 45 (1994)

Selenium and selenium compounds   *9*, 245 (1975) (*corr. 42*, 255);
                                                       Suppl. 7, 71 (1987)

Selenium dioxide (*see* Selenium and selenium compounds)

Selenium oxide (*see* Selenium and selenium compounds)

ortho-Toluidine	*16*, 349 (1978); *27*, 155 (1982) (*corr. 68*, 477); *Suppl. 7*, 362 (1987); *77*, 267 (2000)
Toremifene	*66*, 367 (1996)
Toxaphene	*20*, 327 (1979); *Suppl. 7*, 72 (1987); *79*, 569 (2001)
T-2 Toxin (*see* Toxins derived from *Fusarium sporotrichioides*)	
Toxins derived from *Fusarium graminearum, F. culmorum* and *F. crookwellense*	*11*, 169 (1976); *31*, 153, 279 (1983); *Suppl. 7*, 64, 74 (1987); *56*, 397 (1993)
Toxins derived from *Fusarium moniliforme*	*56*, 445 (1993)
Toxins derived from *Fusarium sporotrichioides*	*31*, 265 (1983); *Suppl. 7*, 73 (1987); *56*, 467 (1993)
Traditional herbal medicines	*82*, 41 (2002)
Tremolite (*see* Asbestos)	
Treosulfan	*26*, 341 (1981); *Suppl. 7*, 363 (1987)
Triaziquone (*see* Tris(aziridinyl)-*para*-benzoquinone)	
Trichlorfon	*30*, 207 (1983); *Suppl. 7*, 73 (1987)
Trichlormethine	*9*, 229 (1975); *Suppl. 7*, 73 (1987); *50*, 143 (1990)
Trichloroacetic acid	*63*, 291 (1995) (*corr. 65*, 549); *84* (2004)
Trichloroacetonitrile (*see also* Halogenated acetonitriles)	*71*, 1533 (1999)
1,1,1-Trichloroethane	*20*, 515 (1979); *Suppl. 7*, 73 (1987); *71*, 881 (1999)
1,1,2-Trichloroethane	*20*, 533 (1979); *Suppl. 7*, 73 (1987); *52*, 337 (1991); *71*, 1153 (1999)
Trichloroethylene	*11*, 263 (1976); *20*, 545 (1979); *Suppl. 7*, 364 (1987); *63*, 75 (1995) (*corr. 65*, 549)
2,4,5-Trichlorophenol (*see also* Chlorophenols; Chlorophenols, occupational exposures to; Polychlorophenols and their sodium salts)	*20*, 349 (1979)
2,4,6-Trichlorophenol (*see also* Chlorophenols; Chlorophenols, occupational exposures to; Polychlorophenols and their sodium salts)	*20*, 349 (1979)
(2,4,5-Trichlorophenoxy)acetic acid (*see* 2,4,5-T)	
1,2,3-Trichloropropane	*63*, 223 (1995)
Trichlorotriethylamine-hydrochloride (*see* Trichlormethine)	
T2-Trichothecene (*see* Toxins derived from *Fusarium sporotrichioides*)	
Tridymite (*see* Crystalline silica)	
Triethanolamine	*77*, 381 (2000)
Triethylene glycol diglycidyl ether	*11*, 209 (1976); *Suppl. 7*, 73 (1987); *71*, 1539 (1999)
Trifluralin	*53*, 515 (1991)
4,4′,6-Trimethylangelicin plus ultraviolet radiation (*see also* Angelicin and some synthetic derivatives)	*Suppl. 7*, 57 (1987)
2,4,5-Trimethylaniline	*27*, 177 (1982); *Suppl. 7*, 73 (1987)
2,4,6-Trimethylaniline	*27*, 178 (1982); *Suppl. 7*, 73 (1987)
4,5′,8-Trimethylpsoralen	*40*, 357 (1986); *Suppl. 7*, 366 (1987)
Trimustine hydrochloride (*see* Trichlormethine)	
2,4,6-Trinitrotoluene	*65*, 449 (1996)
Triphenylene	*32*, 447 (1983); *Suppl. 7*, 73 (1987)
Tris(aziridinyl)-*para*-benzoquinone	*9*, 67 (1975); *Suppl. 7*, 367 (1987)

List of IARC Monographs on the Evaluation of Carcinogenic Risks to Humans*

Volume 1
Some Inorganic Substances, Chlorinated Hydrocarbons, Aromatic Amines, N-Nitroso Compounds, and Natural Products
1972; 184 pages (out-of-print)

Volume 2
Some Inorganic and Organo-metallic Compounds
1973; 181 pages (out-of-print)

Volume 3
Certain Polycyclic Aromatic Hydrocarbons and Heterocyclic Compounds
1973; 271 pages (out-of-print)

Volume 4
Some Aromatic Amines, Hydrazine and Related Substances, N-Nitroso Compounds and Miscellaneous Alkylating Agents
1974; 286 pages (out-of-print)

Volume 5
Some Organochlorine Pesticides
1974; 241 pages (out-of-print)

Volume 6
Sex Hormones
1974; 243 pages (out-of-print)

Volume 7
Some Anti-Thyroid and Related Substances, Nitrofurans and Industrial Chemicals
1974; 326 pages (out-of-print)

Volume 8
Some Aromatic Azo Compounds
1975; 357 pages (out-of-print)

Volume 9
Some Aziridines, N-, S- and O-Mustards and Selenium
1975; 268 pages (out-of-print)

Volume 10
Some Naturally Occurring Substances
1976; 353 pages (out-of-print)

Volume 11
Cadmium, Nickel, Some Epoxides, Miscellaneous Industrial Chemicals and General Considerations on Volatile Anaesthetics
1976; 306 pages (out-of-print)

Volume 12
Some Carbamates, Thio-carbamates and Carbazides
1976; 282 pages (out-of-print)

Volume 13
Some Miscellaneous Pharmaceutical Substances
1977; 255 pages

Volume 14
Asbestos
1977; 106 pages (out-of-print)

Volume 15
Some Fumigants, the Herbicides 2,4-D and 2,4,5-T, Chlorinated Dibenzodioxins and Miscellaneous Industrial Chemicals
1977; 354 pages (out-of-print)

Volume 16
Some Aromatic Amines and Related Nitro Compounds—Hair Dyes, Colouring Agents and Miscellaneous Industrial Chemicals
1978; 400 pages

Volume 17
Some N-Nitroso Compounds
1978; 365 pages

Volume 18
Polychlorinated Biphenyls and Polybrominated Biphenyls
1978; 140 pages (out-of-print)

Volume 19
Some Monomers, Plastics and Synthetic Elastomers, and Acrolein
1979; 513 pages (out-of-print)

Volume 20
Some Halogenated Hydrocarbons
1979; 609 pages (out-of-print)

Volume 21
Sex Hormones (II)
1979; 583 pages

Volume 22
Some Non-Nutritive Sweetening Agents
1980; 208 pages

Volume 23
Some Metals and Metallic Compounds
1980; 438 pages (out-of-print)

Volume 24
Some Pharmaceutical Drugs
1980; 337 pages

Volume 25
Wood, Leather and Some Associated Industries
1981; 412 pages

Volume 26
Some Antineoplastic and Immunosuppressive Agents
1981; 411 pages (out-of-print)

Volume 27
Some Aromatic Amines, Anthraquinones and Nitroso Compounds, and Inorganic Fluorides Used in Drinking-water and Dental Preparations
1982; 341 pages (out-of-print)

Volume 28
The Rubber Industry
1982; 486 pages (out-of-print)

---

* High-quality photocopies of all out-of-print volumes may be purchased from University Microfilms International, 300 North Zeeb Road, Ann Arbor, MI 48106-1346, USA (Tel.: +1 313-761-4700, +1 800-521-0600).

Achevé d'imprimer sur rotative par l'imprimerie Darantiere
à Dijon-Quetigny en janvier 2009

Dépôt légal : janvier 2009
N° d'mpression : 28-1696

Imprimé en France